Praise for *Person and Family Centered Care*

"*Person and Family Centered Care* is an absolute must-have for executives, faculty, and practitioners! The concepts and strategies the authors present will enable cross-disciplinary teams engaged in population health management to create relevant and person-centered programs that meet the Institute of Medicine's definition—care that is respectful, responsive, and inclusive of the values of individuals, families, and communities to be served. Multiple exemplars are presented for readers as they pursue the design of health services that is inclusive of consumers. The models described demonstrate the value of person- and family-centered care in achieving the goals identified by the Institute of Medicine report *The Future of Nursing: Leading Change, Advancing Health*. The book contains wonderful examples for nurses and other health providers on the importance of engaging and working with consumers to lead change that will ultimately improve their health. I highly recommend this fabulous resource to all healthcare practitioners and consumers."

–Linda Burnes Bolton, DrPH, RN, FAAN
Vice President and Chief Nursing Officer
Cedars-Sinai Medical Center
Los Angeles, California

"With the publication of *Person and Family Centered Care*, Barnsteiner, Disch, and Walton, along with an impressive roster of thought leaders, have created a much-needed, valuable resource for twenty-first century healthcare. This book is wonderfully organized with rich, powerful examples and practical guidance to improve healthcare using a person- and family-centered approach."

–Eric S. Holmboe, MD, FACP, FRCP, CAPT, MC, USNR-R
Senior Vice President, Accreditation Council for Graduate Medical Education
Adjunct Professor of Medicine, Yale University School of Medicine

"*Person and Family Centered Care* provides a comprehensive framework for embedding person- and family-centered care into the culture. The authors remind us that for the last 50 years, we have had a physician-directed, acuity-oriented, hospital-based healthcare system, and while that served us well during that period of time, the future of health in this country will need to be radically different."

–Karen Cox, PhD, RN, FACHE, FAAN
Executive Vice President/Co-Chief Operating Officer
Children's Mercy Hospital, Kansas City

"If you think of person-centered care as a 'motherhood and apple pie' concept, this book will surprise you. Each chapter sheds light from a new perspective, leading readers—from novice to expert and across the entire spectrum of healthcare roles—to a deeper understanding of person- and family-centered care. While not minimizing the challenges, the authors offer a rich array of strategies for a different future. We need a copy of this book in every curriculum and workplace!"

–Linda Cronenwett, PhD, RN, FAAN
Co-Director, Robert Wood Johnson Foundation Executive Nurse Fellows Program
Professor and Dean Emeritus, School of Nursing, University of North Carolina at Chapel Hill

Person and Family Centered Care

Jane H. Barnsteiner, PhD, RN, FAAN
Joanne Disch, PhD, RN, FAAN
Mary K. Walton, MSN, MBE, RN

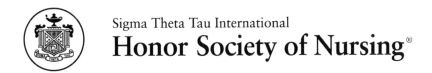

Sigma Theta Tau International
Honor Society of Nursing®

The Honor Society of Nursing, Sigma Theta Tau International (STTI) is a nonprofit organization founded in 1922 whose mission is to support the learning, knowledge, and professional development of nurses committed to making a difference in health worldwide. Members include practicing nurses, instructors, researchers, policymakers, entrepreneurs and others. STTI's 494 chapters are located at 676 institutions of higher education throughout Australia, Botswana, Brazil, Canada, Colombia, Ghana, Hong Kong, Japan, Kenya, Malawi, Mexico, the Netherlands, Pakistan, Portugal, Singapore, South Africa, South Korea, Swaziland, Sweden, Taiwan, Tanzania, United Kingdom, United States, and Wales. More information about STTI can be found online at www.nursingsociety.org.

Sigma Theta Tau International
550 West North Street
Indianapolis, IN, USA 46202

To order additional books, buy in bulk, or order for corporate use, contact Nursing Knowledge International at 888.NKI.4YOU (888.654.4968/US and Canada) or +1.317.634.8171 (outside US and Canada).

To request a review copy for course adoption, e-mail solutions@nursingknowledge.org or call 888.NKI.4YOU (888.654.4968/US and Canada) or +1.317.634.8171 (outside US and Canada).

To request author information, or for speaker or other media requests, contact Marketing, Honor Society of Nursing, Sigma Theta Tau International at 888.634.7575 (US and Canada) or +1.317.634.8171 (outside US and Canada).

ISBN: 9781938835070
EPUB ISBN: 9781938835087
PDF ISBN: 9781938835094
MOBI ISBN: 9781938835100

Library of Congress Cataloging-in-Publication Data

Barnsteiner, Jane Herman, author.
 Person- and family-centered care / Jane Barnsteiner, Joanne Disch, Mary Walton.
    p. ; cm.
 Includes bibliographical references.
 ISBN 978-1-938835-07-0 (book : alk. paper) -- ISBN 978-1-938835-08-7 (EPUB) -- ISBN 978-1-938835-09-4 (PDF ISBN) -- ISBN 978-1-938835-10-0 (MOBI)
 I. Disch, Joanne Marilyn, author. II. Walton, Mary K., author. III. Sigma Theta Tau International, publisher. IV. Title.
 [DNLM: 1. Patient-Centered Care. 2. Nurse-Patient Relations. 3. Professional-Family Relations. W 84.7]
 RT86.3
 610.7306'99--dc23
                        2014016053

First Printing, 2014

Publisher: Renee Wilmeth
Acquisitions Editor: Emily Hatch
Editorial Coordinator: Paula Jeffers
Cover Designer: Rebecca Batchelor
Interior Design/Page Layout: Kim Scott
Indexer: Joy Dean Lee

Principal Book Editor: Carla Hall
Development and Project Editor: Kevin Kent
Development Editor: Jennifer Lynn
Copy Editor: Erin Geile
Proofreaders: Erin Geile, Heather Wilcox

Dedications

To Claire Fagin, PhD, RN, FAAN, eminent nurse leader, whose work on the importance of family presence has served as a lodestar for me throughout my career. In 1970, I read Claire's doctoral dissertation (*The Effects of Maternal Attendance During Hospitalization on the Behavior of Young Children*, 1966, Philadelphia, PA: F.A. Davis) for a paper I was writing in my undergraduate program at the University of Pennsylvania. The notion of the profound importance of family presence and participation has served as a cornerstone for my work the past 44 years.

–Jane H. Barnsteiner

To Rocky Schmitz, my first head nurse, who introduced nursing practices 45 years ago that epitomized person- and family-centered care. These included extensive pre-op and home instructions, teaching patients how to regulate their own Coumadin dosages, and establishing medication self-administration and individualized visiting hours. She created a nursing unit where personalized care, interdisciplinary teamwork, and professional development flourished— and she still today exerts a powerful influence on those of us privileged to have worked with her.

–Joanne Disch

To the children I cared for during my 3 decades of pediatric nursing practice. Children with cystic fibrosis and their parents embodied the healing power of family. Although I shared my knowledge and skills, they shared how to live happy and independent lives despite the need to integrate burdensome care routines into their everyday routine. The privilege of knowing and caring for them is one of the gifts of being a nurse. Their philosophy of life informs my work today.

–Mary K. Walton

Acknowledgments

We would like to express our thanks to Emily Hatch, our book editor, who has provided terrific support and encouragement throughout the process of writing this book. We also thank Carla Hall for her production coordination and Kevin Kent, Jennifer Lynn, and Erin Geile for their unerring and meticulous editing that greatly enhanced our original words. Without this team, there would be no book.

And on a broader scale, we want to acknowledge the daily, often challenging but vitally important contributions that nurses make to deliver person- and family-centered care. Healthcare delivery today can be daunting, and yet these nurses in all settings and situations practice exquisitely. Without them too, this book would not be possible.

About the Authors

Jane H. Barnsteiner, PhD, RN, FAAN, is professor emerita of pediatric nursing at the University of Pennsylvania School of Nursing. Barnsteiner received her diploma of nursing from Misericordia Hospital School of Nursing in Philadelphia, BSN and MSN degrees from the University of Pennsylvania, and PhD from the University of Michigan. In addition to her multiple academic roles in the School, she served as director of nursing for Translational Research at the Hospital of the University of Pennsylvania and as director of nursing practice and research at The Children's Hospital of Philadelphia. Her scholarship focuses on evidence-based practice, translational research, and patient safety, and, with a colleague, she was the first to apply the theory of therapeutic relationships to healthcare professionals in settings other than mental health. Barnsteiner is one of the developers of the Quality and Safety Education for Nurses (QSEN) initiative and is co-author with Gwen Sherwood of the recently published text *Quality and Safety in Nursing: A Competency Based Approach to Improving Outcomes* (Wiley Blackwell, 2012). She currently serves as editor for translational research and quality improvement for the *American Journal of Nursing*. She has received the Distinguished Contributions to Nursing Research Award and the STTI Dorothy Garrigus Adams Award for Excellence in Fostering Professional Standards.

Joanne Disch, PhD, RN, FAAN, is professor ad honorem at the University of Minnesota School of Nursing. She has extensive experience as an educator, chief nurse executive, researcher, leader, policymaker, and spokesperson with degrees from the University of Wisconsin (Madison), the University of Alabama in Birmingham, and the University of Michigan.

Throughout her career, Disch has held numerous national leadership positions, including board chair and board member for AARP, president of the American Association of Critical-Care Nurses, and immediate past president of the American Academy of Nursing. Currently, she is a member of the board of directors for Aurora Health Care and chair of the Chamberlain College of Nursing board of trustees.

For more than 8 years, she was a faculty lead on the Quality and Safety Education for Nurses (QSEN) project, responsible for the content on patient-centered care. She has spoken widely and published extensively on the topic and has created system change in both academic and clinical settings to support the full inclusion of persons and their families in the care relationship.

Mary K. Walton, MSN, MBE, RN, is nurse ethicist and director of patient and family centered care at the Hospital of the University of Pennsylvania. Walton received her BSN and MSN from the University of Pennsylvania and earned a master of bioethics degree and a certificate in clinical ethics mediation from the University of Pennsylvania School of Medicine. She has practiced in academic healthcare settings for over 35 years and has a progressive history of leadership. Roles of clinical nurse specialist and nurse manager included responsibility for clinical ethics committees and ethics consultation services, cultural competency training, and establishment of evidence-based practice standards. Currently, she is responsible for organizational initiatives focused on clinical ethics and improving the patient and family experience of care. She has published in the areas of collaboration, advocacy, healthy work environment, nursing history, and patient-centered care. Recent relevant publications include the chapter on "Patient-Centered Care" in Sherwood and Barnsteiner's book (noted previously) and an *American Journal of Nursing* article on "Communicating with Family Caregivers" (2011).

Contributing Authors

Rita K. Adeniran, DrNP, RN, NEA-BC, serves as director, Office of Diversity and Inclusion, and global nurse ambassador of the Hospital of the University of Pennsylvania (HUP). She provides strategic leadership and direction for diversity, inclusion, and cultural competency for the HUP. Her leadership has brought recognition to the HUP in cultural competence education and as a resource for nurses worldwide. Adeniran was appointed to the Robert Wood Johnson Executive Nurse Fellows (RWJENF) program for 2012–2015. Adeniran is nationally and globally recognized as a consultant, educator, and author in the areas of diversity, inclusion, cultural competency, and development of frontline nursing leadership.

Jehad Z. Adwan, PhD, RN, is a clinical assistant professor at the University of Minnesota School of Nursing. He also serves as a pediatric nurse at the Amplatz Children's Hospital, Minneapolis, Minnesota. Adwan received his undergraduate education in Gaza, Palestine, in 1993, where he practiced nursing in various settings. He came to Minnesota in 1998 as a Fulbright scholar and earned a master's degree in nursing education in 2000. He completed the PhD program in 2010 and a certificate program in healthcare informatics in 2013. Adwan's teaching includes didactic and clinical instruction as part of the BSN and MN pediatric courses. He also co-teaches in the interprofessional Immunization Tour class with colleagues from the School of Nursing and College of Pharmacy. He has been involved in teaching a Massive Online Open Course (MOOC) on interprofessional healthcare informatics. Adwan's research interests include grief among nurses, children with chronic conditions, and health informatics.

Gail E. Armstrong, DNP, ACNS-BC, CNE, is an associate professor at the University of Colorado College of Nursing. Armstrong's early work in quality and safety was in her medical-surgical practice and focused on tracking and working to improve patient outcomes on her unit. Armstrong's increasing focus in quality and safety began in 2007 with her work in the national initiative Quality and Safety Education for Nurses (QSEN). Armstrong worked on the University of Colorado College of Nursing leadership team to update CU's pre-licensure clinical courses to reflect quality and safety trends. Her work in QSEN has focused on curriculum development with an emphasis on threading the competencies and knowledge, skill, and attitude elements across the classroom setting, skills/simulation lab, and clinical rotations.

Amy J. Barton, PhD, RN, FAAN, is professor, Daniel and Janet Mordecai Endowed Chair for Rural Health Nursing, and associate dean for clinical and community affairs at the University of Colorado College of Nursing. As associate dean, Barton is responsible for the continuum of clinical education, which includes oversight of laboratory and simulation experiences, coordination and staffing of over 600 clinical education placements per semester, and leadership of faculty practice. Barton obtained federal funding for Sheridan Health Services, a nurse-managed, federally qualified health center. She has published articles and book chapters on topics including faculty practice, patient outcomes, quality and safety, and informatics. She served as national nursing faculty advisor for the Josiah Macy, Jr. Foundation/IHI Open School initiative, Retooling for Quality and Safety, which involved educating medical and nursing students together. Barton is a member of the 2005 cohort of the Robert Wood Johnson Executive Nurse Fellows, a Distinguished Practitioner in the National Academies of Practice, and a fellow in the American Academy of Nursing.

Carrie Brady, JD, MA, is principal at CBrady Consulting. She is a consultant, author, and speaker who partners with hospitals to develop creative solutions to their operational challenges. For more than 15 years, Brady has worked with clinical and administrative leaders and frontline caregivers to improve the patient and staff experience, engage patients and families, and enhance quality and safety. Brady also has collaborated with policymakers on several national initiatives, including the Agency for Healthcare Research and Quality (AHRQ)/Health Research Educational Trust (HRET), HCAHPS Patient Safety Learning Network program, and Picker Institute's Always Events initiative. She is author of the book *HCAHPS Basics* (HCPro, Inc., 2009) and co-author of book chapters and resource guides on patient-centered care, including the 2013 World Innovation Summit for Health patient engagement report. Brady has held leadership positions in two provider associations, serving as vice president of quality at Planetree and as a vice president of the Connecticut Hospital Association. Brady also has directly served hospital patients and families as a volunteer artist in residence.

Tara A. Cortes, PhD, RN, FAAN, is recognized for her distinguished career spanning executive leadership, nursing education, research, and practice. She is currently the executive director of the Hartford Institute for Geriatric Nursing and a professor in geriatric nursing at the New York University College of Nursing. Cortes has provided significant contributions to advance the health of people, particularly those with limited access to the healthcare system. Importantly, she has developed collaborative models with advanced practice nurses and physicians in traditional as well as nontraditional settings to enhance the care of the American elderly population.

Cortes is a fellow of the American Academy of Nursing and a fellow of the New York Academy of Medicine. She is a past fellow of the Robert Wood Johnson Executive Nurse Fellows program. Cortes serves on several boards, including university boards and boards of healthcare organizations.

Karen Drenkard, PhD, RN, NEA-BC, FAAN, is SVP/chief clinical officer and chief nursing officer at GetWellNetwork, an interactive patient engagement technology solution firm. Her past experience includes serving as executive director at the American Nurses Credentialing Center and as SVP/chief nurse executive of Inova Health System in northern Virginia. Drenkard has published in the nursing literature on topics including strategic planning and leadership, disaster preparedness, and quality and safety in nursing; she was the principal investigator in HRSA-funded research involving the implementation of a human caring model in acute care hospitals. She is an editorial advisor to *Journal of Nursing Administration* and *Nursing Administration Quarterly* (NAQ). She is an active member of many nursing and civic organizations, serves on the board of visitors for the University of Pittsburgh School of Nursing, and is a board of trustees member at Loudoun Hospital. She is a fellow in the American Academy of Nursing.

Autumn Fiester, PhD, is director of education in the Department of Medical Ethics and Health Policy at the Perelman School of Medicine at the University of Pennsylvania. She is director of the Penn Clinical Ethics Mediation Program, which promotes clinical ethics mediation as a conflict-resolution method in both formal clinical ethics consultations and ethics conflicts at the bedside. She has been a member of the American Society for Bioethics and Humanities task force on clinical ethics consultation professionalization (Clinical Ethics Consultation Affairs standing committee). She is also co-director (with Lance Wahlert) of the newly launched Bioethics, Sexuality, and Gender Identity Project that seeks to demarcate a sub-field within bioethics that focuses on the intersection of LGBTQI issues and medical ethics (http://www.queerbioethics.org/). She is author of over 70 publications in the areas of clinical ethics, gender and sexuality, and animal ethics.

Jessie Gruman, PhD, is president and founder of the Center for Advancing Health, a nonpartisan, Washington-based policy institute that, since 1992, has been supported by foundations and individuals to work on people's engagement in their healthcare from the patient perspective. Gruman draws on her experience of treatment for five cancer diagnoses, interviews, surveys, and empirical research as the basis of her advocacy for policies and practices to overcome the challenges people face in finding good care and getting the most from it. She holds a BA from Vassar College and a PhD in social psychology from Columbia University and is a professorial lecturer in the School of Public Health and Health Services at George Washington University. She is a member of the American Academy of Arts and Sciences and the Council on Foreign Relations and a fellow of the New York Academy of Medicine and the Society of Behavioral Medicine.

Mary Koloroutis, MSN, RN, is vice president and senior consultant at Creative Health Care Management. As a co-creator, author, and editor of the *Relationship-Based Care* series of books and seminars, Koloroutis helps healthcare organizations create a framework for delivering world-class care with strong underlying values and principles. One of her most far-reaching programs, Re-Igniting the Spirit of Caring, helps members of the healthcare team transform their workplaces into cultures where responsibility prevails, relationships thrive, and caring and healing are the foundations of each working day.

Her most recent works—the Therapeutic Relationships workshop and the book *See Me as a Person: Creating Therapeutic Relationships with Patients and their Families* (Creative Health Care Management, 2012), co-created with psychologist Michael Trout—emphasize the importance of an authentic therapeutic connection, with every person needing care as a fundamental condition for healing.

Koloroutis has her BSN from the University of Mary-Hardin Baylor in Temple, Texas, and earned an MSN in nursing administration from the University of Minnesota. She currently lives in Champaign/Urbana, Illinois.

Françoise Mathieu, MEd, CCC, is a certified mental health counsellor, compassion fatigue specialist at Compassion Fatigue Solutions Inc. Mathieu is author of *The Compassion Fatigue Workbook,* which was published by Routledge in 2012. She is a leader in compassion fatigue and vicarious trauma education in Canada. Her experience stems from many years working as a crisis counsellor and trauma specialist in various settings, such as healthcare, community mental health, the military, and with victims of crime. Since 2001, she has offered hundreds of seminars on compassion fatigue and vicarious trauma across North America to thousands of helping professionals in the fields of healthcare, trauma services, law enforcement, immigration services, child welfare, palliative care, education, and addiction.

Leslie McLean, MScN, RN, is an advanced practice nurse and project manager with the Capital Health Cancer Care Program in Halifax, Nova Scotia; coordinator of the Capital Health Clinical Ethics Consultation Service; and adjunct professor with Dalhousie University School of Nursing. McLean obtained a bachelor of arts degree from Mount Allison University, a degree in chemistry from the University of Toronto, a bachelor of science in nursing from McMaster University, and a master of science in nursing from Dalhousie University. She has worked for over 30 years in a variety of roles and settings in healthcare, both within Canada and abroad, and is dedicated to helping to create healthy, supportive work environments for healthcare providers.

Shirley M. Moore, PhD, RN, FAAN, is the Edward J. and Louise Mellon Professor of Nursing and associate dean for research at Frances Payne Bolton School of Nursing, Case Western Reserve University. She is past president of the Academy for Healthcare Improvement. She has provided leadership in six national projects addressing the design and test of interdisciplinary curricula on continuous quality improvement and is currently co-director of the VA National Quality Scholars Fellowship Program. Moore was a member of the leadership team of the national Quality and Safety Education for Nurses (QSEN) project and is a leader in the QSEN Institute located at Case Western Reserve University. She is director of a National Institutes of Health-funded Center of Excellence in Self-Management Research. An important dimension of this center is the FIND Lab, a laboratory that is focused on the full inclusion of persons with disabilities in mainstream research.

Wesley Nuffer, PharmD, BCPS, CDE, is assistant director of experiential programs at the University of Colorado Skaggs School of Pharmacy and Pharmaceutical Sciences. Nuffer works in the experiential office of the School of Pharmacy, working to coordinate student activities in pharmacy practice sites during their introductory and advanced pharmacy practice experiences. He is involved in a number of interprofessional education initiatives both on campus and in experiential training sites. His research interests include obesity, diabetes, women's health, and experiential teaching and learning. He practices in the endocrinology department of University of Colorado Hospital, helping to manage patients with diabetes.

Meghan Thornton O'Brien, MBE, is an MD candidate for 2014 at the Perelman School of Medicine, University of Pennsylvania. Thornton is a graduate of the Perelman School of Medicine at the University of Pennsylvania, where she earned her master of bioethics degree. As an undergraduate at Brown University, she studied American studies with a focus on race and ethnicity. Since starting medical school, she has worked extensively with Puentes de Salud, a Philadelphia clinic that serves mostly undocumented Spanish-speaking immigrants. She has also worked on health-policy projects to improve care transitions and looks forward to continuing advocacy work and patient care as she embarks on the next phase of her clinical training.

Margaret Dexheimer Pharris, PhD, MPH, RN, FAAN, is associate dean and professor for nursing at St. Catherine University in St. Paul and Minneapolis, Minnesota. As associate dean, she collaborates with 80+ nurse educator colleagues to serve 800+ nursing students from associate degree to DNP and actively collaborates on interprofessional education with directors of the 30+ health programs within St. Catherine's Henrietta Schmoll School of Health. Her vocation focuses on graduating diverse nurse leaders who are adept at interprofessional team collaboration to provide high-quality patient-centered care, with particular attention on addressing health inequities. Her community-based collaborative action research is inspired by the theory of Margaret Newman. With Susan Bosher, Pharris co-edited the 2008 book *Transforming Nursing Education: The Culturally Inclusive Environment* (Springer, 2008) and she has co-authored with Carol Pavlish *Community-Based Collaborative Action Research: A Nursing Approach* (Jones & Bartlett Learning, 2011), which won a 2011 *AJN* Book of the Year Award in the research category.

Susan A. Phillips, MSN, RN, PMHCNS-BC, is an advanced practice nurse living in Phoenix, Arizona, who worked for Banner Health for 26 years. Phillips is a psychiatric mental health clinical nurse specialist and nurse practitioner who has practiced in both the behavioral health and medical-surgical acute care settings. Most recently, Phillips was senior manager in the Department of Professional Practice at Banner Good Samaritan Medical Center, a Magnet hospital. Phillips co-facilitated the Workplace Violence Committee there and taught crisis intervention to employees for many years. Phillips is passionate about creating safe and healthy work environments so nurses can find joy in their work and provide excellent nursing care. She is also adjunct faculty in the College of Nursing and Health Sciences at University of Phoenix and has taught in a variety of nursing programs.

Victoria L. Rich, PhD, RN, FAAN, is recognized for her leadership in healthcare, business, and nursing education, most notably for her pioneering work in patient safety and cultural diversity. She is the 2013 recipient of the American Organization of Nurse Executives (AONE) Prism Diversity award and was featured on the cover of the national magazine *Nurse Leader*, June 2013 issue.

Rich earned her bachelor of science in biology from Indiana University of Pennsylvania and graduated summa cum laude with a bachelor of science in nursing in 1979 from Indiana University of Pennsylvania. She received a master of science and a doctorate degree in nursing administration from the University of Pittsburgh in 1984 and 1991, respectively. She has developed numerous patient safety initiatives for healthcare systems globally. Rich is an expert in root cause analysis and the development of corrective action plans for hospitals and state and federal agencies; she has provided consultation and expertise in patient safety and nursing leadership practice worldwide.

Rich recently stepped aside as chief nurse executive and associate executive director at the University of Pennsylvania Medical Center, where she directed nursing practice at the 802-bed, quaternary acute care academic center and 47 medical practice sites. Since 2002, she served as a senior hospital administrator to implement the academic center's missions, strategic plans, patient care programs, nursing budgets, resource allocations, and operational plans. She is an associate professor of nursing administration at the University of Pennsylvania School of Nursing.

Cheristi Cognetta Rieke, DNP, RN, is a nurse manager of acute and critical care nursing float pool at the University of Minnesota Amplatz Children's Hospital and the University of Minnesota Medical Center, Fairview. She is a graduate of the doctor of nursing practice program in the specialty of Health Innovation and Leadership. Rieke was the principle investigator and boundary-spanning leader for the MyStory Initiative that was supported by the Picker Institute with an Always Events Grant.

Juliette Schlucter, BS, is a patient- and family-centered care consultant at BRIDGEKEEPER Consulting. For the past 22 years, Schlucter has worked with healthcare professionals in developing systems that support patient- and family-centered care. She came to her work initially as a family advocate, following the diagnosis of cystic fibrosis of her son and daughter in 1991. She has consulted on topics related to quality, safety, and education with numerous healthcare organizations.

From 1995 through 2010, Schlucter provided leadership for patient- and family-centered care at The Children's Hospital of Philadelphia. While there, Schlucter created and served as lead author of The Promise of Partnership, a toolkit used to teach best-practice behaviors for patient- and family-centered care. She co-created the Family as Faculty program, established the Family Advisory Council, created the Family-Centered Intern program, and wrote Partners for Excellence, a workshop to teach parents about using healthcare resources effectively.

Since 1996, Schlucter has served as faculty to the Institute for Patient- and Family-Centered Care.

Gwen D. Sherwood, PhD, RN, FAAN, is professor and associate dean for academic affairs at the University of North Carolina at Chapel Hill School of Nursing. Sherwood has a distinguished record in advancing nursing education locally and globally. She served as co-investigator from 2005–2012 for the Robert Wood Johnson-funded Quality and Safety Education for Nurses (QSEN) project to transform curricula to prepare nurses to be able to lead quality and safety as part of their daily work. Her work to advance nursing education and nursing leadership derives from her research on teamwork to improve patient safety, caring and spirituality, reflective practice, and interactive pedagogy. She is a graduate of Georgia Baptist College of Nursing, North Carolina Central University, the University of North Carolina at Chapel Hill, and the University of Texas at Austin. She is past president of the International Association for Human Caring and past vice president of the Honor Society of Nursing, Sigma Theta Tau International. Among many honors, she is a fellow in the American Academy of Nursing. Her most recent books include *AJN* Book of the Year *Quality and Safety Education: A Competency Approach for Nurses* (Wiley-Blackwell, 2012) and *Reflective Practice: Transforming Education to Improve Outcomes* (Sigma Theta Tau International, 2012).

Carol Taylor, PhD, RN, is a senior research scholar in the Kennedy Institute of Ethics at Georgetown University and a professor of nursing. Taylor has a PhD in philosophy with a concentration in bioethics from Georgetown University and a master's degree in medical-surgical nursing from Catholic University. She chose doctoral work in philosophy with a concentration in bioethics because of a passion to "make healthcare work" for those who need it. She now works closely with healthcare professionals and leaders who are exploring the ethical dimensions of their practice. She lectures internationally, writes on various issues in healthcare ethics, and serves as an ethics consultant to systems and professional organizations. She is the author of *Fundamentals of Nursing: The Art and Science of Nursing Care* (Lippincott, Williams & Wilkins, 2013), which is now in its seventh edition, and co-editor of *Health and Human Flourishing: Religion, Medicine and Moral Anthropology* (Georgetown University Press, 2006) and the fourth edition of *Case Studies in Nursing Ethics* (Jones & Bartlett Learning, 2011).

Michael Trout, MA, is director of The Infant-Parent Institute, Inc. Trout completed his specialized training in infant psychiatry at the Child Development Project, University of Michigan School of Medicine. He directs an institute engaged in research, clinical practice, and clinical training related to problems of attachment. He was founding president of the International Association for Infant Mental Health, was on the charter editorial board of *Infant Mental Health Journal*, served as vice president for the United States for the World Association for Infant Mental Health, and served on the board of directors for the International Society for Prenatal and Perinatal Psychology and Medicine. He currently serves on the professional advisory board for Attachment Parenting International. Trout is author or co-author of three books and producer of 15 documentary films and two meditation CDs. He was the 1984 recipient of the Selma Fraiberg Award and the 2009 recipient of a Lifetime Achievement Award for his clinical work with infants of loss and trauma.

Sarah Vittone, MSN, MA, RN, is assistant professor of nursing at the School of Nursing and Health Studies at Georgetown University, where her teaching assignments include human growth and development and healthcare ethics. Her clinical background is in pediatric nursing. Vittone is an ethics consultant with the Center for Clinical Bioethics at Georgetown University, where she works with interdisciplinary teams. She is also supported through grant funding by the Georgetown-Howard University Clinical and Translational Science Award for work in research ethics, human protection, and advocacy.

Lance Wahlert, PhD, is assistant professor of medical ethics and health policy and director of the master of bioethics program in the Perelman School of Medicine at the University of Pennsylvania. An historian of medicine, literary scholar, queer theorist, and disability scholar by training, Wahlert is also core faculty member in gender, sexuality, and women's studies at Penn and serves as director of the Project on Bioethics, Sexuality, and Gender Identity, which has demarcated a sub-field within bioethics that focuses on the intersections of LGBTQI health issues and medical ethics. Having been funded by the Wellcome Trust Centre for the History of Medicine, the National Institutes of Health, and the Pew Foundation, Wahlert's work on narrative medicine and LGBTQI health has been featured in numerous peer-reviewed publications in the humanities and biosciences, including his serving as guest editor of the *Journal of Medical Humanities* and the *Journal of Bioethical Inquiry*.

Jennifer E. Wason, BA, MLIS, currently is project assistant to Shirley M. Moore, associate dean for research and the Edward J. and Louis Mellon Professor of Nursing at the Frances Payne Bolton School of Nursing at Case Western Reserve University. She was formerly assistant editor for Webster's New World brand products at John Wiley and Sons and Houghton Mifflin Harcourt. She completed her master of library and information science degree at Kent State University and also attended Kenyon College.

Ann S. Williams, PhD, RN, CDE, is research associate professor at Case Western Reserve University. Williams has worked in community-based diabetes education since 1986, initially as a clinician and more recently as a nurse scientist. She designs and conducts self-management research, with particular interest in the self-management needs of persons with disabilities. Her projects have included investigations of the accuracy of dosing with insulin pens by blind persons; the effectiveness of a novel method of nonvisual foot self-examination for people with visual impairment; and the effectiveness of systems-based, community-based support groups for maintaining diabetes self-management behaviors for both fully sighted and visually impaired persons. Williams was lead author of the Disabilities Position Statement for the American Association of Diabetes Educators. She is also co-director of the FIND Lab at Case Western Reserve University, which provides consultation to healthcare researchers promoting **F**ull **IN**clusion of Persons with **D**isabilities in mainstream healthcare research.

David Wright, MPH, brings more than 20 years of experience in healthcare and hospital leadership to his role as senior vice president at GetWellNetwork. Prior to joining the organization, Wright spent 13 years as lead marketing, strategy, and business development executive for the Inova Health System, one of the largest integrated health systems on the Eastern Seaboard. Wright's role at GetWellNetwork centers on assisting clients in achieving their desired outcomes. Greater Washington universities recognize Wright as an outstanding preceptor and adjunct faculty member. He has received numerous awards for communications, advertising, public relations, healthcare strategy, and marketing excellence, including the American Hospital Association's (AHA) national marketing excellence award. Wright has a BS degree from Virginia Polytechnic Institute and State University and a master's degree in public health with an emphasis in healthcare administration from the University of California, Los Angeles.

Lynne Yancey, MD, is an associate professor and associate director of interprofessional education at the University of Colorado School of Medicine. Yancey is an emergency physician and associate director for interprofessional education (IPE) at the Anschutz Medical Campus. She directs two of the three portions of the IPE curriculum. The Clinical Transformations Program serves to bridge the pre-clinical and clinical portions of the curriculum through interprofessional simulation experiences coupled with debriefs by trained facilitators. The Clinical Integrations Program serves as the capstone of the IPE curriculum, where students apply their knowledge of team function and communication to the real world of patient care.

Prior to joining the IPE team, Yancey created the first-ever interprofessional simulation experience within the School of Medicine and served as medical director of the Center for Advancing Professional Excellence, where she supervised development of teaching curriculum and evaluation modules using simulation and standardized patients for multiple healthcare professional education programs. Before entering academic medicine, she learned firsthand the importance of highly functioning teams as an aircrew member and flight surgeon in the U.S. Air Force.

Table of Contents

About the Authors vii
Contributing Authors viii
Foreword xxvii
Introduction xxix

Part I: Person- and Family-Centered Care—Setting the Scene

Chapter 1: The Landscape for Nurturing Person- and Family-Centered Care . . 1
    Definition of Person- and Family-Centered Care (P&FCC) 2
    Understanding Societal Factors That Affect P&FCC 3
        The Medical-Industrial Complex 3
        A Widening Income Gap 4
        Social Values 5
        Consumerism 5
        Time 7
        Incivility 7
    Understanding the Healthcare-Related Factors That Affect P&FCC 8
        The Medical Model of Healthcare Delivery 9
        Mismatch Between What Providers Believe and What Patients Want 10
        Professional Autonomy 10
        Technology 12
        The Education of Health Professionals 12
        Financing of Healthcare 13
    Conclusion 15

Chapter 2: Overview and History of Person- and Family-Centered Care 19
    An Overview of Person- and Family-Centered Care 20
    History of Person- and Family-Centered Care 23
    Demonstrated Outcomes of Person- and Family-Centered Care 24
        Person Outcomes 25
        Financial Outcomes 25
        Family Outcomes 26
    Myths Related to Person- and Family-Centered Care 26
    Standards and Regulations: A Stimulus for Person- and
        Family-Centered Care 28
    Competencies Necessary for Delivering
        Person- and Family-Centered Nursing Care 30
    Conclusion 32

Chapter 3: A Patient's Perspective on Patient- and Family-Centered Care 35

    A Patient's Perspective 35

    Reorganizing Healthcare to Become Patient- and Family-Centered 36

        What Are Our Responsibilities for Our Healthcare? 37

        How Are We Responding to the Need to Participate More Fully in

            Our Care? 38

        How Can Healthcare Be Organized to Support Patients' and Families'

            Active and Knowledgeable Participation in Our Care? 39

    Conclusion 41

Chapter 4: Avoiding the Dark Sides of Patient- and Family-Centered Care 43

    The Dark Sides of Leadership 44

        Making Patient-Centered Commitments Without Planning 45

        Reinforcing Misperceptions 46

        Avoiding the Dark Sides of Leadership 47

    The Dark Sides of the Patient/Family Partnership 48

        Doing Things to/for Patients and Families Instead of in Partnership 48

        Inappropriate Transfer of Responsibility 50

        Avoiding the Dark Sides of the Patient/Family Partnership 50

    The Dark Sides of Staff Engagement 51

        Dismissing Staff Needs 52

        Creating the Expectation That the Patient Is Always Right 53

        Avoiding the Dark Sides of Staff Engagement 54

    The Dark Sides of Patient-Centered Data Use 54

        Losing Sight of the Goal and Chasing Scores 55

        Demoralizing Staff 55

        Avoiding the Dark Sides of Data Use and Performance Improvement 56

    Conclusion 56

Chapter 5: The "Difficult" Patient Reconceived 59

    The Conventional View of the "Difficult" Patient 60

    The "Difficult" Patient Reconceived 62

    Ethical Obligations to the "Difficult" Patient 64

    The "Difficult" Patient and the Role of the Ethics Consultation Service 66

    Conclusion 68

Chapter 6: A Global View of Person- and Family-Centered Care 71

    A Global Concept of Patient- and Family-Centered Care 72

        A Global Definition of P&FCC 72

        Components of P&FCC 74

        Stakeholders in P&FCC 76

    International Perspectives on P&FCC 76

        International Alliance of Patients' Organizations 77

        The World Health Organization 78

The Pan American Health Organization 80
Institute for Healthcare Improvement 80
International Council of Nurses 81
Patients' Experiences With Care 82
Examples of P&FCC in Other Countries 84
Palestine: Family Involvement in Care in Gaza Hospital 85
Sweden 87
Australia 87
The Democratic Republic of the Congo (DRC) 88
Uganda 88
Somalia 88
Interventions to Promote P&FCC 89
Conclusion 92

Part II: Models for Person- and Family-Centered Care

Chapter 7: Patient Engagement and Activation 95
What Is Patient Engagement? 96
Why Is Patient Engagement Important? 97
The Current State of Patient Engagement 100
The Influence of Engagement on Patient Outcomes 100
Patient Activation 101
Focus of Research 102
Patient Engagement and Technology 103
Interactive Patient Care Technology: Improving Patient Engagement 103
Interactive Patient Care Technology: Advancing Nursing Practice 106
Nursing's Role in Patient Engagement 106
Barriers and Challenges to Increasing Patient Engagement 108
Patient Engagement and Population Health 109
Conclusion 110

Chapter 8: Cultivating Mindful and Compassionate Connections 113
Relationship-Based Care 115
Human Caring Research and Theory 117
Knowing 118
Being With 118
Doing For 118
Enabling 118
Maintaining Belief 118
Attunement and Human Attachment 119
The Therapeutic Relationship 120
Presence Through Attunement 121
Wondering 121
Following 122

Holding *122*
Applications in the Field 123
Q&A: Perceiving a Family Member as Aggressive or Controlling *123*
Q&A: Staying Compassionate With Patients Suffering From
Medical Issues Related to Alcoholism *125*
Conclusion 126

Chapter 9: Hallmarks of a Culture of Patient- and Family-Centered
Care in the Care Setting 129
Reconceptualizing Hospital Culture 130
Realigning Organizational Philosophy and Operations 131
Education and Commitment of Providers 133
Patient Engagement: Active Agents in the Hospital Experience 134
Exemplar Models of Care 135
Institute for Healthcare Improvement *135*
Institute for Patient- and Family-Centered Care *136*
The Picker Institute *136*
The Planetree Model *137*
Changing the Culture: Patient-Centered Approaches to Encourage
Patient and Family Engagement 141
Reframing Hospital Processes to Establish a Culture of P&FCC *141*
Resources to Help Change the Culture *142*
Putting It Together: Hallmarks of P&FCC 142
Admission *143*
Interprofessional Patient Rounds *144*
Family Meetings *144*
Flexible Schedules *144*
Patient-Directed Visitation *145*
Patient/Family-Initiated Rapid Response Teams *146*
Spiritual Care *146*
Respectful Partnerships *146*
Nurse-to-Nurse Handoffs (Handovers) *146*
Coordinating Care in Ancillary Departments *147*
Discharge Planning *147*
Healing Environment *147*
Access to Nutrition Resources *147*
Information Resources *148*
Working With Patient and Family Advisors *148*
Conclusion 148

Chapter 10: Family Systems Theory 151
Systems Theory 152
Family Systems Theory 153
Boundary *154*
Differentiation *155*

Balance *155*
Overfunctioning/Underfunctioning *156*
Triangles *156*
Families of Origin *157*
Integrating the Concepts of Family Systems Theory Into Care Strategies 157
A Communication Link for Information Exchange *158*
An Appropriate Communication Care Plan *159*
Family Meetings *159*
Sources of Family Anger and Other Strong Emotions *160*
Sources of Collateral and Historical Information *161*
Family Opinions and Expectations *161*
Applying Family Systems Theory to Foster a Healthy Work Environment ... 162
Therapeutic Relationships 163
Overfunctioning and Underfunctioning in One's Professional Role *164*
Self-Monitoring *166*
Conclusion 166

Chapter 11: Ethical Dilemmas in Person- and Family-Centered Care 169
Nursing and Ethics 170
Nursing *170*
Nursing Ethics *171*
Moral Distress *172*
Theories of Bioethics 173
Person-Centered Care 174
What Makes a Dilemma Ethical in Nature? 175
What Is a Dilemma? *176*
Examples of Ethical Dilemmas *176*
The Role of Values in Ethical Dilemmas 177
Diversity—Discipline and Specialty Values *177*
Identifying and Reflecting on Personal Values *178*
Value-Laden Conflict *179*
Enablers for Voicing Values 180
Things Within Our Own Control *180*
Within the Organizational Context *181*
Resources to Assist With Morally Distressing Situations 181
Conclusion 183

Chapter 12: Patient-Centered Care in the Face of Cultural Conflict 185
The Backbone of Patient-Centered Care in the Face of Cultural Conflict 186
Patient-Centered Care Calls for a Dual Focus on Systems and Individuals .. 187
Averting Cultural Conflict Through Caring Connection 189
Unconscious Bias 192
Patient-Centered Care Across Cultural Care Belief Systems ... 192
Nursing in the Midst of Serious Cultural Conflict 194

Engaging Patient Perspectives to Create Systems of Cultural Care 198
Implications for Practice 199
Conclusion 200

Chapter 13: Special Considerations of Person- and Family-Centered Care Related to Age 203
Population Relevant Statistics 204
Challenges 205
Age-Specific Needs—Children *206*
Age-Specific Needs—Older Adults *206*
Communication With and Integration of All Families 207
Collaboration and Integration With All Families 209
Coordination and Integration of All Families 210
Exemplar of Person-Centered Care for the Special Patient Population 210
Key Points and Practical Implications 211
Communication, Coordination, and Collaboration Across the Care Continuum *211*
Strategies to Ensure Emphasis and Rigor Are Applied to P&FCC Initiative *212*
Leveraging Technology to Provide and Embed P&FCC Within an Organizational Structure *213*
Conclusion 213

Part III: Strategies to Promote Person- and Family-Centered Care

Chapter 14: Advocating for Patients and Families 215
Defining Patient Advocacy 216
The What *of Patient Advocacy* *216*
The Who *of Patient Advocacy* *220*
The How *of Patient Advocacy* *221*
Advocacy Reflection 222
Advocacy as a Skill 225
Critiquing the Adequacy of One's Personal, Team, and Institutional
Ability and Willingness to Advocate for Patients and Families 227
Scenario 1: "Staying the Course" *227*
Scenario 2: "Don't Rock the Boat" *229*
Scenario 3: Compassionate Use…Maybe? *230*
The *When* of Advocacy 231
The *Why* of Advocacy 231
Arguments Debating the Role of the Nurse Advocate 233
Advocating for Advocates 234
Constraining and Facilitating Forces for Advocacy 235
Constraining Forces *235*
Facilitating Forces *236*
Conclusion 239

Chapter 15: Using the Techniques of Mediation to Promote Person- and Family-Centered Care 243

What Is Mediation? 244
Using Mediation in Healthcare 245
The Unique Position of the Clinical Nurse 246
Techniques to Promote Person- and Family-Centered Care ... 247
    Listening for Understanding 247
    Preparing 249
    Summarizing 249
    Distinguishing Between Positions and Interests 250
    Reframing 251
    Questioning 253
    Elevating the Definition of the Problem 254
    Eliciting the Medical Facts 254
    Caucusing 255
    Developing Options and Packaging Proposals 256
    Establishing a Clear Agreement 256
Conclusion 256

Chapter 16: Ethics Consultation 259

Origins of Ethics Consultation Services 260
What Is Healthcare Ethics Consultation? 261
    Literature Regarding Ethics Consultation 261
How Does Ethics Consultation Promote P&FCC? 262
    Quality in Ethics Consultation 262
    Bringing the Patient Voice Forward 263
    Recognition of the Important Role of the Family 264
Identifying the Value-Laden Concerns 266
    What Are Values? 266
Formulating an Ethics Question 268
    Transparency 270
The Nursing Role in Using Ethics Consultation to Promote P&FCC ... 271
    Initiating an Ethics Consultation 271
    Assisting in the Ethics Consultation Process 273
    Identify the Key Stakeholders 273
    Illustrate the Patient's Daily Life 274
    Support the Patient and Family 274
    Participate in Consult Meetings 274
Learning From the Consultation Process 275
Conclusion 275

Chapter 17: High-Intensity Situations That Provoke Conflict ... 279

Defining Conflict 280
    Prevalence of Conflict in Healthcare 280

Causes and Sources of High-Intensity Conflict in Healthcare 281
Preventing, Resolving, and Managing High-Intensity Conflict 284
   Gracious Space. 285
   Effective Communication. 285
   Conflict Management 290
Consequences of Unresolved Conflict in Healthcare 291
A Patient- and Family-Centered Approach to Preventing Conflict
   in Healthcare. 292
Conclusion 293

**Chapter 18: Working With Abusive, Bullying, or Violent Patients
and Families** 297
What Is Workplace Violence? 298
   Workplace Violence Statistics. 298
   Why Patients and Families Exhibit Violent Behavior. 299
   Factors That Contribute to Violence 299
Why Are Nurses Vulnerable? 301
   The Nature of the Relationship. 301
   A Lack of Skill 302
   An Assumption That It's Part of the Job 302
   Underreporting 302
   Environmental Influences 303
   Impact of Violence 303
   Healthcare Professional's Responses 303
Proactive Organizational Strategies to Counter Workplace Violence 305
Working With Disruptive Family Members 307
Individual Strategies to Counter Workplace Violence 308
Setting Limits 310
Treatment Team Strategies 311
   Behavioral Contracts. 311
   Debriefing 311
Conclusion 312

**Chapter 19: Narrative Approaches to Understanding Patient and
Family Perspectives** 315
The Relationship Between Storytelling and Healthcare. 317
How Stories Work and Why They Are Important in Clinical Settings 318
   Active Listening. 319
   Close Reading. 319
   Close Listening. 319
   Telling Stories. 320
   The Healing Power of Hearing. 321
Types of Narrative. 321

What to Do With Stories 322
   To Bear Witness 322
   To Share 323
   To Interpret and Authenticate 324
The Narrative in Clinical Practice 325
   Close Reading 326
   Telling Stories 326
   Eliciting the Patient's Story 327
   Writing the Patient's Story 328
   Writing With Patients and Their Families 328
Narrative Pitfalls 329
Case Scenarios 330
   Healthcare Scenario 1: Narrative in an Emergency Care Setting 330
   Healthcare Scenario 2: Narrative in a Chronic Care Setting 331
   Healthcare Scenario 3: Narrative in a Pastoral Care Setting 332
Conclusion 334

Chapter 20: Managing Compassion Fatigue, Burnout, and Moral Distress 337
Burnout 339
   Burnout in Physicians Affects Patient Care 340
   The Challenge of Increased Interaction With Family Members 340
Role Overload 341
Compassion Fatigue 343
   What Is Compassion Fatigue? 343
   The Impact of Compassion Fatigue and Burnout on
     Patient-Centered Care 347
An "Ethical Climate" 348
Moral Distress 348
   What Is Moral Distress? 349
   Three Causes of Moral Distress 349
   The Connection Between Compassion Fatigue and Moral Distress 352
Strategies for Creating a Positive Ethical Climate 352
   Reducing Compassion Fatigue and Burnout—What Works? 353
   Individual Strategies 355
   Professional Strategies 356
   Organizational Strategies 359
Conclusion 360

**Chapter 21: Patient- and Family-Centered Care and the
Interprofessional Team** 365
P&FCC and the Interprofessional Mandate for All Healthcare Professions . . 366
Strategies to Enhance Team Functioning 368
   Open and Direct Communication 368
   Shared Decision-Making 370

Collegial Trust *371*
"Swift" Trust *372*
Virtual Teams and Trust *373*
Humility *373*
Barriers to Effective Team Functioning 374
Failure to Understand and Respect Each Other's Strengths 374
Team Conflict 374
The Persistently Dynamic Makeup of Healthcare Teams 375
Authority Gradients 376
Avoiding Confrontation 377
Is the Difficult Patient Really the Complex Patient? 378
Contemporary Models for Care Provision with the Patient and
    Family as Integral Partners 379
Outpatient Patient-Centered Medical Home Model 379
Inpatient P&FCC Models 381
Case Scenario 1: At the Pharmacy 381
Case Scenario 2: Palliative Care 383
Conclusion 386

Chapter 22: Healing Environments **389**
What Is a Healing Environment? 390
The Use of Evidence-Based Design to Promote Healing Environments 391
Patient Comfort and Control 391
Reduction of Stress Through Environmental Features 393
Access to Social Support From Family and Friends 393
Healing Environments Are Safe Environments 394
Design for Inclusion 395
Key Points for Practice 399
Conclusion 400

Chapter 23: System Change for Patient- and Family-Centered Care 403
Leadership Commitment 404
Patient and Family Engagement: A Call to Action 406
Formal Patient and Family Advisory Roles 407
Patient, Family, and Youth Advisory Councils 407
Patient and Family Faculty 407
Peer-to-Peer Mentors 407
Patients and Families in Paid Professional Roles 408
A Model of Collaboration 408
An Example to Appreciate Separate Realities 410
Domains of System Change and Key Questions 412
Vision, Mission, and Strategy 412
Communication 412
Training, Tools, and Resources 413

      Human Resources 413
      Honoring Excellence 414
   Conclusion 414

**Chapter 24: The Role of Leaders in Assuring Person- and
Family-Centered Care** 415
   The Role of Leaders in Promoting Person-Centered Care 416
   Gaining Organizational Buy-In for P&FCC 419
   Strategies for Achieving P&FCC 422
   Activities for Incorporating Patients and Families 423
      Conduct an Organizational Assessment 424
      Invite Clinicians and Leaders to Conduct Self-Assessments 424
      Establish a Person and Family Advisory Council 425
      Create a Healthy, Person-Centered Environment 425
      Select and Implement Specific Programs and Initiatives 427
   Analysis of the Vignette 427
   Establish Ways to Contribute to Policy Development 428
   Conclusion 430

Chapter 25: The Call for a Change to Person- and Family-Centered Care 433
   New Ways of Thinking 433
      *A Move From Patient-Centered Care to Person- and
        Family-Centered Care* 434
      P&FCC Is Not an "Add-On" 434
      Patients and Families as Partners With the Healthcare Team 435
      Moving From the Notion of a Family Spokesperson to a Spokesgroup 435
      Understanding Culture and Diversity 436
      Reconceptualizing Work Processes 437
      *Understanding the Health Insurance Portability and
        Accountability Act* 439
      Creating a Culture, Not a Program 439
      Increasing Use of Technology 440
   Cutting-Edge Initiatives That Illustrate P&FCC 440
   Conclusion 441

Appendix: Resources 443

Index 453

Foreword

One of the privileges of my role at the Institute for Healthcare Improvement (IHI) is the opportunity to witness, firsthand, inspiring innovations in person- and family-centered care. I have seen many examples—both here in the USA and in healthcare systems around the world. As a result, I know that when we *truly* partner with patients and their families, we can radically transform the way healthcare is delivered.

Christian Farman of Sweden is a patient who transformed the way his personal care was delivered and led the way for others. Farman was on dialysis, and in frustration, he said to staff nurse Britt-Mari Banck, "You have to help me treat myself. I need to have control in my life." Banck courageously agreed to help. She went to the head nurse on the unit, and together they approached the hospital's CEO to plan how to meet Farman's needs. With him playing a central role, the team set up a new *self-dialysis* unit. It takes this kind of full collaboration—patients working with frontline staff, managers, and senior leaders—to transform care.

Years later, patients in Jönköping County participate and collaborate in teaching each other how to self-dialyze. They attend dialysis when it suits their schedule, rather than following the hospital's schedule. This control and freedom make it easier for them to find jobs, and they experience fewer complications and infections. This is just one example, but it perfectly illustrates how person- and family-centered care not only reduces the burden of treatment but also produces better health and outcomes.

I have respected and followed the work of Jane Barnsteiner, Joanne Disch, and Mary Walton for many years. As editors of this book, they have created a comprehensive guide for nurses. This indispensable volume reveals an important truth—that person- and family-centered care is a journey, not a destination.

The authors expertly take us through many aspects of person- and family-centered care. Each chapter begins with a patient story or a case study and then provides the relevant theoretical frameworks and strategies to improve how we address the specific area. They cover wide-ranging themes—from culture to strategy and from patient perspectives to the challenges staff members face in delivering direct care.

I thoroughly agree with the authors when they say that true engagement will be "highly disruptive." We need nurses who are willing to partner with patients and their families to lead these disruptive innovations to transform the delivery of care.

One of the issues I've been thinking about lately is, how do we take up the challenge of meeting the healthcare needs of the so-called Millennial generation? Last year, I met Trevor Torres, a young man with diabetes. He described to me how *he* is the expert in managing his own diabetes. When Trevor has a query for his healthcare team, he doesn't want an appointment for a face-to-face visit in a couple of weeks. He wants his team to be as accessible as other parts of his life are. He wants a video call, or an email conversation, or text messages with prompt responses. We need the kinds of disruptive innovations described in this book if we are to meet the challenge of caring for a new generation of patients.

Those who may have heard me speak over the years about this crucial issue know that person- and family-centered care is very close to my heart. Whether I'm sitting in a boardroom full of senior healthcare professionals, or speaking to large audiences at IHI Forums, or visiting healthcare teams, I always try to bring the conversation back to the patients and their families. As my colleagues Michael Barry and Susan Edgman-Levitan powerfully expressed, we need to know and ask *"What matters to you?"* and not *"What's the matter?"* We need to be ready to listen when we receive the answer and to partner with patients and their families to meet their needs and co-produce better health.

In our new information age, with online specialists and e-journals, some may ask why we need a physical textbook at all. This book precisely answers those questions. In a single, easily accessible volume, you have at your fingertips not just a string of facts and evidence, but the distillation of the personal experiences of multiple gifted authors. Their voices bring to life, and set in a real context, the road map to person- and family-centered care.

All around the world, nurses are at the forefront of delivering person- and family-centered care. This book is an essential resource for all nurses—whether they are delivering direct care, managing services, or advocating for patients in the boardroom. I know you will enjoy it and learn from it, just as much as I have.

Maureen Bisognano
President and CEO
Institute for Healthcare Improvement

Introduction

The impetus for this book arose from a series of experiences we each have encountered over the years as nurses, patients, and family members. We have worked with frustrated nurses, other healthcare providers, and administrators who complained about angry patients and demanding family members. Additionally, each of us has experienced being a patient and at the bedside of a loved one and recognized the power of and the need for person-centered care. At one point, someone suggested that "a book needs to be written—to help nurses know how to deal with these difficult people." When this suggestion was made to us, we agreed that a book needed to be written—but not to put "these people" in their place. Rather, we thought it would be helpful to view the concept of patient-centered care in a broader, more contemporary light and to offer strategies for effectively working with patients and their families.

Along the way, we gained several insights that shaped this book. First, and most importantly, the word "patient" is no longer adequate for representing a recipient of care. Increasingly, in today's healthcare environment, individuals receiving care are not only patients in hospitals but also individuals in ambulatory facilities, clinics, schools, community centers, and in their own homes or as residents in long-term care facilities. They may be ill, they may be healthy with a chronic condition, or they may be seeking preventive healthcare. And healthcare is being delivered in all manner of environments, not just hospitals, so the word patient is insufficient.

Furthermore, there is growing recognition that caregivers need to "engage the person to treat the patient" (Schenck & Churchill, 2012, p. 138), even if the person is a patient in a hospital. In their award-winning book, Koloroutis and Trout (2012) give voice from the patient's perspective: *See me as a person*. No matter the setting, patients teach us that individuals seeking healthcare are vulnerable, and effective clinicians are able to recognize, validate, and lessen their vulnerability through partnerships aimed at healing (Churchill, Fanning, & Schenck, 2013). Because this change from patient to person is evolutionary, you will note that some chapters retain the use of the term *patient* and some use *person*. Both terms are used, at times for clarity and depending on the situation and the author.

Second, the person needs to be less a recipient of care and more "a source of control and full partner," according to the QSEN definition (Cronenwett et al., 2007, p. 123). This is congruent with the Institute of Medicine (2001) definition of patient-centered care: "To create systems, processes and structures for providing care that is respectful of and responsive to individual patient preferences, needs, and values and ensuring that patient values guide all clinical decisions" (p. 40). This shift in perspective—from healthcare provider as expert to complementary expertise between healthcare provider and the person—is profound when the full implications are considered. Several chapters in this book speak to the necessary changes that will have to occur to fully achieve this change.

Third, the person exists within the context of a family, however he or she defines it. Family provides the connection to one's identity beyond any illness or health crisis. Actually, this perspective is one very familiar to nurses who use a holistic approach and traditionally include the person's significant others in planning, delivering, and evaluating care. Working with a person to achieve any health outcome requires full inclusion of and engagement by the family. Yet our healthcare environment does not fully encourage, support, or even sometimes allow this. This must change.

As a result of these insights and our beliefs and experiences, we have organized the book into three parts:

- **Part I, "Person- and Family-Centered Care—Setting the Scene,"** provides a series of contexts for thinking about person- and family-centered care, ranging from the current environment in the United States to a global appreciation to an individual person's perspective. In this section, the evolution of the concept is provided, along with examples of ways in which the concept has been reconceived or even misconceived.

- **Part II, "Models for Person- and Family-Centered Care,"** offers a number of models and frameworks that have emerged to help healthcare providers understand key elements in person- and family-centered care and to guide practice. Models such as patient engagement and activation, therapeutic relationships, and mindful and compassionate connection are just a few that are covered. Also in this section is an exploration of ethical dilemmas in healthcare today.

- **Part III, "Strategies to Promote Person- and Family-Centered Care,"** contains several pragmatic chapters with strategies that can be used to establish or improve a person- and family-centered approach to care. Included here is content on ethics consultation, mediation, the use of narratives, organizational support systems and healing environments, the power of the interprofessional team, and the role of leaders in creating needed change. Also in this section are strategies for working with patients, family members, and visitors who are bullies or abusive, as well as suggestions for helping nurses avoid compassion fatigue. The final chapter presents emerging trends in person- and family-centered care—what should we be thinking about now to prepare for tomorrow's healthcare environment?

Healthcare today is so very different from even 25 years ago: the sites, the personnel, technology, treatment options, and resources. Yet the goal of nursing remains constant. As proposed by Virginia Henderson long ago, that goal is relevant yet today and to this book: *To help people (sick or well) perform activities that contribute to health, recovery, or a peaceful death* (Henderson, 1966, p. 15). We hope that this book reminds all nurses of the powerful work that they do on a daily basis, offers encouragement and recognition of their successes, and provides a resource for achieving person- and family-centered care.

Jane H. Barnsteiner
Joanne Disch
Mary K. Walton

References

Churchill, L. R., Fanning, J. B., & Schenck, D. (2013). *What patients teach—The everyday ethics of health care*. New York, NY: Oxford University Press.

Cronenwett, L., Sherwood, G., Barnsteiner, J., Disch, J., Johnson, J., Mitchell, P.,…Warren, J. (2007). Quality and safety education for nurses. *Nursing Outlook, 55*(3), 122-131.

Henderson, V. (1966). *The nature of nursing: A definition and its implications for practice, research, and education*. New York, NY: Macmillan Publishing.

Institute of Medicine (IOM). (2001). *Crossing the quality chasm: A new health system for the 21st century*. Washington, D.C.: National Academies Press.

Koloroutis, M., & Trout, M. (2012). *See me as a person: Creating therapeutic relationships with patients and their families*. Minneapolis, MN: Creative Healthcare Management

Schenk, D., & Churchill, L. (2012). *Healers: Extraordinary clinicians at work*. New York, NY: Oxford University Press.

Chapter 1

The Landscape for Nurturing Person- and Family-Centered Care

Joanne Disch, PhD, RN, FAAN

Jane H. Barnsteiner, PhD, RN, FAAN

Mary K. Walton, MSN, MBE, RN

They had been together for 34 years, and she was dying. They had tried to support her at home through the visiting nurse service, but this eventually became inadequate. Her pain had become so intense, unrelieved by the medications, that the nurse practitioner coordinating her care believed she needed to be admitted to the hospital for pain management. After a lengthy stay in the emergency department, she was finally admitted to the inpatient unit, and intravenous medication was started. The nurse on the unit explained the plan of care to the woman's husband and encouraged him to go home and get some rest. "She is in good hands now."

But he was reluctant to leave and, in fact, said he would stay the night. "That really isn't necessary." But he persisted. "Alright, if you must, we can bring in a chair to put at her bedside." He thanked the nurse but indicated that that wasn't what he had in mind. They had been together almost 35 years and had slept together every night since they were married. That's what he had in mind. The nurse pointed out the visiting hours and the fact that the man needed his sleep. He persisted; she replied: "There is no way that we can do this. It wouldn't be right." The man asked to talk with the "next higher-up nurse" and then to the doctor (a resident on call), but to no avail.

Just as he was wondering whom to talk with next—and thinking he would just climb into her bed—the evening supervisor appeared. [One of the new nurses on the unit had overheard the nurse and doctor talking and had called him.] He listened to the man's story, understood the importance to him and his wife of sleeping together and helped the nurse see why this was important, and showed how it could be done. The man settled in next to his wife, and they both fell asleep.

The beginning portion of the preceding vignette is commonplace in many hospitals in the United States today—that is, a patient or family member encountering resistance to some personalized approach to care. Organizational rules, regulations, historical practices, and traditional ways of thinking are some of the reasons for this resistance. Yet with the publication of the Institute of Medicine (IOM) report *Crossing the Quality Chasm* in 2001, a rising crescendo of voices from individuals, communities, and organizations has advocated for improving the quality and safety of care and for actively engaging patients, and then patients and their families, into that process. The new nurse and the supervisor in the vignette reflect this new way of thinking and acting that will eventually become the norm. However, these efforts to change the current reality are occurring against a backdrop of strong traditional forces within society and the healthcare industry that must first be addressed.

Experts observe that we have not made much progress in improving either safety or patient engagement. A report from the Consumers Union, *To Err Is Human—To Delay Is Deadly*, noted: "Despite a decade of work, we have no reliable evidence that we are any better off today" (2009, p. 12–13). And Kathleen Sebelius, secretary of the U.S. Department of Health and Human Services, concluded: "If we only improve care as much in the next decade as we have in the past, we are failing the American public" (Sebelius, 2011, p. 5). Much work remains to be done.

This chapter explores the societal context of healthcare delivery and the social and healthcare-related factors that make person- and family-centered care (P&FCC) challenging to achieve yet are essential to address if we are to be more successful over the next decade. We begin the chapter with definitions of person- and family-centered care.

Definition of Person- and Family-Centered Care (P&FCC)

Although we advance many definitions of P&FCC throughout this book, we use two as our foundation. The first comes from the IOM (2001): "Providing care that is respectful of and responsive to individual patient preferences, needs, and values and ensuring that patient values guide all clinical decisions" (p. 40). The second is an extension of this that was developed for the QSEN (Quality and Safety Education for Nurses) work: "Recognize the patient or designee as the source of control and full partner in providing compassionate and coordinated care based on respect for patient's preferences, values and needs" (Cronenwett et al., 2007, p. 123).

However, as is noted in the Introduction, this book uses the concept of *person* rather than *patient* for several reasons:

- Many individuals engaging in a care relationship are not patients in hospitals but are receiving care in ambulatory facilities, clinics, community centers, and their own homes.

- Some individuals are residents in long-term care or living facilities rather than patients receiving care for a particular illness.

- Even if someone is in a hospital, Schenck and Churchill urge "engaging the person to treat the patient" (2012, p. 138).
- Koloroutis and Trout, the authors of Chapter 8, give the individual's point of view: *See me as a person.*

However, you will note that, although this is the direction toward which we believe the emphasis needs to move, at times the concept of patient seems to fit better, or the wording is so awkward when using *person* that we retain the use of *patient*. Thus, you will see that both terms are used, depending on the situation and the author.

Understanding Societal Factors That Affect P&FCC

Several strong forces are operating within society today, some that advance the concept of P&FCC, but more that obstruct its adoption. All need to be addressed if P&FCC is to become the standard of care. These factors include:

- The medical-industrial complex
- A widening income gap
- Social values
- Consumerism
- Time
- Incivility

Each of these factors is discussed in more detail in the following sections.

The Medical-Industrial Complex

Perhaps the greatest challenge to adopting a person-centered approach to healthcare is the powerful influence that the medical-industrial complex exerts on society. Introduced as a concept in 1971 (Ehrenreich & Ehrenreich), it refers to the vast healthcare industry that encompasses the multiple, multibillion-dollar enterprises of hospitals, health systems, drug companies, supply and equipment vendors, drug manufacturers, insurance companies, physicians and their practices, nursing homes, convenient care organizations, real estate and construction, consulting and accounting firms, technology innovators, banks, and any other business or industry that is touched by and benefits from the delivery of healthcare.

An original premise, and one that seems very evident today, is that an important function of the healthcare system, if not the main one, is to make a profit, with research and education being a secondary responsibility of certain segments. Estes, Harrington, and Pellow (1999) point out several implications arising from the corporatization of healthcare:

- Healthcare is no longer provided in small individual hospitals, much less the home as it historically had been, but in large corporate enterprises, with physicians more likely to be employed in group practices than as solo practitioners.

- Healthcare corporations are increasingly diverse, large, complex, and complicated. The number of hospitals is declining, but comprehensive healthcare systems are growing in size and influence. Nick Turkal, president and CEO of Aurora Health System in Milwaukee, predicts that "in about six years, there will be 100 'super-regional' systems, with further consolidation five years after" (2013, para. 12).

- The distinction between for-profit and nonprofit health systems is blurring, because both are pursuing greater operating margins and revenues through cost cutting and mergers.

- The rapidly growing healthcare industry is placing significant financial pressures on individuals, organizations, the government, and society—with the result that healthcare outcomes are significantly poorer in the United States than in countries spending far less on healthcare.

- Investments in softer services, such as patient care or human capital, are increasingly difficult to justify, because their cost-benefit analysis is often skewed toward a short-term benefit calculation, which unfairly undervalues their long-term impact. This is also true when evaluating other investments, such as preventive health versus surgical interventions or adequate education for school children versus joblessness later in life.

Against this backdrop, healthcare has become increasingly *im*personal and treated as a commodity. Productivity and efficiency drive much of the decision-making. Interactions that take up too much time are less valued.

A Widening Income Gap

Over the past 50 years, the income gap between the poorest and the wealthiest Americans has dramatically widened. One Pulitzer Prize–winning journalist found that income for the bottom 90% of Americans grew only $59 (adjusted for inflation) from 1966 to 2011, while income for the top 10% rose by $116,071 (Gilani, 2013). To offset this, assistance programs at the federal level equaled $746 billion; adding state spending brought the total to $1.03 trillion.

Today, more is spent on welfare than on Social Security or defense (Gilani, 2013). Sharing the wealth, or narrowing the gap, is an intensely political issue, with many Americans saying that this is what a just society should do, and others vehemently opposed. In addition, the growing evidence that an income gap is associated with a two-tiered healthcare system and health disparities directly challenges the ability for all persons to get healthcare that meets their particular needs.

Social Values

Americans seem to be espousing more polarized views and values. This is apparent in Washington, D.C., in the media, in our local communities, and in our organizations. A 2007 survey by Jacobs (2010), which was a repeat of one conducted in 1976 and 1986, asked 1,500 Americans to prioritize eight values. The values were:

- Self-respect ("to be proud of yourself and confident in who you are")
- Security ("to be safe and protected from misfortune and attack")
- Warm relationships with others
- A sense of accomplishment
- Self-fulfillment
- Being well respected
- A sense of belonging
- Fun-enjoyment-excitement ("to lead a pleasurable, happy life; to experience stimulation and thrills")

Self-respect led the list in all three surveys, by an increasing percentage each survey, while security dropped in importance. The value of warm relationships increased, while a sense of belonging dropped greatly, replaced by fun-enjoyment-excitement. Jacobs believes that this value for independence and self-respect underscores a more individualistic spirit today than ever before.

We see this reflected in the large divide between those who believe that healthcare is a right and those who believe it is a privilege, and those who believe we have a responsibility to help those less fortunate and those who believe people should fend for themselves. When traveling in other countries, we have heard citizens there often express their disbelief that so many Americans are without insurance or adequate healthcare. How can we close the gap in health disparities and ensure that everyone receives needed services if we continue to value independence and self-sufficiency in all situations, even in the face of severe resource imbalances?

Consumerism

There are two ways to think about consumerism. One is that it is a push for purchasing things in ever-greater amounts, often in excess of what is needed; the other is that it is a movement centered around consumer protection or consumer activism.

Several implications and beliefs are associated with consumerism:

- Consumers should be fully informed about choices and their costs.
- The "marketplace" should be fair and just, not advantaging one individual or group over another with the same information.

- The active engagement of individuals in selecting goods and services puts pressure on organizations and industries to radically revise traditional ways of practice.

- Advertising and information sharing escalate greatly—and create challenges in ensuring that information is accurate, usable, and formatted in a way that the consumer can understand.

- Gaps among groups as to the availability of goods and services can widen due to disparities in access to information or to the desirable items and services.

- The boomer generation is exerting significant pressure in consumers' being able to be engaged in all aspects of their lives.

This latter bullet is a very positive outcome of the consumer movement. Separate from governmental or healthcare organizations, what may be the greatest opportunity for input from patients and families into shaping policy is the multitude of consumer organizations that press for either broad social change or change related to specific populations, diseases, or issues.

NOTE

Perhaps the most well known of these consumer groups is AARP, formerly known as the American Association of Retired Persons (AARP, 2013). With its solid policy and advocacy infrastructure and its 37 million members, it serves as a powerful advocate for individuals over 50, their dependents, and their caregivers of any age. Whether it is an issue related to housing, insurance, consumer fraud, or accessible healthcare and prescription drugs, AARP encourages members and consumers to speak loudly for all Americans at both the state and national levels.

Similarly, groups with a more direct focus, such as the American Heart Association, American Cancer Society, Mothers Against Drunk Driving, and the Josie King Foundation, comprise consumers who joined together to advance a particular cause. Most of these have been incredibly influential in shaping policy.

But even individuals can make a difference, such as Helen Haskell, who galvanized the healthcare industry when her son, Lewis Blackman, died as a result of medical error. She communicated her story directly to consumers, healthcare providers, and the general public. This powerful story can be accessed at http://qsen.org/videos/the-lewis-blackman-story/.

Another very influential individual is e-Patient Dave (deBronkart), a former marketing executive who actively speaks up in numerous national forums, exhorting that patients be included in every aspect of planning and implementing their healthcare. After his experience with cancer and becoming self-knowledgeable about all the resources available to people, he questions: "How can it be that the most useful and relevant information can exist outside the traditional medical literature?" (Versel, 2013, para. 9). His book *Let Patients Help* (CreateSpace Independent Publishing Platform, 2013) is a useful guide to getting persons more engaged in their care. (He notes that the "e" in his title refers to *equipped*, *engaged*, *empowered*, or *enabled*, depending on the context.)

Quinlan (2013) describes the e-Patient Manifesto:

> Nothing about us without us. If you're planning a healthcare industry event that is focused on patient engagement, patient-centered design, patient-centered care, patient-centered technology, or touches on patient care in any part of the healthcare setting or system, you have to include patients on your program or be judged "Patients Excluded." (para. 11)

It is interesting to note that consumers are often able to exert the greatest influence *outside* formal healthcare organizations, which tend to maintain a bureaucratic hierarchy with their traditions and mechanisms of control.

Time

The pressures of time in today's constantly multitasking society place a greater burden on everyone, but particularly on healthcare. Much of this is due to how healthcare is financed, with shorter lengths of stay and more clinic appointments per day. At the same time, individuals seeking healthcare are encouraged to be active, engaged, informed, and ready to partner. This creates challenges for healthcare providers.

Don Brady is a physician and president of the American Academy on Communication in Healthcare, an organization that was founded in 1978 to "improve health care by enhancing communication skills among clinicians and across health care teams and systems" (2013, p. 8). He notes that one of the biggest obstacles to successful communication is the time factor: "Even with improved skills, 10 minutes with one patient is a very short time" (2013, p. 8). Indeed. This pressure is compounded when dealing with individuals with multiple chronic illnesses—and perhaps limited health literacy. It saps energy from clinicians, most of whom go into healthcare to connect with and help others.

Krichbaum and colleagues (2007) describe the phenomenon of *complexity compression*, where nurses describe the unexpected (and unstaffed for) responsibilities that nurses must assume in a given shift. These pressures to do more, or the same, within a shortened time frame take a toll on clinicians, as "it is the power of the human encounter in response to illness that keeps them going" (Schenck & Churchill, 2012, p. 9). These relationships can take time to develop and nurture. Adequate time is also important for patients and their families. Patients worry: "Will the doctor listen to me?" or "When will I get interrupted?" Families wonder: "What am I expected to do to help?" and "How can I learn it all?"

Incivility

Contrary to what many individuals might believe, violent crime in America has actually declined over the past 20 years, from 757 per 100,000 people in 1992 to 386 in 2011. This trend occurred in spite of the fact that the population rose from 255 million to more than 310 million. Despite a stunning number of high-profile shootings, less than 2% of Americans said that crime was the nation's most important problem, as opposed to more than 50% who said it was in 1994 (Fisher, 2013).

What has not declined, however, is *incivility,* or rude or impolite attitude or behavior (Incivility, n.d.). Porath and Pearson (2013) have polled thousands of workers over the past 14 years and found that 98% have experienced uncivil behavior. In 2011, approximately half of those polled said that they were treated rudely at least once a week, compared to about 25% in 1998.

There are similar trends in nursing, with numerous studies reporting on horizontal violence, defined as any unwanted abuse or hostility, in the range of 65–85% (Lewis & Malecha, 2011; Stagg, Sheridan, Jones, & Speroni, 2011; Stanley, Martin, Nemeth, Michel, & Welton, 2007; Vessey, Demarco, Gaffney, & Budin, 2009; Wilson, Diedrich, Phelps, & Choi, 2011). In 2008, The Joint Commission issued a Sentinel Event Alert on behaviors that undermine a culture of safety, and in 2009, it issued a new leadership standard that addresses disruptive and inappropriate behaviors (TJC, 2008, 2009). Becher and Visovsky (2012) describe the wide array of consequences that affect nurses, care team members, and ultimately the patient and family. How can healthcare providers focus on the needs of individuals and their families and provide respectful, personalized care if they are sniping at or undermining the performance and sense of pride of their colleagues?

Understanding the Healthcare-Related Factors That Affect P&FCC

According to the *Future of Nursing* report by the IOM (2011), the U.S. healthcare system is characterized by

> a high degree of fragmentation across many sectors, which raises substantial barriers to providing accessible, quality care at an affordable price. In part, the fragmentation in the system comes from disconnects between public and private services, between providers and patients, between what patients need and how providers are trained, between the health needs of the nation and the services that are offered, and between those with insurance and those without…. Communication between providers is difficult, and much care is redundant because there is no way of sharing results. (p. 21)

Thus, in addition to the sample of societal factors already identified that affect the delivery of respectful, person-centered care, there are factors related to the healthcare industry and health professionals' educational programs that either compromise or enhance the ability to deliver P&FCC. These factors include:

- The medical model of healthcare delivery
- Mismatch between what providers believe and what patients want
- Professional autonomy

- Technology
- The education of health professionals
- Financing of healthcare

The following sections describe each of these factors in more detail.

The Medical Model of Healthcare Delivery

Healthcare delivery is still largely shaped and delivered around the medical model of care delivery (that is, physician-directed, acuity-oriented, and hospital-based). Its origins stem from the work by Pasteur and others in formulating the germ theory of disease around the late 19th century: Illness is caused by disease and can be treated. Diseases have symptoms and, wherever possible, can be tackled, and a cure or improvement can be achieved. This model relies heavily on knowledge of pathophysiology, biology, chemistry, pharmacology, and other core sciences, and because physicians are trained heavily in these sciences, they are the experts.

Within the profession of medicine, there exists "specialty dominance" (Starfield, 2011), which has two meanings: a greater value for specialty physician practice and a predominant interest in individual diseases. Even chronic care management, as opposed to primary care, usually operates from the view of the management of a single long-term illness, such as cancer, HIV, cardiac diseases, and so forth. *Chronic* has been interpreted to relate to chronic disease; guidelines are based on algorithms, even in primary care, focusing on single, discrete diseases—"an outmoded concept of health problems in populations" (Starfield, 2011, para. 14). All these factors make it difficult to see the individual holistically and as part of a bigger family unit, with intersecting problems unless care coordination is exquisitely done. This is rare. In much of society, there still exists the idea that the physician is "the captain of the ship" and equipped to lead in all situations.

Chesney (personal communication, November 21, 2013) refutes this view, noting the overlapping nature of the roles of nurses and physicians, particularly with advanced practice nurses (APNs), and yet the distinct differences that equip nurses to lead in many situations. Nurses have a holistic orientation (mind-body-spirit) and view individuals in the context of their environment, including concern for the social determinants of health. The nature of the relationship is care that is grounded in "a culturally sensitive, caring interpersonal relationship" (American Nurses Association, 2004, p. 8), and the focus includes individuals, their families (as individuals define them), communities, and populations. Physicians, on the other hand, practice medicine, or "the science that deals with preventing, curing, and treating diseases" (Medicine, n.d.).

Eisler and Potter (2014) describe the differences in this way:

> [T]he medicine of physicians is primarily based on only two domains: active caring and evidence based in science. By contrast, nursing's medicine is primarily based on four domains: being present, active caring, stories/narrative evidence, and evidence based in science. Comparing these two paradigms, you see that consistently being present and consistent use of stories or narrative-based evidence differentiates the medicine of nursing from the medicine of physicians. (p. 23)

There are growing challenges to the patriarchal medicine of physicians. Leape and a group of his colleagues who are leaders in the quality care movement observe: "Many physicians do not know how to be team players and regard other health workers as assistants. Outmoded hierarchical structures inhibit collaboration and learning" (2009, pp. 424–425).

In 2012, Nutting, Crabtree, and McDaniel noted a physician-centric mind-set that exists within primary care that compromises the capability of small primary-care practices to move to a new care model. Over a period of 15 years, this group of researchers closely examined more than 400 primary care practices and found that they were "extremely physician-centric, lacked meaningful communication among physicians, were dominated by authoritarian leadership behavior, and were underserved by midlevel clinicians who had been cast into unimaginative roles" (p. 2417). Their sense was that, unless these aspects changed, they would not be able to move toward a model that would effectively meet person/family needs or provide satisfaction to the physicians or others in these practices.

Mismatch Between What Providers Believe and What Patients Want

There is a growing mismatch between what providers believe their patients want and what patients say they want. Healthcare providers believe that individuals want high clinical value. Patients want "whole-person" care, comprehensive communication and coordination, patient support and empowerment, and ready access (Bechtel & Ness, 2010). Naturally they also want competent practitioners who are knowledgeable—but they expect that as a baseline. Frank (2002) shared this quote from patients: "I do not want my questions answered: I want my experiences shared" (p. 133). Schenck and Churchill (2012), after dozens of interviews with exceptional clinicians, reported that patients said, "technical alone is insufficient" and "I may not expect emotion or intimacy from physicians and nurses, but I do expect recognition" (p. 136).

Spath (2008) cites the IOM's 2006 report *Preventing Medication Errors,* which outlines patients' expectations: "being listened to and respected as a care partner, being told the truth, having care and information sharing coordinated with all members of the team, and partnering with staff who are able to provide both technically and emotionally supportive care" (p. 133). Yet a visit to most healthcare settings would reflect practices that do not deliver on these requests and expectations. As reflected in the quotes, what individuals want varies. The solution is to ask them.

Professional Autonomy

Amalberti, Auroy, Berwick, and Barach (2005) examined five system barriers that prevent ultra-safe patient care. These are (1) allowing decision-making without regulation or constraints; (2) clinging to professional autonomy; (3) being stuck in the mind-set of craftsmen; (4) having no system-level processes to optimize safety strategies; and (5) adhering to complex and counterproductive professional rules and regulations. In addition to preventing safe patient care, these barriers also can compromise person-centered care.

Instead the authors propose the following changes in strategy:

- Accept limits on the extent to which individuals can make solo decisions.
- Abandon professional autonomy.
- Transition from the mindset of craftsman to equivalent actor.
- Install system level arbitration to optimize safety strategies.
- Simplify professional rules and regulations.

Two of these five have particular implications for healthcare professionals (HCPs), especially physicians. The proposed changes offered by these authors would require profound culture change.

The first recommendation that they make is the abandonment of professional autonomy. One example that they give is how drivers, in order to get to their goal, have to relinquish some of their preferred patterns of driving, and that there are certain "rules of the road" that people in a civilized society follow. In the aviation industry, for safety purposes, regulations have limited the unilateral authority and autonomy that pilots had previously enjoyed and mandated training in communication and crew resource management. Training in teamwork and communication has changed the thinking and practices of many physicians, affirming that all members have something that is needed by the team and that the decisions one person makes have implications for the work of others. A surgeon and an anesthesiologist may have excellent partnership skills, for example, but if they fail to take into consideration communication with the hospitalist, intensive care physician, or circulating nurse, care will be compromised. So HCPs must not only work well together, but they also must broadly consider the full team—which has to include patients and their families.

The second recommendation that they make is the movement of HCPs from being craftsmen to equivalent actors: "Healthcare professionals must face a very difficult transition: abandoning their status and self-image as craftsmen and instead adopting a position that values equivalence among their ranks" (Amalberti et al., 2005, p. 759). They cite the examples of an airline pilot who is not concerned if, at the last minute, a new co-pilot is assigned, or in an operating room, a patient who is not concerned if an anesthesiologist has to be replaced. The pilot and the patient have confidence that the people replacing the original professionals are competent and equipped to do their jobs. The issue of equivalent actor is a proxy for equivalent care: A certain standard of practice should be expected from each HCP.

Within medicine, this analogy works only part of the time. In highly specialized cases, or where there is instability in the environment, a certain amount of latitude and professional expertise is needed. Some practitioners in certain situations are not interchangeable with others. However, in many situations, there is more stability and predictability as to what should be done according to evidence-based practice than HCPs acknowledge. In these situations, unnecessary variability is unhelpful and leads to greater sources of error, inefficiency, and confusion.

Technology

The explosive growth in technology is both a blessing and a curse. It has saved millions of lives, enabling the smallest premature infants to survive and extending the life of older adults for decades. It was not too long ago that patients over the age of 55 could not receive a transplant; today patients into their 80s, and older, can undergo complex surgical procedures of all kinds. With sophisticated high-resolution imagery, extensive diagnostic tests can be performed and beamed around the world for interpretation. Nurses can monitor patients in their homes without being there, and physicians can conduct complex physical assessments from across the country. We are seeing the emergence of e-ICUs and tele-hospice. The words of cardiovascular surgeon C. Walton Lillehei in the 1950s come to mind: "What mankind can dream, research and technology can achieve" (Lillehei Heart Institute, 2010).

Yet with this technology comes extraordinary complexity in learning how to use the equipment, in operating it, and in addressing the unintended consequences. A November 2013 report from the ECRI Institute (Brown) identifies the top 10 technology hazards for 2014:

1. Alarm hazards

2. Infusion pump medication errors

3. Radiation exposures in pediatric patients

4. Data integrity failures in electronic health records (EHRs) and other health information technology systems

5. Occupational radiation hazards in hybrid operating rooms

6. Inadequate reprocessing of endoscopes and surgical instruments

7. Neglecting change management for networked devices and systems

8. Risks to pediatric patients from "adult" technologies

9. Robotic surgery complications due to insufficient training

10. Retained devices and unretrieved fragments

Consumers are increasingly being invited, some would say mandated, to become actively involved in using technology for care, and for communication. To the extent that technology can close the gap between providers and patients, it can be helpful. To the extent that it creates a bigger barrier, or a burden for patients and their families, it is a factor that requires attention.

The Education of Health Professionals

How health professionals are educated, and the extent to which they develop competencies in delivering personalized care, should be of paramount importance to individuals and their significant others. The traditional models of healthcare education have not served us well, and many advocate that health professionals' education must change: "There is a growing sense nationally that exclusive reliance on the paradigm of the Flexner report, with its narrow focus on biological functions, no longer serves us well" (Schenck & Churchill, 2012, p. 186).

Within nursing, Cronenwett and her colleagues (2007), who launched a national initiative to prepare nurses with the competencies necessary for improving the quality and safety of patient care, found that faculty had significant gaps in their knowledge: "[T]he ideas for what to teach, how to teach, and how to assess learning of the competencies are sorely lacking, and there are few, if any, examples of schools claiming to execute a comprehensive quality and safety curriculum" (p. 124).

Moreover, in a focus group of new graduates, "[n]ot only did these nurses report that they lacked learning experiences related to the [needed content], they did not believe their faculties had the expertise to teach some of the content." One of the specific areas that required a total reconceptualization was in "patient-centered care," with a need to move from "doing for" the patient to "including the patient or designee as the source of control or full partner in providing compassionate and coordinated care" (Cronenwett et al., 2007, p. 123).

The subsequent national movement known as QSEN (Quality and Safety Education for Nurses), funded by the Robert Wood Johnson Foundation for 8 years, addressed these gaps with stunning success. Current attention is being focused on ensuring that clinical nurses also understand these competencies and that academic-practice partnerships strengthen the learning experiences of students and clinical staff alike.

However, improving the education of health professionals still exists mostly in silos, and many prominent individuals and organizations are working to change this. The Lancet Commission report *Health Professionals for a New Century: Transforming Education to Strengthen Health Systems in an Interdependent World* calls for significant educational reform in healthcare. What is needed is to promote "interprofessional and transprofessional education that breaks down professional silos while enhancing collaborative and non-hierarchical relationships in effective teams" (Frenk et al., 2010, p. 1924).

George Thibault (2013), president of the Josiah Macy Jr. Foundation, has specified the areas that need significant reform: interprofessional education, new models for clinical education, new content to complement the biological sciences, new educational models based on competency, new educational technologies, and faculty development for teaching and educational innovation.

Financing of Healthcare

Corrigan (2012) notes that we have a payment system that continues "to reward the volume of services rather than patient outcomes and the absence of integrated delivery systems that possess the necessary scale, breadth, and depth of expertise to identify and remove waste while preserving necessary services that enhance patient outcomes and experience" (p. 2588). We also have a system that continues to favor medical interventions instead of preventive care and health promotion, and one that values specialists over generalists.

Reid (2009), author of *The Healing of America*, suggests that there is no one system. Depending on your age and circumstances, your options in the United States vary greatly. For most working people under 65, a model similar to that used in Germany is used, whereby private initiatives provide most of the healthcare, and insurance companies are also private. However, in

Germany, the insurance companies are nonprofit and are required to sign up individuals without consideration of preexisting conditions. For those older than 65, the U.S. system is similar to the Canadian single-payer system. For Native Americans, military personnel, and veterans, the government is both the payer and provider, similar to Britain. And for those uninsured, the "system" is similar to what exists in underdeveloped countries (i.e., healthcare is too expensive, and they often cut back or cut out).

Partly because of this disjointed and complicated *non*system in the United States, up until the past few years, healthcare spending has exceeded the rate of inflation. The United States is now spending approximately 18% of its gross domestic product on healthcare, or about $8,500 a year per person (the next two highest countries are Switzerland and Norway at ~ $5,700, the Netherlands ~ $5,000, and France at less than half, or $4,100 per person; Lehigh, 2013).

Economists have said that the problem is not how much is spent—for wouldn't a developed country appropriately spend a good amount for the health of its people—but the outcomes we achieve. In a study funded by the Commonwealth Fund, Schoen, Osborn, Squires, and Doty (2013) report on a survey of adults in the United States and 10 other developed nations concerning access and affordability of care and insurance complexity. The 10 other countries are Australia, Canada, France, Germany, the Netherlands, New Zealand, Norway, Sweden, Switzerland, and the United Kingdom. Among their findings:

- The United States has the most citizens *not* seeing a doctor because of cost (32% vs. the next highest countries, the Netherlands and New Zealand at 20%).

- The United States has the most citizens who have not filled a prescription or skipped drugs due to the costs (21%; all other countries < 10%).

- Almost half of Americans said that the system needs "fundamental change," with 27% saying "completely rebuild."

Kellerman (2013) in a *Health Affairs* commentary points out some interesting implications for individuals who are trying to make sense of the system and its perverse incentives and byzantine structure. First, there is *information asymmetry*:

> Although the internet and social media have provided modern consumers with greater access to information than ever before; the bewildering number of websites and the variable quality of information has left many consumers confused. As a result, many patients still look to their personal physician, a trusted family member, or a friend for advice. Sometimes this works; sometimes it doesn't. (para. 10)

There are resources that may be helpful, such as *Consumer Reports*, one's health plan, a trusted website, or a *patient navigator*. But the complexity and volume of information are daunting to the average individual.

Second, there is the growing presence of cost sharing, both by the employer and by employees if they still have benefit coverage. This is one area that is particularly confusing, with terms such as *consumer directed*, which is not person-oriented at all but a high-deductible health plan. If an individual makes a poorly informed choice, there can be significant financial consequences.

Third, innovation, although normally a positive thing, in the healthcare industry often favors "highly expensive drugs, biologics, devices, and tests rather than highly effective technologies that could improve health at lower cost" (Kellerman, 2013, para. 13). Until significant incentives can be developed to encourage the medical industrial complex to change its priorities, consumers will continue to be in jeopardy by the current financing of healthcare. It is unclear at this point what the long-term impact of the Affordable Care Act will be; experts note that it is, at least, offering options for coverage for millions more people.

The whole issue of costs in healthcare is one that hospital administrators or doctors do not like to talk about. Chen, in a 2012 article in *The New York Times,* quotes Dr. Robert Truog about the lack of full transparency between physicians and their patients, which is particularly true when the issue of the costs of healthcare come up:

> I think that the biggest challenge by far is the need to make choices that are efficient or, to use a word that has come up a lot recently, parsimonious. That is something physicians don't want to say, and patients don't want to hear. Everyone wants to believe that decisions are all based on medical criteria. In my field of practice, for example, when a patient is transferred out of the ICU or not admitted to the ICU, it's our practice not to disclose that these decisions may be based on limitations of resources. Those decisions are completely opaque. And no one wants to hear that their loved one is not getting the best because of resource restraints, even if it's true. (para. 9)

Conclusion

Within the United States at the present time, several societal forces and healthcare-related factors are in play at the same time that a national mandate has been issued for including persons and their families as "the source of control and full partner" (Sherwood & Barnsteiner, 2012, p. 341) in their healthcare. Many of these forces and factors can be simultaneously helpful and harmful, such as the growth in information yet the difficulty in making sense of all that is available, or the benefits of some of the new innovations in healthcare yet their unavailability. What will be required for harnessing these multiple forces and factors is far greater than finding financial solutions to our problems.

Although the costs of healthcare are high, the solution is not in finding ways to finance the current system. As Disch notes in a letter to the editor of *Health Affairs* (2008), "[F]inding better ways to finance, access or measure results within the current paradigm is not the good news—or the right answer. What is needed is to move from the physician-dependent, hospital-based, acuity-oriented system to one that is safe, convenient, effective, efficient and personalized." This requires leadership, culture change, a profound rethinking of priorities and, within healthcare, fully engaging the persons and their families who seek healthcare in ways that matter to them.

References

AARP. (2013). Advocacy. Retrieved from http://www.aarp.org/politics-society

Amalberti, R., Auroy, Y., Berwick, D., & Barach, P. (2005). Improving patient care: Five system barriers to achieving ultrasafe health care. *Annals of Internal Medicine, 142*(9), 756-764.

American Nurses Association. (2004). *Scope and standards of nursing.* Silver Springs, MD: Author.

Becher, J., & Visovsky, C. (2012). Horizontal violence in nursing. *MedSurg Nursing, 21*(4), 210-232.

Bechtel, C., & Ness, D. L. (2010). If you build it, will they come? Designing truly patient-centered health care. *Health Affairs, 29*(5), 214-220.

Brady, D. W. (2013). Improving patient-physician communication. *Minnesota Physician, 27*(7), 8-9.

Brown, T. (2013, November). Top 10 healthcare technology hazards for 2014. *Medscape Medical News.* Retrieved from http://www.medscape.com/viewarticle/814043

Chen, P. W. (2012, March 8). What doctors and patients don't want to talk about. *The New York Times.* Retrieved from http://well.blogs.nytimes.com/2012/03/08/what-doctors-and-patients-dont-want-to-talk-about/?emc=eta1&_r=0

Consumers Union. (2009). Safe patient project. Retrieved from www.safepatientproject.org/pdf/safepatientproject.org-to_delay_is_deadly-2009_05.pdf

Corrigan, J. (2012). We've only just begun to make headway on patient safety. *Health Affairs, 31*(11), 2588-2589.

Cronenwett, L., Sherwood, G., Barnsteiner, J., Disch, J., Johnson, J., Mitchell, P.,…Warren, J. (2007). Quality and safety education for nurses. *Nursing Outlook, 55*(3), 122-131.

Disch, J. (2008). [Letter to the Editor.] *Health Affairs, 27*(2), 585.

Ehrenreich, B., & Ehrenreich, J. (1971). *The American health empire: Power, profits, and politics.* New York: Vintage Books.

Eisler, R., & Potter, T. M. (2014). *Interprofessional partnerships in practice, education and research.* Indianapolis, IN: Sigma Theta Tau International.

Estes, C. L., Harrington, C., & Pellow, D. N. (1999). Medical-industrial complex. In E. F. Borgatta & R. J. V. Montgomery (Eds.), *Encyclopedia of sociology* (2nd ed.). Retrieved from http://edu.learnsoc.org/Chapters/21%20health%20and%20medicine/12%20medical-industrial%20complex.htm

Fisher, M. (2013, March 3). Gun deaths, violent crime overall are down in District and U.S., but reasons are elusive. *The Washington Post.* Retrieved from http://www.washingtonpost.com/national/gun-deaths-violent-crime-overall-are-down-in-district-and-us-but-reasons-are-elusive/2013/03/03/7455ccde-7d24-11e2-a044-676856536b40_story.html

Frank, A. (2002). *At the will of the body: Reflections on illness.* Boston, MA: Houghton Mifflin.

Frenk, J., Chen, L., Bhutta, Z. A., Cohen, J., Crisp, N., Evans, T.,…Zurayk, H. (2010). Health professionals for a new century: Transforming education to strengthen health systems in an interdependent world. *The Lancet, 376*(9756), 1923-1958.

Gilani, S. (2013, September). Income inequality is what's destroying America. *Forbes.* Retrieved from http://www.forbes.com/sites/shahgilani/2013/09/27/income-inequality-is-whats-destroying-america/

Incivility. (n.d.) In *Merriam-Webster's online dictionary* (11th ed.). Retrieved from http://www.merriam-webster.com/dictionary/incivility

Institute of Medicine (IOM). (2001). *Crossing the quality chasm: A new health system for the 21st century.* Washington, DC: National Academy Press.

Institute of Medicine (IOM). (2011). *The future of nursing: Leading change, advancing health.* Washington, DC: National Academies of Science. Retrieved from http://www.nap.edu/openbook.php?record_id=12956&page=21

Jacobs, D. (2010, May). Self-respect tops list of American social values. *Pacific Standard.* Retrieved from http://www.psmag.com/culture/self-respect-tops-list-of-american-social-values-16121/

The Joint Commission (TJC). (2008). Sentinel event alert: Behaviors that undermine a culture of safety. Retrieved from http://www.jointcommission.org/assets/1/18/SEA_40.PDF

The Joint Commission (TJC). (2009). Leadership standard clarified to address behaviors that undermine a safety culture. Retrieved from http://www.jointcommission.org/assets/1/6/Leadership_standard_behaviors.pdf

Kellerman, A. L. (2013). Health care spending: What's in store? The Rand Corporation. Retrieved from http://www.rand.org/commentary/2013/07/16/HA.html

Krichbaum, K., Diemert, C., Jacox, L., Jones, D., Koenig, P., Mueller, C., & Disch, J. (2007). Complexity compression: Nurses under fire. *Nursing Forum, 42*(2), 86-94.

Leape, L., Berwick, D., Clancy, C., Conway, J., Gluck, P., Guest, J., …Isaac, T. (2009). Transforming healthcare: A safety imperative. *Quality & Safety in Health Care, 18*(6), 424-428.

Lehigh, S. (2013, November 20). Best health care system? Not in the US. *The Boston Globe.* Retrieved from http://www.bostonglobe.com/opinion/2013/11/20/health-care-not-world-best/lYaLDSJNLZGczOH9SNYmkO/story.html

Lewis, P. S., & Malecha, A. (2011). The impact of workplace incivility on the work environment, manager skill, and productivity. *Journal of Nursing Administration, 41*(1), 41-47.

Lillehei Heart Institute (LHI). (2010). Retrieved from https://www.facebook.com/lhi.umn

Medicine. (n.d.). In *Merriam-Webster's online dictionary* (11th ed.). Retrieved from http://www.merriam-webster.com/dictionary/medicine

Nutting, P. A., Crabtree, B. F., & McDaniel, R. R. (2012). Small primary care practices face four hurdles—including a physician-centric mind-set—in becoming medical homes. *Health Affairs, 31*(11), 2417-2422.

Porath, C., & Pearson, C. (2013). The price of incivility. *Harvard Business Review, 91*(1/2), 115-121.

Quinlan, C. (2013, November 18). e-Patient manifesto: "Patients Included." Retrieved from http://e-patients.net/archives/2013/11/e-patient-manifesto-patients-included.html

Reid, T. F. (2009). *The healing of America.* New York: Penguin Books.

Schenck, D., & Churchill, L. (2012). *Healers: Extraordinary clinicians at work.* New York: Oxford University Press.

Schoen, C., Osborn, R., Squires, D., & Doty, M. M. (2013). Access, affordability, and insurance complexity are often worse in the United States compared to ten other countries. *Health Affairs, 32*(11). Retrieved from http://content.healthaffairs.org/content/early/2013/11/12/hlthaff.2013.0879.full

Sebelius, K. (2011). The Richard and Hinda Rosenthal lecture: New frontiers in patient safety. Washington DC: Institute of Medicine, National Academies Press. Retrieved from http://www.iom.edu/Reports/2011/The-Richard-and-Hinda-Rosenthal-Lecture-2011-New-Frontiers-in-Patient-Safety.aspx

Sherwood, G., & Barnsteiner, J. (2012). *Quality and safety in nursing: A competency approach to improving outcomes.* West Sussex, UK: Wiley-Blackwell.

Spath, P. L. (2008). *Engaging patients as safety partners.* Chicago, IL: American Hospital Association.

Stagg, S. J., Sheridan, D., Jones, R. A., & Speroni, K. G. (2011). Evaluation of a workplace bullying cognitive rehearsal program in a hospital setting. *Journal of Continuing Education in Nursing, 42*(9), 395-401. doi: 10.3928/00220124-20110823-45

Stanley, K. M., Martin, M. M., Nemeth, L. S., Michel, Y., & Welton, J. M. (2007). Examining lateral violence in the nursing workforce. *Issues in Mental Health Nursing, 28*(11), 1247-1265.

Starfield, B. (2011). Is patient-centered care the same as person-focused care? *The Permanente Journal, 15*(2), 63-69. Retrieved from http://www.ncbi.nlm.nih.gov/pmc/articles/PMC3140752/

Thibault, G. E. (2013). Reforming health professions education will require culture change and closer ties between classroom and practice. *Health Affairs, 32*(11), 1928-1932.

Turkal, N. (2013, November). Healthcare's transformation is inevitable. *Modern Healthcare.* Retrieved from http://www.modernhealthcare.com/article/20131109/MAGAZINE/311099982/

Versel, N. (2013, November). "e-Patient Dave" tells medical informatics group to let patients help. *Mobi Health News.* Retrieved from http://mobihealthnews.com/27464/e-patient-dave-tells-medical-informatics-group-to-let-patients-help/

Vessey, J. A., Demarco, R. F., Gaffney, D. A., & Budin, W. C. (2009). Bullying of staff registered nurses in the workplace: A preliminary study for developing personal and organizational strategies for the transformation of hostile to healthy workplace environments. *Journal of Professional Nursing, 25*(5), 299-306.

Wilson, B. L., Diedrich, A., Phelps, C. L., & Choi, M. (2011). Bullies at work: The impact of horizontal hostility in the hospital setting and intent to leave. *The Journal of Nursing Administration, 41*(11), 453-458.

Chapter 2

Overview and History of Person- and Family-Centered Care

Jane H. Barnsteiner, PhD, RN, FAAN

News Story: Patient-Centered Care Redistributes Responsibility

Betty A. Marton, April 2012, HealthLeaders

In 2008, a 23-year-old woman with severe cystic fibrosis successfully carried and delivered a healthy, full-term baby girl at Long Island Jewish Medical Center, in New Hyde Park, NY. Despite that major achievement, the complex regimen of daily medications that Christina Marie McDonald needed to manage her disease created challenges. "On the maternity ward, no one understood anything about CF," says Ruben Cohen, MD, director of the adult CF program and co-director of the asthma center for the 888-bed tertiary care teaching hospital. "She didn't receive her medications when she needed them."

"After that experience, the patient's father wrote a letter asking, 'Why does the hospital tie our hands and put these routine measures in the hands of busy medical personnel when the patients and their families know the illness very well and are experts in their own care?'" explains Fatima Jaffrey, MD, director of outcomes research at LIJ Medical Center. The hospital realized they needed a new way of doing things. LIJ Medical Center embarked on a process to explore how to improve the in-hospital delivery of daily medications to CF patients.

In February 2009, Jaffrey began coaching an interdisciplinary team of all the frontline caregivers, including Cohen, and a respiratory therapist, dietician, nurse, pharmacist, CF social worker, and Christina's father, in how to apply the methods of improvement science to improving CF care. The team focused on how it could support and empower the patient while still meeting regulatory requirements. "The goal," says Jaffrey, was to go from "a system of care that wasn't deeply connected to patients' experiences to one that is incredibly connected." Six months after it was established, the team met its first two goals of reducing the length of time patients had to wait for the delivery of the medications for which they were admitted—to two hours (from 15 or more) for the first breathing treatment and four hours (from 18) for IV antibiotics.

The program went live in March 2010, with patients who opt to self-administer receiving special locked boxes containing all of their medications. Patients keep a log of what they take and when, and nurses review the log to determine if medications are being taken correctly. The nurses also work with the hospital's pharmacists to keep the box replenished. "The process gives the nurses oversight so we can still manage the documentation," says Margaret Murphy, RN, senior administrative director of patient care services. "It all seems so simple in retrospect, but at the time it required a lot of coordination and education. It offers a tremendous amount of efficiency while ensuring that the patients who know their medications are administering them correctly."

Having dramatically reduced the time it takes to provide the care CF patients need has reduced the average length of stay in the hospital for CF patients to 7 days from 11. The success of self-administration is also reflected in patient and professional satisfaction surveys: Satisfaction rates for both groups rose from less than 20% before the intervention to above 95%. "What's remarkable is that this sophisticated work can only be done at ground level," explains Jaffrey. "People who do the day-to-day work can get through these issues with so much velocity. When we empower them to be the change agents, we're leveraging the largest untapped resource we have in healthcare."

The steady movement toward person- and family-centered care (P&FCC) has occurred for reasons of safety, quality, and person and family preference (Disch, 2010). As the preceding scenario demonstrates, the primary drivers of P&FCC are respectful partnerships and a commitment to the shared values of P&FCC as well as the engagement of the "hearts and minds" of all healthcare providers (Balik, Conway, Zipperer, & Watson, 2011).

This chapter describes the history of P&FCC and the positive individual, financial, and family outcomes to implementation. Multiple myths related to P&FCC are explored and the evidence explained to refute the myths. National standards and various organizational regulations that may serve as a stimulus for implementation of P&FCC are introduced. Lastly, the competencies necessary for all healthcare providers for delivering P&FCC are presented.

An Overview of Person- and Family-Centered Care

Dimensions of P&FCC include (Gerteis, Edgman-Levitan, Daley, & Delbanco, 1993):

- **Respect for patients' values, preferences, and expressed needs:** freely sharing information with the person and family, actively partnering to establish care priorities and a plan, adjusting the plan as needed, and modifying the level of involvement according to the person and family preferences

- **Coordination and integration of care:** bringing together the people and resources necessary to create smooth transitions across the continuum of care

- **Information, communication, and education:** individualizing explanations and presentation of materials to people's preferences, ensuring that communication and information are presented in a way that makes sense to them and accommodates their levels of literacy

- **Physical comfort:** ensuring comfort and freedom from pain

- **Emotional support:** assessing the person and family for anxiety and distress and identifying and addressing the underlying causes

- **Involvement of family and friends:** structuring family and friend presence to meet the needs of the person regardless of age

Sullivan (2003), discussing the view of medicine—which can easily be expanded to all of healthcare—notes that the role of clinicians needs to change to focus on patients' lives rather than their bodies. Outcome measures in the future will focus less on physiologic function and disease severity measures and more on person-centered quality-of-life measures. A person's values and preferences will shape the goals of healthcare.

> **NOTE**
>
> As noted in Chapter 1, there is still variability among authors and organizations as to whether the concept is appropriately titled *person-centered* or *patient-centered*. This chapter uses the phrases interchangeably.

P&FCC does not negate the person's rights to privacy or control, but rather recognizes that this is a choice that the person can make. It is a philosophy that considers the person as the unit of attention within the individual's network of relationships. It should not be equated with any one intervention, such as open visiting hours or the family having equal say in the decision-making.

Rather, "[p]atient and family-centered care is a term describing a philosophy and culture that emphasizes partnerships between patients, family members, and health care providers" (Walton & Barnsteiner, 2012, p. 68). It comprises not only a one-to-one relationship with a healthcare provider but also partnerships across all levels and components from task forces to governing boards. Sherwood, in Chapter 9 of this book, lists the 10 categories that Planetree designates an organization can use to assess where they are on the continuum from being disease-centered and clinician-focused to person-centered and promoting health and wellness. This entails changes in operations, strategic planning, resource allocation, and the environment of care (Frampton & Guastello, 2010).

The 2011 Institute of Medicine (IOM) report *The Future of Nursing: Leading Change, Advancing Health* notes the need for patient-centered care (PCC) to improve quality, access, and value yet recognizes that "practice still is usually organized around what is most convenient for the provider, the payer, or the health care organization and not the patient" (p. 51). "Patients who receive individualized care and who are part of the decision making process have reduced anxiety and stress, and have shorter lengths of stay in hospital" (Balik et al., 2011, p. 6). Person-centered care demands that the ways in which individuals are cared for should always be under their control. They, not others, should direct their own care, and everyone in a healthcare system should know and honor what they want (Berwick, 2011).

As you learned in Chapter 1, the definitions of P&FCC vary depending on the organization, but the myriad definitions do share common elements. The IOM, in its landmark book *Crossing the Quality Chasm* (2001), defines *patient centered* as "providing care that is respectful of and responsive to individual patient preferences, needs, and values and ensuring that patient values guide all clinical decisions" (p. 40). Patient-centered care is one of the six dimensions of quality espoused by the IOM (2001, pp. 39–40):

- Safe
- Timely
- Effective
- Efficient
- Equitable
- Patient-centered

The IOM (2001) report, among others, calls for a redirection of care from provider-centric to person- and family-centric with full engagement of the person and family members, as the person wishes, calling it a "partnership among practitioners, patients and families (when appropriate) to ensure that decisions respect patient wants, needs and preferences and that patients have the education and support they require to make decisions and participate in their own care" (p. 40).

The Joint Commission (TJC) has adopted the definition of P&FCC that the Institute for Patient- and Family-Centered Care (IPFCC) established. This is

> an innovative approach to plan, deliver, and evaluate health care that is grounded in mutually beneficial partnerships among health care providers, patients, and families. Patient- and family-centered care applies to patients of all ages, and it may be practiced in any health care setting. (TJC, 2010, p. 92)

Recently, the Quality and Safety Education for Nurses (QSEN) initiative has defined PCC as recognizing "the patient or designee as the source of control and full partner in providing compassionate and coordinated care based on patient's preferences, values and needs" (Cronenwett et al.,

2007; Cronenwett et al., 2009). It is the most inclusive of the definitions, calling for the patient and/or designee to be the source of control and full partner in care decisions.

Berwick (2009) further articulates PCC as the experience (to the extent the informed individual patient desires it) of transparency, individualization, recognition, respect, dignity, and choice in all matters without exception, related to one's person, circumstances, and relationships in healthcare.

History of Person- and Family-Centered Care

P&FCC may seem like a relatively recent movement to many; however, Hippocrates taught the first medical students "to provide by listening to the patient" (Guastello, 2012, p. 4). The literature often cites that the beginning of patient-centered medicine as a concept was introduced in a publication by Balint in 1969; Balint asserts that allowing patients to state their stories and what they want in their own words results in more positive patient outcomes.

In actuality, there are many earlier examples of P&FCC. In the early days of hospitals, only the poor were admitted, as hospitals were seen as places that were unclean and infection was a likely outcome. Instead, family and private-duty nurses cared for people in their homes if at all possible. This practice changed for children when a hospital dedicated to their care was established in 1855 with the opening of the Children's Hospital of Philadelphia. Many children's hospitals followed soon thereafter.

All the early children's hospitals were founded by reformers and philanthropists who shared a dual purpose of improving the medical and moral status of children. It was hoped that during a hospital stay, children, away from their families, would learn the rules of health and ways of middle-class life. Visiting hours for parents, if any, were generally restricted to a few hours on Sundays (Barnsteiner, 2005; Barnsteiner & Walton, 2005). Limiting contact of hospitalized children with their families continued through the first half of the 20th century. Nurses believed that children were better off, as they got upset when parents left. The thought was that children should settle in.

A number of research studies converged to begin a change in parent visiting, leading to what we know today as parent participation and family-centered care. Spitz coined the term *hospitalism* and documented the decline in the health of children due to long confinement in the hospital (1952). Robertson (1952), motivated by observations of his own child's hospital stay, filmed *A Two-Year-Old Goes To the Hospital*, demonstrating the withdrawing behavior of children who were left without their parents. And lastly, Fagin (1966) did her doctoral dissertation on the post-hospital effects of children with and without parents during a hospital stay. Her research demonstrated that children whose parents stayed with them had fewer regressive behaviors post-discharge.

Changes came slowly. In the 1970s, we saw increased visiting hours and, finally, provisions for parents to stay overnight. When visiting hours changed and mothers were allowed to stay at the bedside, nurses needed to learn new skills on how to work with anxious, questioning parents. Despite a mountain of theoretical and empirical evidence, staff were reluctant, and change was slow and fragmented. We continue to see some restrictions today in many neonatal and critical care areas.

In 1982, the President's Commission for the Study of Ethical Problems in Medicine and Biomedical and Behavioral Research criticized the extent to which medical decisions were being made in a paternalistic way, with physicians essentially controlling the decision-making. The commission took the position that patients must be provided with the information they needed to form their own opinions about what should be done and that their voices should be well reflected in the resulting decisions.

The changes witnessed in pediatric nursing have gradually taken hold in the care of adults and their families. Patients and families have been engaged for decades in various activities that have equipped them to be partners in their own care. Examples include receiving pre-operative and discharge-to-home instructions, learning to take medications and perform treatments, monitoring vital signs, and watching for complications. Over the past three decades, we have witnessed people being discharged to home with ever-more-complicated care, including home dialysis and the use of ventilators.

More recently, patients and family members are also being invited to actively participate on health system boards, committees, and task forces. In 1986, the Picker family, based on a hospitalization experience of Jean Picker, decided to focus their family foundation on research to determine the factors most important to patients and whether healthcare providers are sufficiently responsive to patient preferences. Harvey Picker is credited with having coined the phrase *patient-centered care* in 1988. "Patient and family centered care places an emphasis on collaborating with patients and families of all ages, at all levels of care, and in all health care settings" (Conway et al., 2006).

Demonstrated Outcomes of Person- and Family-Centered Care

PCC leads to improved physical, emotional, and social well-being (Beadle-Brown, 2006; McCormack & McCance, 2006) for the individual. As an approach to nursing, it is respectful, humanitarian, and ethical (Edvardsson & Innes, 2010). Families may also benefit from P&FCC by being present to support their loved ones and being better prepared to support care as a result of being active participants. Additionally, the Planetree experience has demonstrated positive financial outcomes for the healthcare organization (Charmel & Frampton, 2008). "Engaging patients as partners in their care and recognizing them as multidimensional human beings also drives patient satisfaction, which positions an organization in the marketplace as a provider of choice" (Charmel, Stone, & Otero, 2013, p. 28).

Person Outcomes

A growing body of evidence demonstrates that improving the patient experience and developing partnerships with patients correlates with improved health outcomes. For example, evidence shows that patients who are more involved in their care are better able to (Jarousse, 2011):

- Manage complex chronic conditions
- Seek appropriate assistance
- Have reduced lengths of stay and avoidable readmissions and emergency department (ED) visits
- Experience increased patient satisfaction and employee engagement

As noted in Chapter 1, patients want "whole-person" care, and this results in improved health outcomes and increased satisfaction with the healthcare delivery system.

Financial Outcomes

Hospitals that provide PCC have demonstrated numerous financial benefits. The more than 100 healthcare institutions practicing the Planetree model of P&FCC have reported many clinical and operational benefits resulting from a PCC approach, including (Charmel & Frampton, 2008):

- Increased patient satisfaction
- Increased staff retention
- Enhanced staff recruitment
- Decreased length of stay
- Decreased ED return visits
- Decreased adverse events including fewer medication errors
- Reduced operating costs' and a lower cost per case
- Increased market share
- Improved liability claims experience

Eighteen months into implementing a structured approach to PCC, Stamford Hospital, a 305-bed tertiary care center in Stamford, Connecticut, demonstrated an increase in employee satisfaction from the 33rd to the 60th percentile (Charmel & Frampton, 2008). Hospital leadership credited the increase, in part, to a number of initiatives, including the attendance of all staff at a series of retreats focused on boosting employee morale and community building.

In the context of an increasingly competitive marketplace, growing healthcare consumerism, and the trend toward greater transparency, these benefits make a compelling business case for P&FCC. However, there is a long way to go in reaching the mandate for P&FCC. A recent study by Fowler and colleagues (Fowler, Gerstein, & Barry, 2013) reported that physician discussions with patients about common tests, medications, and procedures as reported by patients do not reflect a high level of shared decision-making. Responses from more than 2,000 persons indicated the majority of physicians do not solicit patient preferences or values when ordering common healthcare interventions.

Family Outcomes

Families also benefit from being more fully involved in the care of their loved ones, or in the care of those for whom they have volunteered to serve as advocates or designees. Henneman and Cardin (2002) note that family members have to be "active participants in planning the care of their loved ones" and that being involved enables them to be better prepared for an "ever-increasing role as direct caregivers" (p. 12).

As an example of how this can be helpful, Meyers (2008) reports the experience of Hollis Ryan, the mother of a patient, who was actively engaged in her son's care process: "In the past, I felt like I was always standing on the outside, looking in…. Suddenly I was a part of the care process. They removed that veil of mystery that had shrouded my health care experiences for most of my life" (p. 14).

In addition to the benefits that family members themselves receive, there are many additional positive outcomes that can also be realized:

- Improved communication between the patient and the medical staff (Agency for Healthcare Research & Quality [AHRQ], 2012; Aronson, Yau, Helfaer, & Morrison, 2009; Rotman-Pikielny et al., 2007)
- The family's belief that their presence on rounds would improve the medical staff's attitude toward the patient (Rotman-Pikielny et al., 2007)
- The discovery of new information from family members (Aronson et al., 2009)
- Clarification of orders and discharge instructions (Aronson et al., 2009)

Despite the evidence that P&FCC has numerous positive outcomes for the person, family members, healthcare organizations, and providers, multiple myths are often stated as reasons for the inability to implement many of the components of P&FCC. These myths and the countering explanations are described in the following section.

Myths Related to Person- and Family-Centered Care

Over the past 20 years, a number of organizations have proposed strategies for engaging patients and families, many of which are cited in this book. Fraenkel (2013) outlines strategies for bringing patients and their family members into the decision-making process, including the use of questionnaires to assess knowledge specific to their disease processes and values related to escalation in treatments to assist in incorporating their preferences into point-of-care decision support. Many healthcare providers and leaders think P&FCC strategies are too difficult to put into place. The Picker Foundation dispels a number of myths associated with P&FCC (see Table 2.1).

TABLE 2.1   Myths Related to Person- and Family-Centered Care

MYTH	REFUTING THE MYTH
It is too costly.	A 5-year study of units that implemented the Planetree principles and those who had not found the Planetree units less costly, with a shorter length of stay, lower cost per stay, and higher patient satisfaction. Another myth related to cost is that major facility renovations are necessary. Although making physical changes to accommodate persons and family members may increase comfort, it is not a requisite of P&FCC.
P&FCC is nice but not important.	One major benefit to P&FCC is error prevention. Patient- or family-initiated rapid-response teams can prevent patient deterioration as a result of errors from occurring. Medication reconciliation with every person may avert costly errors due to lack of information about allergies or inaccurate listing of current medications. Giving people access to their healthcare records provides an opportunity to correct any mistakes, perhaps preventing future errors. My own experience of viewing my electronic health record (EHR) enabled me to correct my record, which stated a family history of GU cancer when in fact it was GI cancer. This had ramifications not only for potential treatment decisions but also for the potential denial of service costs due to my need for more frequent than usual colonoscopy.
Providing P&FCC is the job of nurses.	Everyone working in a healthcare organization (HCO) contributes to the P&FCC experience. It requires a changed culture with involvement of everyone at all levels of an HCO, from the board of trustees to all frontline staff.
Providing P&FCC takes more staff.	There are no data to support this. When compared with non-P&FCC organizations, staffing costs are similar.
It can only be effective in small, independent hospitals.	There are no data to support this. Aurora Health System and Cleveland Clinic are examples of HCOs that have successfully implemented P&FCC.
There is no evidence that this is an effective model of care delivery.	Planetree and Picker provide a lot of evidence that P&FCC is effective (Frampton, 2009).

continues

TABLE 2.1 *continued*

MYTH	REFUTING THE MYTH
It increases infection.	There is no evidence to support this. Evidence indicates that open visiting, pet visitation, and other innovations do not result in increased infection.
Implementing P&FCC will necessitate renovation or construction.	Many organizations have demonstrated that capital improvements, such as building renovations, are nice but not necessary.
It is a magic bullet to better patient satisfaction.	It is not a magic bullet. It is about changing culture, not ratings.
It is a Health Insurance Portability and Accountability Act (HIPAA) violation.	Not so. Access to information is a patient right, and patients can also designate who among their family and friends may also have access to their healthcare information and records.

Standards and Regulations: A Stimulus for Person- and Family-Centered Care

Accreditation standards and federal regulations provide a powerful stimulus to motivate organizations to move toward a culture of P&FCC. Over the past decade, national regulatory agencies have weighed in on P&FCC. TJC, the National Committee for Quality Assurance (NCQA), and the Centers for Medicare & Medicaid Services (CMS) have become involved in stating expectations and monitoring performance.

The federal government uses the Hospital Consumer Assessment of Healthcare Providers and Systems (HCAHPS) survey to measure patients' perceptions of their inpatient and ambulatory experience and posts public results (www.hospitalcompare.hhs.gov). This tool allows consumers to compare hospitals nationally on key variables that include communication, responsiveness, cleanliness, noise, and pain management. Some questions, such as pain management and call-bell response time, specifically relate to nursing performance. CMS has created an incentive program to reward facilities that use the tool and, more importantly, report their data (www.cms.gov).

CMS has also established federal regulations for patient rights as a result of a presidential memorandum focused on hospital visitation and specifically noting the issues of lesbian, gay, bisexual, and transgender patients and their families (The White House Office of the Press Secretary, 2010). Based on the memorandum, which was introduced in January 2011, CMS issued a new Condition of Participation standard, requiring hospitals to inform patients of visitation rights and the patients' right to receive visitors whom they designate, including spouses, domestic partners, family members, or friends. These regulations were an outgrowth of an egregious care situation in a Florida hospital where a woman was not permitted to be at the bedside of her same-sex partner, who was dying from a ruptured cerebral aneurysm.

On April 15, 2010, President Barack Obama issued a moving presidential memorandum on hospital visitation and patient representation that begins:

> There are few moments in our lives that call for greater compassion and companion-ship than when a loved one is admitted to the hospital. In these hours of need and moments of pain and anxiety, all of us would hope to have a hand to hold, a shoulder on which to lean—a loved one to be there for us, as we would be there for them.
>
> Yet every day, all across America, patients are denied the kindnesses and caring of a loved one at their sides—whether in a sudden medical emergency or a prolonged hospital stay. Often, a widow or widower with no children is denied the support and comfort of a good friend. Members of religious orders are sometimes unable to choose someone other than an immediate family member to visit them and make medical decisions on their behalf. Also uniquely affected are gay and lesbian Americans who are often barred from the bedsides of the partners with whom they may have spent decades of their lives—unable to be there for the person they love, and unable to act as a legal surrogate if their partner is incapacitated….
>
> [This means that] all too often, people are made to suffer or even to pass away alone, denied the comfort of companionship in their final moments while a loved one is left worrying and pacing down the hall (White House, 2010).

The National Quality Forum (NQF) is a voluntary consensus standards-setting body that uses its influence to promote patient and family involvement. It has endorsed more than 500 measures of quality and safety. Through its National Priorities Partnership (NPP; 2011), it has identified six priorities with the greatest potential for improving care, reducing disparities, and eliminating waste. One of the six is Patient and Family Engagement. NQF is working to ensure that all patients:

- Will be asked for feedback on their experience of care, which healthcare organizations and their staff will then use to improve care
- Will have access to tools and support systems that enable them to effectively navigate and manage their care
- Will have access to information and assistance that enables them to make informed decisions about their treatment options

TJC issued *Advancing Effective Communication, Cultural Competence and Patient- and Family-Centered Care: A Roadmap for Hospitals* (2010) to provide specific methods to improve quality and safety initiatives and implement new accreditation standards. The document outlines strategies and practices for care improvement, with a summary checklist focused on points along the care continuum: admission processes, assessment, treatment, end-of-life care, discharge, and transfer (TJC, 2010, pp. 5–6). Specific recommendations on assessment and approaches to elicit and understand the patient's values and perspectives are included (TJC, 2010, pp. 13–16).

TJC standards include the patient's right to identify a support person and have access to that person throughout an inpatient admission. Accreditation site surveyors review the process for notifying patients of their rights and identifying the support persons. The identified support person, based on the patient's preference, may be involved in patient care rounds, education, and discharge planning. Patients in intensive-care units (ICUs) are particularly vulnerable, with complex communication needs: "These patients must have unrestricted access to their chosen support person while in the ICU to provide emotional and social support" (TJC, 2010, p. 22).

These TJC and CMS requirements recognize the vulnerability of hospitalized individuals and formally establish the role of a "support person" in the hospital setting in the CMS Conditions of Participation (CMS, 2010). Persons may choose to have allies at their bedsides to ensure that their preferences, needs, and values are respected and assist in guiding clinical decision-making.

External pressure is also coming from many other groups that are promoting P&FCC. Consumers Advancing Patient Safety, the Institute for Patient- and Family-Centered Care, and AARP are examples of consumer advocacy groups. AARP is advocating for quality initiatives including the use of evidence-based shared decision-making to improve care (AARP, 2012). The World Health Organization (WHO) encourages partnerships among patients, their families, and healthcare workers to promote various quality initiatives in healthcare settings (WHO, 2005). The NPP, a group of 28 organizations with an interest in improving healthcare, also identified patient and family engagement as a national priority (NPP, 2011). The advocacy of these and other groups creates an environment in which doing anything less than full implementation of P&FCC is poor-quality healthcare.

Competencies Necessary for Delivering Person- and Family-Centered Nursing Care

QSEN is a four-phase initiative, funded by the Robert Wood Johnson Foundation. In Phase 1 (2005–2007), a group of experts developed competency definitions and learning objectives for the quality and safety domains outlined in the IOM (2003) report on health professions education; PCC is one of the competencies. Table 2.2 lists the PCC knowledge, skills, and attitudes (KSAs) needed by pre-licensure nurses to function in today's healthcare settings. Increasingly, nursing leaders in practice have been using the KSAs as a framework for clinical practice.

TABLE 2.2 Patient-Centered Care Knowledge, Skills, and Attitudes

PATIENT-CENTERED CARE

Definition: Recognize the patient or designee as the source of control and full partner in providing compassionate and coordinated care based on respect for patient's preferences, values, and needs.

KNOWLEDGE	SKILLS	ATTITUDES
Integrate understanding of multiple dimensions of PCC: Patient/family/community preferences, values Coordination and integration of care Information, communication, and education Physical comfort and emotional support Involvement of family and friends Transition and continuity	Elicit patient values, preferences, and expressed needs as part of clinical interview, implementation of care plan, and evaluation of care Communicate patient values, preferences, and expressed needs to other members of the healthcare team	Value seeing healthcare situations "through patients' eyes" Respect and encourage individual expression of patient values, preferences, and expressed needs Value the patient's expertise with own health and symptoms
Describe how diverse cultural, ethnic, and social backgrounds function as sources of patient, family, and community values	Provide PCC with sensitivity and respect for the diversity of the human experience	Seek learning opportunities with patients who represent all aspects of human diversity Recognize personally held attitudes about working with patients from different ethnic, cultural, and social backgrounds Willingly support PCC for individuals and groups whose values differ from your own

continues

TABLE 2.2 *continued*

KNOWLEDGE	SKILLS	ATTITUDES
Examine how the safety, quality, and cost-effectiveness of healthcare can be improved through the active involvement of patients and families	Remove barriers to presence of families and other designated surrogates based on patient preferences	Value active partnership with patients or designated surrogates in planning, implementating, and evaluating of care
Examine common barriers to active involvement of patients in their own healthcare processes	Assess level of patient's decisional conflict and provide access to resources	Respect patient preferences for degree of active engagement in care process
Describe strategies to empower patients or families in all aspects of the healthcare process	Engage patients or designated surrogates in active partnerships that promote health, safety and well-being, and self-care management	Respect patient's right to access to personal health records

Source: Cronenwett et al., 2007, p.122–123. Reprinted with permission from Elsevier, Ltd.

The KSAs are competencies that should be demonstrated by every graduating pre-license nurse as well as all practicing nurses. Numerous strategies have been used to teach the competencies in education and practice settings, and many can be found on the QSEN website (www.qsen.org). Strategies include inviting patients and family members to classes, new employee orientation sessions, and grand rounds to share patients' and families' narratives about their healthcare experiences and what they would like to see from healthcare providers. Other strategies include developing case studies and discussing all decisions from the patient's point of view, including the scheduling of treatments and medications, and analyzing how this looks different from the traditional, provider-centric view.

Conclusion

P&FCC is supported by numerous individuals, groups, and organizations. There is widespread evidence of a compelling business and quality case for P&FCC, but it requires a paradigm shift. Nursing leaders and frontline clinicians must partner with consumers and other health professionals to intentionally lead the necessary culture shift by integrating the person and family voice into not only direct care but also all improvement efforts, leadership committees, and newly designed programs.

We also need to help healthcare professionals be equipped with the resources, knowledge, skills, and attitudes to deliver P&FCC through comprehensive education programs and adequate resources to deliver such care. There is increasing momentum and support. Healthcare providers, administrators, and policymakers are recognizing the importance of "nothing about me without me" (Berwick, 2009, p. w560).

References

AARP. (2012). Moving toward person and family centered care. Retrieved from http://www.aarp.org/content/dam/aarp/research/public_policy_institute/ltc/2012/moving-toward-person-and-family-centered-care-insight-AARP-ppi-ltc.pdf

Agency for Healthcare Research and Quality (AHRQ). (2012). *Guide to patient and family engagement: Environmental scan report.* Rockville, MD: Author.

Aronson, P. L., Yau, J., Helfaer, M. A., & Morrison, W. (2009). Impact of family presence during pediatric intensive care unit rounds on the family and medical team. *Pediatrics, 124*(4), 1119-1125.

Balik, B., Conway, J., Zipperer, L., & Watson, J. (2011) *Achieving an exceptional patient and family experience of inpatient hospital care.* IHI Innovation Series white paper. Cambridge, MA: Institute for Healthcare Improvement. Retrieved from www.IHI.org

Balint, E. (1969). The possibilities of patient-centered medicine. *Journal of the Royal College General Practitioners, 17*(82), 269-276.

Barnsteiner, J. H. (2005). *Pediatric nursing: 150 Years of Caring for Children and Families.* Keynote Address: Society of Pediatric Nursing Conference, Philadelphia, PA (April 15).

Barnsteiner, J. H., & Walton, M. (2005). Milk depots, yarn trusses and pediatric nurses. *Journal of Urologic Nursing, 25*(3), 160-161.

Beadle-Brown, J. (2006). Person-centred approaches and quality of life. *Tizard Learning Disability Review, 11*(3), 4-12.

Berwick, D. (2009). What patient-centered should mean: Confessions of an extremist. *Health Affairs, 28*(4), w555-w565.

Berwick, D. (2011, December). The moral test. Keynote address: Institute for Healthcare Improvement National Forum, Orlando, FL.

Centers for Medicare and Medicaid Services (CMS). (2010). Changes to the hospital and critical access hospital conditions of participation to ensure visitation rights for all patients, 75 Fed. Reg. 70,831 (Nov. 19, 2010) (to be codified at 42 CFR pts. 482 and 485). Retrieved from http://www.gpo.gov/fdsys/pkg/FR-2010-11-19/pdf/2010-29194.pdf

Charmel, P. A., & Frampton, S. B. (2008). Building the business case for patient-centered care. *Healthcare Financial Management, 62*(3), 80-85.

Charmel, P. A., Stone, S., & Otero, D. (2013). The patient-centered care value equation. In S. B. Frampton, P. A. Charmel, & S. Guastello (Eds.), *The putting patients first field guide: Global lessons in designing and implementing patient-centered care* (pp. 19-44). Hoboken, NJ: Wiley-Blackwell.

Conway, J., Johnson, B., Edgman-Levitan, S., Schlucter, J., Ford, D., Sodomka, P., & Simmons, L. (2006). Partnering with patients and families to design a patient- and family-centered care system. Retrieved from http://www.hsi.gatech.edu/erfuture/images/c/c2/Family.pdf

Cronenwett, L., Sherwood, G., Barnsteiner, J., Disch, J., Johnson, J., Mitchell, P., … Warren, J. (2007). Quality and safety education for nurses. *Nursing Outlook, 55*(3), 122-131.

Cronenwett, L., Sherwood, G., Pohl, J., Barnsteiner, Moore, S., Sullivan, D., …Warren, J. (2009). Quality and safety education for advanced practice nurses. *Nursing Outlook, 57*(6), 338-348.

Disch, J. (2010). Patient-centered care. Enhancing Quality and Safety in Nursing Education: Preparing Nurse Faculty to Lead Curricular Change. CDROM, Vol. 1, Version 7A. *Quality and Safety Education for Nurses/*American Association of Colleges of Nursing.

Edvardsson, D., & Innes, A. (2010). Measuring person-centered care: A critical comparative review of published tools. *The Gerontologist, 50*(6), 834-846.

Fagin, C. (1966). *The effects of maternal attendance during hospitalization on the behavior of young children: A comparative survey.* Philadelphia, PA: F. A. Davis.

Fowler, F. J., Gerstein, B. S., & Barry, M. J. (2013). How patient centered are medical decisions? Results of a national survey. *JAMA Internal Medicine, 173*(13), 1215-1221.

Fraenkel, L., (2013). Incorporating patients' preferences into medical decision making. *Medical Care Research and Review, 70*(1), 80S-93S.

Frampton, S. B. (2009). Creating a patient-centered system. *American Journal of Nursing, 109*(3), 30-33.

Frampton, S. B., & Guastello, S. (2010). Patient-centered care: More than the sum of its parts. *American Journal of Nursing, 110*(9), 49-53.

Gerteis, M., Edgman-Levitan, S., Daley, J., & Delbanco, T. L. (1993). *Through the patient's eyes: Understanding and promoting patient-centered care.* San Francisco, CA: Jossey-Bass.

Guastello, S., (2012). Advancing patient centered care across the continuum of care. Retrieved from http://planetree.org/wp-content/uploads/2012/01/Advancing-PCC-Across-the-Continuum_Planetree-White-Paper_August-2012.pdf3/1/14

Henneman, E. A., & Cardin, W. (2002). Family-centered care: A practical approach to making it happen. *Critical Care Nurse, 22*(6), 12-19.

Institute of Medicine (IOM). (2001). *Crossing the quality chasm: A new health system for the 21st century.* Washington, DC: National Academies Press.

Institute of Medicine (IOM). (2003). *Health professions education: A bridge to quality.* Washington, DC: National Academies Press.

Institute of Medicine (IOM). (2011). *The future of nursing: Leading change, advancing health.* Washington, DC: National Academies Press.

Jarousse, K. (2011). Putting patients first. *Trustee, 64*(10), 26.

The Joint Commission (TJC). (2010). *Advancing effective communication, cultural competence, and patient- and family-centered care: A roadmap for hospitals.* Oakbrook Terrace, IL: Author.

Marton, B. A. (2012, April). Patient-centered care redistributes responsibility. *Health Leaders.* Retrieved from http://www.healthleadersmedia.com/content/PHY-279857/PatientCentered-Care-Redistributes-Responsibility##

McCormack, B., & McCance, T. V. (2006). Development of a framework for person-centred nursing. *Journal of Advanced Nursing 56*(5), 472-479.

Meyers, S. (2008, April). Take heed: How patient and family advisors can improve quality. *Trustee,* 14-22.

National Priorities Partnership. (2011). National Quality Forum. National Priorities Partnership 2011. Retrieved from http://www.qualityforum.org/Setting_Priorities/NPP/National_Priorities_Partnership.aspx

President's Commission for the Study of Ethical Problems in Medicine and Biomedical and Behavioral Research. (1982). *Making health care decisions.* Washington, DC: Government Printing Office.

Robertson, J. (1952). A 2 year old goes to the hospital. Retrieved from http://www.ncbi.nlm.nih.gov/pmc/articles/PMC1918555/pdf/procrsmed00418-0060.pdf

Rotman-Pikielny, P., Rabin, B., Amoyal, S., Mushkat, Y., Zissin, R., & Levy, Y. (2007). Participation of family members in ward rounds: Attitude of medical staff, patients and relatives. *Patient Education and Counseling, 65*(2), 166-170.

Spitz, R. (1952). Psychogenic disease in infancy. Retrieved from https://archive.org/details/PsychogenicD

Sullivan, M. (2003). The new subjective medicine: Taking the patient's point of view on health care and health. *Social Science and Medicine, 56*(7), 1595-1604.

Walton, M., & Barnsteiner, J. (2012). Patient centered care. In G. Sherwood and J. Barnsteiner (Eds.), *Quality and safety in nursing: A competency approach to improving outcomes* (pp. 67-90). Hoboken, NJ: Wiley-Blackwell.

White House Office of the Press Secretary. (2010). *Presidential Memorandum for the Secretary of Health and Human Services—Hospital visitation.* Released April 15, 2010. Retrieved from http://www.whitehouse.gov/the-press-office/presidential-memorandum-hospital-visitation

World Health Organization (WHO). (2005). Preparing a health care workforce for the 21st century. Retrieved from http://www.who.int/chp/knowledge/publications/workforce_report.pdf

Chapter 3

A Patient's Perspective on Patient- and Family-Centered Care

Jessie Gruman, PhD

"Your pathology report indicates that you have stomach cancer." With those words, I felt, for the fourth time since age 20, as though I had been dropped into a foreign country. After a series of four life-threatening diagnoses, starting with Hodgkin's when I was 20, once again, I didn't know the language, I didn't understand the culture, I had no map, and I desperately wanted to find my way home. On that day 3 years ago, I was once again vividly reminded that my active participation in responding to this diagnosis wasn't just a nice thing to do if I had a little extra time and a feisty spirit. It would be necessary for my care to have its optimal effect.

We patients heartily endorse the shared aim of the healthcare enterprise to improve the health of individuals and populations. Increasingly, however, achieving it requires active, knowledgeable participation in our care by us and our family caregivers. Care that is patient- and family-centered reduces barriers and supports our efforts to participate in caring for ourselves and thus to make the best possible use of the tools of medicine. This chapter explores from the patient's perspective the challenges we face and provides suggestions that might give more of us the opportunity to actively engage in caring for ourselves and those we love.

A Patient's Perspective

Each of the five times I have been diagnosed with cancer, I have been challenged by the need to participate actively and knowledgeably in all aspects of my healthcare if I am to benefit fully from it. Advances in medicine increasingly shift responsibilities for care from healthcare clinicians to patients and our families. Thus, patient- and family-centered care (P&FCC) must be built around our central role in our health and in our care and be organized to guide and support us as we take on new, unfamiliar, and complicated tasks to get better and stay well.

As a patient with far too much experience finding and using healthcare, I reflect on three questions:

- What are our responsibilities for our healthcare today?
- How are we reacting to the need for greater participation in our care?
- How can healthcare be organized to support our and our families' active and knowledgeable participation in our care?

Only by interviewing three surgeons did I learn that my choice of one of them would make a permanent and profound difference in my quality of life, the difference between a partial and a complete gastrectomy. Only by careful listening did I discover that their varied surgical approaches would not affect the risk of recurrence. Only through a series of tough conversations did my oncologist and I come up with a chemotherapy regimen that balanced likely benefits against long-term risks and immediate side effects. Only by understanding my insurance benefits and working with my plan provider was I able to ensure that the care I needed was covered.

This responsibility was a heavy lift for me, even with the experience of three previous cancer diagnoses, a career in advocating patient engagement in healthcare, and good connections. It is sobering to consider how people who have less experience and less access to support and information could do the same.

Despite the millions of dollars worth of research that had been distilled into treatments, technologies, and drugs requiring thousands of dollars to purchase and many hours of time to deliver, the success of my care largely rested on me, the patient. If I did not participate actively and knowledgeably, I would squander this enormous investment. And although I would be the one to suffer most from my lack of active participation, I almost certainly would have wasted resources that could help others.

I am not alone in feeling challenged by what I, as a patient, must know and do to find the healthcare I need to stay healthy and treat my illnesses. I have interviewed hundreds of people about their experiences with healthcare. They—caregivers and patients alike—tell similar stories of being surprised and burdened by what they have to do to find good care that provides the greatest benefit and is consistent with their goals and values.

Reorganizing Healthcare to Become Patient- and Family-Centered

The primary aim of reorganizing healthcare to become patient- and family-centered is to ensure that we are able to make the best possible use of the tools of medicine available to us. Again, it is important to ask three key questions: Just what are our responsibilities when we seek healthcare that make such reorganization necessary? What affects our ability to take on those tasks? And how can healthcare be organized to support patients' and families' active and knowledgeable participation in our care? The following sections describe the answers to these important questions.

What Are Our Responsibilities for Our Healthcare?

Advances in medicine promise better health outcomes but often shift considerable responsibilities to patients if we are to fully realize their effects. New surgical procedures, combined with institutional reimbursement incentives, mean that we often return home from the hospital quicker but sicker (National Center for Health Statistics [NCHS], 2012a). Tasks that were once carried out by health professionals in hospitals now fall to us and our family caregivers. These tasks include managing symptoms, medications, wound care, and rehabilitation (Fex, Ek, & Soderhamn, 2009; Lerret & Weiss, 2011). Similarly, new medications make it possible for those of us with chronic conditions, such as HIV, cancer, heart disease, and diabetes, to live long and well but only if we are able to maintain the complicated drug regimens and lifestyle changes required to make them effective (Kobin & Sheth, 2011). And the proliferation of specialists and treatment sites makes care coordination a tricky business that often falls to patients and families due to fragmented care, spotty inter-clinician communication, and a lack of interoperable electronic health records (Jamoom et al., 2012; NCHS, 2012b).

These shifts in responsibility for our care result not only from advances in healthcare but also from the drive to make treatment more efficient by delivering equivalent or superior care while minimizing demands placed on professionals' time (Lewis, 2012; Varma, 2009). Skyrocketing healthcare costs drive health insurance plans to require that patients and caregivers shop for care options, compare quality of providers, and absorb higher deductibles and co-pays (Mayne, Girod, & Weltz, 2012). Research demonstrating that we do better when we have a say in our own care also supports a shift from a paternal, often authoritative style of medicine toward a more patient- and family-centered approach (Katon et al., 1995).

Because most of us are mostly well most of the time, we are often unaware of these changes in healthcare delivery and the changes in our responsibilities. What seems obvious to healthcare professionals is often a mystery to us. Just the simplest basics of getting care can be challenging.

After my stomach cancer diagnosis, it was only with competent, consistent help from my husband that I was able to remember, understand, and share in decisions about my care. And only with a sizable investment of precious energy was I able to make and keep all those appointments, get the tests, take the drugs, and make sure all my doctors got the appropriate test results and notes so they could advise me accurately and help me make it safely to where I am today.

Yet even my best efforts to stick to my chemotherapy regimen were discouraged by my chemo nurse, who thought I could do nothing right. She scolded me for sending an email when she thought I should have called and vice versa. She scolded me for going home before my next appointment was scheduled. She scolded me for asking whether my clinical information and questions were shared between my oncologist and the staff of the chemo suite. I could go on…

My concern isn't the scolding *per se*. When patients start chemotherapy or have a heart attack, brain injury, stroke, or a serious chronic condition, we sign on to a long-term relationship with a whole crew of people—receptionists, nurses, aides, physical therapists, phlebotomists, pharmacists, and doctors—that is likely to require a lot of back-and-forth if we are to complete the multitude of tasks involving tests, drugs, procedures, appointments, and general follow-through. Chances are that these professionals have figured out ways to work together pretty efficiently. But few of them let us in on the action: They rarely provide us with clear verbal and written directions and guidance that would help us communicate with them more easily. Instead, they leave us to guess, and often we guess wrong. This, of course, frustrates us. And it makes those public health messages encouraging us to "ask more questions" or "compare treatment options" seem out of touch with the reality of our confusing experiences with healthcare.

Print and electronic media flood us with a steady stream of health messages. Drug advertisements and public service announcements for cancer screenings are just two examples of a daily cascade of pitches. Yet many of us—and many of the clinicians who care for us—lack a clear picture of the significance of our own behaviors in ensuring that we get the full benefit from the healthcare available to us (Madde & Zickuhr, 2011). Patients and caregivers who lack the perseverance, capacity, resources, or ability to seek out information, navigate their way, and fulfill these responsibilities will benefit less.

How Are We Responding to the Need to Participate More Fully in Our Care?

The measure most commonly used to assess patient engagement is the Patient Activation Measure, which focuses on respondents' confidence in fulfilling their clinical responsibilities for healthcare (Hibbard, Stockard, Mohaney, & Tusler, 2004). Judith Hibbard, who developed this measure, has repeatedly found that between one-quarter and one-third of respondents surveyed about their level of activation are confident that they know what to do, that they can safely act, and that their actions will make a difference to their health. The other two-thirds of respondents believe they can (or should) remain passive recipients of care, lack basic facts about their health or their recommended treatments, or, even if they have some knowledge, lack the confidence and skill to act on it (Hibbard & Cunningham, 2008).

Data from the 2007 Medicare Current Beneficiary Survey show that about only 30% of older people reported feeling confident that they possessed both the motivation and skills to engage fully in their healthcare (Williams & Heller, 2007). A 2010 assessment by the Center for Advancing Health of people's performance on a wide range of engagement behaviors found that for the vast majority of behaviors, one-third or fewer respondents reported performing them (Center for Advancing Health, 2010).

A variety of factors influences the likelihood that we are willing and able to perform these behaviors to improve and maintain our health. We vary in our ability to act on our own behalf. Those of us who are seriously ill or cognitively impaired find it difficult to coordinate our care among multiple clinicians (Bayliss, Edwards, Steiner, & Main, 2008; Noel et al., 2007). People with limited education or skills in health literacy and numeracy, for example, cannot understand the information on medication packages or the risk/benefit trade-offs of different treatment options (Katz, Jacobson, Veledar, & Kripalani, 2007; Shrank, Avorn, Rolon, & Shekelle, 2007). Low English-language proficiency and lack of familiarity with U.S. healthcare also impede the participation of some (Sudore et al., 2009). And a good number of us are fully engaged in our health using approaches outside the U.S. healthcare system: We seek treatment from alternative and religious healers and eschew the drugs and technologies of Western medicine (Institute of Medicine [IOM], 2005) until an emergency arises.

Characteristics of healthcare organizations and health professionals can also affect our participation in our care. Many of us find it daunting to ask questions or discuss our preferences with clinicians who cut us off or are unresponsive (Meguerditchian et al., 2012). Although we are urged to be good consumers of healthcare, we often find that the irrelevance (to many of us) of comparative quality information of facilities and doctors, the lack of price information, and the incomprehensible presentation of insurance benefit information renders futile any intentions we might have to shop around (Ginsberg & Glasmire, 2011).

In addition, we are on the receiving end of media warnings about alarming failures of U.S. healthcare. Messages about the number and seriousness of medical errors, the dangers of harmful tests, and frequency of overtreatment, fraud, and cost-shifting remind us that we must be vigilant, that we cannot rely on the safety of the care we receive or the trustworthiness of those who deliver it (Ornstein & Weber, 2011; Pear, 2012). We often experience these reports, whether accurate or exaggerated, as overwhelming additional burdens, especially when we are ill and anxious.

Clearly, we face many barriers to getting the greatest benefit from our healthcare. What can be done to orient care toward ensuring that all patients and families are able to act effectively on behalf of themselves or family members in order to achieve the best possible outcomes?

How Can Healthcare Be Organized to Support Patients' and Families' Active and Knowledgeable Participation in Our Care?

Some professional health stakeholders have awoken to our vital role in our healthcare by introducing and implementing new policies that tie payment for healthcare services to outcomes, such as:

- Pay-for-performance programs
- Shared savings via accountable care organizations
- Medicare payment policies to prevent rehospitalizations
- Use of patient experience of care surveys as part of reimbursement plans

Each of these policies reminds clinicians and institutions that they cannot be successful without our participation in our care, and in some cases this knowledge has prompted them to establish practices that support our efforts.

My recent experience as a patient reminded me that the cultural shift required to build a healthcare system that supports our engagement in our care means that the behavior of everyone—not just that of patients—must change. This will be highly disruptive for each of us. But I do not believe that there is an alternative, given the complexity and price/cost of care and what is at stake. If our participation is this critical to the results we all seek, patients and caregivers simply must be more actively and knowledgeably engaged in our care, whether we—or our clinicians—want this or not.

How will we accomplish this? It is outside the scope of my expertise to make specific recommendations about how to restructure healthcare to be patient- and family-centered. Generally, however, the implementation of some policies could expedite and institutionalize the shift:

- Regulators could specify the inclusion of patients and families in the governance of health systems, hospitals, clinics, and group practices.

- Public agencies that regulate professional licensure and organizations that certify specialists could require that clinicians demonstrate competence in communicating and sharing decisions.

- Medical, nursing, and allied health professional schools and teaching hospitals could recruit faculty who can model the new orientation and restructure curricula to prepare students to practice in collaboration with their patients.

- The trend of public and private payers' holding hospitals and systems accountable for specific outcomes could expand the number and types of outcomes that measure our participation in our care.

But such policies can have a positive impact only if they are accompanied by a focus on values. Based on interviews with fellow patients and family members, three principles emerged. If used to guide this transformation in care generally, these principles could contribute greatly to our ability to participate as fully as we are able in our personal care:

- **We need to know that it is *important* to participate on our care.** We will probably do better if we are engaged in our care and worse if we are not. Our clinicians can communicate directly the importance of our participation. They can seek our involvement in decisions about our care, discuss the risks and benefits of treatments (and no treatment), help us understand the stakes of our participation, and support us in our efforts to care for ourselves.

- **We need to believe that it is *possible* to participate in our care.** There are specific things we can do that make it more likely that we will recover with less difficulty. We need to know that it is within the abilities of people like us to perform these tasks successfully and improve our chances for a good outcome. Our clinicians can ensure that we possess the knowledge and skills to care for ourselves once we are home from the hospital stay or a clinic visit and that we have easy access to advice and guidance when we have doubts or questions.

- **We must be confident that it is *safe* for us to do these things.** We will not be given responsibilities that we cannot handle, given our age, resources, and cognitive and health status, and we will not be punished for asking questions. Our clinicians can work with us to develop treatment plans that we agree are feasible and then revisit those plans over time, allowing for modifications as our illness and life demands shift.

All of us, as patients, need to know that our knowledge and behavior have a significant influence on how much we benefit and how much we risk when we receive healthcare. Our families and close friends should also know how much their actions can benefit us and could decrease our risk of being harmed when we are unable to make our own decisions about the care we receive. We must be willing to make the effort and ask for help (and receive it) when we are unable to manage the responsibilities. And all of us who are willing should be able to do these things and not be hindered by, for example, lack of relevant, clear, and timely information or uncooperative clinicians and staff.

Conclusion

I am profoundly concerned about those who cannot or will not engage in their care; they will suffer unnecessarily. The current system has few safeguards to ensure that if we are unable to act on our own behalf, we will not be harmed.

I am, however, encouraged by the creativity and drive of so many of us who are taking on these new responsibilities as patients, parents, children, spouses, siblings, and friends. P&FCC has the potential to enable more of us to overcome the formidable barriers we face in working with our clinicians to plan our treatments and then, day after day, take the actions that could help us and the people we love live as well as we can for as long as we can.

References

Bayliss, E. A., Edwards, A. E., Steiner, J. F., & Main, D. S. (2008). Processes of care desired by elderly patients with multimorbidities. *Family Practice, 25*(4), 287-293. Retrieved from http://fampra.oxfordjournals.org/content/25/4/287.full

Center for Advancing Health (CFAH). (2010). Snapshot of people's engagement in their health care. Washington, D.C. Retrieved from http://www.cfah.org/engagement/research/snapshot

Fex, A., Ek, A. C., & Soderhamn, O. (2009). Self-care among persons using advanced medical technology at home. *Journal of Clinical Nursing, 18*(20), 2809-2817. Retrieved from http://www.ncbi.nlm.nih.gov/pubmed/19747254

Ginsberg, M., & Glasmire, K. (2011). *Consumers' priorities for hospital quality improvement and implications for public reporting.* Sacramento, CA: California Health Care Foundation. Retrieved from http://www.chcf.org/~/media/MEDIA%20LIBRARY%20Files/PDF/C/PDF%20ConsumerPrioritiesHospitalQIImplicationsPubReporting.pdf

Hibbard, J. H., & Cunningham, P. J. (2008). How engaged are consumers in their health and health care, and why does it matter? (HSC Research Brief No. 8). Washington, DC: Center for Studying Health System Change. Retrieved from http://www.hschange.com/CONTENT/1019/

Hibbard, J. H., Stockard, J., Mahoney, E. R., & Tusler, M. (2004). Development of the Patient Activation Measure (PAM): Conceptualizing and measuring activation in patient and consumers. *Health Services Research, 39*(4 Pt 1), 1005-1026. Retrieved from http://www.ncbi.nlm.nih.gov/pmc/articles/PMC1361049/

Institute of Medicine (IOM), Committee on the Use of Complementary and Alternative Medicine by the American Public. (2005). Prevalence, cost, and patterns of CAM use. *Complementary and alternative medicine in the United States.* Washington, DC: National Academies Press. Retrieved from http://www.ncbi.nlm.nih.gov/books/NBK83794/

Jamoom, E., Beatty, P., Bercovitz, A., Woodwell, D., Palso, K., & Rechtsteiner, E. (2012). Physician adoption of electronic health record systems: United States, 2011. (NCHS Data Brief No. 98). Hyattsville, MD: National Center for Health Statistics. Retrieved from http://www.cdc.gov/nchs/data/databriefs/db98.pdf

Katon, W., Von Korff, M., Lin, E., Walker, E., Simon, G. E., Bush, T., … Russo, J. (1995). Collaborative management to achieve treatment guidelines: Impact on depression in primary care. *Journal of the American Medical Association, 273*(13), 1026-1031. Retrieved from http://www.ncbi.nlm.nih.gov/pubmed/7897786

Katz, M. G., Jacobson, T. A., Veledar, E., & Kripalani, S. (2007). Patient literacy and question-asking behavior during the medical encounter: A mixed-methods analysis. *Journal of General Internal Medicine, 22*(6), 782-786. Retrieved from http://www.ncbi.nlm.nih.gov/pmc/articles/PMC2583801/

Kobin, A. B., & Sheth, N. U. (2011). Levels of adherence required for virologic suppression among newer antiretroviral medications. *Annals of Pharmacotherapy, 45*(3), 372-379. Retrieved from http://www.ncbi.nlm.nih.gov/pubmed/21386024

Lerret, S. M., & Weiss, M. E. (2011). How ready are they? Parents of pediatric solid organ transplant recipients and the transition from hospital to home following transplant. *Pediatric Transplantation, 15*(6), 606-616.

Lewis N. (2012, July). Remote patient monitoring market to double by 2016. *Information Week*. Retrieved from http://www.informationweek.com/healthcare/mobile-wireless/remote-patient-monitoring-market-to-doub/240004291

Madde, M., & Zickuhr, K. (2011). 65% of online adults use social networking sites: Women maintain their foothold on SNS use and older Americans are still coming aboard. Pew Research Center. Retrieved from http://pewinternet.org/~/media//Files/Reports/2011/PIP-SNS-Update-2011.pdf

Mayne, L., Girod, C., & Weltz, S. (2012). Healthcare costs for American families in 2012 exceed $20,000 for first time. Milliman Research Report. Retrieved from http://publications.milliman.com/periodicals/mmi/pdfs/milliman-medical-index-2012.pdf

Meguerditchian, A. N., Dauphinee, D., Girard, N., Eguale, T., Riedel, K., Jacques, A.,…Tamblyn, R. (2012). Do physician communication skills influence screening mammography utilization? *BMC Health Services Research, 12*, 219-226. Retrieved from http://www.ncbi.nlm.nih.gov/pubmed/22831648

National Center for Health Statistics (NCHS). (2012a). Health, United States, 2011: With special feature on socioeconomic status and health. Table 106, 341-343. Retrieved from http://www.cdc.gov/nchs/data/hus/hus11.pdf#listtables

National Center for Health Statistics (NCHS). (2012b). Health, United States, 2011: With special feature on socioeconomics and health. Tables 109, 110, 349-350. Retrieved from http://www.cdc.gov/nchs/data/hus/hus11.pdf#listtables

Noel, P. H., Parchman, M. L., Williams, J. W., Cornell, J. E., Shuko, L., Zeber J. E.,…Pugh, J. A. (2007). The challenges of multimorbidity from the patient perspective. *Journal of General Internal Medicine, 22*(Suppl 3), 419-424. Retrieved from http://www.ncbi.nlm.nih.gov/pmc/articles/PMC2150619/

Ornstein, C., & Weber, T. (2011, May). Doctors' groups welcome medical company dollars. *USA Today*. Retrieved from http://www.usatoday.com/money/industries/health/2011-05-05-medical-societies-sell-access-to-manufacturers_n.htm

Pear, R. (2012, January 6). Report finds most errors at hospitals go unreported. *The New York Times*. Retrieved from http://www.nytimes.com/2012/01/06/health/study-of-medicare-patients-finds-most-hospital-errors-unreported.html

Shrank, W., Avorn, J., Rolon, C., & Shekelle, P. (2007). Effect of content and format of prescription drug labels on readability, understanding, and medication use: A systematic review. *Annals of Pharmacotherapy, 41*(5), 783-801. Retrieved from http://www.ncbi.nlm.nih.gov/pubmed/17426075

Sudore, R. L., Landefeld, C. S., Pérez-Stable, E. J., Bibbins-Domingo, K., Williams, B. A., & Schillinger, D. (2009). Unraveling the relationship between literacy, language proficiency, and patient-physician communication. *Patient Education and Counseling, 75*(3), 398-402. Retrieved from http://www.ncbi.nlm.nih.gov/pubmed/19442478

Varma, N. (2009). Therapeutic implications of automatic home monitoring of implantable cardiac devices. *Current Treatment Options in Cardiovascular Medicine, 11*(5), 366-372. Retrieved from http://www.ncbi.nlm.nih.gov/pubmed/19846034

Williams, S. S., & Heller, A. (2007). Patient activation among Medicare beneficiaries: Segmentation to promote informed decision making. *International Journal of Pharmaceutical and Healthcare Marketing, 1*(3), 199-213. Retrieved from http://www.emeraldinsight.com/journals.htm?articleid=1623724&show=html

Chapter 4

Avoiding the Dark Sides of Patient- and Family-Centered Care

Carrie Brady, JD, MA

Patients often ask, "Shouldn't all healthcare be patient-centered? How could anyone argue with that?" Yet patients and families are often left out of decision-making in their own care and in organizational planning. Doing things to and for patients instead of in partnership is ineffective, as one hospital discovered when it decided to improve the physical environment by painting one wall of every patient room a bright color. After the painting was completed, the feedback from staff was very positive. The hospital was briefly pleased with the decision, until it realized that not only had it excluded patients and families from the decision-making process, but also it had fundamentally failed to consider the patient perspective. The hospital had painted the wall behind each patient's bed!

To the public, the need for patient-centered care (PCC) seems obvious and undeniable. Who can argue with putting the patient at the center of the healthcare team and building services that are designed to most effectively meet each patient's needs? The concept makes perfect sense but is often overlooked in practice, as the preceding painting vignette demonstrates. PCC is rooted in the ancient history of medicine, as you can see in this quote, perhaps apocryphal, which is often attributed to Hippocrates, "It is more important to know what sort of person has a disease than to know what sort of a disease a person has." More recently, the concept has been formally recognized as one of the pillars of a high-performing healthcare system (Institute of Medicine [IOM], 2001) and embedded in healthcare policy through incentives and penalties devised to foster it.

As with any concept, however, sometimes things get lost in the translation between an idea and its execution. In some hospitals, the essence of PCC has been misunderstood and replaced with a version that pits patients against providers. When it is misapplied, PCC can have the opposite effect of what is intended. Rather than building effective partnerships between patients and providers, it erodes them, breeding distrust, frustration, and, in some cases, outright hostility. These are the dark sides of PCC.

The purpose of this chapter is to help healthcare providers recognize when they are heading toward or have reached the "dark sides" and show them how to redirect their efforts in a manner that will achieve the many benefits of patient- and family-centered care (P&FCC). It is important to acknowledge these dark sides, because they are fairly ubiquitous in healthcare organizations. Fortunately, they can be avoided through careful attention to building and maintaining core foundations of patient-centered organizations, including leadership, patient and family partnerships, staff engagement, and effective data use for quality improvement (Balik, Conway, Zipperer, & Watson, 2011; Luxford, Safran, & Delbanco, 2011; Shaller, 2007). Because dark sides can erode any one of these foundations, this chapter describes common dark sides related to each of the four foundations as well as strategies to avoid them.

The Dark Sides of Leadership

Consider the following scenario:

> *Every meeting we heard the same thing from management: "Our HCAHPS scores are low; they need to get better. Let's tell all the nurses to implement scripted hourly rounding and pass out script cheat-sheet cards to nurses. That will fix our scores."*
>
> *So then we sprinkle some pixie dust and write a policy—and there's no improvement.*
>
> *Then we hear, "Hold them [the staff] accountable."*
>
> *We've changed our approach now. Staff engagement and ownership are fostered by education focusing on why and how. We brainstorm barriers and strategies to address the barriers. The nurses are the experts, and they design the improvement initiatives. We monitor and provide positive feedback. These are the keys to success. Pixie dust is not the answer.*

As you can see in the above scenario, patient-centered leaders set the tone for positive partnership. Patient-centered leaders:

- Lead by example
- Align priorities
- Communicate the why (not just the what and how)
- Remove roadblocks
- Inspire others

Good leaders realize that PCC is not easy; it requires careful planning and an allocation of resources. In many organizations, however, well-intentioned leaders unwittingly derail PCC by:

- Making commitments without planning
- Reinforcing misperceptions
- Not partnering with patients, families, or frontline staff

The first two leadership dark sides are discussed in this section of the chapter. Failure to partner is discussed in more detail in both "The Dark Sides of the Patient/Family Partnership" and "The Dark Sides of Staff Engagement" sections later in the chapter.

Making Patient-Centered Commitments Without Planning

PCC is a top priority for most healthcare leaders, but considerable gaps exist between intention and execution. In a 2013 survey of more than 1,000 hospital and health system leaders, 70% identified patient experience/satisfaction as a top priority for the next 3 years, even higher than quality and safety (63%) (The Beryl Institute, 2013). Although many leaders say their organizations are patient-centered, they could not tell you what that means in practice. Some take the approach that PCC is so obvious they do not need to invest resources in planning and execution, or they "struggle with integrating efforts to improve the patient experience into the strategic work of the hospital, treating these efforts instead as an array of good ideas" (Balik et al., 2011, p. 1).

Not surprisingly, the key drivers of patient-centered success depend on leadership (Balik et al., 2011). In fact, the results of 2013 Beryl survey identified "strong visible support 'from the top'" as the most important driver (The Beryl Institute, 2013, p. 21). Identified roadblocks include leaders' being pulled in too many directions and other organizational priorities that reduce the emphasis on patient experience. Twenty-six percent of the respondents identified "lack of sufficient budget or other necessary resources" as a significant barrier (The Beryl Institute, 2013, p. 21).

Organizations need to define what PCC means to them and how it relates to other organizational priorities, not relegate PCC to vague requests to staff to "be nicer to patients." Over the past 2 years, the percentage of healthcare organizations creating formal definitions, structures, and mandates to support PCC has grown, but more than half still lack a formal definition (The Beryl Institute, 2013). Personnel assigned to patient experience are often tasked with multiple responsibilities and so are not able to devote full time to patient experience, and they have few or no staff members to support them (The Beryl Institute, 2013).

Healthcare staff face a daily barrage of responsibilities, and healthcare leaders must make sense of these potentially competing priorities. Efforts to improve healthcare quality, for example, may paradoxically result in limiting and/or interrupting staff time with patients rather than increasing it (Disch & Sinioris, 2012). Patient experience efforts support other organizational goals, such as quality and safety, financial viability, and employee engagement, but most organizations do not connect the dots between these initiatives at a staff level. As one CEO notes, "Right now, there are so many goals—we need to strategize where we want to leverage ourselves. It gets embraced on the senior side, foggy in the middle—when it gets to the staff level, it's overwhelming" (Disch & Sinioris, 2012, p. 400). Professional education often also fails to reinforce patient and family partnership skills, although efforts are underway to more deeply embed patient- and family-centered care into medical education (Philibert, Patow, & Cichon, 2011).

Alignment Exercise

What is the highest priority in your organization? How is that priority set and reinforced? How does patient experience relate to that priority?

If you asked 10 staff members to identify the highest organizational priority, would you get the same answer? Does everyone in the organization understand the relationship between the highest priority and patient experience? How is that relationship described and reinforced?

Reinforcing Misperceptions

Although improving the patient experience has been linked to many positive clinical outcomes (Doyle, Lennox, & Bell, 2013), in many organizations the patient experience is still viewed as a "customer-service" initiative only, not a clinical initiative. If patient experience is positioned as customer service, clinicians are less likely to want to get involved, and yet their active involvement is essential to the success of any patient-centered initiative.

In the Beryl Institute survey, the existence of clinical managers who visibly support patient experience was the second-most-important driver of patient-centered success, and lack of physician involvement was one of the commonly cited barriers (The Beryl Institute, 2013). Leaders should focus on making linkages between PCC and patient safety and quality rather than creating silos. One way to do this is by creating structures that reinforce the connection, such as assigning primary responsibility for quality, safety, and patient experience to the same organizational department.

Leaders also should be careful not to emphasize nonclinical amenities, such as more cable TV channels (Adamy, 2012), as the key to improving the patient experience. A focus on amenities distracts from the relationship-building core tenets of PCC and can alienate clinicians who are interested in better care and outcomes, not luxury hospitalizations. As any organization that has built a new hospital or new department can attest, changing the environment and amenities does not automatically improve the patient experience if the same poor relationships among providers, patients/families, and ineffective or inefficient processes exist in the new space.

Finally, leaders should avoid "whack a mole"–like approaches to improving the patient experience. A "whack a mole" approach to improvement involves leadership chastising staff for poor Hospital Consumer Assessment of Healthcare Providers and Systems (HCAHPS) survey scores and ordering them to "get those scores up" without providing any information or support that would help staff achieve that objective. As in the earlier example, improvement does not happen by exhortation, command, or pixie dust. Leaders must provide staff with the education, resources, and time necessary to devote to patient experience improvement and respect the expertise of frontline staff.

Avoiding the Dark Sides of Leadership

Leaders are responsible for setting the course toward PCC, and leaders can help their organization's progress in many ways. Three key steps are:

- **Commit.** Leaders should remember the Pentagon's wisdom that "a vision without resources is a hallucination" (Kotkin, 2008, p. BU8). The concept of PCC may be easy to understand, but it is not simple to execute. Leaders should apply the same level of planning, time, and resources to PCC as they do to other key initiatives in the organization, such as budget formulation. PCC must be embedded at every level and in every activity of the organization (Balik et al., 2011). Frontline staff should be involved in every step of the process and given the training, skills, and tools to support their work. Some organizations, for example, provide quality-improvement training to all staff. Avoid the situation described by one nurse leader: "We constantly hold people accountable for things we haven't taught them to do." A few of the many tools designed to assist leaders in building successful patient-centered organizations are described in this chapter's section in the Resource appendix at the end of the book.

- **Connect the dots.** Leaders should set the appropriate context by explicitly making the connection between patient experience, quality, and safety and formally aligning patient experience with other organizational priorities (e.g., mission statement, strategic plan; Balik et al., 2011).

- **Engage patients, families, and all staff.** Leaders should explicitly commit to building partnerships and act on that commitment by regularly engaging patients and families at all levels, including in organizational governance (e.g., as board members; Johnson & Abraham, 2013). Leaders should consider the impact on the patient experience to be a key part of every organizational decision (Balik, 2011). Leaders should also set expectations for how staff treat each other and reinforce that PCC is the responsibility of all staff members, not a select few.

The Dark Sides of the Patient/Family Partnership

A patient presented to the emergency department with shingles and was admitted by a hospitalist. Due to her recent chemotherapy, the patient was placed on neutropenic precautions. Staff placed a large sign to that effect on the patient's door, along with a caddy of supplies. Despite the sign and ready access to supplies, many staff members entered the room without using gowns, gloves, or masks. During a call to the oncologist's office, the family expressed concern that the sign was not being followed. The oncology nurse told the patient's family, "It is your job to tell the staff they must use appropriate precautions. Physically block them at the door if you have to, but don't let them near the patient."

The Institute for Patient- and Family-Centered Care (IPFCC) defines P&FCC as "an approach to the planning, delivery, and evaluation of health care that is grounded in *mutually beneficial partnerships* among health care providers, patients, and families" (emphasis added; Johnson et al., 2008, p. vi). In some organizations, however, the concept of partnership has been distorted, as demonstrated by the example at the start of this section. At one extreme, healthcare providers say they are committed to PCC and work hard to do things to improve the patient experience, but they rarely directly involve patients and families in those efforts. Providers still do all the decision-making. At the other extreme, PCC is used as justification to give patients and families inappropriate levels of responsibility for their care. This section describes both extremes:

- Doing things to/for patients and families instead of in partnership
- Inappropriate transfer of responsibility

Doing Things to/for Patients and Families Instead of in Partnership

Most hospitals are working to improve the patient experience, but many are doing it in a way that misses the core concept. Instead of working *with* patients and families, these organizations are doing more things *to* or *for* their patients. No matter how wise, passionate, and committed healthcare providers are, they cannot achieve the same results on their own as they can by partnering with patients and families.

If you are a healthcare professional, you may be thinking that because you have been a patient before and your loved ones have probably been patients, you know what it is like to be a patient or family member. But if you work in healthcare, you have lost the ability to see the same way patients do, even though you may not realize it. As a simple demonstration of this point, please count the number of times the letter *f* appears in the following sentence:

> The foundation of patient and family engagement
> is full recognition of the power
> of patient and of family expertise.

Consider how confident you are that you can complete this simple task of counting letters. If you are with other people as you are reading this, please show the sentence to colleagues, friends, even children, and ask them to count the number of times the letter *f* appears. You may be surprised by the different answers to a seemingly simple question. (You can find the answer and explanation for this exercise in the sidebar at the end of this section.)

Improving the patient experience requires that healthcare providers invite others who can still see a situation with fresh eyes into the dialogue. The "experts" do not have all the answers. In fact, they are sometimes blinded by their expertise. To improve the patient and family experience, providers need to put patients and families on the team. The Institute for Healthcare Improvement (IHI) has identified putting patients and families on improvement teams as one of seven key leadership leverage points for improving healthcare, noting that "leaders often cite this change—putting patients in a position of real power and influence, using their wisdom and experience to redesign and improve care systems—as being the single most powerful transformational change in their history" (Reinertsen, Bisognano, & Pugh, 2008, p. 17).

The IHI, the IPFCC, and others have extensively documented the power of patient and family partnerships, yet many providers are still reluctant to directly engage patients and families as partners and advisors. Even patient-centered medical homes rarely put patients on quality-improvement teams (Han, Scholle, Morton, Bechtel, & Kessler, 2013), and the majority of hospitals reporting data to the Centers for Medicare & Medicaid Services (CMS) Partnership for Patients have not met the patient-engagement criteria for that program, which include active patient and family advisory committees or a former patient serving on a patient-safety or quality committee or team.

In the absence of such partnerships, providers not only miss enormous opportunities for improvement but also run the risk of investing huge sums of money and time only to find out that they were chasing the wrong goal. Administrators at one hospital reported, for example, that they had been working to improve physician communication with little success. After the hospital personnel began speaking with patients about their experiences, rather than just relying on survey data, they learned that patients were delighted with the inpatient communication; the source of the patients' frustration was the communication between the hospitalist and the primary care physician. If the hospital staff had not asked the patients, they would have continued to work on the inpatient communication, which was already working well.

Explanation of the *F* Exercise

There are eight occurrences of the letter f *in this sentence: "The foundation of patient and family engagement is full recognition of the power of patient and of family expertise."*

Many people will miss one or more of the fs *because when we learn to read, we begin to skip over words that are unimportant, like "of," and we blend double letters together. We also may overlook the* f *in "of" because it makes a v sound, not an f sound. We have built-in blinders based on the way we process information that we do not even realize we have.*

Healthcare is infinitely more complex than this sentence. To improve the patient experience, you need to engage people who can view it from a variety of perspectives, including patients and families, not just staff members who may share certain blinders by virtue of their training and/or experience.

Inappropriate Transfer of Responsibility

As the healthcare pendulum swings from a provider-centered model of care to a patient-centered model of care and roles are redefined, it is important not to let the pendulum swing so far that providers abdicate their responsibility. For example, an emergency department (ED) physician, presumably in an attempt to implement "shared decision-making," said to a patient who was being evaluated, "You can have a CT scan or not have a CT scan, do you want one?" without giving the patient any basis on which to make that decision.

Inappropriate shifts of responsibility are particularly troubling in the patient-safety arena (Entwistle, Mello, & Brennan, 2005). Many hospitals encourage patients or families to take action to improve safety, but these messages are often not well designed to achieve the desired result. For example, patients are given buttons to wear asking, "Have you washed your hands?" or they receive materials encouraging patients to ask all healthcare providers this question. Patients and families frequently are not involved in creating these messages and in many cases are not willing to act on the recommendations, in part because they are concerned about negative responses from providers (Maurer, Dardess, Carman, Frazier, & Smeeding, 2012). Family members report that they feel responsible for protecting their loved ones from healthcare harm and feel intense guilt if they are not successful (Delbanco & Bell, 2007).

Another inappropriate transfer of responsibility occurs when providers confuse patient engagement with compliance or adherence and "imply that patients are said to be engaged when they do what physicians, nurses… and others want them to do" (Sofaer & Schumann, 2013, p. 10). Some organizations abdicate their responsibility to patients by branding them as "noncompliant" without making any effort to engage them in developing shared care plans or to understand their perspectives and then blame their patients for poor outcomes.

It is equally important, however, that P&FCC is not interpreted as encouragement for staff to take on too much responsibility for patients, such as by becoming "like a member of the family." Maintaining therapeutic boundaries is important, and organizations should take care to develop programs to ensure that staff members are fostering independence of patients and families rather than promoting dependence (Barnsteiner & Gillis-Donovan, 1990).

Avoiding the Dark Sides of the Patient/Family Partnership

There are several ways that healthcare providers can build effective patient/family partnerships instead of misapplying the concept of PCC:

- **Recognize the expertise of patients and families.** Patients and families have expertise about themselves, their care, and the healthcare experience that is essential both to caring for individual patients and to building a better healthcare system. Healthcare professionals must recognize that they cannot get that expertise any other way than by directly engaging patients and families at every level.

- **Never engage in a patient-experience initiative that does not directly involve patients and families.** When undertaking any patient-experience initiative, always do it *with* patients and families, not just *for* them. There are many roles for patients and families (e.g., as advisors, faculty, or peer mentors; Johnson & Abraham, 2013). If patients and families are not already involved in an initiative underway in your organization, bring them into the initiative. Their participation will not only improve the effectiveness of the initiative but also help build a culture in which such partnerships are the norm rather than the exception.

- **Develop shared models of responsibility in conjunction with your patients and families.** To avoid inappropriate transfer of responsibility, engage patients and families directly in the development of guidelines for shared responsibility. Distinguish provider roles from patient roles and plan for a variety of patient roles, recognizing that patients' ability to engage will vary. The Center for Advancing Health, for example, encourages medical practices to develop a patient-clinician pact identifying respective responsibilities and provides a model pact (Gruman, Jeffress, Edgman-Levitan, Simmons, & Kormos, 2011b) as well as sample patient guides to orient patients to their healthcare practice (Gruman, et al., 2011a). Do not label patients "noncompliant" for failing to accept a provider recommendation; respect the patient's autonomy (Olson, 2013). Work to understand the patient and to develop a shared treatment plan through such techniques as shared decision-making and other communication competencies (*AHRQ Guide*, 2013; The Joint Commission, 2010).

The Dark Sides of Staff Engagement

During a hospital consultation, the first stop on the facility tour was the staff bathroom. It was an ordinary bathroom—one toilet, one sink, relatively small. I asked my nurse tour guide why that was the first stop and was told, "For years we didn't have a bathroom on the labor and delivery unit. We were told to use the bathroom on another unit, but it takes a few minutes to walk there. We provide 1:1 coverage for laboring moms. Rather than leave our patients, we used to dehydrate ourselves so we wouldn't need to go to the bathroom. We love having this bathroom."

Imagine if you were told that the only way to read this book was to do it in one sitting without taking a break to eat, drink, or use the restroom. No matter how good the content is, you probably would not enjoy it, might find it difficult to process the information you were reading, and likely would resent whoever was making you do it. Two of the common dark sides of staff engagement produce the same frustration:

- Dismissing staff needs
- Creating the expectation that the patient is always right

Dismissing Staff Needs

It is stunning how often organizations demand that staff be more attentive to patients' and families' needs while simultaneously becoming less attentive to the needs of their own staff. Staff is a healthcare organization's most important resource. Staff members will not be able to meet the needs of their patients if their own needs are not being met.

The preceding bathroom example may sound extreme, but it appears to be fairly typical. Even if staff members have access to a bathroom, they may not have time to use it. Or they may not take a break to eat. It is not difficult to understand compassion fatigue and burnout under these circumstances. Even the basic needs of staff on Maslow's hierarchy are not being met consistently, not to mention the more complex emotional needs.

In many cases, organizations roll out initiatives designed to improve the patient experience without including frontline staff in the planning or even considering the impact of the initiative on frontline staff. With so many things already on their to-do lists, staff members are naturally skeptical of any new initiatives that they may perceive as adding difficulty without meaningful benefit. This situation typically results in "arm wrestling," during which staff resists implementation and leadership intensifies efforts to force compliance. Arm wrestling is counterproductive; everyone is pushing as hard as possible, and no one wins.

A dramatic example of arm wrestling occurred in a hospital implementing hourly rounding. When staff did not consistently participate, administration tried unsuccessfully to find new ways to hold staff accountable and ultimately designed a function to force staff participation. Every hour a loud buzzer sounded in each patient's room, and the only way to turn it off was for the nurse to enter the patient's room and press the reset button. This guaranteed that the nurse was in the room every hour, but it was entirely counterproductive. The nursing staff was angry, and the patients could not figure out why periodically a loud alarm went off and an exasperated nurse would walk in, press the button, and leave. Patient care did not improve, and staff morale deteriorated. In arm-wrestling situations, it is easy for staff members to perceive PCC as anti-provider.

Frontline staff should always be involved in designing, implementing, and evaluating patient-centered initiatives. Not only do frontline staff members have the best perspective on what will work effectively to improve the patient experience, but also they often can simultaneously improve the staff experience. For example, while the Picker Institute was developing its Always Events initiative, we interviewed patients and hospital staff to identify what they thought should always happen for patients. Patients wanted to always know the name of their hospital physician.

When we spoke with nursing staff about this request, we discovered that the staff members did not know either. The nurses were very enthusiastic about developing a process to consistently identify the doctor responsible for the patient, because it would save them time calling multiple specialists to determine who had responsibility for a clinical decision.

Often, the things that are the most frustrating for patients are the same things that are frustrating for staff, so a solution designed by frontline staff will benefit everyone. A comparison of the Agency for Healthcare Research and Quality (AHRQ) patient-safety culture survey of staff and the HCAHPS survey of patients demonstrates some of the common sources of frustration for patients and staff, including teamwork and communication. Improving the staff experience as reflected in the culture survey will likely have a positive effect on the patient experience (Sorra, Khanna, Dyer, Mardon, & Famolaro, 2012).

Creating the Expectation That the Patient Is Always Right

Many hospitals communicate to staff that patients are always right and that staff must comply with every patient request or demand. Staff members know this is unrealistic. At times, some patients and family members are disruptive and/or abusive to staff members, ask for things that are unsafe, or engage in behaviors that interfere with other patients. Patients are not always right, and a patient-centered approach to care does not mean that whatever the patient says goes.

Failure to distinguish between reasonable and unreasonable requests and to support staff in challenging situations tends to result in staff's feeling abandoned and perceiving all patients/families as potentially unreasonable. For example, patients have the right to involve loved ones in their care, but that right is not unlimited. It would be unreasonable for a stable patient in a shared room to have five family members stay overnight.

> **NOTE**
>
> Staff members often lament that one isolated patient comment can adversely affect their performance review, even if most patients have given positive feedback. As one physician remarked, "I've had patients whose family members have been arrested in the emergency department for their violent behavior, but the patient still gets a survey." If one negative patient comment has the power to affect a staff member's evaluation months later, it is not surprising for providers to be somewhat hostile toward PCC.

Instead of communicating that PCC means that every patient or family member is right, patient-centered organizations explicitly acknowledge that is not true. One way in which they support their staff is by teaching communication techniques to assist in preventing or managing challenging situations. Patient-centered organizations also provide staff with backup processes, such as patient advocates whom they can turn to for support.

Avoiding the Dark Sides of Staff Engagement

To effectively engage staff in the patient experience, it is important to set the right expectations. Staff members need to know that the organization respects their expertise and will involve them in every step of designing and implementing patient-experience initiatives. Staff members also need to know that meeting their needs is a priority and that the organization will support them in situations where it is challenging to meet patient and family needs or difficult to maintain appropriate professional boundaries.

Healthcare providers can do a couple things to effectively engage staff in PCC:

- **Build better teams.** Many organizations choose to build their patient-experience initiatives by first strengthening teamwork among staff, implementing programs that emphasize teamwork throughout the organization to ensure that staff feel supported. When staff needs are being met, staff members are able to more effectively meet patient and family needs. Involve frontline staff in every aspect of patient-experience work from planning to execution and evaluation. Take staff concerns seriously and ensure that programs not only improve the patient experience but also are designed to improve the staff experience as well.

- **Plan for challenging situations.** Staff members who feel safe and secure in the organization will be better able to meet patient and family needs. Staff members need to know that if there is a difficult situation with a patient or family member, there is someone they can go to for help. Identify and/or develop organizational resources to address both staff and patient/family needs, such as social work, guest relations, and ethics consultants. Build staff communication skills, including de-escalation techniques, and provide ongoing coaching. Recognize that any change has the potential to be challenging for overwhelmed staff, even when there are clear benefits to staff. Ask staff members to share their concerns both before and after implementation, take the expressed concerns seriously, and work through solutions together. For example, the *AHRQ Guide to Patient and Family Engagement* includes a bedside shift report implementation handbook and training presentation, which identify and address common staff concerns and surface other concerns through role-playing practice and discussion.

The Dark Sides of Patient-Centered Data Use

"When I walk into the staff lounge at the beginning of my shift and see the new HCAHPS report posted with a sea of red, I know it's going to be a bad day. I'm working as hard as I can, and no one seems to appreciate my efforts. Am I doing anything right?"

In a data-driven industry, such as healthcare, it is not surprising that as attention to PCC has increased, many new metrics have been developed to measure it. The HCAHPS survey and other patient-experience survey tools are one method for patients to share their perspective on how well providers are meeting patient needs, but they may have unintended consequences, such as demotivating staff, as described in the scenario at the beginning of this section. Although these surveys are designed to amplify patient voices and channel them into quantitative data, the way the metrics are used can become a barrier to success in PCC if organizations either:

- Lose sight of the goal and chase scores; or
- Demoralize staff with the data.

Both of these barriers are discussed in the following sections.

Losing Sight of the Goal and Chasing Scores

HCAHPS is a performance metric and tool, but in many organizations, improving HCAHPS scores has become the key goal rather than improving patient care. Staff members do not want to chase numbers or "game" surveys—they want to provide better care. Many staff members react poorly when value-based purchasing or public reporting is emphasized as the reason for focusing upon HCAHPS performance. As one physician group told hospital administrators, "HCAHPS is a reimbursement initiative, not a patient-care initiative."

The goal of patient-experience initiatives always should be grounded in providing better patient care, not raising scores for reimbursement. The survey is merely a tool that can help achieve that goal. Patient experience should be integrated and aligned with other organizational goals, and the connection between patient experience, quality, and safety should be explicitly discussed.

Demoralizing Staff

With the advent of value-based purchasing, patient perceptions as reported on the HCAHPS survey have become increasingly important to hospitals' financial well-being. In an effort to improve HCAHPS scores, many hospitals bombard staff with "red" data signifying that the hospitals have not met their performance goals. Patient complaints or negative comments are emphasized, while compliments are largely ignored.

Dissemination of the data alone, without any accompanying improvement priorities or strategies, is counterproductive. A data report that shows only current performance compared to the benchmark is like asking staff to pole vault without giving them the pole. You have established that the organization is here (current performance) and you want scores to go higher (over the benchmark "bar"), but you have not provided any tools to facilitate improvement.

Like the nurse in the scenario at the beginning of this section, managers and staff who are constantly told that they are "failing" quickly become exhausted. Organizations that continually reinforce the message that patients do not appreciate staff or that use isolated nonrepresentative patient comments in performance reviews erode relationships rather than strengthen them. Staff members may begin to feel that their patients will never be satisfied, so why bother to try?

Avoiding the Dark Sides of Data Use and Performance Improvement

There are several additional steps that organizations can take to avoid the dark sides of patient-centered data use:

- **Emphasize and learn from the positive.** Staff members need to be reminded that they are making a difference in patients' lives. Consider implementing a compliment hotline. When presenting patient-experience data, include compliments and spotlight innovations and improvement. Analyze compliments to understand what makes a difference to patients and families. Identify high performers within your own organization (individuals or departments) and learn from them. One effective strategy is to have a staff member from a lower-performing unit trade places for a few hours with a staff member from a higher-performing unit and then have the two staff members meet to discuss the differences.

- **Never present data without strategies for improvement.** Staff members often note that data are presented as a failure rather than as an opportunity to work together to develop a better process. Data should be part of a robust performance-improvement system that supports teams in identifying, deploying, and evaluating strategies for improvement. Emphasize why patient experience is important to outcomes, not how it is connected to reimbursement.

- **Integrate other perspectives.** HCAHPS is only one way of measuring the patient experience. Hospitals have many other ways of getting feedback from patients, including important qualitative data gained from such activities as post-discharge phone calls, rounding, advisors, focus groups, and daily patient interactions. Staff perspectives are critically important as well. Frontline staff members have a much richer knowledge and understanding of patient care than any survey can provide. Patient-experience improvement efforts should be based on a synthesis of all this information.

- **Design better, more timely, reports.** Staff members do not have time to waste, so make sure that any data report shared with them is worthy of the time they spend reviewing it. Engage frontline staff members in designing reports that will be most useful to them. Ensure that all the data included are timely and relevant. It is incredibly frustrating for staff to get reports of incidents that occurred 6 months ago or to be asked to respond to last year's data.

Conclusion

A growing body of evidence validates that PCC is better care (Boulding, Glickman, Manary, Schulman, & Staelin, 2011; Doyle et al., 2013; Glickman et al., 2010; Isaac, Zaslavsky, Cleary, & Landon, 2010; Saman, Kavanagh, Johnson, & Lutfiyya, 2013). To achieve these benefits, organizations must pay careful attention to building solid foundations, including leadership, patient and family partnership, staff engagement, and effective use of data for quality improvement. Acknowledging the existence of the dark sides helps organizations avoid them and builds credibility with staff, who is well aware of their prevalence. Working together in respectful partnerships, organizations can develop systems and processes that provide mutual benefits for patients, families, and staff.

References

Adamy, J. (2012, October 12). U.S. ties hospital payments to making patients happy. *Wall Street Journal*, p. A1.

AHRQ Guide to Patient and Family Engagement in Hospital Quality and Safety. (2013, June). Agency for Healthcare Research and Quality, Rockville, MD. Retrieved at http://www.ahrq.gov/professionals/systems/hospital/engagingfamilies/index.html

Balik, B. (2011, July/August). Leaders' role in patient experience. *Healthcare Executive, 26*(4), 76-79. Available at http://www.ihi.org/resources/Pages/Publications/LeadersRoleinPatientExperience.aspx

Balik, B., Conway, J., Zipperer, L., & Watson, J. (2011). *Achieving an exceptional patient and family experience of inpatient hospital care.* IHI Innovation Series white paper. Cambridge, MA: Institute for Healthcare Improvement. Retrieved from http://www.ihi.org/resources/Pages/IHIWhitePapers/AchievingExceptionalPatientFamilyExperienceInpatientHospitalCareWhitePaper.aspx

Barnsteiner, J. H., & Gillis-Donovan, J. (1990). Being related and separate: A standard for therapeutic relationships. *Maternal Child Nursing, 15*(4), 223-228.

The Beryl Institute. (2013). *The state of patient experience in American hospitals 2013: Positive trends and opportunities for the future.* Retrieved from http://www.theberylinstitute.org/?page=PXBenchmarking2013

Boulding, W., Glickman, S. W., Manary, M. P., Schulman, K. A., & Staelin, R. (2011). Relationship between patient satisfaction with inpatient care and hospital readmission within 30 days, *American Journal of Managed Care, 17*(1), 41-48.

Delbanco, T., & Bell, S. K. (2007). Guilty, afraid, and alone: Struggling with medical error. *New England Journal of Medicine, 357*(17), 1682-1683.

Disch, J., & Sinioris, M. (2012). The quality burden. *Nursing Clinics of North America, 47*(3), 395-405.

Doyle, C., Lennox, L., & Bell, D. (2013). A systematic review of evidence on the links between patient experience and clinical safety and effectiveness. *BMJ Open, 3,* e001570. doi:10.1136/bmjopen-2012-001570

Entwistle, V. A., Mello, M. M., & Brennan, T. A. (2005). Advising patients about patient safety: Current initiatives risk shifting responsibility. *Joint Commission Journal on Quality and Patient Safety, 31*(9), 483-494.

Glickman, S. W., Boulding, W., Manary, M., Staelin, R., Roe, M. T., Wolosin, R. J., … Schulman, K. A. (2010). Patient satisfaction and its relationship with clinical quality and inpatient mortality in acute myocardial infarction. *Circulation: Cardiovascular Quality and Outcomes, 3*(2), 188-195. Retrieved from http://circoutcomes.ahajournals.org/content/3/2/188.long

Gruman, J., Jeffress, D., Edgman-Levitan, S., Simmons, L. H., & Kormos, W. A. (2011a). *Creating a patient guide for a clinic or medical practice.* Center for Advancing Health. Retrieved from http://www.cfah.org/file/CFAH_PACT_GUIDE_Medical_Practice_Clinic.pdf

Gruman, J., Jeffress, D., Edgman-Levitan, S., Simmons, L. H., & Kormos, W. A. (2011b). *Supporting patients' engagement in their health and health care.* Center for Advancing Health. Retrieved from http://www.cfah.org/file/CFAH_PACT_Special_Current-2011.pdf

Han, E., Scholle, S. H., Morton, S., Bechtel, C., & Kessler, R. (2013). Survey shows that fewer than a third of patient-centered medical home practices engage patients in quality improvement. *Health Affairs, 32*(2), 368-375.

Institute of Medicine (IOM). (2001). *Crossing the quality chasm: A new health system for the 21st century.* Retrieved from http://www.iom.edu/Reports/2001/Crossing-the-Quality-Chasm-A-New-Health-System-for-the-21st-Century.aspx

Isaac, T., Zaslavsky, A. M., Cleary, P. D., & Landon, B. E. (2010). The relationship between patients' perception of care and measures of hospital quality and safety. *Health Services Research, 45*(4), 4-10.

Johnson, B. H., & Abraham, M. R. (2013). *Partnering with patients, residents, and families: A resource for leaders of hospitals, ambulatory care settings, and long-term care communities.* Bethesda, MD: Institute for Patient- and Family-Centered Care.

Johnson, B., Abraham, M., Conway, J., Simmons, L., Edgman-Levitan, S., Sodomka, P.,…Ford, D. (2008). *Partnering with patients and families to design a patient- and family-centered health care system: Recommendations and promising practices.* Bethesda, MD: Institute for Patient- and Family-Centered Care in collaboration with the Institute for Healthcare Improvement. Available at http://www.ipfcc.org/pdf/PartneringwithPatientsandFamilies.pdf

The Joint Commission (TJC). (2010). *Advancing effective communication, cultural competence, and patient- and family-centered care: A roadmap for hospitals.* Oakbrook Terrace, IL: Author. Retrieved from http://www.jointcommission.org/assets/1/6/aroadmapforhospitalsfinalversion727.pdf

Kotkin, S. (2008, September 6). A call to action, for earth and profit. *The New York Times.* Retrieved from http://nytimes.com

Luxford, K., Safran, D. G., & Delbanco, T. (2011). Promoting patient-centered care: A qualitative study of facilitators and barriers in healthcare organizations with a reputation for improving the patient experience. *International Journal for Quality in Healthcare, 23*(5), 1-6. Retrieved from: http://pickerinstitute.org/wp-content/uploads/2011/06/Luxford-etal-Promoting-patient-centered-care-20111.pdf

Maurer, M., Dardess, P., Carman, K. L., Frazier, K., & Smeeding, L. (2012). *Guide to patient and family engagement: Environmental scan report.* (Prepared by American Institutes for Research under contract HHSA 290-200-600019.) AHRQ Publication No, 12-0042-EF. Rockville, MD: Agency for Healthcare Research and Quality. Retrieved from http://www.ahrq.gov/research/findings/final-reports/ptfamilyscan/index.html

Olson, D. P. (2013). Helping patients who don't help themselves. *American Journal of Nursing, 113*(7), 66-68.

Philibert, I., Patow, C., & Cichon, J. (2011). Incorporating patient- and family-centered care into resident education: Approaches, benefits, and challenges. *Journal of Graduate Medical Education, 3*(2), 272-278.

Reinertsen, J. L., Bisognano, M., & Pugh, M. D. (2008). *Seven leadership leverage points for organization-level improvement in health care (2nd ed.).* IHI Innovation Series white paper. Cambridge, MA: Institute for Healthcare Improvement. Retrieved from http://www.ihi.org/knowledge/Pages/IHIWhitePapers/SevenLeadershipLeveragePointsWhitePaper.aspx

Saman, D. M., Kavanagh, K. T., Johnson, B., & Lutfiyya, M. N. (2013). Can inpatient hospital experiences predict central-line bloodstream infections? *PLOS One, 8*(4), e61097. Retrieved from http://www.plosone.org/article/info%3Adoi%2F10.1371%2Fjournal.pone.0061097

Shaller, D. (2007). Patient-centered care: What does it take? Picker Institute. Retrieved from http://www.commonwealthfund.org/Publications/Fund-Reports/2007/Oct/Patient-Centered-Care--What-Does-It-Take.aspx

Sofaer, S., & Schumann, M. J. (2013). Fostering successful patient and family engagement: Nursing's critical role. *Nursing Alliance for Quality Care.* Retrieved from http://www.naqc.org/WhitePaper-PatientEngagement

Sorra, J., Khanna, K., Dyer, N., Mardon, R., & Famolaro, T. (2012), Exploring relationships between patient safety culture and patients' assessments of hospital care. *Journal of Patient Safety, 8*(3), 131-139.

Chapter 5

The "Difficult" Patient Reconceived

Autumn Fiester, PhD

Joanna is a 23-year-old patient with a history of substance abuse. Her drugs of choice are heroin, Oxy, and ethanol. A few weeks ago, she was injured in a car accident, and she is now paralyzed from the neck down. She has what she describes as a fairly constant level "10" pain in her neck and shoulder areas, and she complains of frequent headaches. The nursing staff observes that she does not sleep much. Because of excruciating pain, she cannot fully participate in her PT/OT sessions. She tells the nursing staff that the pain meds she is receiving do nothing for her pain despite the fact that many changes have been made. When nurses encourage her to get out of bed, she refuses.

She claims that the nurses in charge of her care believe she is a "liar" because she has a history of drug abuse. She overheard one of the physicians describe her as "drug seeking." She calls out to the nursing station, demanding pain meds an hour and a half before it is time for her next dose. The nurses and the physicians on her case have repeatedly explained why she cannot get her meds early. Joanna takes this out on the whole staff. She sits in the hallway crying and demanding the nurses provide her with immediate attention. Nurses are refusing to work with her because she is so difficult.

Like Joanna, many patients are considered "difficult" by their nurses and physicians. Although the figure for nurses is unknown, between 15% and 60% of treating physicians label their patients as "difficult" (Hahn, 2001; Hahn, Thompson, Wills, Tern, & Budner, 1994; Jackson & Kroenke, 1999). Given that nurses routinely spend significantly more time with patients than physicians do, it is reasonable to expect that the figures are at least comparable. Even at the lower end of those estimates, the implication is that a significant portion of nurse-patient and physician-patient relationships are fraught with conflict, negative feelings, and unsatisfying interactions, as in the case of Joanna.

There is no shortage of nursing and physician literature highlighting the harmful consequence of a dysfunctional treating relationship to both providers and patients (Koekkoek, Hutschemaekers, van Meijil, & Schene, 2011; Lin et al., 1999; Miksanek, 2008; Podrasky & Sexton, 1988; Sheldon, Barrett, & Ellington 2006; Smith & Hart 1994; Steinmetz & Tabenkin, 2001; Wasan, Wootton, & Jamison, 2005). So the moral imperative to resolve such conflicts is clear. But the remedy, of course, depends on the cause.

The conventional explanation for these conflicts lays the blame squarely at the feet of the patient, typically via mental disorders or maladaptive personality traits, and the specter of flawed moral character lurks as well. But the prevalence of the problem either serves as a psychological and moral indictment for up to 60% of our citizenry or suggests the possibility of a less pathological cause. In fact, the behaviors that saddle a patient with the label "difficult" can better be explained as responses to problematic interactions or negative experiences related to the delivery of healthcare. If there are grounds to reconceive the "difficult" patient as someone reacting to the perception of ill treatment in the healthcare setting—someone who feels morally wronged—then there is an ethical obligation to address this perception of harm.

Resolution of such conflicts currently lies solely in the dyad of provider and patient. But the ethical stakes place this species of conflict into the province of the Ethics Consultation Service (ECS). (Refer to Chapter 16 for further discussion of ECS.) As the resource for addressing ethical dilemmas that occur at the bedside or clinic, there is a moral mandate to offer assistance in the resolution of this pervasive type of ethically charged conflict that is no less pressing or consequential than the more familiar terrain of clinical ethics consultation.

This chapter explores the conventional ways of understanding why patients are deemed "difficult" by their treating team, an alternative explanation for challenging patient behaviors in the clinic, a myriad of approaches to diffuse difficult patient-nurse situations, and the corresponding ethical obligations we have to make patient-provider interactions function more productively.

The Conventional View of the "Difficult" Patient

Research on the "difficult" patient generally defines the problem exclusively from the provider's perspective, and this is true of both the nursing and physician literature (Gerrard & Riddell, 1988; Haas, Leiser, Magill, & Sanyer, 2005; Kahn, 2009; Lin et al., 1991; Miksanek, 2008; Podrasky & Sexton, 1988; Smith & Hart, 1994; Steinmetz & Tabenkin, 2001; Wilkinson, 1991). On the physician side of the equation, "difficult" patients are typically described as "those who raise negative feelings within the clinician," presumably due to behaviors deemed "inappropriate" in a treatment setting (Wasan et al., 2005, p. 185). On the nursing side of the issue, "difficult" patients are those patients who challenge nurses' control of patient care (Sheldon, et al., 2006; Smith & Hart, 1994). The nurses' and physicians' experiences of frustration, anxiety, guilt, or dislike in interactions with the patient frame the research that explores the causal explanation of the dysfunctional dynamic.

The causal mechanisms that produce the "difficult" patient are largely unaddressed in the nursing literature. But the conclusion that most studies in the healthcare literature reach is that a set of patient-centered problems or flaws accounts for the inappropriate behavior. The most commonly attributed cause of the "difficult" patient is the presence of a psychiatric disorder. Concludes one study, "The difficult or frustrating patient… often has unrecognized psychiatric problems" (Haas et al., 2005, p. 2065). Others concur (Hahn et al., 1996; Lin et al., 1991). The candidates for such psychiatric diagnoses range from depression and anxiety to "comorbid psychopathology, hostility, suicidality, aberrant drug behavior, and chronic noncompliance" (Wasan et al., 2005, p. 186).

What seems to go unnoticed in these physician-centered studies is that some of what is couched as mental illness falls well inside the range of "normal" for individuals faced with significant life-stressors, such as illness or the perception of ill treatment. Hostility, anger, depression, anxiety, and even noncompliance are common reactions to difficult circumstances, even among the psychologically healthy and typically well adjusted. Even if we grant that *some* patients who exhibit behaviors that get them labeled "difficult" have diagnosable psychiatric disorders, there will be others who exhibit these same behaviors who do not. Although there may be a correlation in some patients of psychiatric diagnosis and "difficult" behaviors, this does not demonstrate causation. In fact, even among those patients who have *both* a psychiatric diagnosis *and* are perceived as "difficult," it is not clear that the patient's psychiatric condition *causes* negative behaviors.

A closer look at one of the studies that confidently claims that "significant psychopathologic disorders" (Hahn, 2001, p. 898) is the root cause of the "difficult" patient reveals how spurious that conclusion really is. Hahn's own study finds two other significant factors that correlate strongly with physician-perceptions of "'hateful,' 'heartsink,' 'problem,' or 'difficult' patients" (2001, p. 899):

- First, 90% of the patients described as "difficult" were found to have an "abrasive personality style" (Hahn, 2001, p. 899), which is practically a tautological conclusion. The meek and mild would not be forceful enough to earn the title "difficult," so it is definitionally true that temperament plays a large role in landing a patient in this category.

- Second, the most significant predictor of being labeled "difficult"—and one that could not be explained away by association with psychopathology—was having multiple symptoms, five in particular: "stomach pain, fainting, sleep problems, loose stools/diarrhea, and palpitations" (Hahn, 2001, p. 900).

Physicians reported these patients as being both "time consuming" and "manipulative," and they garnered high levels of physician frustration. Although there is little data in the nursing literature about the precise behaviors associated with being labeled "difficult" by the nursing staff, we could easily surmise that parallel behaviors to those listed above would generate significant frustrations for nurses: frequent use of the call light, constant demands, abusive language, disruption of other patients, and so forth.

Although Hahn takes great pains to convince the reader that patients with psychopathologies have a predilection for psychosomatic complaints and that somatoform disorders might thus account for the correlation between "difficult" and "multiple symptoms," he admits that physicians are "frustrated by the symptoms' 'vagueness' and their own inability to make a diagnosis" (2001, p. 900). In other words, physicians may label a patient "difficult" because of their own inability to effectively diagnose or treat the problem, or because of a patient's reaction to this failure. There are similar findings in the nursing literature (Podrasky & Sexton, 1988; Smith & Hart, 1994).

All told, then, the foregoing explanations for the "difficult" patient are partial at best and specious at worst.

The "Difficult" Patient Reconceived

The studies designed to detect the causes of the problematic patient expend almost no attention defining the set of patient behaviors that provokes the label "difficult." Although one author defends this lack of precision by claiming that it is "intuitively understood" (Hahn, 2001, p. 898), it turns out that there is a wide range of behaviors falling under this rubric in the literature, many of which do not even seem inappropriate, let alone pathological. In the laundry list of one study, the "difficult" patient includes "patients who make repeated visits without apparent medical benefit, patients who do not seem to want to get well, patients who engage in power struggles, and patients who focus on issues seemingly unrelated to medical care" (Haas et al., 2005, p. 2066).

In contrast to this relatively benign list, a different study identifies the set as: "[i]nvalidating, demanding, disruptive, attention-seeking, annoying, and manipulative behavior" (Knesper, 2007, p. 247). To make the case that we need to reconceive the "difficult" patient, I want to focus on the worst of what might invite this label—namely, behaviors that include:

- Raising one's voice or shouting
- Using foul language
- Making accusatory remarks or insulting comments
- Using racial or ethnic slurs
- Using sexist, homophobic, racist, or anti-Semitic epithets

If these incontrovertibly inappropriate behaviors lend themselves to a more compelling explanation than patient pathology, then the arguably more benign set surely will. To make the argument, then, that we have misdiagnosed the underlying cause of the "difficult" patient, let's look at the following case of Fred:

> Fred is a 17-year-old man with an incomplete C-4 injury to his spinal cord as the result of a gunshot wound. He is currently unable to move his arms or legs, although he does have sensation in his lower extremities. Before his injury, Fred attended school intermittently and was on probation for heroin possession. Fred was admitted to an inpatient rehabilitation unit after 2 weeks in acute care. His mother is unable to visit during the week because of her work schedule, and the patient's only other living relative is an elderly grandmother who is homebound.

> *Since he has come to the rehab hospital, Fred has been verbally abusive to the nursing staff, frequently using racial slurs. His cursing, often loud, distresses the other patients as well as the nurses. Fred often complains of pain and screams loudly when moved, although the clinical team members insist he is on the highest dose of narcotics that they feel comfortable prescribing. Because of Fred's language and derogatory comments, the nursing staff members have requested he be transferred to another unit, saying they should not have to put up with his treatment of them.*

Fred is most certainly difficult.

What makes Fred an ideal patient to discuss in this context is that he obviously has an "abrasive personality style"; indisputably has multiple symptoms, some of which are being presumed to be exaggerated or imagined; and likely has at least one psychiatric diagnosis. And yet…we could put ourselves in Fred's shoes and envision myriad interactions that he might experience on a daily basis at this rehab hospital that would seriously test our equanimity and self-possession, although we may have none of the hypothesized causes for being difficult. Consider the treatment, situations, and dynamics that would provoke anyone's ire as a patient:

- How often has Fred felt patronized, dismissed, demeaned, or humiliated?
- How many needless indignities has he been subjected to?
- Does he feel powerless and emasculated, and, if so, from the injury or the treatment they are giving for it?
- Does he feel heard, validated, and respected?
- Does he believe that staff members are treating him as well as they treat all other patients, or does he sincerely believe that their view of him is prejudiced by his past truancy and heroin use?
- Does he feel victim to being branded "drug-seeking," "gang member," "high school dropout," or "junkie"?
- Does he believe that the clinical team members really care about him? Do they?

The key to Fred's escalating bad behavior lies in the answers to the question: Does Fred feel mistreated or wronged? Persons who feel indignation, resentment, or offense are susceptible to manifesting their moral grievance in counterproductive ways. Only the most self-controlled consistently work through moral offense by calm, rational, productive means. Fred's behavior should be first and foremost understood as a reaction to a therapeutic situation that is malfunctioning for him, failing to meet his needs and perhaps undermining his sense of self and self-esteem.

But you might object: Which came first, his bad behavior or his perception that he is being treated badly? Let's assume that he treated the nursing staff badly from the moment of his intake, motivated not by a loss of faith in the medical establishment from his stay at the acute-care hospital but sourced solely in the horrific situation he finds himself in. He was merely angry at fate, God, the person who shot him, his family—who knows?—but there was no culpability on the part of any clinical provider. Let's grant all of that. Consider the following:

- What reactions did Fred get at the rehab hospital to his understandable anger and frustration?
- What stereotypes or biases lie underneath the attitudes or perceptions of his current caregivers?
- What sources of support did they offer him?
- How did they reassure him that his mental, spiritual, emotional, and physical well-being would be safeguarded with them?

Lending credence to this reconceived view of the "difficult" patient is an older nursing study that looked at the perspectives of patients that clinical teams deemed "difficult." The study participants claimed that if they were given more respect and decision-making power, their potent feelings of anger would be significantly reduced (Breeze & Repper, 1998). Another physician-based study found that causal explanations for the behavior of the "difficult" patient differed markedly between physician and patient (Lin et al., 1991). Tellingly, physicians who scored lower on scales measuring empathy were more likely to perceive their patients as "difficult" than those who scored higher (Jackson & Kroenke, 1999). The moral of this study, then, is that the behaviors patients are exhibiting are less objectively "difficult" and more vulnerable to the "eye of the beholder" problem that may overstate or exacerbate those negative behaviors.

The conventional view that locates the source of patient-provider conflict in the patient's mental or physical pathologies is not only weak as an explanatory model but also ethically irresponsible for the way it undermines our resolve to explore more nuanced causal dynamics and redress them. The reconceived view of the "difficult" patient calls for that exact reexamination, viewing the fractured patient-provider relationship not only as amendable to repair but as demanding that level of moral attention.

Ethical Obligations to the "Difficult" Patient

Reframing the "difficult" patients as people who perceive themselves as wronged in the healthcare encounter—perceive being treated unfairly, disrespectfully, dismissively, condescendingly, or offensively—generates an ethical duty to address, validate, repair, or assist in making amends. And those obligations to assist are binding, whether the ethical harm is perceived or real. In other words, whether there is any true culpability on either side misses the point; if my behavior toward you is reactive, the solution for altering it is for me to change my perceptions.

Take as an example: If a patient's perceptions shift from feeling dismissed to feeling validated, the original intentions, dynamics, or actions on the part of the provider are irrelevant. The nurse may have had the very best of intentions, and the perception of the nurse's being dismissive could have been pure misunderstanding. But what matters in resolving "difficult" behavior is that a new understanding of mutual respect has been forged, and that new understanding will translate into transformed conduct on the part of the patient.

Lest this analysis itself seem condescending to the "difficult" patient, consider the case of Susan:

> Susan is the mother of an 8-year-old daughter, Emily, who has come to a children's hos-
> pital for a possible fracture of a growth plate in her ankle. Emily's injury is a week old,
> but it took that long to get an appointment with the pediatric orthopedic surgeon, and
> she could not be treated by her general pediatrician. Emily has been in significant pain
> all week. Susan and Emily arrive on time for their 1:00 appointment, where they are
> shown into a small, sparse exam room with no toys or books. After an hour of waiting,
> Susan goes to speak with an unfriendly receptionist, who tells her she has no idea how
> much longer it will be. Another hour goes by, and Emily is in pain, bored, cranky, and
> hungry. When the nurse practitioner (NP) finally arrives at 3:30, she is brusque, offers
> no apology for the extensive wait, and starts to complain that her busy day has allowed
> her time to eat only two energy bars. Susan begins to yell loudly at the NP.

Susan's case is instructive because there is clear culpability on the care delivery side. At the very least, there is a systems-level problem in both appointment scheduling and adequate infrastructure for pediatric patients, but also the NP seems to bear some responsibility for Susan's outburst by her failure to acknowledge the institutional issues, her brusque bedside manner, and the mention of her own needs before addressing Emily's. Susan has compelling grounds for taking offense; this is no mere misunderstanding. But the approach to remedying Susan's negative reaction—that is, the means to resolve or alter her "difficult" behavior—does not differ or depend on the moral fact pattern of the case. She is offended and feels wronged on behalf of her daughter, and when she believes that her concerns have been heard, validated, and addressed, she will surely stop yelling.

The moral salve needed in such cases is the basic set of conflict resolution techniques, and this is not lost on the authors of research about the "difficult" patient. One author after another advises an approach to resolving the problems in the doctor-patient relationship through a process either implicitly or explicitly identified as mediation and negotiation. For example, one nursing study is tellingly titled "Nurses and 'Difficult' Patients: Negotiating Noncompliance" (Russell, Daly, Hughes, & Hoog, 2003).

Similarly, in the piece "My Favorite Tips for Engaging the Difficult Patient on Consultation-Liaison Psychiatry Services," the author is quite upfront about borrowing his solutions from the Harvard Negotiation Project (Knesper, 2007). Knesper suggests, first, a strategy of mediation and finding "the third story," a key concept from a well-known book by Harvard Negotiation Project instructors of developing a version of the events that both disputing parties can agree on (Stone, Patton, & Heen, 1999, p. 4); and, second, a process of "negotiating, concession making, and control sharing" (Knesper, 2007, p. 250), a classic next step in the mediation method.

In a *New England Journal of Medicine* piece on dealing with the "difficult" patient, the author advocates gleaning insights from conflict-resolution methodology, for example arguing, "Successful negotiation begins with some basic understanding of the other side's position" (Kahn, 2009, p. 443). Others writing on the "difficult" patient allude to mediation methods, although not by name (Bellet, 1994; Haas et al., 2005), and one author generates a didactic mnemonic that could have been plucked straight from classic negotiation texts (see sidebar).

Five *As* for Dealing With Hostile Patients

1. ***Acknowledge*** *the problem.*

2. ***Allow*** *the patient to vent uninterrupted in a private place.*

3. ***Agree*** *on what the problem is.*

4. ***Affirm*** *what can be done.*

5. ***Assure*** *follow-through.*

Source: Wasan, 2005

The recommendations and guidance these authors offer are intended for the nurses or physicians directly involved in conflicts with their patients. They are meant to help the providers cope more effectively with patients they view as "'hateful,' 'heartsink,' 'problem,' or 'difficult'" (Hahn, 2001, p. 898). But although a mediation skill set is very handy to have and may indeed forestall problems or even rectify a provider-patient relationship gone bad, it is asking a lot of a stakeholder in a conflict to also be that conflict's mediator.

In fact, although the authors cited here accurately represent the relevant mediation techniques, they fail to grasp one of the fundamental principles of mediation: It is a process conducted by a neutral third party. Physicians or nurses embroiled in a provider-patient conflict are dealing with negative feelings of anger, frustration, anxiety, or guilt—after all, the definition of the "difficult" patient is someone who engenders those very feelings. Providers in these conflicts are partisans, and as such, it is not easy for them to bracket those negative feelings in order to conduct a conversation that is impartial or lacks an intrinsic bias. If they can, they deserve a great deal of credit.

But having that ability or skill set in such situations should not be an expectation. Think about Knesper's suggestion of creating a "third story." As the Harvard Negotiation Project authors write, "The Third Story is one an impartial observer, such as a mediator, would tell; it's a version of events both sides can agree on" (Stone et al., 1999, p. 4). Anything short of being able to generate that third story undercuts the usefulness and value of what a mediation process could bring to these conflicts. Nurses and physicians not able to achieve that in a conflictual interaction with a patient need a resource external to the dyad of provider and patient.

The "Difficult" Patient and the Role of the Ethics Consultation Service

The institution in American healthcare charged with both addressing ethics-infused conflicts and possessing the skill set to mediate them is the Ethics Consultation Service (ECS). Required by The Joint Commission (TJC), each hospital must have "a process that allows staff, patients, and families to address ethical issues" (TJC, 2011), and most institutions operationalize this through an ethics committee and/or clinical ethicist. It is the ECS that should provide the resource for resolving the ethically charged conflicts between "difficult" patients and their clinical teams that have not been able to be successfully managed within those relationships.

That this species of conflict legitimately falls within the sphere of the ECS can be clearly seen in the self-described mission of those ethics bodies. In a highly regarded national study of ECSs, participants were asked about the primary goals of their ethics consultation service (Fox, Myers, & Pearlman, 2007). Assisting in the repair of the relationships between patients deemed "difficult" and the providers reluctant to continue working with them meets many of the most frequently cited goals of ECSs in that study (Fox et al., 2007):

- 77% of ECSs viewed their charge as "resolving real or imagined conflicts"
- 75% as "changing patient care to improve quality"
- 68% as "increasing patient/family satisfaction"
- 50% as "meeting a perceived need of the staff"

Not only does addressing these conflicts fit well within those explicit goals, I am arguing the stronger point that ECSs actually shirk their duty by failing to recognize this obligation as being part of their self-identified mandate. Without a serious response to the real or imagined ethical offenses and injuries involved in these conflicts, patient care will necessarily remain substandard in the patients' perspective; therefore, they could not possibly feel satisfied with the care they have received. Correspondingly, staff needs will also go unmet.

If it is granted that conflicts involving the "difficult" patient fall under the purview of the ECS, do ECSs possess the skill set to navigate them? There are two separate issues embedded in this important question:

- What skills should an ECS have?
- What skills do most ECSs actually possess?

Taking the latter question first, it is well known that ECSs in general have little training (Fox et al., 2007), and a task force created by the national bioethics organization—the American Society of Bioethics and Humanities (ASBH)—was formed to address this pervasive problem (Clinical Ethics Consultation Affairs Committee, 2010). Although this may appear as a glib dodge to a very worrisome problem, my answer to the second question is that ECSs are currently no less qualified to navigate this type of ethics conflict than any other.

The former question—what skills *should* an ECS have?—has a more straightforward answer, and these skills make them the ideal body to resolve conflicts between patients labeled "difficult" and the providers they work with. Universally, the various task forces charged with determining this key skill set deem mediation techniques—from facilitation to other modes of conflict resolution—as essential process skills. For example, the National Working Group for the Clinical Ethics Credentialing Project lays out the "Fundamental Elements of Clinical Ethics Consultation," writing:

> Clinical ethics consultation is an intervention in which a trained clinical ethics professional:...employs expert discussion of bioethical principles, practices, and norms and uses reason, facilitation, negotiation, or mediation to seek a common judgment regarding a plan of care going forward. (Dubler et al., 2009, p. 25)

Similarly, ASBH recently revisited, and largely reaffirmed, its earlier report (Aulisio, Arnold, & Youngner, 2000) on the necessary qualifications of ECSs, what are known as the "Core Competencies" (ASBH, 2011). Its members write, "We believe an ethics facilitation approach is most appropriate for HCEC [healthcare ethics consultation]," and they list, as an indispensable skill of facilitation, the ability to "apply mediation or other conflict resolution techniques" (ASBH, 2011, p. 10–11). Further clarifying, they write:

> Bioethics mediation is a well-tested conflict resolution technique. It combines the clinical substance and perspective of clinical ethics consultation with the tools of the mediation process, using the techniques of mediation and dispute resolution to promote a principled resolution, compatible with the principles of bioethics and the legal rights of patients and families. (Dubler & Liebman, 2011, cited in ASBH, 2011, p. 11)

Others have made similar arguments on the essential role mediation plays in resolving clinical ethics disputes (Caplan & Bergman, 2007; Dubler & Liebman, 2011; Fiester 2007a; Fiester, 2007b; Fiester, 2011).

Conclusion

If adequately trained in the compulsory competencies outlined by various clinical ethics working groups, the ECS is the ideal resource to provide assistance in mediating these ethics-related conflicts when they have proven intractable to the efforts of the treating providers. This work is not only commensurate with the mission and function of the ECS, but the resolution of these conflicts is universally recognized as requiring a very particular skill set that is rare among clinical providers and obligatory for members of ECSs.

Although the "difficult" patient and the dysfunctional patient-nurse or patient-doctor relationship that is its sequela are currently not explicitly named as cause for calling an ethics consult, this problematic dynamic likely undergirds the vast majority of the consults requested. Explicitly identifying this type of conflict as a legitimate reason for prompting a consult would enable caregivers to initiate the resources of the ECS early in the conflict, before it has irreparable consequences for the patient-provider relationship or a detrimental impact on provider morale. We need to expand the moral mandate of the ECS to include addressing the conflicts between the "difficult" patient and the nurses and physicians who treat them.

References

American Society for Bioethics and Humanities (ASBH). (2011). *Core competencies for healthcare ethics consultation* (2nd ed.). Glenview, IL: Author.

Aulisio, M. P., Arnold, R. M., & Youngner, S. J. (2000). Health care ethics consultation: Nature, goals, and competencies. [A position paper from the Society for Health and Human Values-Society for Bioethics Consultation Task Force on Standards for Bioethics Consultation.] *Annals of Internal Medicine, 133*(1), 59-69.

Bellet, P. (1994). How should physicians approach the problems of their patients? *Pediatrics, 94*(6), 928-931.

Breeze, J. A., & Repper, J. (1998). Struggling for control: The care of experiences of "difficult" patients in mental health services. *Journal of Advanced Nursing, 28*(6), 1301-1311.

Caplan, A., & Bergman, E. (2007). Beyond Schiavo. *Journal of Clinical Ethics, 18*(4), 340-345.

Clinical Ethics Consultation Affairs Committee. (2010). *Certification, accreditation, and credentializing of clinical ethics consultants.* CECA report to the Board of Directors, ASBH. Retrieved from http://www.asbh.org/uploads/files/ceca%20c-a%20report%20101210.pdf

Dubler, N. N., & Liebman, C. (2011). *Bioethics mediation: A guide to shaping shared solutions.* Nashville, TN: Vanderbilt University Press.

Dubler, N. N., Webber, M. P., Swiderski, D. M., & the Faculty and the National Working Group for the Clinical Ethics Credentialing Project. (2009). Charting the future. *Hastings Center Report, 39*(6), 23-33.

Fiester, A. (2007a). The failure of the consult model: Why "mediation" should replace "consultation." *American Journal of Bioethics, 7*(2), 31-32.

Fiester, A. (2007b). Mediation and moral aporia. *Journal of Clinical Ethics, 18*(4), 355-356.

Fiester, A. (2011). Ill-placed democracy: Ethics consultations and the moral status of voting. *Journal of Clinical Ethics, 22*(4), 23-32.

Fox, E., Myers, S., & Pearlman, R. A. (2007). Ethics consultation in United States hospitals: A national survey. *American Journal of Bioethics, 7*(2), 13-25.

Gerrard, T. J., & Riddell, J. D. (1988). Difficult patients: Black holes and secrets. *British Medical Journal, 297*(6647), 530-532.

Haas, L., Leiser, J., Magill, M., & Sanyer, O. (2005). Management of the difficult patient. *American Family Physician, 72*(10), 2063-2068.

Hahn, S. (2001). Physical symptoms and physician-experienced difficulty in the physician-patient relationship. *Annals of Internal Medicine, 134*(9 Pt 2), 897-904.

Hahn, S. R., Kroenke, K., Spitzer, R. L., Brody, D., Williams, J. B., Linzer, M., & Verloin deGruy III, F. (1996). The difficult patient: Prevalence, psychopathology, and functional impairment. *Journal of General Internal Medicine, 11*(1), 1-8.

Hahn, S. R., Thompson, K. S., Wills, T. A., Tern, V., & Budner, N. S. (1994). The difficult doctor-patient relationship: Somatization, personality and psychopathology. *Journal of Clinical Epidemiology, 47*(6), 647-657.

Jackson, J. L., & Kroenke, K. (1999). Difficult patient encounters in the ambulatory clinic: Clinical predictors and outcomes. *Archives of Internal Medicine, 159*(10), 1069-1075.

The Joint Commission (TJC). (2011). *The comprehensive accreditation manual for hospitals (CAMH) and homecare (CAMH).* Oakbrook, IL: Author.

Kahn, M. (2009). What would Osler do? Learning from "difficult" patients. *New England Journal of Medicine, 361*(5), 442-443.

Knesper, D. (2007). My favorite tips for engaging the difficult patient on consultation-liaison psychiatry services. *Psychiatric Clinics of North America, 30*(2), 245-252.

Koekkoek, B., Hutschemaekers, G., van Meijel, B., & Schene, A. (2011). How do patients come to be seen as "difficult"? A mixed-methods study in community mental health care. *Social Science and Medicine, 72*(4), 504-512.

Lin, E. H., Katon, W., Von Korff, M., Bush, T., Lipscom, P., & Russo, J. (1991). Frustrating patients: Physician and patient perspectives among distressed high users of medical services. *Journal of General Internal Medicine, 6*(3), 241-246.

Miksanek, T. (2008). On caring for "difficult" patients. *Health Affairs, 27*(5), 1422-1428.

Podrasky, D., & Sexton, D. (1988). Nurses' reactions to difficult patients. *Journal of Nursing Scholarship, 20*(1), 16-21.

Russell, S., Daly, J., Hughes, E., & Hoog, C. O. (2003). Nurses and "difficult" patients: Negotiating noncompliance. *Journal of Advanced Nursing, 43*(3), 281-287.

Sheldon, L., Barrett, K., & Ellington, L. (2006). Difficult communication in nursing. *Journal of Nursing Scholarship, 38*(2), 141-147.

Smith, M. E., & Hart, G. (1994). Nurses' responses to patient anger: From disconnecting to connecting. *Journal of Advanced Nursing, 20*(4), 643-651.

Steinmetz, D., & Tabenkin, H. (2001). The "difficult patient" as perceived by family physicians. *Family Practice, 18*(5), 495-500.

Stone, D., Patton, B., & Heen, S. (1999). *Difficult conversations: How to discuss what matters most.* New York: Penguin Books.

Wasan, A. D., Wootton, J., & Jamison, R. N. (2005). Dealing with difficult patients in your pain practice. *Regional Anesthesia and Pain Medicine, 30*(2), 184-192.

Wilkinson, S. (1991). Factors which influence how nurses communicate with cancer patients. *Journal of Advanced Nursing, 16*(6), 677-688.

Chapter 6

A Global View of Person- and Family-Centered Care

Joanne Disch, PhD, RN, FAAN

Jehad Z. Adwan, PhD, RN

Mr. Elmasri, 75 years old, is being treated at a surgical ward in Shifa hospital of Gaza, Palestine. He has undergone a bowel resection due to colon cancer. Mr. Elmasri's wife, three sons, three grandsons, and four of his extended family members have escorted him from the recovery room to the surgical ward. Mr. Elmasri shares the room with another surgical patient who has several relatives at the bedside as well. The two families exchange greetings, pleasantries, and health stories as the day goes by.

Isam, the nurse assigned to the room, is also taking care of 20 other patients along with four other nurses based on a team nursing model of care at Shifa hospital. Mrs. Elmasri, her children, and grandchildren stay at the bedside overnight to look after Mr. Elmasri. They take initiative in looking after Mr. Elmasri's basic needs, such as positioning, making his bed, and alerting the nurses when he seems to be in pain or when he needs a new IV bag. It's becoming cumbersome for Isam to deliver timely nursing interventions. The Elmasris have many questions regarding the care of their patient, and Isam tries to answer as many of these questions as possible, but he feels overwhelmed and is running behind in taking care of other patients. The room tends to be noisy most of the time due to the presence of multiple visitors and helpers at any one time. The Elmasris find themselves catering to their visitors and guests from out of town who come to visit at the hospital.

Person- and family-centered care (P&FCC) is being adopted in many countries of the world, regardless of physical, cultural, or technological barriers or geographic boundaries. For patients and families, the desire for respectful care, continuity of provider, and effective treatment is universal. How it plays out in different cultures and countries varies, as shown in the preceding vignette. The role of the individual and community, the availability of healthcare providers and treatments, and the settings in which healthcare is provided differ and are important consider-ations in designing and offering personalized care.

The interconnected world in which we live today enables educators, researchers, and clinicians to be connected instantly without the need to travel or experience the hassles and financial burdens of re-creating relevant and needed knowledge to provide P&FCC. Providing individualized care requires that we incorporate elements of culture, gender, age, and other fundamental dimen-sions into care, and that we partner with a wide array of individuals, groups, and communities to develop and implement these plans of care. However, geopolitical forces within different coun-tries and the sufficiency of resources are realities that can thwart efforts to deliver P&FCC, even when the commitment is strong,

In this chapter, the concept of P&FCC is examined through a global lens:

- Is there a global definition of patient- or person-centered care?
- What do prominent international health and consumer organizations say about P&FCC, and what are they doing to advance the concept?
- What issues do persons and their families in different countries have in receiving care that is safe, timely, effective, efficient, equitable, and patient-centered?
- What other aspects of healthcare do providers who are providing P&FCC need to consider?

This chapter provides perspectives of P&FCC from organizations with a global health mission, examines the concept of P&FCC from the lens of different countries, and suggests implications for practice that should be considered when providing healthcare within different countries. Although many terms are used globally, this chapter uses *patient- and family-centered care (P&FCC)*, unless quoting from specific sources.

A Global Concept of Patient- and Family-Centered Care

Although the world is increasingly becoming a smaller community, vast differences still exist in such important concepts as healthcare and the individual's role in healthcare delivery. This section explores the extent to which a global definition of P&FCC exists and examines several components that are universal. In addition, numerous stakeholders interested in promoting the concept are identified.

A Global Definition of P&FCC

Although substantial work is being done internationally to address the issue of patient-centered care, no universal definition has been adopted. Furthermore, of those definitions proposed, all are from the Western hemisphere; no examples of non-Western definitions have been found, according to the International Alliance of Patients' Organizations (IAPO). IAPO (2007) uses the term *patient-centred healthcare* to "describe healthcare that is designed and practiced with the patient at the centre" (p. 2). Furthermore, IAPO (2007) asserts that "the patient is the only person in a position to make the decision on what patient-centred healthcare means to them, as an individual in the treatment of their condition and the living of their life" (p. 5). In every almost every country where work is being done, the phrase used is *patient-centered care*.

> **NOTE**
>
> One noteworthy exception to the use of the term *patient-centered care* is in Sweden, which has legislated the use of the term *"person"-centered care*. This is covered in greater detail in Chapter 25.

While acknowledging that priorities for healthcare differ greatly among countries and disease conditions, IAPO believes that all healthcare must be based on five principles:

- Respect
- Choice and empowerment
- Patient involvement in health policy
- Access and support
- Information

These key elements must be included with the IAPO definition because the definition by itself, given above, could reflect a form of patient-centered care in which healthcare providers, usually well intentioned, design the system with their own perspective as to what the patient and/or family wants.

The importance of a precise and universal definition cannot be overstated. Although the concept of P&FCC is being discussed more throughout the world, there continues to be a difference of opinion as to whether P&FCC is "about" the patient and family or "with" the patient and family. Such terms as *patient-focused*, or even *individualized* or *personalized care*, can leave the patient and family on the periphery. One extreme example of this type of thinking is the surgeon who said, "I'm patient-centered. I take care of patients."

The Institute of Medicine (IOM, 2001) explicitly includes the patient in the care process, as reflected in its definition of P&FCC: "Providing care that is respectful of and responsive to individual patient preferences, needs, and values and ensuring that patient values guide all decisions" (p. 40). The competency for the nursing practice of P&FCC, developed through the Quality and Safety Education for Nurses (QSEN) initiative, takes this definition one step further: "Recognize the patient or designee as the *source of control and full partner* [emphasis added] in providing compassionate and coordinated care based on respect for patient's preferences, values and needs" (Cronenwett et al., 2007, p. 123).

Components of P&FCC

Rather than providing a definition of P&FCC, many scholars and organizations offer a set of components or elements that are associated with the concept. For example, through a comprehensive review and analysis of the literature, Mead and Bower (2002) have developed a model of the components of this relationship and identified five elements:

- Biopsychosocial perspective (consideration of the full range of difficulties affecting patients)
- The "patient-as-person" (the personal meaning of the situation)
- Sharing power and responsibility
- Therapeutic alliance
- The "doctor-as-person" (the personal qualities of the physician)

Little et al. (2001), in a study of 865 patients in the waiting room of three doctors' offices in the United Kingdom, found that three domains were identified as reflective of patient-centeredness from the patients' perspective: communication, partnership, and an emphasis on health promotion. Relatively few patients believed that an examination or prescription was essential for a patient-centered approach.

Similarly, Stewart (2001) describes the concept as follows:

> Patients want patient-centred care which (a) explores the patients' main reason for the visit, concerns and need for information; (b) seeks an integrated understanding of the patients' world—that is, their whole person, emotional needs, and life issues; (c) finds common ground on what the problem is and mutually agrees on management; (d) enhances prevention and health promotion; and (e) enhances the continuing relationship between the patient and the doctor. (p. 444)

Gerteis, Edgman-Levitan, Daley, and Delbanco (1993) identify several dimensions of patient-centered care:

- Respect for patients' values, preferences, and expressed needs
- Coordination and integration of care
- Information, communication, and education
- Physical comfort
- Emotional support
- Involvement of family and friends

This work shaped the framework developed by the Picker Institute, which has done substantial work in the United States, Canada, and Europe to improve the quality of healthcare through enhancing the patient experience (see Table 6.1). The definition that it uses is "improving health care through the eyes of the patient" (Walton & Barnsteiner, 2012, p. 69). Work by the Picker Institute has widely influenced the development of care models and served as a framework for research in evaluating P&FCC.

TABLE 6.1   Patient-Centered Care Principles From the Picker Institute

Effective treatment delivered by staff you can trust

Involvement in decisions and respect for patients' preferences

Fast access to reliable healthcare advice

Clear, comprehensive information and support for healthcare

Physical comfort and a clean, safe environment

Empathy and emotional support

Involvement of family and friends

Continuity of care and smooth transitions

The U.S. Agency for International Development (as cited in IAPO, 2007) offers a set of components also incorporating the Gerteis team's concepts:

> [A]n approach to care that consciously adopts a patient's perspective. This perspective can be characterized around dimensions such as respect for patients' values, preferences, and expressed needs in regard to coordination and integration of care, information, communication and education, physical comfort, emotional support and alleviation of fear and anxiety, involvement of family and friends, transition and continuity. (p. 9)

This set of elements has been included in the glossary of the World Health Organization European Observatory on Health Systems and Policies.

In summary, several points about the global concept of P&FCC can be made:

- At this time, there is no universal definition of P&FCC.
- Most of the work surrounding P&FCC has been done in the United States and European countries.
- There is some convergence around the concepts that Gerteis and colleagues have developed.
- There is still variability around the extent of patient/family involvement (e.g., ranging from actively included, to one where their perspectives are strongly considered, to one where systems and processes are designed with the patient and family in mind).

Stakeholders in P&FCC

Many individuals with valid views, expertise, and perspectives have a stake in how P&FCC is defined and operationalized. Patients, families, patient organizations, healthcare providers, governmental agencies, researchers, and policymakers have valid points of view. However, patient and family voices, as well as caregivers who are not physicians, are often underrepresented. As reflected in some of the earlier examples, much of the earlier international literature and research on P&FCC focuses on the relationship between the physician and patient.

More recently, researchers and those setting up care models are beginning to recognize and use the concept of the healthcare provider (HCP) as the focus of interest. This is particularly appropriate in considering global health and assessing the effectiveness of various models of care delivery. Differences as to who is the primary care provider within and among countries exist because there may be few physicians in a region or country, or the historical tradition may be that care is provided by others.

In a study conducted in the United Kingdom, Gillespie, Florin, and Gillam (2004) speak about the attitude of healthcare professionals, in general, as a barrier to true patient-centered care. They suggest that "[a]ttitudinal change is needed to redistribute the power between professionals and patients." Another example is the work of Mirzaei and colleagues (2013), who used the Wagner model of chronic care management to conduct in-depth interviews with patients ($n=52$), their caregivers ($n=14$), and HCPs ($n=63$) in the Australian Capital Territory and New South Wales. Patients reported a wide range of concerns, including:

- A need for improved communication and information delivery by HCPs
- Well-organized health services and reduced waiting times to see HCPs
- Greater recognition by HCPs of the need for holistic and continuing care
- Including patients and caregivers in decision-making
- Help with self-care

Whether the focus of attention is the physician or the HCP, it is most important to recognize that evaluating the success of P&FCC has to include the patient and family perspective. Not only must patients and families be fully included in evaluating the care, but they need to be active participants in its delivery and, actually, in helping define measures that are meaningful to them. This can vary from population to population, and from country to country.

International Perspectives on P&FCC

Included in this section is an introduction to several international organizations whose missions relate to improving the health of individuals globally and a description of some specific initiatives that they have launched to include the patient and family more fully in decision-making.

International Alliance of Patients' Organizations

IAPO was founded in 1999 by 40 patients' organizations from around the world as "the only global alliance representing patients of all nationalities across all disease areas and promoting patient-centred healthcare worldwide" (2013, para. 1). Its mission is to build patient-centered healthcare globally through:

- Partnerships with patients' organizations

- Using a strong patient voice to advocate on healthcare policy to influence policy agendas and policies at regional, national and international levels

- Building cross-sector alliances and working collaboratively with those of similar goals, including healthcare providers, policymakers, educators, researchers, and industry leaders

NOTE

IAPO also formed a World Health Professions Alliance in 1999 to represent the world's 23 million nurses, physicians, and pharmacists in addressing global health issues and in delivering improved healthcare to global populations.

In 2006, IAPO developed a Declaration on Patient-Centred Healthcare. The goal was to guide healthcare systems in designing and delivering healthcare through greater patient engagement and optimal usage. The Declaration is excerpted in the accompanying sidebar.

The IAPO Declaration on Patient-Centred Healthcare

"To achieve patient-centred healthcare we believe that healthcare must be based on the following Five Principles:

1. *Respect—Patients and carers have a fundamental right to patient-centred healthcare that respects their unique needs, preferences and values, as well as their autonomy and independence.*

2. *Choice and empowerment—Patients have a right and responsibility to participate, to their level of ability and preference, as a partner in making healthcare decisions that affect their lives. This requires a responsive health service which provides suitable choices in treatment and management options that fit in with patients' needs, and encouragement and support for patients and carers that direct and manage care to achieve the best possible quality of life. Patients' organizations must be empowered to play meaningful leadership roles in supporting patients and their families to exercise their right to make informed healthcare choices.*

3. *Patient involvement in health policy—Patients and patients' organizations deserve to share the responsibility of healthcare policy-making through meaningful and supported engagement in all levels and at all points of decision-making, to ensure that they are designed with the patient at the centre. This should not be restricted to healthcare policy but include, for example, social policy that will ultimately impact on patients' lives. See IAPO's Policy Statement at: www.patientsorganizations.org/involvement.*

4. *Access and support—Patients must have access to the healthcare services warranted by their condition. This includes access to safe, quality and appropriate services, treatments, preventive care and health promotion activities. Provision should be made to ensure that all patients can access necessary services, regardless of their condition or socio-economic status. For patients to achieve the best possible quality of life, healthcare must support patients' emotional requirements, and consider non-health factors such as education, employment and family issues which impact on their approach to healthcare choices and management.*

5. *Information—Accurate, relevant and comprehensive information is essential to enable patients and carers to make informed decisions about healthcare treatment and living with their condition. Information must be presented in an appropriate format according to health literacy principles considering the individual's condition, language, age, understanding, abilities and culture. See IAPO's Policy Statement at www.patientsorganizations.org/healthliteracy."*

(IAPO, 2009)

Retrieved from http://www.patientsorganizations.org/declaration and reprinted with permission from the International Alliance of Patients' Organizations.

The World Health Organization

The World Health Organization (WHO, 2014a) is

the directing and coordinating authority for health within the United Nations system. It is responsible for providing leadership on global health matters, shaping the health research agenda, setting norms and standards, articulating evidence-based policy options, providing technical support to countries and monitoring and assessing health trends. (para. 1)

WHO uses a six-point agenda to guide its activities and measure its success. The six points are:

1. Promoting development
2. Fostering health security

3. Strengthening health systems

4. Harnessing research, information and evidence

5. Enhancing partnerships

6. Improving performance (WHO, 2014d)

In 2004, WHO launched a program targeted at "bringing significant benefits to patients in countries rich and poor, developed and developing, in all corners of the globe" (WHO, 2014c, para. 1). This effort, called WHO Patient Safety, was in response to a resolution that had been adopted in 2002 by WHO's 55th World Health Assembly, encouraging member states to pay close attention to patient safety and to implement evidence-based systems to make patient safety a public health priority. Historically, healthcare providers and policymakers had thought that patients and families were unable to comprehend the complexities of healthcare, yet they often have invaluable insights into system failures along the trajectory of care and certainly do know the individual patients best and what they prefer.

One of the main components of WHO Patient Safety is an initiative called Patients for Patient Safety (PFPS), designed to ensure that the views of patients, families, consumers, and citizens (however a country wishes to term the participants) are incorporated into the safety efforts. Safety "can be improved if patients are included as full partners in reform initiatives" (WHO, 2014c, para. 2). Ways in which patients and families can contribute include:

- Sharing stories of preventable injuries and their impact

- Contributing knowledge gained or lessons learned

- Serving as partners in aspects of care delivery

- Contributing to policymaking bodies

The London Declaration of 2005 (WHO, 2014b) crystallized the vision for PFPS:

> A world in which patients are treated as partners in efforts to prevent all avoidable harm in healthcare. PFPS calls for honesty, openness and transparency, and aims to make the reduction of healthcare errors a basic human right that preserves life around the world. (para. 1)

To achieve this vision, WHO Patient Safety created a Global Network with PFPS Champions who advocate for patient engagement in patient safety improvement efforts at international, national, and local levels. The original group of Champions numbered 21; today there are 250 representing 50 countries. WHO has also created a number of educational tools, such as the Multi-Professional Patient Safety Curriculum Guide, for use in health professions programs, such as dentistry, midwifery, nursing, medicine, and pharmacy, and the Patient Safety Quiz to test health professionals' knowledge about safety science. In 2012, it began offering workshops in a number of countries to help educate health professionals in essential patient safety principles and concepts.

The Pan American Health Organization

The Pan American Health Organization (PAHO), founded in 1902, serves as the Regional Office for the Americas of WHO and is a member of the United Nations system (http://www.paho.org). PAHO is the specialized health agency of the Inter-American System and is the world's oldest international public health agency, providing technical cooperation and partnerships to improve health and quality of life in the countries of the Americas.

PAHO provides a number of publications and modules on specific topics affecting health and safety, such as violence against women; gender, diversity, and human rights; environmental surveillance; and the participation of men and women in monitoring maternal and child health in a rural segment of Peru. In its *Improving Chronic Illness Care Through Integrated Health Service Delivery Networks* (Barcelo et al., 2012), it advocates for patient-centered care as the way to more effectively prevent and control chronic conditions. For this group, P&FCC involves:

- "Ensuring the accessibility and continuity of care;

- Strengthening patient involvement in care by making it easier for patients to express their concerns and for health care service providers to respect their patients' values, preferences and needs and offer emotional support, especially to relieve their anxieties and fears;

- Supporting self-management across all levels of the system by facilitating therapeutic goal-setting and boosting the confidence of patients and their families in self-care;

- Establishing more efficient mechanisms for inter-unit cooperation and integration." (p. 23)

PAHO also suggests specific responsibilities for health providers, such as to operate in consideration of these principles; to define roles and assign tasks among all members of the team; to use evidence-based care; to ensure patient monitoring; and to "provide care that patients can understand and that is culturally appropriate" (p. 23). PAHO calls for a role of care coordinator to improve communication and help the patient navigate the system and encourages the use of collaborative—not directive—counseling approaches in working with the patient.

Institute for Healthcare Improvement

The Institute for Healthcare Improvement (IHI) was founded in the late 1980s by Don Berwick, Paul Batalden, and a number of visionary leaders in the United States who were committed to designing an entirely new healthcare system without errors, waste, delay, impersonal service, and untenable costs (IHI, 2014). IHI's vision and mission are "a future in which everyone has the best care and health possible" (para. 2) and a "resolve to approach them with optimism grounded in rigorous science, hard work, and a relentless drive for results" (para. 3).

Based in Cambridge, Massachusetts, IHI has partnered with countries, organizations, and individuals around the world and has a significant footprint in many countries, including Canada,

England, Scotland, Denmark, Sweden, Singapore, Latin America, New Zealand, Ghana, Malawi, and South Africa. It has revolutionized safety and quality improvement efforts through such programs as:

- The 5 Million Lives Campaign
- The use of bundles in aggregating evidence-based practices
- Rapid-cycle testing
- The Breakthrough Series Collaborative
- The Open School for health professional students' education
- The Triple Aim framework for simultaneously addressing the three key goals of healthcare (improving the patient experience with healthcare, improving the health of populations, and reducing the cost)

On its website and through its programming, IHI offers a wide array of tools for achieving patient-centered care, one of its core values. Specific initiatives targeted toward incorporating the patient as an active partner in healthcare decision-making and delivery include:

- The Conversation Project, working to ensure that every person's end-of-life wishes are expressed and respected
- The Patient Experience Seminar, which brings global leaders together to learn how to provide an extraordinary patient care experience
- Patient Experience collaboratives, projects to identify and address systemic barriers to patient-centered care

As an overarching statement, IHI's Framework for Public and Patient Engagement recognizes that engaging patients in their own healthcare is critically important in achieving the Triple Aim of an improved patient experience, better outcomes, and lower costs.

International Council of Nurses

The International Council of Nurses (ICN), founded in 1899, is the world's first and broadest reaching organization for health professionals (ICN, 2013). A federation of more than 130 national nurses associations, it represents more than 16 million nurses worldwide. ICN works to "ensure quality nursing care for all, sound health policies globally, the advancement of nursing knowledge, and the presence worldwide of a respected nursing profession and a competent and satisfied nursing workforce" (para. 1). It addresses these goals through a wide range of initiatives, including regional and national conferences, policy statements, publications, research, awards, networks and platforms, and advocacy for such initiatives as the Girl Child Education Fund, Wellness Centres for Health Care Workers, and the International Centre for Nurse Migration.

In 2003, it adopted a position statement (revised in 2008) on Informed Patients, noting that "informed patients are crucial for ensuring patient safety and should be part of the efforts to improve quality and safety of health care" (ICN, 2008, p. 2). Within the document, ICN outlined several rights of individuals, including

> the right to up-to-date information related to health promotion and maintenance of health and the prevention and treatment of illness…the right to access to information, in an appropriate format and to the level of their understanding that enables them to make informed choices and decisions regarding their health…and the right to privacy and to confidentiality of their information about their health. (2008, p. 1)

Healthcare providers are encouraged to work in partnership with patient organizations, self-care groups, and other interested parties to ensure that these rights are being met. To assist in this effort, ICN hosts a Patient Talk website that provides health information and support to patients in choosing health options that work best for them.

Patients' Experiences With Care

In 2001, Coulter and Cleary reported on an analysis of Picker patient surveys conducted in Germany, Sweden, Switzerland, the United Kingdom (UK), and the United States (U.S.), revealing many problems with sharing of information, coordination of care, respect for patient preferences, inclusion of family and friends, continuity and transition of care, and adequate physical and emotional support. According to the authors, there were several particularly striking findings:

- Although the tool used was developed in the United States, there was strong similarity in the responses of patients in all of the countries.

- The most commonly reported problems in all countries were associated with continuity and transition of care.

- There was great variation among hospitals within the same country (e.g., among 272 U.S. hospitals, the percentage of patients who said they were given inadequate information in the emergency department [ED] ranged from 7% to 73%).

- Methodological issues posed a significant challenge when trying to compare across countries due to differences in interpretation, translation, demographics, cultural and health system differences, and differences in sampling processes. (Coulter & Cleary, 2001)

Schoen and colleagues (2007) conducted several surveys across many countries to identify differences in processes, patient/family satisfaction, and outcomes. In 2005, they surveyed adults with health conditions in six countries regarding safety risks, poor care coordination, and deficiencies in care for chronic conditions. Although the study highlighted a number of problems, findings related to the patient experience and particularly related to aspects of P&FCC:

- Between 19% and 26% reported communication gaps.

- One in six of the patients would have liked greater involvement in decisions about their care.

- One in three patients did not receive instructions about symptoms to watch for, did not know whom to contact with questions, or did not know follow-up arrangements for care.

- If errors occurred, 61% to 83% in each country reported that the HCP did not alert them about the mistake.

- Although no country was uniformly best or worst in the findings, patients in the United States most frequently reported coordination gaps (one of three patients; Schoen et al., 2005).

In 2007, Schoen and her team reported on adults' healthcare experiences in seven countries: Australia, Canada, Germany, the Netherlands, New Zealand, the UK, and the U.S. As could be expected, there were some similarities and some differences across the experiences in the various countries:

- For elective surgery, German and U.S. respondents reported the most rapid access to care, with the UK and Canadian respondents the least. Few respondents in any country reported waiting more than a year.

- The majority of patients in every country (with 100% in the Netherlands) reported having a regular doctor. Half or more of Dutch or German respondents noted that their regular primary care practice (PCP) had early morning hours; Australians reported weekend hours most frequently, while more than one-third of the respondents from Canada, the UK, and the U.S. reported that their doctors were not available outside a 9 a.m. to 5 p.m. schedule.

- For same-day appointments, half or more of the German, Dutch, and New Zealand adults reported that they were able to receive same-day appointments when they were sick. Canadian and U.S. respondents were most likely to report long waits (6 days or more) to see a doctor when sick.

- In every country, a significant majority of adults said that their doctors always explained things clearly, and the majority of adults rated highly the quality of care they received. However, British patients were least likely to report that their doctors included them in care decisions, and patients in the UK, the U.S., and Canada were less likely to report that their physicians always spent enough time with them (Schoen et al., 2007).

As with the 2005 study, no one country had the best care processes or outcomes, nor did any one country have the worst. Consistent with other reports, the United States "spends by far the highest share of national income on healthcare yet is the only country that leaves a high percentage of the population uninsured or poorly protected in the event of illness" (Schoen et al., 2007, p. w718).

In 2013, Faber and several European colleagues surveyed more than 6,400 chronically ill patients and 152 primary care providers in five countries (Belgium—Flanders only, Denmark, Germany, the Netherlands, and England) to assess the extent to which aspects of the U.S. model of the patient-centered medical home (PCMH) were present. Although titled the *patient-centered medical home*, it is interesting to note that the seven components of the system do not necessarily include the key concepts described earlier as being consistent with patient- or person-centered care, such as patient or designee as active partner, patient involvement, and information. In the PCMH, the seven components are personal physician, physician-directed medical practice, whole-person orientation, care that is coordinated or integrated, quality and safety, enhanced access, and payment reform. Depending on how these components are operationalized, they can indeed be congruent with patient/person-centered care or be physician-driven. Findings included the following:

- 100% of practices, except for Germany, had computerized medical record systems.

- 91% of Danish practices offered patients direct access to their medical records, but almost no patients in the other countries had this option.

- Approximately 60% of patients had written instructions for self-management (in Belgium, 84% did).

- Up to 40% of patients reported that their expectations of care were not met or that the physicians did not show interest in their psychological well-being or home situations.

- Patients and physicians differed in their perceptions of aspects of care. For example, Dutch and Belgian physicians reported less frequent handouts of self-management material than did their patients (35% vs. 59% in the Netherlands; 52% vs. 84% in Belgium). However, in England, 79% of physicians (vs. 63% of patients) reported the provision of handouts, and 91% reported that their patients' expectations were met (vs. 79% of patients; Faber et al., 2013).

As interesting as these comparisons can be, cross-country findings need to be interpreted with caution. As noted earlier, differences among countries can be the result of differences in care expectations, insurance schemes, cultural norms, and care practices. There also may be demographic differences, translation problems, and differences in the sampling processes. They do illustrate, however, that patient expectations and perspectives can be similar and yet differ within and across countries, and are multifactorial.

Examples of P&FCC in Other Countries

The following section contains an in-depth analysis of nursing and P&FCC in Palestine, drawing from the example in the vignette at the beginning of the chapter. In addition, a few observations are shared relating to P&FCC in other countries that illustrate the great variability in the implementation of P&FCC, even if there is commitment to the concept.

Palestine: Family Involvement in Care in Gaza Hospital

The following narrative in this section is from Jehad Adwan: The Gaza Strip is a very small (360 km^2) and highly populated strip of land with 5,000 people per square kilometers. (CIA, 2013). It is located on the southeast corner of the Mediterranean Sea and has been politically unstable since 1967, when it was occupied by Israeli forces. It has gone under partial Palestinian Authority control following the Oslo peace accords in 1993. In 2006, the Palestinian Authority lost control of the Gaza Strip to its political rival, the Hamas movement, which currently governs the tiny strip of land with almost two million inhabitants. Consequently, healthcare in the Gaza Strip has been as turbulent as the geopolitical circumstances around it. Fragmentation of health-care delivery systems evidenced by the multiple systems (governmental, private, nongovern-mental organizations, and charities, among others) renders the strip into a state of unidentifiable central healthcare infrastructure to be referred to or used for long-term planning. This multiple system predictably lacks coordination and a mutually helpful national plan of healthcare.

As a new nurse in Gaza's Shifa hospital in 1995, I served in adult and pediatric surgical and emergency units. In Palestine, a majority of the nurses are male (56%, Palestinian Central Bureau of Statistics, 2013), and the healthcare system is chaotic, with very crowded clinics and hospitals. Most patients are typically accompanied by several family members throughout the hospital stay. Although nurses are responsible for providing care for these patients, family members offer many benefits by being at the bedside. They provide care and assistance to their loved one similar to what a nursing assistant would, such as activities of daily living (ADLs), making beds, feeding, and cleaning the environment around their patient. They serve an important role by acting as advocates or representatives for their patient on a consistent basis.

Palestinian and Islamic cultures put a great emphasis on the immediate family in specific and the extended family in general. Religion plays a big role in encouraging family members, neighbors, and friends to make visitation to the sick and helping their family financially or otherwise. In fact, visiting the sick is considered a spiritual charity and is highly rewarded in the Islamic tradition. As a patriarchal society, Palestinian families respect their elders to make sound decisions when it comes to health matters if the patient is unable to consciously make these decisions in emergency situations. The family as a whole participates in sharing thoughts regarding the health of a loved one, while community leaders and *imams* (religious leaders) have respected input when their counsel is needed.

Team nursing is the predominant nursing care delivery model. When I practiced in Gaza, there was usually a fixed number of nurses on the floor during day, evening, and night shifts. Nurses are led by a charge nurse, who delegates task-specific rather than patient-centered assignments for the nurses. For example, one nurse will administer all meds to all patients, while another will change all the dressings, and so on. This helps run the unit in a more efficient and cost-effective fashion due to the high patient-to-nurse ratio.

That is where family chaperones came in handy for doing tasks for the patient that the nurse would not have the time to perform, including basic personal care and feeding. This proved to be useful during the night shift when staffing was very short—two nurses for night shift, as opposed to five to seven during days, took care of up to 24 patients. One night, I—along with one other nurse—was responsible for taking care of 32 patients in a 12-hour night shift. My partner had to go home sick at 4 a.m. that night, and my supervisor could not find me any help for the remaining busiest 3 hours of the shift. I had to continue alone until the shift ended at 7:00 a.m. I was thankful that family members were available to help with patient care.

This practice, however, can create problems for the healthcare providers in delivering care to the patient. The number of relatives or visitors was often overwhelmingly large—although visiting hours are established and strictly enforced in many hospitals. To solve this issue, the hospital administration issued one or two family members passes to be chaperones who could stay with the patient at all times, especially overnight. During open visiting hours, which took place during the early evening, it became impossibly challenging for the nurse or other healthcare team members to enter the patient's room or deliver care as needed.

An illustrative example happened while I was working in the ED at Shifa in 1996. When a seriously ill person was received in the hospital's 11-bed ED, several other family members arrived at the same time to ensure the well-being of their loved one. As time went by, more neighbors, extended family members, and friends arrived at the relatively small and always busy ED. This situation seriously undermined our ability to deliver care effectively and safely. Reaching the patient to conduct a physical assessment, take vital signs, and administer medication was a difficult and time-intensive task. And occasionally the healthcare team had to call security for help to remove visitors from the patient's room in order to enable the nurses or the physicians to reach the patient and deliver necessary care. It is understandable that family presence at the bedside helps the patient overcome physical and psychological adversity while in the hospital (Emergency Nurses Association, 2009). The patient can benefit from the family's assistance and advocacy by ensuring that he or she receives the care in timely fashion, and the family ensures that their loved one is kept up-to-date and involved in the care delivery as well as the decision-making process.

In Palestinian culture, family-centered care is a highly valued concept. Families tend to have numerous members—I come from a family of 11 members—and I would probably follow the same tradition if one of my siblings or parents were admitted to the hospital. This sense of togetherness is prevalent throughout Palestinian society. Although the healthcare team appreciated, collaborated with, and utilized the family willingness to help, the fact that the family is present and involved can provide a challenging double-edged sword to care providers if not managed well.

Nurses practicing in an intensely family-focused environment, such as Palestine, have to keep some tools at their disposal to deal with either aspect of the heavy family presence and influence on patient care. Nurses may ask the family to appoint a spokesperson or a leader to bring questions or requests to the nurses or attend rounds and patient care conferences. They can ask the family to create a list of family helpers who can work together to divide labor and responsibilities or specific chunks of time that they can carry out these tasks. By doing this, the family would feel like active participants in their loved one's care and the decision-making process while being close enough to the patient to act as a link to the healthcare team.

Shifa hospital administration did try to enforce the chaperone policy, but it was not effective all the time due to the lack of personnel; the nurses had a lot to do and had no time to police the visitors. And so, the challenge continued.

Sweden

The Gothenburg University Centre for Person-Centred Care (GPCC) is an interdisciplinary research center, established in 2010 and supported by the Swedish government's strategic investment in health and care research initiative (http://www.gpcc.gu.se). The basis of person-centered care (PCC), which guides the development of the care plan, is "the patient's experience and PCC emanates from the individual's resources and restraints. PCC is a partnership between patients and professional care givers, with the starting point *the patient narrative*."

In Sweden, the emphasis is becoming stronger toward *person*-centered care rather than *patient*-centered care, as it conveys a more holistic approach to the person(s) involved in the care experience. The Swedish Society of Nursing recently published the *Quality and Safety in Nursing* textbook and revised references to *patient*-centered care to read *person*-centered care.

Australia

The vision of the Australian Institute for Patient and Family Centred Care (AIPFCC; n.d.) is to "transform the quality and safety of the Australian healthcare culture by developing effective and innovative partnerships between patients, families and healthcare professionals" (para. 1). This organization supports a paradigm where patients and their families are equal partners in the healthcare process, as they have a central role in the healthcare team. A new model of care has been proposed, which is seen as a radical departure from the patient's being a passive recipient of healthcare. According to the AIPFCC, the patient gets a place at the table.

In 2010, the Australian Commission on Safety and Quality in Health Care (ACSQHC) issued a discussion draft report for public consultation (ACSQHC, n.d.) that extensively examined the concept of patient-centered care, overviewed supportive evidence for patient-centered care, and detailed international approaches and initiatives to patient-centered care, including policy-level drivers, emerging views on appropriate outcomes for service, and approaches and strategies to promote patient-centered care.

Policy-level recommendations of this paper include advocating for policies that promote patient-centered care, collecting data about quality of patient experiences nationally, funding performance-based payments that should include patient experience as one clinical quality measure, and improving transparency by having policymakers and regulators make patient experience data publicly available. It makes 11 organizational-level recommendations, including systems for reporting patient care experience, quality measures that include patient feedback regarding services received, and organizational contributions to the evidence base on patient-centered care.

The Democratic Republic of the Congo (DRC)

According to IMA World Health (2010):

> In much of DRC, living conditions are dismal, access to health care is minimal and violence still erupts in unstable areas. Rape and violence against women may be more common in DRC than anywhere else in the world. Though rich in resources that allow hope for a bright future as a thriving country, DRC is still in dire need of economic and social reconstruction. (para. 2)

Consequently, healthcare in the Congo is very unstructured and often based on a "pay as you go" premise: Because there are so few resources, patients, family members, or sometimes nurses must go out to the black market to try to buy necessary medications and supplies. Although resources are few, there is a high value placed on "Western medicine." Patients seeking care might go to both a traditional healer and a traditional healthcare clinic.

There are very few doctors, particularly in rural areas, so nurses and community caregivers provide most of the care. Family members may stay at the patient's side and provide some of the care. There is no licensing system for nurses; two or three individuals working as nurses might care for several hundred patients in one of the urban hospitals. Patients are rarely involved in decision-making because there are so few treatment options. Physicians usually make the decisions, although again there are few physicians in the country (C. Robertson, personal communication, October 30, 2013).

Uganda

In Uganda, care can be quite different, depending on whether it is provided in an urban or rural area or whether it is public or private. In the urban area, there are more caregivers, including both nurses and physicians. In both areas, the whole family may be at the bedside. Family members will bring their own mattresses and bedding, with at least one person staying with the patient, feeding him or her with food from home. Nurses can prescribe here without a license. In private hospitals, particularly those supported by USAID, where wealthier people go, the care could be comparable to Western levels. In religious healthcare systems, there are fewer supplies or resources (C. Robertson, personal communication, October 30, 2013).

Somalia

The country of Somalia is a clan-based society where membership in a patrimonial clan family shapes all aspects of daily life, including economic, political and social welfare, and physical safety (Carroll et al., 2007). Most Somalis are Muslim, with gender-specific roles and responsibilities, and traditions are the norm.

Prior to the civil war in 1991, healthcare was designed along Western-style lines, especially in urban areas, with "cultural" doctors more common in rural areas. More than 3,000,000 Somalis were displaced as a result of the war, with more than 100,000 coming to the United States. Somalis are familiar with Western healthcare concepts, such as vaccination, antibiotics, rehydration, and infectious diseases. They also incorporate more traditional approaches to treating illness, such as prayer, religious ceremonies, healing spirits, and the use of herbs and botanicals.

In their survey in 2007, Carroll and her team found positive themes related to patient-centered communication, such as positive nonverbal communication and signs of the clinician's personality, the importance of feeling valued and respected as a person, and an interest by the clinician in understanding the individual's psychosocial context. For women, female interpreters were key, as were female clinicians providing care.

Interventions to Promote P&FCC

Numerous factors must be considered in delivering P&FCC, such as the individual's race/ethnicity, gender, age, religion, sexual orientation, socioeconomic status, and political affiliation, among many others. In delivering P&FCC in a different country, however, these challenges exist, as well as others that are indigenous to the particular country, requiring greater consideration when planning and providing healthcare in one country as opposed to another. Table 6.2 provides a list of considerations for personalizing care within different countries.

TABLE 6.2   Cultural and Social Factors Differentiating Person- and Family-Centered Care

Who is the family?
What role does the family play in healthcare? What role does the community play?
Who is the decision-maker in major decisions?
What is the role of men and women?
Who can provide healthcare? To whom?
What is the role of children?
What are the food preferences? Who is permitted to cook for the patient?
What are treatment options? How available are they to all patients?
What are the value and reward systems?
What is the meaning of illness to the family?
What is the worldview of the family?
What is the family's religion? How influential is it in their daily lives?
What communication patterns are used? Who speaks in important matters?

continues

TABLE 6.2 *continued*

What language(s) does the patient speak? What is the predominant language?

What language is spoken at home?

What is the patient's/family's concept of time (e.g., specific or general)?

What are the "rules" about healthcare (e.g., first come/first seen; only the wealthy deserve it)?

What are the structural dimensions within the family and community (e.g., hierarchical, collaborative)?

When preparing to practice in a different country, several steps are recommended:

1. First, and of primary importance, is to understand fundamental norms and practices that reflect the country's or region's cultural values. Also note the geopolitical situation and implications as to who is providing care and what resources are available. In many Western countries, although there are probably never enough resources, there are certainly more than in countries where there are extremely inadequate resources. In these countries, a decision about patient- or person-centered care may be almost moot because there are so few treatment options, supplies, or medications. However, treatment for the individual as a person in any country warrants respect and compassion, and that can be delivered regardless of the extent of resources available.

2. Conduct an assessment of the factors outlined in Table 6.3 from one or more of the following resources: the patient, family, healthcare providers, professional colleagues, religious groups, governmental agencies, or online resources. Having an appreciation for the challenges faced by patients and families, as well as nurses and other healthcare providers who may philosophically support the concept of P&FCC but be unable to deliver it, is crucial.

3. Develop a set of realistic, priority goals that can be accomplished in working with individual patients and their families, or in efforts to promote P&FCC.

4. Identify allies within and outside the country with whom you can work to achieve a greater level of P&FCC, and create or strengthen relationships with them in pursuit of your common goal of P&FCC. These can include individuals, local groups, community organizations, and nongovernmental support agencies.

In Chapter 12 of this book, Dexheimer-Pharris points out two dichotomies that identify key components that differentiate cultures and that suggest approaches that might work. These dichotomies apply to global cultures as well as to cultures that exist within countries or even organizations. First is the individualistic-collectivist value orientation. Individualistic cultures emphasize personal goals, individuality, autonomy, and independence. Individuals within this culture often acts on their own, making decisions that fit their view of the world. Collectivist cultures focus on harmony, interconnectedness, relationships, and communal well-being rather than personal gain. Individuals operating within a collectivist framework might use the group as a major resource in decision-making or seek consensus rather than speak their own mind.

A second dichotomy relates to power differences among members of the group. In a small power-distance culture, individual credibility, democratic decision-making, and speaking one's thoughts are valued—even between children and adults. Another example would be among members of the healthcare team: The belief is that everyone has a role to play and something valuable to offer. However, in a large power-distance culture (again taking healthcare as an example), seniority, rank, age, and other status factors impede open communication, and those younger or with perceived less power must defer to those who may have more seniority or rank but perhaps less knowledge of a particular situation. In large power-distance cultures, it is very difficult to get people to speak up, even if they have vitally important information to share. In many cultures, there is a clear hierarchy as to who is valued; sometimes this extends to gender and, certainly, religion and political affiliation.

One can envision the importance of understanding other dichotomies or differing perspectives, as suggested in Table 6.2. How does the individual perceive time? Is it something that has to be tightly adhered to or generally considered? Who makes the decisions in the group—is there consensus or even an opportunity for the individual to speak up? How are priorities determined—first come/first served or according to severity of the problem? Although we may have our own ideas about each of these concepts, they are likely heavily influenced by our Western (or Eastern) philosophies of thought.

With all these factors operating, it is impossible to develop interventions that fit all countries. Although it is challenging enough to offer sensitive, person-centered care to a person from a different culture within one country (e.g., the United States), what is needed here is to first understand the context and culture of the relevant country in which the person is seeking care and then tailor care that meets the person's preferences within the context of the country's norms.

The one exception that may be universally appropriate is to ask the patient and spokesperson in the particular culture their perspectives or recommendations. The questions in Table 6.2 can serve as a guideline for concepts to cover. Another resource that has become invaluable in many cultures is Kleinman's framework of eight questions for patients and families to understand the meaning of illness, its cause, and acceptable treatments. The questions are listed in Table 6.3.

TABLE 6.3 Kleinman's Questions

What do you think has caused your problem?
Why do you think it started when it did?
What do you think your sickness does to you? How does it work?
How severe is your sickness? Will it have a short or long course?
What kind of treatment do you think you should receive?

continues

TABLE 6.3   *continued*

What are the most important results you hope to receive from this treatment?

What are the chief problems your sickness has caused you?

What do you most fear from your sickness?

Source: Kleinman, Eisenberg, & Good, 1978

Regardless of the country of origin or culture, we have to remember that global healthcare brings different perspectives on human rights and different views of social justice as well. Sherwood (2012) reminds us of our responsibility for ethical practice and our moral commitment to do no harm. What this may look like—and what actions it may require—will vary among countries and cultures. We need to be able to recognize the profound differences that exist throughout the world in how care is delivered, and how that may be very different from what we are used to and yet be within acceptable ranges. However, in situations where we believe that threats to patient safety exist, we are obligated to work with the appropriate leaders to address the situation.

Conclusion

In considering a global approach to person-centered care, one size does not fit all individuals or all countries. However, although there is no universally accepted definition, there are some common goals that can be pursued, such as those outlined in the IAPO Declaration on Patient-Centred Healthcare (2006): respect, choice and empowerment, patient involvement in health policy, access and support, and information. Several internationally oriented organizations have launched significant initiatives to strengthen the concept of P&FCC. Within these countries, serious efforts are underway to establish programs that fit their particular values and priorities. And finally, at the individual level, this chapter offers two frameworks for obtaining the person's or family's perspectives on what would constitute P&FCC in whichever country they reside. As we seek to develop a global definition, for now we can perhaps follow the suggestion of Berwick (2008) to adopt these useful maxims to guide us: (1) "The needs of the patient come first"; (2) "Nothing about me without me"; and (3) "Every patient is the only patient" (p. w560).

References

Australian Commission on Safety and Quality in Health Care (ACSQHC). (n.d.). Retrieved from http://www.safetyandquality.gov.au/

Australian Institute for Patient and Family Centered Care (AIPFCC). (n.d.) Retrieved from http://www.aipfcc.org.au/vision.html

Barcelo, A., Luciani, S., Agurto, I., Ordunez, P., Tasca, R., & Sued, O. (2012). *Improving chronic illness through integrated health service delivery networks.* Washington, DC: PAHO.

Berwick, D. (2008). What "patient-centered" should mean: Confessions of an extremist. Retrieved from http://content.healthaffairs.org/content/28/4/w555.full

Carroll, J., Epstein, R., Fiscella, K., Gipson, T., Volpe, E., & Jean-Pierre, P. (2007). Caring for Somali women: Implications for clinician-patient communication. *Patient Education and Counseling, 66*(3), 337-345.

Central Intelligence Agency (CIA). (2013). The world factbook: Gaza Strip. Retrieved from https://www.cia.gov/library/publications/the-world-factbook/geos/gz.html

Coulter, A., & Cleary, P. D. (2001). Patients' experiences with hospital care in five countries. *Health Affairs, 20*(3), 244-252.

Cronenwett, L., Sherwood, G., Barnsteiner, J., Disch, J., Johnson, J., Mitchell, P.,…Warren, J. (2007). Quality and safety education for nurses. *Nursing Outlook, 55*(3), 122-131.

Emergency Nurses Association. (2009). Emergency nursing resource: Family presence during invasive procedures and resuscitation in the emergency department. Retrieved from http://www.ena.org/Research/ENR/Documents/FamilyPresence.pdf

Faber, M., Voerman, G., Erler, A., Eriksson, T., Baker, R., DeLepeleire, J.,…Burgers, J. (2013). Survey of 5 European countries suggests that more elements of patient-centered medical homes could improve primary care. *Health Affairs, 32*(4), 797-806.

Gerteis, M., Edgman-Levitan, S., Daley, J., & Delbanco, T. (Eds.). (1993). *Through the patient's eyes: Understanding and promoting patient-centered care*. San Francisco: Jossey-Bass.

Gillespie, R., Florin, D., & Gillam, S. (2004). How is patient-centred care understood by the clinical, managerial and lay stakeholders response for promoting this agenda? Health Expectations, 7(2), 142-148. Retrieved from http://www.ncbi.nlm.nih.gov/pubmed/15117388

IMA World Health. (2010). Democratic Republic of Congo. Retrieved from http://www.imaworldhealth.org/where-we-work/democratic-republic-of-congo.html.

Institute for Healthcare Improvement (IHI). (2014). Vision, mission and values. Retrieved from http://www.ihi.org/about/Pages/IHIVisionandValues.aspx

Institute of Medicine (IOM). (2001). *Crossing the quality chasm: A new health system for the 21st century*. Washington, DC: National Academies Press.

International Alliance of Patients' Organizations (IAPO). (2007). What is patient-centred healthcare? A review of definitions and principles. Retrieved from http://www.patientsorganizations.org/attach.pl/547/494/IAPO%20Patient-Centred%20Healthcare%20Review%202nd%20edition.pdf

International Alliance of Patients' Organizations (IAPO). (2009). Declaration on patient-centred healthcare. Retrieved from http://www.patientsorganizations.org/declaration

International Alliance of Patients' Organizations (IAPO). (2013). About IAPO. Retrieved from http://www.patientsorganizations.org/showarticle.pl?id=7&n=101

International Council of Nurses (ICN). (2008). Position statement: Informed patients. Geneva, Switzerland: Author. Retrieved from http://www.icn.ch/images/stories/documents/publications/position_statements/E06_Informed_Patients.pdf

International Council of Nurses (ICN). (2013). About ICN. Retrieved from http://www.icn.ch/about-icn/about-icn/

Kleinman, A., Eisenberg, L., & Good, B. (1978). Culture, illness and care. *Annals of Internal Medicine, 88*, 251-258.

Little, P., Everitt, H., Williamson, I., Warner, G., Moore, M., Gould, C., … Payne, S. (2001). Preferences of patients for patient centred approach to consultation in primary care: Observational study. *British Medical Journal, 284*, 468-472.

Mead, N., & Bower, P. (2002). Patient-centred consultations and outcomes in primary care: A review of the literature. *Patient Education and Counseling, 48*(1), 51-61.

Mirzaei, M., Aspin, C., Essue, B., Jeon, Y., Dugdale, P., Usherwood, T., & Leeder, S. (2013). A patient-centred approach to health service delivery: Improving health outcomes for people with chronic illness. *BMC Health Services Research, 13*, 251. doi:10.1186/1472-6963-13-251

Palestinian Central Bureau of Statistics. (2013). Retrieved from http://www.pcbs.gov.ps/site/507/default.aspx

Pan American Health Organization. (2012). Improving chronic illness care through integrated health service delivery networks. Retrieved from http://www.paho.org/hq/index.php?option=com_docman&task=doc_view&gid=21403&Itemid=

Schoen, C., Osborn, R., Doty, M. M., Bishop, M., Peugh, J., & Murukutla, N. (2007). Toward higher-performance health systems: Adults' health care experiences in seven countries, 2007. *Health Affairs, 26*(6), w717-w734. doi:10.1377/hlthaff.26.6.w717

Schoen, C., Osborn, R., Huynh, P. T., Doty, M., Zapert, K, Peugh, J., & Davis, K. (2005). Taking the pulse of health care systems: Experiences of patients with health problems in six countries. *Health Affairs, 24*, W5-509525. doi:10.1377/hlthaff.wf.f09

Sherwood, G. (2012). Quality and safety: Global issues and strategies. In G. Sherwood & J. Barnsteiner (Eds.), *Quality and safety in nursing: A competency approach to improving outcomes* (pp. 323-340). West Sussex, UK: Wiley-Blackwell.

Stewart, M. (2001). Towards a global definition of patient centred care: The patient should be the judge of patient centred care. *British Medical Journal, 322*, 444-445.

Walton, M., & Barnsteiner, J. (2012). Patient-centered care. In G. Sherwood & J. Barnsteiner (Eds.), *Quality and safety in nursing: A competency approach to improving outcomes* (pp. 67-90). West Sussex, UK: Wiley-Blackwell.

World Health Organization (WHO). (2014a). About WHO. Retrieved from http://www.who.int/about/en

World Health Organization (WHO). (2014b). Patients for patient safety. Retrieved from http://www.who.int/patientsafety/patients_for_patient/en/

World Health Organization (WHO). (2014c). Patients for patient safety—Statement of case. Retrieved from http://www.who.int/patientsafety/patients_for_patient/statement/en/

World Health Organization (WHO). (2014d). The WHO agenda. Retrieved from http://www.who.int/about/agenda/en/index.html

Chapter 7

Patient Engagement and Activation

Karen Drenkard, PhD, RN, NEA-BC, FAAN
David Wright, MPH

Carrie, age 54, learns in her visit with her primary care physician that she will need knee-replacement surgery. Upon referral, Carrie's surgeon accesses the GetWellNetwork ambulatory solution on her tablet and reviews with Carrie an educational video on the planned procedure. Completion of that education is automatically documented in the electronic medical record (EMR). The office nurse practitioner shows Carrie how to sign up for the network, which is accessible through the hospital's portal. The surgeon prescribes further education and preparation activities for Carrie to complete on her smartphone, tablet, or personal computer once at home. The surgeon is notified when Carrie completes these prescribed interventions, and her activities and results are automatically documented in the EMR.

Once at the hospital, on the day of the procedure, the pre-operative nurse provides Carrie with a tablet so that she can access further education about the knee-replacement procedure and complete the necessary informed consent forms. Following the procedure, once admitted to the inpatient room, Carrie will complete education prescribed for her to prepare her for discharge and follow-up care through a series of automated workflows, known as patient pathways, that will measure her understanding and comprehension along the way. Additionally, her pain will be automatically reassessed through technology at the appropriate time following administration of the medication. Carrie will be periodically invited to provide real-time feedback about her experience, enabling rapid service recovery, and she will be guided about the steps she must take and items to complete to be discharged on time through a discharge readiness pathway. Carrie also has access to tools empowering her to have control over her environment, connecting her to food services or housekeeping when a need arises.

During mid-shift communication and hand-offs, nurses access the digital whiteboard in Carrie's room to see how she has progressed in completing her tasks and meeting the goals for the day. They work together to establish new goals for the next shift. This is also a great opportunity for nurses to address questions Carrie or her family members have posted on the digital whiteboard for the patient care team.

Prior to discharge, Carrie receives three prompts on her television that inquire whether she would like to have her discharge medications filled at the hospital pharmacy before she leaves, provide information to schedule her home health visit with physical therapy, and inquire whether she has had a mammogram in the past 12 months and would like to schedule an exam following her discharge. The nurse also helps Carrie access the network via the hospital portal to show her where she can find the education she received and her list of medications and discharge instructions.

Once at home, Carrie's mobile device or personal computer reminds her of follow-up appointments, physical therapy appointments, and when to take her medications. She also knows that she and/or her family can access additional information and education as needed.

True transformation of healthcare requires that people take a more active role in managing their health status. People receiving healthcare along the continuum from wellness to chronic disease management will need to become active participants in their care and decision-makers about the care they receive, just as Carrie did in the preceding vignette. They will need to become central members of the healthcare team rather than be passive recipients of care. The concept of *patient engagement* is the term most frequently used to describe the level of interaction that people have with their healthcare journeys.

Likewise, healthcare providers, especially nurses, will need to shift their focus from being providers of care to a new role and a new emphasis. Nurses will need to more fully engage patients in their care so that they can be active partners and so that the locus of control shifts to a truly patient-driven delivery model.

This new paradigm of care delivery is still unfolding, and there are many external forces driving these changes. These forces include the changes in the U.S. care delivery system as envisioned by the Affordable Care Act (ACA), the boom of technology to assist care processes, the change in expectations of the next generation of Americans, and the explosion of knowledge available to people about healthcare conditions and treatment options.

The purpose of this chapter is to examine patient engagement and activation and their placement within the framework of healthcare policy priorities. The role of the nurse in promoting these initiatives is covered, as are the barriers, challenges, and opportunities in more fully engaging people in contributing to their own health outcomes.

What Is Patient Engagement?

Definitions of patient engagement vary considerably. Patient engagement as a concept sits within the broader term of *patient- and family-centered care* (P&FCC) as a vision for what healthcare should be—a true partnership between care providers and patients and families, where care is based on the respect of patients' preferences, values, and beliefs. Coulter (2011) offers that patient engagement is "the relationship between patients and healthcare providers as they work together to promote and support active patient and public involvement in health and healthcare and to strengthen their influence on healthcare decisions, at both the individual and collective levels" (p. 10).

Patient engagement leads to a "broader concept that includes patient activation" (Hibbard & Greene, 2013, p. 216). Patient activation is measurable and represents the likelihood that patients or health consumers will take the necessary actions to comply with their care plans or maintain positive health status. Patient engagement can be viewed as the means to activate health consumers, to help them be more involved in their care journey (Hibbard & Greene, 2013).

Although there is no widely accepted definition of patient engagement, the concept of engagement captures the notion that patients are involved in their care—actively processing information, deciding how best to fit care into their lives, and acting on decisions (Gruman et al., 2010). P&FCC encompasses patient and family engagement in care, including shared decision-making, and preparation and activation for self-care management, and the outcomes of interest to patients receiving healthcare services, including health-related quality of life, functional status, symptoms and symptom burden, and experience with care (National Quality Forum [NQF], 2013a).

Why Is Patient Engagement Important?

Since the National Quality Forum (NQF) defined Patient and Family Engagement as one of the top six national health priorities (National Priorities Partnership, 2008), there has been a dramatic shift in the interest, and now benefits of a more active focus on patient engagement. Table 7.1 describes these national priorities and expands on the goals for patient engagement. Increasingly, patient engagement is at the forefront of healthcare transformation discussions.

TABLE 7.1   The NQF's Top Six National Priorities and Goals for Patient Engagement

1. Engage patients and families in managing their health and making decisions about their care.

   All patients will be asked for feedback on their experience of care, which healthcare organizations and their staff will then use to improve care.

   All patients will have access to tools and support systems that enable them to effectively navigate and manage their care.

   All patients will have access to information and assistance that enables them to make informed decisions about their treatment options.

2. Improve the health of the population.

3. Improve the safety and reliability of America's healthcare system.

continues

TABLE 7.1 *continued*

4. Ensure patients receive well-coordinated care within and across all healthcare organizations, settings, and levels of care.

5. Guarantee appropriate and compassionate care for patients with life-limiting illnesses.

6. Eliminate overuse while ensuring the delivery of appropriate care.

Source: National Priorities Partnership, 2008

According to the NQF, the extent to which patients and their families are involved in making decisions and feel prepared to manage their conditions is critical to improving the quality and the reducing cost of healthcare. Commonwealth Fund research has shown that P&FCC that incorporates shared decision-making can reap potential healthcare savings of $9 billion over 10 years (NQF, 2013a). The NQF has outlined several goals to ensure P&FCC across the healthcare landscape:

"1. Improve patient, family, and caregiver experience of care related to quality, safety, and access across settings.

2. In partnership with patients, families, and caregivers—and using a shared decision-making process—develop culturally sensitive and understandable care plans.

3. Enable patients and their families and caregivers to navigate, coordinate, and manage their care appropriately and effectively." (NQF, 2013a, para. 3–5)

It is common to see standards or references to patient engagement in new policies and regulations. Research is being actively conducted to measure the impact of patient engagement on performance outcomes. Even more, payment practices are reflecting the need for and importance of patient engagement.

Patient engagement can be described as "the actions that people take to improve their health and benefit from care" (Sandy, Tuckson, & Stevens, 2013, p. 1440) or "actions individuals must take to obtain the greatest benefit from health services available to them" (Center for Advancing Health (CFAH), 2013) so that patients become the central force in achieving health. In this era of patient safety and quality outcomes, the patient as a full partner is essential to maximize the likelihood that safe patient care is provided and that high-quality outcomes are achieved. This happens through patient involvement in care decisions and care delivery, such as the following:

- A patient who fully understands his medications and what they look like can serve as a double check when medications are administered in the hospital.

- A patient who fully understands her pain medications and can identify her needs will have better pain control.

- A patient who is engaged and involved in identifying his discharge needs and plans will be more likely to be in charge of his post-hospital care, resulting in better quality of care. This could result in a lower chance of his readmission.

It is logical to think that the more informed, involved, and active patients are in managing their own health statuses, the better the patient outcomes will be.

Patient Engagement as Part of the Affordable Care Act and Federal Healthcare Strategy

The 2010 ACA requires the secretary of the Department of Health and Human Services (HHS) to establish a National Strategy for Quality Improvement in Health Care, also known as the National Quality Strategy (CFAH, 2013). The strategy establishes three objectives:

- *Better care*

- *Affordable care*

- *Healthy people and communities*

In an effort to meet these objectives in a coordinated and aligned effort, the National Quality Forum identified patient engagement as a key strategy for improving quality and safety. There are several key drivers of emphasis on these concepts:

- *The ACA includes provisions requiring patient experience measures, new models of care and how they are evaluated, quality measures, and incentive payment based on outcomes.*

- *The National Committee for Quality Assurance (NCQA; www.ncqa.org) released standards for accountable care organizations, and they identified patient experience as one of three dimensions of accountable care organization performance.*

- *HHS, in 2010, published the meaningful use Health Information Technology (HIT) requirements. These requirements stipulate that hospital and physician IT systems funded by the Health Information Technology for Economic and Clinical Health (HITECH) Act incorporate demographic criteria into data-collection efforts. This will make a substantial contribution to population health management improvement efforts.*

- *The Hospital Consumer Assessment of Healthcare Providers and Systems (HCAHPS) survey, identified by Centers for Medicare & Medicaid Services (CMS) as a core measure set linked to reimbursement for hospitals and healthcare organizations, is driving attention to the patient experience and more broadly engaging patients in their care (National Priorities Partnership, 2010).*

The Current State of Patient Engagement

The evidence linking patient-engagement interventions to patient outcomes is still emerging. "In 2012, an NQF's Measure Gap Analysis identified that measures of P&FCC are significantly lacking across the care continuum, particularly patient-reported outcomes, defined as 'any report of the status of a patient's health condition that comes directly from the patient, without interpretation of the patient's response by a clinician or anyone else'" (NQF, 2013c, para. 1). In October 2013, NQF launched a two-phased project to review P&FCC measures for endorsement. Phase 1 will focus on experience with care measures; Phase 2 will examine measures of health-related quality of life, including functional status and clinician-assessed function (NQF, 2013b). A future phase of this project will review measures on patient communication and symptom/symptom burden.

There are barriers and challenges to improving a patient's level of engagement. A key challenge for nursing leaders is to design frameworks and models of nursing care that match patient-engagement interventions with key assessment criteria—including health literacy, cultural competence, socioeconomic factors, and willingness to be engaged. One such model has three key levels of patient engagement (Carman et al., 2013), which includes the following:

- **Consultation**: Patients receive information about a diagnosis.
- **Involvement**: Patients are asked about their preferences in treatment plans.
- **Partnership and shared leadership**: Treatment decisions are made based on patients' preferences, medical evidence, and clinical judgment.

Factors influencing patient engagement include their beliefs about their role as a patient, their health literacy, and their education as well as their socioeconomic status, psychosocial status, and willingness and motivation to be a part of their health dynamic. The challenge for the nurse is to move patients along this continuum of engagement to increase the level of activation and move to a shared decision-making model. Determining which interventions will assist in moving a patient's level of engagement is a body of research that is in its infancy.

The Influence of Engagement on Patient Outcomes

Early outcome studies (Balik, Conway, Zipperer, & Watson, 2011) show that better-quality outcomes are achieved when the patients partner with their care providers and assume greater responsibility for managing their own health. Patients who are actively engaged by their care providers are more likely to comply with their care plans. Those who are educated about their conditions and understand their treatment options and plans are more likely to take an active role in decisions regarding their care. As patients and their families become active participants in their care, they are more likely to effectively manage their own care, engage in healthy behaviors, and for those with chronic conditions, actively monitor and manage health status while making necessary changes in everyday lifestyle activities. Patients' participation in chronic care self-management programs can lower underuse or overuse of healthcare services and have a substantial impact on their health and the cost to care for these patients.

Patient Activation

A relatively new concept in the emerging space of patient engagement is the concept of patient activation. One of the leaders in identifying and measuring patient activation is Dr. Judith Hibbard (Hibbard & Greene, 2013; Hibbard, Greene, & Overton, 2013), and her work on developing a measurement tool to better understand patient activation is promising.

Patient activation can be described as "understanding one's role in the care process and having the knowledge, skills and confidence to take on that role" (Hibbard, et al., 2013, p. 216). Patient activation includes assessing the level of "the skills and confidence that equip patients to become actively engaged in their healthcare" (Hibbard, et al., 2013, p. 216). Hibbard has begun to explore the difference that patient activation makes in the Triple Aim: health outcomes, cost, and the patient experience. Patient activation emphasizes patients' willingness and ability to take independent actions to manage their health and care. The concept equates patient activation with understanding one's role in the care process and having the knowledge, skill, and confidence to manage health and care.

Dr. Hibbard has developed a Patient Activation Measure (Hibbard, Mahoney, Stockard, & Tusler, 2005), which is a 13-item tool that measures a person's level of activation through direct questions that assess a person's self-concept as a manager of health and healthcare. The tool has a scale that measures from 0 to 100 and categorizes responses into four levels of activation (1 = least and 4 = highest). The 13-item questionnaire incorporates questions that assess patients' beliefs, their confidence in management of health-related tasks, and self-assessed knowledge of their clinical state. Examples of the Patient Activation Measure (PAM) questions include the following:

- "I am confident that I can tell whether I need to go to the doctor or whether I can take care of a health problem myself."
- "I know what treatments are available for my health problems."
- "I am confident that I can tell a doctor my concerns, even when he or she does not ask." (Hibbard et al., 2005)

Responses are degrees of agreement or disagreement. As a patient completes the questionnaire, the baseline level of activation is determined. To increase the level of activation, interventions need to be identified and implemented. Examples of interventions to increase patient activation are outlined in Table 7.2. The interventions include patient skill development, changes to the social environment, and tailoring support to a person's activation level.

TABLE 7.2   Interventions to Improve Patient Activation Scores

INTERVENTION CATEGORY TO INCREASE PATIENT ACTIVATION	EXAMPLES OF INTERVENTIONS TO IMPROVE PATIENT ACTIVATION
Patient skill development, including problem solving and peer support	Self-management programs, helping chronically ill patients handle problems, communicate with caregivers, engage in exercises
	Skill development—intervention focuses on importance of taking an active role in managing condition, teaching strategies to be more active, asking questions
Changing the social environment	Change social environment to facilitate people's change in beliefs, social norms, skills, and engagement in health behavior
	Health classes, posters, information campaigns, personal coaching for high-risk persons
Tailoring support to person's activation level	Individual coaching designed to help patients develop self-management skills
	Interventions that outline small manageable steps
Innovation in care delivery	Improving care by tailoring coaching, education, and care protocols to patients at different levels of activation
	Stratified support—more support to less-activated patients with heavy care burdens

Source: Hibbard & Greene, 2013

Focus of Research

In all areas of patient engagement and patient activation, the evidence is just emerging. Promising evidence demonstrates the power of improving patient engagement and patient activation and its impact on patient outcomes and population health management (Phytel, 2012). However, further research needs are being identified, including expanding the evidence base about the efficacy of different patient engagement strategies in different settings.

Currently, there are no indications of which interventions are the most effective or which will work best with specific patient populations. For example, web-based interventions and portals are showing promise in actively engaging patients in management of their healthcare activities, but more rigorous studies are needed to determine the direct impact on outcomes of care. Research is also needed to identify strategies that increase participation of less-activated patients. Models of care to more actively engage people and to assist care providers in patient engagement strategies need to be developed and tested. Measurement tools for evaluating patient engagement strategies need to continue to be developed and tested. The research arena is wide open for creative and innovative studies, and the creation of a nursing research agenda in this area of patient engagement is a potential area for study and further development.

Patient Engagement and Technology

The Medicare and Medicaid Electronic Health Record (EHR) Incentive Programs include two "meaningful use" objectives focused on patient engagement as part of their Meaningful Use Program (CMS, 2013):

- The first objective is to encourage providers to offer patients and families health information and clinical summaries so they are better equipped to manage their care at home and throughout their everyday lives.
- The patient and family engagement objectives also promote the sharing of patients' medical information among care providers in an effort to strengthen coordination of care.

The Meaningful Use Program guidelines require that patients are provided copies or have access to their health information so that they may share this information with their other healthcare providers.

> **NOTE**
>
> The healthcare industry has invested a lot of time and resources on finding ways to deliver more patient-centered care over the last 10 years. Many different strategies have been tried and tested—some successful, many not. Many of those efforts were focused on strategies working around the patient rather than with the patient as the leader in the care. In order to realize the benefit of patient engagement, we will have to change the way we deliver care. We must move from a model where care is delivered to and around the patient to one in which the care is delivered with the patient.

Interactive Patient Care Technology: Improving Patient Engagement

There is also an emerging care delivery model known as Interactive Patient Care (IPC). IPC is based on the premise that a more engaged patient is a satisfied patient with better outcomes. There is a growing body of outcomes data (Hibbard & Greene, 2013) associated with this innovative care delivery model demonstrating that patient engagement through IPC is a proven strategy for performance improvement. As the responsibility of nursing advances to one of building and sustaining patient activation and the role of nursing moves to be more consultative across care settings, technology will play a vital role for both the nurse and the patient.

Today, IPC technology enables active engagement of the patient in any setting. Nurses can use IPC technology to proactively engage the patient and shift the responsibility for completing certain care interventions. These interventions range from education about discharge care plans and medications in the inpatient setting to the patient's checking and documenting daily assessment of signs and symptoms from work or home. Further, care providers are using IPC technology to send daily reminders about taking medications or the need for follow-up visits with the physician when data and input from the patient indicate the need to do so.

The use of this innovative technology in and of itself serves to evaluate patient capacity and likelihood of compliance while creating new efficiencies for nursing. There are many forms of technology and many applications available today for clinicians and the health consumer to manage their health. The most effective use of technology is one that enables patient engagement through personalized, dynamic, and purposeful interaction between the care team and the patient. IPC technology has emerged as a powerful means to facilitate patients' responsibility for their own care management by providing the tools and resources the patients need to understand their conditions, keep track of their medications, make their daily care interventions routine, and remain current and informed on their health statuses.

IPC technology is also designed to foster two-way communication between patients and their care teams. It enables clinicians to monitor patient health status over time, to make changes in patients' care plans based upon dynamic feedback from the patients, and to allow for real-time or rapid interventions that will boost patients' ability to improve and maintain their health statuses.

Meaningful use of technology will enable more informed collaborative decisions about patients' care needs. The increasing interoperability of technology allows for the merging of information and data to create a more continuous, complete picture of patients' health, and competency in complying with and responding to their care plans. The ability to integrate and interface technologies allows clinicians to capture data in real time from home monitoring devices, patient input, and patient activity, which informs the need for changes to care plans or new interventions that will boost patients' response to care interventions.

One exciting application of this technology can be seen in the work being done by Florida Hospital Celebration Health, in partnership with GetWellNetwork (Knych, 2013). They utilized a four-phase interactive heart-failure care plan built on the principles of patient activation to proactively engage and activate heart-failure patients to best prepare them to manage their condition once discharged. See the accompanying sidebar for further information.

An Application of Patient Activation Measure

Florida Hospital Celebration Health has been leveraging bedside technology and an interactive patient care delivery model to reduce heart-failure readmissions 30 days post-discharge. Recognizing the importance of patient engagement in care management, Celebration Health embarked on a project to implement a new program of patient activation and assess its impact, particularly on reducing readmissions. This 182-bed hospital is known as a pioneer in many areas of healthcare delivery, bringing best practice and many "firsts" to the industry as it continually leverages people, processes, and technology to advance the quality and safety of care it provides.

In this project, Celebration Health utilized a four-phase interactive heart-failure care plan available through GetWellNetwork, an interactive patient-care technology solution, to proactively engage and activate heart-failure patients to best prepare them to manage their condition once discharged. GetWellNetwork is available at the bedside through the patient's in-room television and navigated through use of an integrated pillow speaker and/or wireless keyboard. The Interactive Heart Failure Care plan, prescribed by the cardiologist and activated by the nurse at the bedside once a diagnosis is confirmed, begins with an explanation of the patient's diagnosis and care plan and the use of the PAM (developed by Dr. Judith Hibbard) to establish a baseline patient activation level. An Interactive Heart-Failure Care Plan is developed that the patient and family or caregiver can move through at their own pace, enabling the patient to learn and absorb what is necessary to manage this condition and health status as the patient is ready.

This Interactive Heart-Failure Care Plan structures teaching, evaluates understanding, and measures patient competency in monitoring this condition and taking action to control symptoms and condition flare-up. The four phases include education for the patient and family about the condition, medications, symptoms to watch for, and early warning signs. The care plan includes education and resources to help the patient develop a plan and comply with necessary lifestyle changes in diet, fluid intake, exercise, and medication compliance. At the end of each education session, the patient completes a comprehensive questionnaire. Throughout the care plan, there are checkpoints for the clinical team to assess the patient's competency in managing the condition, and at the end of each phase, there is a recap of what the patient has learned and completed during that session. During the final phase, often completed just before discharge, the patient is educated on how to cope with any needed changes in lifestyle and a post-intervention assessment of the patient's activation level is completed.

Findings from this innovative approach to reducing heart-failure readmissions are impressive. They include a significant increase in the level of patient activation and a corresponding decrease in heart-failure readmissions 30 days post-discharge of almost 50% in those patients with a higher activation level following completion of the care plan.

Interactive Patient Care Technology: Advancing Nursing Practice

IPC technology is advancing nursing practice in several ways. This innovative technology creates new efficiencies by automating important nursing activities and responsibilities, such as patient teaching and comprehension assessment, pain assessments, medication teaching, and documentation of results. The interactivity and use of mobile technology enables real-time interaction and communication with the patient, regardless of location, fostering and enabling a more longitudinal, consultative relationship with the patient. Increasingly, IPC technology employs algorithms to automatically prescribe standard care paths or data-triggered care interventions, creating greater consistency and standardization in care. The experience of utilizing IPC technology is also an effective way to continuously evaluate patient capability and likely compliance with the care regime.

The use and application of IPC technology will continue to advance. It can be leveraged in ways that support the advancement of nursing practice while creating efficiencies in workflow that have a very positive effect on nursing satisfaction and operational effectiveness.

Nursing's Role in Patient Engagement

Nursing has always been and will always be about the relationship and interaction with the patient. Traditionally, nursing care has been centered on episodic care management. Efforts to engage the patient and the family occurred primarily by educating them about the condition and care plan during an episode of care. Today, new payment models are requiring a shift away from an episodic approach to care management to a model of care that is continuous, longitudinal, and centered on managing the health of the patient over time rather than at one point in time (Drenkard, 2014). As this shift occurs, the role of nursing must evolve as well. In a population health management model, nurses must take on the important role of activating patients to assume more responsibility for their health statuses and continuing health management. This requires different skills, resources, and an expanded viewpoint about the nurse's interaction with the patient.

Nursing care is no longer just about stabilizing and supporting patients' health needs while in our direct care. The role of nursing must move beyond the traditional approach to managing care to a role that is more consultative—guiding and leading patients to better health for themselves. This advanced role requires even more emphasis on a relationship-based care model. To be effective in activating patients, nurses must be able to better assess and understand patient beliefs, values, and needs. They must be able to influence patients rather than completing patient care interventions for them.

Nurses must also have the ability to assess patients' levels of motivation to care for themselves, their understanding of their conditions and care plans, and their competency in knowing what, when, and how to manage their health. The nurse must have the time and resources to ensure adequate education and comprehension assessment. The nurse must have tools that measure and demonstrate patients' likelihood and ability to care for themselves. They must have the skill and knowledge to design care plans that are based upon what they have learned and assessed about patients' levels of activation, their response to their care plans, and their resulting health statuses.

Nursing serves an important role in creating and building patient interest and motivation and in creating a level of activation that results in increased patient involvement and responsibility in managing health over time rather than one episode a time. That means that the role of the nurse will become less transactional and more focused on supporting continuity through an interactive, continuing patient care management model.

To be most effective in engaging patients, and particularly in activating patients, the nursing role must evolve and advance. The need for change and adaptation is certainly not new to our profession. However, there is a pivotal opportunity today to shift the role of the nurse away from a more task-oriented, episodic, care management function to one that is more centered on building, sustaining a care management relationship with a population of patients with the effective use of IPC technology. This shift in the nursing role requires an advanced set of skills. It requires more time in care planning and adaptation, and it necessitates a different mindset for the nurse and other members of the care team about the patient's versus the provider's role.

The nurse of the future must have the skills, resources, and work environment to enable and support a continuous approach to managing the health of patients. The nurse's care of patients who are part of an assigned or attributed population needs to be continuous rather than episodic. There is a need for efficiencies and interoperability of technologies and information in order to make better informed decisions and in order to scale and deliver care in a cost-effective manner.

To that end, there is a need to establish a nursing model that employs and leverages the nurse's critical thinking skills within a relationship-based care delivery environment. We must determine and design changes in clinical (and specifically nursing) practice to effectively and continuously assess the level of activation and the ability for patients (and their families) to care for themselves. The role of the nurse will move from "doing for" the patient to focusing on managing health with the patient. The Nursing Alliance for Quality Care (NAQC) released *Guiding Principles for Patient Engagement,* a list of core principles designed to support nurses and other healthcare providers in delivering high-quality, patient-centered care. These principles are outlined in accompanying sidebar.

Guiding Principles for Patient Engagement

"1. There must be an active partnership among patients, their families, and the providers of their healthcare.

2. Patients are the best and ultimate source of information about their health status and retain the right to make their own decisions about care.

3. *In this relationship, there are shared responsibilities and accountabilities among the patient, the family, and clinicians that make it effective.*

4. *While embracing partnerships, clinicians must nevertheless respect the boundaries of privacy, competent decision making, and ethical behavior in all their encounters and transactions with patients and families. These boundaries protect recipients as well as providers of care. This relationship is grounded in confidentiality, where the patient defines the scope of the confidentiality.*

5. *This relationship is grounded in an appreciation of patient's rights and expands on the rights to include mutuality. Mutuality includes sharing of information, creation of consensus, and shared decision making.*

6. *Clinicians must recognize that the extent to which patients and family members are able to engage or choose to engage may vary greatly based on individual circumstances, cultural beliefs and other factors.*

7. *Advocacy for patients who are unable to participate fully is a fundamental nursing role. Patient advocacy is the demonstration of how all of the components of the relationship fit together.*

8. *Acknowledgment and appreciation of culturally, racially or ethnically diverse backgrounds is an essential part of the engagement process.*

9. *Health care literacy and linguistically appropriate interactions are essential for patient, family, and clinicians to understand the components of patient engagement. Providers must maintain awareness of the language needs and health care literacy level of the patient and family and respond accordingly."*

Source: Sofaer & Schumann, 2013

The release of the principles is the first component of the alliance's effort to enhance nurses' attitudes and behaviors that foster the engagement of patients in their care. During 2013, NAQC discussed how to implement the principles with the nation's leading nursing organizations, patient advocates, and other provider groups. More information is available at www.naqc.org.

Barriers and Challenges to Increasing Patient Engagement

In all the early literature describing patient engagement and the models to improve patients' participation in their care process, it is clear that the provider must adopt interventions, attitudes, and behaviors to support and encourage patients to become more engaged. However, there are barriers and challenges to increasing patient engagement. These barriers include (Friedberg, Van Busum, Wexler, Bowen, & Schneider, 2013; Legare & Witteman, 2013):

- **Primary care provider's time constraints**: The need for increased access is stressing the time limits during and between primary care visits, and as a result, there is less time for visits and for patient-engagement interventions. Technology may assist in overcoming this barrier as primary care providers serve as a referral source for technology supports that may help patients access increased information and knowledge.

- **Insufficient provider training**: The fundamental shift for care providers to move from providers of care "doing to" to a strong shared decision-making model where patients are active and engaged participants in their care decisions requires that providers be educated about patient engagement. Providers may not have the latest information about how to assess patient-engagement levels and may not know what interventions are available to patients to increase their participation in their care processes.

- **Inadequate clinical information systems**: Although there is a systematic push for increased information systems in healthcare, there are still widely inconsistent levels of adoption of IT systems across the United States.

- **Patient willingness and lack of knowledge**: The benefits of patient engagement and patient activation are emerging and seem favorable to patient outcomes, but there are patient barriers as well. These include inability and unwillingness of certain patients for various reasons to actively engage in their care. Such factors to be considered include health literacy, health disparities, socioeconomic considerations, and level of interest in engaging in care.

- **Clinical situations**: Patient clinical situations clearly affect patients' ability to be engaged in their care. Patient-engagement models for all level of acuity and disease conditions will need to be developed.

Although the barriers may seem formidable, the work of the interprofessional team needs to be focused on identifying those barriers and working together to overcome them. The team needs to develop a strategy to systematically overcome any barriers to more actively involving patients in their own healthcare journeys.

Patient Engagement and Population Health

As our industry shifts to more of a population health management model and as providers assume risk for the cost and efficiency of care delivery, it is more important than ever to strengthen patients' role in managing their own health as a means to increase compliance with their care plans. As the population ages, the prevalence of chronic conditions also increases. Today, nearly 75% of all healthcare expenditures are related to management of chronic conditions that can often be controlled through lifestyle changes and better management of health behaviors, which require patient activation (Centers for Disease Control and Prevention [CDC], 2009).

Patient activation will be a key to reducing the cost of healthcare over time.

In a white paper on "Provider-Based Patient Engagement: An Essential Strategy for Population Health" (Phytel, 2012), the authors argue that patient engagement is essential for improved health outcomes. A variety of interventions, including technology tools, will be critical to increasing engagement of patients in their care. In particular, chronic disease management, complicated treatment protocols, lifestyle requirements, and managing as the leader of the care process all make for a heavy burden on patients. Emerging outcomes identified that patients who are engaged and active in their care have better outcomes and lower cost of care.

A population healthcare management model requires a more informed and dynamic relationship with the patient. It requires access to and interpretation of more extensive, real-time data in order to make informed and rapid changes in care plans to avoid unnecessary utilization of more expensive services. It requires an assessment of the physical, social, emotional, and behavioral attributes of the patient in order to fully understand the factors that will motivate the patient to remain responsible for care management.

Conclusion

To move to a full model of patient engagement, the provision of nursing care needs to change to more fully engage and activate patients. Nurses cannot solely, and in isolation, provide care to patients. Our role is changing, and we must work to more actively engage patients in managing their care based on their individual needs, beliefs, values, and preferences. To truly engage patients, we need a whole new mind-set of our role, moving from provider of care to partner in care.

As this shift to increased patient control of their care occurs, the role of nursing must evolve as well. As we move to a population health management model, nursing must take on the important role of activating patients to assume more responsibility for their care, health statuses, and continuing health management.

This is a fundamental shift in nursing practice. As nurses, we are going to need to develop and utilize improved tools to help us assess a patient's state of engagement and then implement a plan to improve that level of engagement. Patient engagement is a key factor to improving quality, obtaining better patient clinical and satisfaction outcomes, and managing population health.

References

Balik, B., Conway, J., Zipperer, L., & Watson, J. (2011). Achieving an exceptional patient and family experience of inpatient hospital care. IHI Innovation Series white paper. Cambridge, MA: Institute for Healthcare Improvement.

Carman, K. L., Dardess, P., Maurer, M., Sofaer, S., Adams, K., Bechtel, C., & Sweeney, J. (2013). Patient and family engagement: A framework for understanding the elements and developing interventions and policies. *Health Affairs, 32*(2), 223-229.

Center for Advancing Health (CFAH). (2013). What is patient engagement? Retrieved from http://www.cfah.org/engagement/

Centers for Disease Control and Prevention (CDC). (2009). Chronic disease prevention and health promotion. Chronic diseases: The power to prevent, the call to control: At a glance 2009. Retrieved from http://www.cdc.gov/chronicdisease/resources/publications/aag/chronic.htm

Centers for Medicare & Medicaid Services (CMS). (2013). Meaningful use. Retrieved from http://www.cms.gov/Regulations-and-Guidance/Legislation/EHRIncentivePrograms/Meaningful_Use.html

Coulter, A. (2011). Engaging patients in healthcare. New York, NY: McGraw-Hill Education.

Drenkard, K. (2014). Patient engagement: Essential partnerships to improve outcomes. *Journal of Nursing Administration, 44*(1), 3-4. doi:10.1097/NNA.0000000000000022

Friedberg, M. W., Van Busum, K., Wexler, R., Bowen, M., & Schneider, E. C. (2013). A demonstration of shared decision making in primary care highlights barriers to adoption and potential remedies. *Health Affairs, 32*(2), 268-275.

Gruman, J., Rovner, M. H., French, M. E., Jeffress, D., Sofaer, S., Shaller, D., & Prager, D. J. (2010). From patient education to patient engagement: Implications for the field of patient education. *Patient Education and Counseling, 78*(3), 350-356.

Hibbard, J. H., & Greene, J. (2013). What the evidence shows about patient activation: Better health outcomes and care experiences: Fewer data on costs. *Health Affairs, 32*(2), 207-214.

Hibbard, J. H., Greene, J., & Overton, V. (2013). Patients with lower activation associated with higher costs: Delivery systems should know their patients' scores. *Health Affairs, 32*(2), 216-219.

Hibbard, J. H., Mahoney, E. R., Stockard, J., & Tusler, M. (2005). Development and testing of a short form of the patient activation measure. *Health Services Research, 40*(6), 1918-1930.

Knych, S. A. (2013). Committing to the one constant of care: The patient. *Transformative health: Expert insights into the future of health care.* GetWellNetwork, Inc. Retrieved from http://www.celebrationhealth.com/digital_assets/TransformativeHealthTrailblazers.pdf

Legare, F., & Witteman, H. O. (2013). Shared decision making: Examining key elements and barriers to adoption into routine clinical practice. *Health Affairs, 32*(2), 276-284.

National Priorities Partnership. (2008). *National priorities and goals: Aligning our efforts to transform America's healthcare.* Washington, DC: National Quality Forum.

National Priorities Partnership. (2010). *Patient & family engagement convening meeting synthesis report.* Washington, DC: National Quality Forum. Retrieved from https://www.qualityforum.org/Publications/2010/05/Patient_and_Family_Engagement_Convening_Meeting_Synthesis_Report.aspx

National Quality Forum (NQF). (2013a). Person- and family-centered care. Retrieved from https://www.qualityforum.org/Topics/Patient_and_Family_Engagement.aspx

National Quality Forum (NQF). (2013b). Person and family centered care measures. Retrieved from https://www.qualityforum.org/projects/person_family_centered_care/

National Quality Forum (NQF). (2013c). Prioritizing measure gaps: Person-centered care and outcomes. Retrieved from https://www.qualityforum.org/projects/prioritizing_measures/person_centered_care/

Phytel. (2012). Provider-based patient engagement: An essential strategy for population health. Retrieved from http://www3.phytel.com/Libraries/Whitepaper-PDFs/Provider-Based-Patient-Engagement---An-Essential-Strategy-for-Population-Health.sflb.ashx

Sandy, L. G., Tuckson, R. V., & Stevens, S. L. (2013). United Healthcare experience illustrates how payers can enable patient engagement. *Health Affairs, 32*, 1440-1445.

Sofaer, S., & Schumann, M. J. (2013). Guiding principles for patient engagement. *Fostering successful patient and family engagement: Nursing's critical role.* George Washington School of Nursing, Washington, DC: Nursing Alliance for Quality Care (NAQC). Retrieved from http://www.naqc.org/WhitePaper-PatientEngagement

Chapter 8

Cultivating Mindful and Compassionate Connections

Mary Koloroutis, MSN, RN
Michael Trout, MA

"I am finding that I have a choice in every moment to keep my heart open or closed, to live in love or in fear. More than any specific practice, I have found that maintaining this awareness of choice is the most important factor in keeping an open heart, for every action, every thought, every moment contains the potential for bringing us closer to either connection and healing or isolation and suffering."

–Dean Ornish, MD (1997, p. 99)

A young nurse manager (in his late 20s, at the most) came in early for his shift, hoping to get some extra work done. He was quickly shuttled into a room in which a patient's son was "dropping the F-bomb" over and over. His mother had sickle cell anemia, and she was in severe pain. The young nurse manager already heard at the nurses' station that a mistake had been made in pharmacy, delaying the arrival of the much-needed pain meds. The son, who had been called by the patient, who wanted him with her, was worried when he found his mother in so much pain, but furious when he discovered that the delay was due to a clinician's error.

The manager and the nurse who had been taking care of the mother divided responsibilities: He would talk with the patient and son while she pursued the problem in pharmacy. His first instinct was to do whatever it took to quiet this man and defuse the situation, and he was feeling defensive and somewhat protective of the nurse who had been caring for the patient and had taken the brunt of this man's rough treatment. But something allowed him to go one step further. Something allowed him not to get caught up in the chaos and the rage and to avoid defensiveness. Instead, he "got it." Something shifted in him, and he thought, "If she were my mom, I would be feeling the same way." He actually heard the pain of this son whose helplessness to relieve his mom of pain made him flail. The young manager's internal shift enabled him to become a sturdy presence for both the young man and his mother. He spoke kindly and gently to both of them. He let them know that he was going to stay right there until the medication arrived and that the nurse was "on it" with the pharmacy.

The nurse manager never resorted to directing the son to quiet down, but, mysteriously, he did. The three of them sat together. Everyone's anxiety subsided, and peace returned to the room. The mother and son talked openly about how difficult it had been, and the young manager offered them nothing more and, more importantly, nothing less than his attuned and compassionate presence.

When it was all done and the medication arrived, the son followed the manager into the hallway, thanked him, and hugged him. He said, "I know I was out of line, but I couldn't stand it anymore."

The people in our care need us, it turns out. Certainly they need us to carry out instrumental care with precision and competence. But they need us, too. They need us to be present with them as people, just as the nurse manager was there for the mother and son in the preceding vignette. We as nurses achieve this presence through the practice of attunement. Through our own open-hearted attunement to others, we create a field in which connection can happen. Within that field, when we apply three practices—wondering, following, and holding—connection does happen.

Our attunement creates a sense of connection and, therefore, security. Our wondering on their behalf allows us to pick up on cues essential to the provision of safe, person-centered care (accurate nursing diagnoses, inviting cooperation through clear communication in which we partner with patients in their care, and noticing modest shifts in the patient's state). Our authentic presence, particularly when combined with our devotion to listening closely and to following the cues that our patients provide, allows patients to relax, to regulate themselves, to demand less, and to report greater satisfaction with their care. When we are present and attuned, wondering and conveying genuine interest, and following their cues, our patients and their loved ones feel seen and held in our care.

This chapter defines and describes these elements of a therapeutic relationship and demonstrates how transformational a commitment to this elevated level of care can become in an organization. We begin by introducing Relationship-Based Care as a framework that helps align the organization's commitment to person- and family-centered care (P&FCC) with a culture that supports it. We suggest that something as simple as mindfulness about how nurses connect with others can transform the experience of patients and the experience of clinicians. And, finally, we tell stories about the efficacy of this sort of practice in real-life, chaotic, time-pressured environments.

Reflection on the Vignette

In the midst of his busy and demanding day, and caught quite off-guard, how had this young clinician, described in the vignette at the beginning of this chapter, managed not to take any of it personally? How was he so able to get himself out of the way and focus his thoughts and care instead on the patient and her son? When he shared this story, weeks later, still in wonder about the whole thing, he told us that it was as if something came over him, allowing him to see the son. He saw this man's outrage for what it really was: pain coming from his love for his mother, pushing through a powerful desire to help her, mixed with utter hopelessness at not being able to do so.

How is it possible to emulate this nurse manager's behavior in our everyday work as clinicians? Are we required to "take it" when patients or family members blow up or we experience them as uncooperative or demanding? What facilitated the internal shift that resulted in this young manager's being able to see the fear and helplessness behind the angry behavior? Was the manager's capacity for compassion unique to his personality, or is it something that can be learned and practiced by any clinician? And what does any of this have to do with the provision of nursing care? What difference does it really make?

We have come to see that it makes all the difference. Just as a distracted or misattuned parent changing his baby's diaper is soon greeted by escalating efforts on the part of the baby to get him to become present, so do vulnerable patients escalate efforts to assure that they are seen. And just as these babies eventually give up and disengage, our patients may do the same. A patient who feels misunderstood, unseen, disregarded, or under-attended-to will seek to rectify that situation in a variety of ways, many of which will become disruptive or disheartening for us.

Relationship-Based Care

Relationship-Based Care (RBC) is a philosophical and operational framework that creates a sense of connection throughout an organization. RBC is customized to reflect each organization's unique mission, purpose, and values, so that all caregivers can align and engage in authentic connection with the patients and families in their care. Because RBC is an organization-wide initiative, the term *caregiver* is expanded to include everyone in the organization engaged in the care of patients and families. In an RBC setting, it is common for people in such departments as laundry, engineering, and dietary services to see themselves as being in direct service to patients and their loved ones. Those implementing RBC in organizations all over the world have consistently seen that a cultural transformation must be inclusive if it is to be sustainable, and that a caring and healing culture recognizes and values the contribution of every member of the team (Koloroutis, 2004).

RBC is a philosophy (a way of being) and a methodology (a way of doing) that strengthens three key relationships in an organization:

- **Relationship with self:** Compassion for others begins with an acceptance and compassion for self. This comes through cultivating self-awareness and self-care. This balances us as caregivers, which enables us to bring an attuned and healing presence to others.

- **Relationships with colleagues:** Healthy colleague relationships are built on trust, mutual respect, consistent and visible support, and open and honest communication. These healthy relationships lead to improved patient safety and an engaged and committed work team.

- **Relationships with patients and their families:** Compassionate therapeutic relationships with patients and their loved ones are the central relationships. When we care for ourselves and cultivate healthy and committed teamwork, we create environments in which relationships with patients and families thrive.

Figure 8.1 shows an illustration of the RBC model.

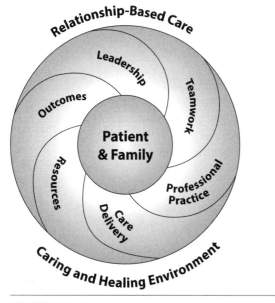

FIGURE 8.1

A Model of Relationship-Based Care. Reprinted with permission of Creative Health Care Management.

The RBC framework and principles help us bring our full attention and skills to the privileged work of connecting authentically with patients and their loved ones as the unique people they are. It provides the culture and infrastructure that empower us to customize our care to what each individual patient and family member teaches us about who they are and what this experience of care means to them.

The most profound gift of RBC is that it creates the conditions for every person in the organization to use time more intentionally and proactively to forge authentic human connections with patients, families, and their team members.

The therapeutic relationship is the heart of RBC. Although therapeutic relationships can and do occur in all healthcare cultures, it is notable that taking time to listen deeply, spending adequate time to inform and prepare patients, and offering your attuned, unhurried presence to a frightened patient are far more likely to happen when a culture actively encourages and supports such actions.

Human Caring Research and Theory

Swanson conducted three sequential research studies to develop a mid-range theory of caring (1991). Swanson says that her research was motivated by the lack of a universal conceptualization of caring. The result of this void was a significant limitation to teaching about caring, evaluating its effectiveness, and consistently bringing it to life in the nursing care of people.

The population for the first study was 20 women who had recently miscarried. The research question that guided the study was, "What constitutes caring in the instance of miscarriage?" The outcome of the miscarriage study was the identification of five caring processes:

- Knowing
- Being With
- Doing For
- Enabling
- Maintaining Belief

Two follow-up studies included clinicians and parents caring for neonates in the neonatal intensive care unit (NICU) and young at-risk mothers being cared for in a public health setting. The subsequent studies served to validate and refine the definitions and the subdimensions of the five caring processes.

Swanson's theory has been foundational to the work presented in the *See Me as a Person* book and workshop and to the evolution of the therapeutic practices. Both of those resources present the therapeutic practices as a means to bring the caring processes to life, as the practices are both a way of thinking and tangible behaviors to put into action. The therapeutic practices align with the five processes as follows:

- **Presence through Attunement:** Being With
- **Wondering:** Knowing, Enabling, Maintaining Belief
- **Following:** Knowing, Doing For, Enabling
- **Holding:** Knowing, Doing For, Enabling, Maintaining Belief

Knowing

It is curious to note that what Swanson (2007) calls *Knowing*, she goes on to describe as "trying to avoid assumptions about patients…. [I]t means that we check out what we know and find out if it happens to be true for this individual" (p. 324). The pathway to *Knowing* is by recognizing that *we do not know,* and that the sense of not knowing is what propels those of us who are intent on forging therapeutic relationships to *wonder* and *follow* with our patients. We begin with a genuine curiosity and interest in the other and gain understanding by suspending our own agendas and allowing the patients to instead teach us. We remember that wisdom does not come from what we already know; it comes from discovering what we do not know.

Being With

Swanson (1991) describes *Being With* as "being emotionally present with another" (p. 162). *Attuning* is a mindful action that leads us to the state of being emotionally present. When we *attune,* we intentionally "tune in" to the person in front of us. We consciously focus on the other with an understanding that such undivided attention is crucial for therapeutic connection.

Doing For

Doing For is described as "doing for the patient what they would do for themselves if it were possible, but not doing more than that" (Swanson, 1991, p. 162). We can only do for others by *following* their lead; otherwise, we would be uninformed about what is effective and therapeutic and what is not. *Doing For* also requires that we *hold* the other with respect and dignity, recognizing that physical contact must be recognized as privileged and sacred.

Enabling

Swanson (1991) describes *Enabling* as "facilitating the other's passage through difficult events and life transitions" (p. 162). The way we can facilitate another's passage is through *following* their lead and supporting their capacity to cope. It requires determining what matters most to them by *wondering* about who they uniquely are and what this experience means to them and to their loved ones. And of course it requires that we advocate for them, inform them consistently, and involve them in all care decisions. These are all acts of *holding.*

Maintaining Belief

Finally, Swanson (1991) describes *Maintaining Belief* as "sustaining faith in the capacity of patients to get through an event or transition and face the future with meaning" (p. 162). This requires that we maintain a state of *wondering.* It means that we recognize that every person has a backstory, a life beyond what we can begin to comprehend during this brief care experience.

When we *wonder,* we stay open and compassionate about the person and are less likely to engage in judgments and assumptions. When we honor the inherent dignity of each person, we are *holding* them in our care.

NOTE

Swanson's work, along with the work of others on the neurobiology of attunement and human attachment, has been a source of inspiration for the *See Me as a Person* work. Concepts as simple as Being With are a fundamental aspect of caring; and still, we struggle sometimes with how to do that. The work of forging therapeutic relationships using the therapeutic practices invites us to consider, for example, that attuning is an action word. This action, therefore, can be taught, modeled, and felt. The practice of attuning to another is a method and discipline that can be cultivated, refined, and deepened.

Attunement and Human Attachment

Consider the following:

A father sits with his agitated, all-adults-are-SO-stupid adolescent daughter. She is an adoptee with developmental delays and mild autism. She is angry most of the time, and she rages against the limits the family tries to impose on her out-of-control behavior. He says he wants to tell her a story. Usually she hates even hearing her parents talk, but something about her dad's demeanor seems different tonight, so she softens momentarily. She agrees when he asks whether she would mind lying on her bed (a favorite place of hers), while he sits on a chair beside the bed. They do not look at each other as the dad begins his story—one that is based on a dream he has just had about his precious little girl.

He says that in his dream she was just a tiny speck, and she was inside a place that was tight, enclosed, and wet—sort of like a uterus. There were quite a number of other people there, too. Soon he realized that this was her first family (her biological family), but that none of them seemed aware that she was there among them. She seemed invisible to them. They were standing in a circle, but she was on the outside of the circle. She was very tiny, but he could see her, in his dream. No one else could.

The daughter lies quietly on her bed. A few tears roll down her cheeks. She hopes no one would notice.

For the next several days her attitude toward her parents and about herself seem changed. She is actually approachable. She leans on her dad's shoulder in the kitchen the next evening, and she tells her mom that dinner was good. The next night, at bedtime, she tells her father that his story is true; this is how it happened.

Who knows what prenatal life was like for this child, whose mom decided, in the 35th week of pregnancy, that she did not want her? Dad had no real facts. So what was it about this very simple story that brought on such profound behavior change?

The story probably did ring true for this little girl, but we wonder whether the overriding element in the interchange between dad and daughter was not the content of the story but the amazing level of presence and *attunement* this dad demonstrated when he sat beside his precious-but-rejecting daughter and told it to her.

At that moment, nothing else existed for the dad, and, to his amazement, this usually bouncing-off-the-wall daughter seemed fully present as well. He tuned in to the very soul of his girl before he ever even knew her—into a moment when some pretty significant damage was probably being done to her very being. And then he sat with her, years later, and talked about it. Our guess is that her tears were about feeling that her father was completely with her. Maybe she could even wonder what it would have been like if he had been with her back then.

That's the way human connection seems to work. We actually enter each other's worlds. We regulate each other's emotions. A nurse enters a world of chaos on the unit, palpates that world, and begins to "tune in" to what is actually happening. If she gets it right, she finds that her attunement to the situation gives her information about what the problem really is. Then her attunement to an individual at the heart of it tells her what that person needs and why he is creating such a ruckus (or pressing the call light 10 times per hour). Then she delivers her*self*, creating a connection with the patient that brings calm and restores neurological regulation to the person who was so out of control. The patient becomes available for healing again. That's the power of attunement. That's the power of nursing.

The Therapeutic Relationship

To be *therapeutic* (from the Greek *therapeuein*) is to minister or attend to another. To be in a *therapeutic relationship* with another means to establish a connection with the other for the purpose of ministering or attending to that person (therapeutic, n.d.).

Such a relationship, of course, is not merely social, because it has a specific purpose (to minister, to attend to another). It is not reciprocal, in the social sense. It rises above the usual rules of social exchange. Nothing is expected in return. It is, therefore, not easy; you may even conclude that it is not "natural." But it makes possible the acceptance, on the part of the patient, of astonishing and really quite shocking demands that nurses make, such as our asking total strangers to take off their clothes.

What would it be like if we asked in words what we so often ask silently of our patients? For example:

- "Allow me to cause you great pain."
- "Lie there quietly, trusting that I will not abandon you when I walk away to be with others."

The unique nature of the relationship we have with patients makes possible the acceptance, on the part of the clinician, of astonishing behavior in the patient as well. Resistance, anger, regression, neediness, and demandingness need not be the "last straw" for us; they are instead symptoms, reasons to wonder.

The practices subsumed under the notion of a therapeutic relationship are imminently practical. They are not additions to your workload. They are a *way of being,* a state of mind with respect to the patient, that will actually ease your burden, increase your efficacy, and allow you to make contact, every day, with the reasons you became a caregiver. These practices are not tasks; they are a way of thinking, understanding, and acting, even in the face of the most-challenging human responses to illness and trauma. When patients experience you in attunement with them, they may be surprised; they may feel comforted. Their confidence in you, and, therefore, their cooperation, may actually increase. You have done nothing extra; it has taken no more time. It's just that you did what you normally do with a slightly different emphasis: You were fully *present,* you *wondered*, you *followed*, you *held*. You did the four things that allow human beings to experience connection with each other.

Presence Through Attunement

A therapeutic relationship, in contrast with everyday, social engagements, requires a particularly high level of presence. Just as we do when we minister to our babies, when we engage in a therapeutic relationship with a patient, we bring our fullest attention, our complete empathy, a kind of disregard for our own needs at the moment, a willingness to suspend wherever our heart happens to be at the moment. We do this so we can be fully *with* the patient. And when we are fully present, the patient experiences us not merely as dispensers of instrumental care but as available, accessible, trustworthy caregivers who understand him and who will look after him because we have *seen* him.

A therapeutic relationship, in contrast with everyday, social engagements, is characterized by a strange connection we call *attunement.* When we are in a state of attunement with another, we find we can read their cues; perhaps we can more easily catch on to pain status, emotional responses, even neurological responses, or rising fear or anger. The patient feels comfortable because he senses our capacity for palpation. And we are able to use ourselves to actually regulate the patient's emotional state.

Wondering

A therapeutic relationship, in contrast with everyday, social engagements, is characterized by *wonder* on our part. We agree, for the sake of ministering or attending to another, to commit ourselves to a state of open-minded curiosity about the patient. We do not presume to know more than we do (a scientifically documented trait of everyday exchanges, in which we make ourselves feel more comfortable by categorizing people, by comparing them to others who *seem* like them, so they appear more predictable to us) (Damasio, 1994; Siegel, 1999; Siegel, 2007).

When we engage in the therapeutic practice of *wonder,* we enter the room of every patient, every time, eager to learn from them, on this day, in this moment. We ask more open-ended questions than closed-ended questions. We are too genuinely curious to resort to "pat" questions that invite "pat" answers ("How are we feeling today?"…"Fine."). Instead, we choose questions that are meaningful, that will actually increase our fund of information about the patient, and that transmit to the patient that we are actually interested in them.

Following

A therapeutic relationship, in contrast with everyday, social engagements, is characterized by a commitment to the magical, complementary act of *following* the patient. This commitment suggests that we believe the patient is a capable guide to his own condition, even when he appears not to be. It suggests we believe we have an unusual capacity for palpation: We have, as clinicians, the wealth of experience (and the high level of sensitivity) required to allow us to "read" the room, to "feel" the patient, to hook onto the words and affect of the patient in ways that allow us a special knowing of the patient (or family member). Even more, we have the discipline needed (in contrast, again, with everyday, social interactions) to make us be quiet, to let the patient lead. Our ministering changes in accord with the perceived fears or other affective responses of the patient as well as our growing knowledge (we have, after all, already committed to *wondering*!) of the patient's history, culture, beliefs, and perspectives. The interaction adjusts itself along the way, in accord with what the patient has just said or done. The interview adapts itself to the new data emerging from the patient. We are not lost. We have a guide; our guide is our patient.

Holding

A therapeutic relationship, in contrast with everyday, social engagements, is characterized by a variety of acts of *holding.* Most of us can remember holding our children; if we are honest, we can also remember that there were days when we held…sort of (without real presence, without much intimacy, eager to move on, maybe even a little bored or agitated) and there were days when we *held.* On the days when we really held, we could feel our devotion to this child, and so could he. On those days, we were ready to defend him; we would go to bat for him; we somehow understood him better; and it was easy to remember exactly how thick he liked the peanut butter on his sandwich. In response to those days of real holding, the strangest thing happened to our children: They grew up confident, secure, and able to take on the world on their own terms.

On the unit, holding may mean remembering something a patient said the day before, which allows her to relax in the belief that you have her back. It may mean defending the patient at the nursing station, where it is clear a label has been appended to a human being to whom you have become devoted. Holding means being guided by what you have discovered through *attunement, wondering,* and *following*: making sure the young mom is covered when the residents come into the room, because you sense that someone may have once sexually misused her; or making eye contact with the patient who seems to be perseverating on the same questions, but who really just needs reassurance about tomorrow's procedure. Holding is what is accomplished invisibly when we pull up a chair for a moment, or make a physical connection, or really attend, each act requiring no additional time commitment on our part, but each one potentially resulting in the patient's feeling the way he did when he was young and vulnerable and scared, and someone who loved him ministered to him simply by holding him dear.

Applications in the Field

We set up a website at www.SeeMeAsAPerson.com as a resource to engage our colleagues in the field in conversations about the things that can make it difficult to remain therapeutic with patients and their families. We thought that some of the questions and answers found on our site might serve to bring the practices to life for you. Here is a sampling of the questions we have received:

- What would a therapeutic relationship look like when one person is angry beyond the ability to be soothed?

- When RNs and techs work together, the techs inevitably feel indignant no matter how you treat them. Can you think of anything I can do to make these relationships better?

- What are your thoughts concerning how to deal with healthcare workers who are detached and apathetic and do the bare minimum for patients and families?

- I find it very stressful to care for patients who do not trust my opinion. How can I stay present with people when I believe they are outright dismissing me?

Our answers to these questions are as specific as the questions themselves, yet we consistently find that the core of our advice is "attune, wonder, follow, and hold," simply because we have discovered that these guides never fail to help matters. Here are two more examples, this time with their complete answers.

Q&A: Perceiving a Family Member as Aggressive or Controlling

Question: I have trouble staying therapeutic when a patient is passive and his or her family member is aggressive and controlling. I find myself advocating for the patient, becoming a little defensive of my patient, and even subtly positioning myself against the family member.

Answer: It might be helpful to remember that you have probably just entered a family dynamic that has been operational for some time. You are not going to be able to change it, and in the short time you interact with the family system, you may not even come to understand it. But it may help you keep frustration and/or aggravation low to hold in mind that you are probably witnessing a version of how things have been for your patient for many years. It is the right thing to attend to your patient, even to advocate for your patient. But don't set as a goal straightening all these people out before discharge!

Use *wondering* to see what you can pick up about this family dynamic into which you have just walked. Replace judgment or aggravation with curiosity about it. Consider:

- What makes it work?
- Who are the key players, and what are their roles?
- Is the patient always this passive, or is there something about the patient's illness or the patient's state (vulnerability, for example) that brings out those characteristics of passivity?
- Does this dynamic arise out of an unspoken (but very clear) agreement between the patient and family member about who gets to be in charge or who gets taken care of or who controls the "gate" into the family?
- Is the family member always this assertive, controlling, or intrusive?
- What function might such behavior serve for the family?

As you *wonder,* remember that your aim is not to figure out the answers to these questions. *Wondering* is about *wondering;* it's not about finding answers or reaching conclusions. Just stay curious.

Use *following* to create a thoughtful question or statement:

- "I see that you're very worried about whether I'll be able to care for Pat. Tell me about your best experience in Pat's previous care?…Tell me about your worst experience!… Oh, my. I see why you might be watching so closely."
- "I see why you might be worried that Pat couldn't speak up well for himself."
- "I see why you would feel protective."

Then use *holding* to reassure, to show respect, to show that you have "caught on" to the family member's concern. If you perceive that the family member is overadvocating, perhaps answering for the patient when the patient could answer for herself, gently clarify why you need to hear directly from the patient on this particular question.

> **NOTE**
>
> As with other examples of using the therapeutic relationship, none of these actions needs to take even a moment of extra time. You do it while you're doing other things in the room. You don't do it as add-on behavior, but as the center of everything else you're doing with the patient.

Q&A: Staying Compassionate With Patients Suffering From Medical Issues Related to Alcoholism

Question: A patient comes to us with medical issues but is also suffering from alcoholism. He has been hospitalized many times in the past for medical issues, most related to his chronic alcoholism. The patient has gone through detoxification many times at our facility, and when he is discharged, he begins drinking again. The patient becomes combative during detoxification and is very verbally abusive toward the team caring for him. How do we ensure that we are not becoming angry and judgmental of this man and instead remain compassionate and caring for this human being who has entrusted us to care for him?

Answer: This is a tough one. You may be vomited upon, swung at, and cursed at by a (momentarily, at least) raving lunatic. You don't deserve this sort of treatment. The patient is not participating in or cooperating with his own treatment. It's maddening. How easy is it to have compassion for people whose own chronic behavior is the cause of their suffering and the suffering of countless others? In these instances, for many of us, judgment comes far more easily.

It may or may not help to know this, but each time you try to engage with this patient, you join a very large group of friends, partners, and family members who have nearly caused themselves head injury from ramming into this same wall, over and over.

You have already taken an enormously important first step in naming the problem. You did not name it "disrespect" or "rudeness," even though those labels seem to apply. You named the problem "alcoholism," and as soon as you used that word, answers began to emerge. Whether we like it or not (and certainly alcoholics don't like it and routinely deny it), alcoholics tend to have a few characteristics in common:

- They drink. (Hmmm…)
- They say they don't drink (or at least not excessively).
- When they have been drinking, they treat most people around them (including those they love) with utter disregard for human courtesy, much less love or respect.
- They neglect their health, eat badly, forget to eat or take certain meds, yell, neglect many of their responsibilities, and act badly even toward people they really love.
- They drink. (Did we already say that?)

We mentioned "they drink" twice because it turns out that an obvious-but-elusive truth is contained therein. Quite naturally (but irrationally, as it turns out), we sometimes expect people not to be who they are. In an Al-Anon meeting, it is commonplace for new members to go on about the drinking and drinking-related behaviors of their partners. Usually everyone is quiet for a while, until finally one of the more seasoned members states the obvious: "Yup, drunks drink."

For some, this is truly a revelation: not that their partners do indeed drink, but that the person living with this behavior is everlastingly surprised and reactive to the fact. Sometimes this is a moment of genuine healing, when a person decides to stop being surprised. This is not a moment of condoning the drinking, but a moment of deciding to stop being surprised and stop reacting.

We in healthcare are not spared this challenge. Alcoholism tends to come with certain features in addition to the drinking itself. Those features are as inevitable (and resistant to rational discourse, or healthcare education, impatience, irritation, or demand) as the drinking itself. These folks are going to be resistant, depressed, and withdrawn, and they are going to be Olympic gold medal champs at denial. And, as if we needed this to be more confusing and confounding, they will also occasionally be incredibly charming, compliant, and articulate. At these moments, we are at great risk of imagining that the other characteristics we saw just a few hours ago are not inherent and therefore may not return. We think: This person *can* be all the things we want him to be! At that moment, we just fell into the trap that the patient's partner, family member, or friend has likely fallen into a hundred times.

So what's the answer for the clinician caring for this person? Acceptance of our inability to make the patient behave better is a terrific first step. This can happen when we pause to *wonder:* Why is my patient acting this way? And then it dawns on us: She's acting this way because that is the nature of the illness she has. Hemophiliacs bleed. Alcoholics drink. At that moment of acceptance, we stop feeling obligated to take on the impossible work of changing the person's behavior, and our frustration can ease.

From there, it gets easier. We're less triggered, and we can focus on the few things we can do: to be *attuned* and compassionate, to show genuine interest by *following* the cues the patient gives us about who he is and what he is going through, and we can *hold* by remembering what he has taught us about who he is in this moment and consciously adjusting our care to meet his specific needs. We can accept this person for exactly who he is—a person suffering from alcoholism—rather than who we want or need him to be.

This doesn't mean we start liking the behaviors being exhibited, and we may still find ourselves susceptible to irritation, dismay, and even disgust. But there's an opening now, through which compassion might find its way into your heart and to your patient's experience of you. Although this won't cure him, it might make you both able to cope just a little better and open the possibility of genuine human connection.

Conclusion

It is very common for people hearing or reading about this work for the first time to say, "But don't we already do this?" And our response is, "Of course you do…when you are intentionally connecting with a person." In a clinician's best moments, he or she is *attuned, wondering, following,* and *holding.* After all, these practices are not things we made up; they are practices we have observed clinicians doing. They are practices that evolved from the research on human caring. They are the kind of interactions patients describe when they talk about truly feeling cared for. They are ways of thinking and being that we have noticed in ourselves and in each other in our most rewarding therapeutic relationships. These best practices that compose the therapeutic relationship are worth describing, reflecting upon, and talking about, because that is the only way they will become more visible, accessible, and formalized in our day-to-day healthcare cultures.

In our best therapeutic moments, when we as clinicians find ourselves *attuning, wondering, following,* and *holding,* we may or may not be fully cognizant that we are doing these things. If you are a natural or intuitive wonderer, for example, you may or may not be conscious of the power of that practice. And if you're not fully aware of it, it is also not available to you to mentor and teach others the practice itself or to help convey the importance it has to safe, quality care. For these reasons, it is essential that the therapeutic practices become visible, teachable, and concrete enough that we can hold each other responsible and accountable to "relational standards" in the same way we expect clinicians to meet technical standards.

Think back to the story that opened this chapter. The young nurse manager certainly had little time to devise a plan to get the irate family member to quiet down and "comply," and it's likely that no such plan would have worked anyway. Instead, in what he experienced as a moment of illumination, he found the wisdom to simply attend to the irate man's suffering. He saw him as a person, and everything shifted. Seeing the man as a person certainly didn't take any more time than any other action would have taken. In *attuning* to this man, he could see him for what he was: a son tormented by worry about his mother's suffering and who-knows-what-else. The young manager *wondered* what it would be like if he were in this man's shoes. He listened, and in his willingness to be led by what the man said and did, he *followed,* showing the man (although unintentionally) his devotion to his mother's care and the son's well-being. And in all these actions, the irate son saw that someone had his back. He felt *held,* perhaps for the first time in a long time. It is unlikely that the nurse manager will ever find out all the details of this man's backstory. The details do not matter. What matters is that he cared enough to wonder, and in so doing, he connected.

Lessons Learned Writing *See Me as a Person*

We learned a great many things during the dual adventure of writing See Me as a Person *and developing the* See Me as a Person *workshop, and here is some of what we learned:*

- *The provision of healthcare cannot be done effectively outside of human connection and relatedness.*
- *Empathy heals wounds.*
- *Attunement supports the patient's capacity to regulate himself, which improves healing, makes the tasks of data collection and administration of treatment more efficient, and makes our job easier.*
- *Patients and their loved ones have a great deal to teach us; without learning about them, we cannot provide high-quality care.*

- *The ultimate compliment to another human being—indeed, the ultimate intimacy—is to attune to him, thereby seeing and accepting him exactly where he is. Once that happens, we have a bond that significantly increases the likelihood of cooperation.*

- *Modern, technology-driven healthcare is marvelous, and at the same time, it's a potential impediment to human connection. It is up to us to make technology work for us in the service of human connection.*

- *The relational aspects of healthcare are as much a part of our discipline as the instrumental aspects. Healing is threatened if the relational aspect is missing (Koloroutis & Trout, 2012, pp. 380–381).*

References

Damasio, A. (1994). *Descartes' error: Emotion, reason and the human brain.* New York, NY: Quill.

Koloroutis, M. (Ed.). (2004). *Relationship-Based Care: A model for transforming practice.* Minneapolis, MN: Creative Health Care Management.

Koloroutis, M., & Trout, M. (2011). The "see me as a person" workshop: Four practices to improve quality, safety, and the patient experience. Minneapolis, MN: Creative Health Care Management.

Koloroutis, M., & Trout, M. (2012). *See me as a person: Creating therapeutic relationships with patients and their families.* Minneapolis, MN: Creative Health Care Management.

Ornish, D. (1997). *Love and survival: The scientific basis for the healing power of intimacy.* New York, NY: HarperCollins.

Siegel, D. (1999). *The developing mind: Toward a neurobiology of interpersonal experience.* New York, NY: The Guilford Press.

Siegel, D. (2007). *The mindful brain: Reflection and attunement in the cultivation of well-being.* New York, NY: W. W. Norton.

Swanson, K. M. (1991). Empirical development of a middle range theory of caring. *Nursing Research, 40*(3), 161–166.

Swanson, K. M. (2007). Caring made visible. In M. Koloroutis (Ed.), *Relationship-based care: Visions, strategies, tools and exemplars for transforming practice* (pp. 323–328). Minneapolis, MN: Creative Health Care Management.

therapeutic. (n.d.). m-w.com. Retrieved from http://www.merriam-webster.com/dictionary/therapeutic

Chapter 9

Hallmarks of a Culture of Patient- and Family-Centered Care in the Care Setting

Gwen D. Sherwood, PhD, RN, FAAN

Ten-month-old Lindy finally was sleeping at 8 p.m. after having serious surgery earlier that day in a large teaching hospital. Her tired, tense father stretched on the narrow fold-out bed beside her in the Pediatric ICU. Suddenly the light came on, and a perky voice greeted them, "Hi, I'm Kathy, your nurse here to assess Lindy and help you through the night." The father rubbed his eyes, squinting in the bright lights while Lindy began crying, softly at first and louder as the nurse worked with her.

The bandages covered almost all of her head; only her eyes, nearly swollen shut, were visible. It was a frightening sight, and the father remained concerned about what was normal post-operative progression. The nurse completed her check of vital signs and other assessments, turned out the light, and departed. The father quieted Lindy, comforting her as best he could through the tubes and bandages that surrounded her.

The scenario was repeated two more times over the next 2 hours as the nurse came in first to administer medication and then to check the IV. Finally, in total fatigue, the father asked the nurse, "Could we talk about what other things you will need to do tonight? Could we think about what things could be clustered together so that we do not have to awaken Lindy so often? What can we do to make this an easier night for all of us?"

In the current mainstream, patients and their families enter healthcare settings as guests; the environment, policies, and procedures are provider-centric and are often incongruent with patient and family preferences and needs. The hospital culture, familiar to healthcare workers, may feel like another world to patients. Providers become accustomed to the maze of hallways, constant noise, and shared, tight rooms, forgetting how strange the environment may feel to those who come for treatment and care. In addition:

- Physical design in many institutions gives little consideration to the impact on staff and even less consideration for how patients and families will navigate hallways and seek ways to be near their loved one.

- Orientation to help patients and families upon admission is often limited or hurried, and they are often treated as if they have no rights or opinions about their care.

- Schedules and procedures are set to accommodate staff rather than minimize impact on patients and their families, as described in the preceding vignette in which the nurse believed she was delivering patient-centered care, but the patient's father did not perceive it that way.

However, planning ahead could have minimized the disruption for Lindy and her father, there could have been discussion during the care transition on what care would be needed during the night, and goals could have been set for mutual benefit. A hospital culture based on patient- and family-centered care (P&FCC), or care that seeks to improve health through the eyes of the patient, would have provided a different experience for Lindy and her father.

The 2001 Institute of Medicine (IOM) report *Crossing the Quality Chasm: A New Health System for the 21st Century* identifies patient engagement as a key to P&FCC (IOM, 2001), with a direct link to quality and safety outcomes. Emerging evidence is further identified in the follow-up IOM report in 2003 (Greiner & Knebel, 2003); patient-centered care is one of the critical competencies for all health professionals in achieving optimal care and patient safety goals. Objectives to achieve patient-centered care are identified in the Quality and Safety Education for Nurses (QSEN) project (Cronenwett et al., 2007; Walton & Barnsteiner, 2012). This emphasis has led numerous organizations to issue white papers and resources to guide patients and families, healthcare workers, and organizations wishing to change (see the resources in the appendix toward the end of the book).

Regulations and payment systems are recalibrating to require considerations of patients and families in how hospitals are designed and operated. How does a philosophy of P&FCC affect the fundamental aspects of the patient experience, such as patient assessment, inclusion in care planning, information access, provider handovers, routing through ancillary departments, and the overall environmental design? This chapter explores the hallmarks of a culture of P&FCC and examines system changes for implementation. Successful models that demonstrate transformation in care delivery, environmental design, and orientation to patients and families, primarily based on Planetree and Picker Institute guidelines, offer ways to rescript how patients and families become partners in care in achieving overall goals for quality and safety.

Reconceptualizing Hospital Culture

Hospitals have largely followed the same structure and process of care delivery throughout modern times, with little consideration for the impact on patients. Some systems have reconsidered policies about family presence based on research, but in many situations, families may still feel unwelcome with few provisions for their comfort, may be excluded from decisions about care, and may not be allowed access to the patient's medical record (Frampton, Horowitz, & Stumpo, 2009). Admission is accomplished via a checklist; belongings are stashed as patients enter the chaotic hospital environment, and families are allowed limited access. Many hospitals have found it difficult to know how to improve the patient and family experience or, when they have improved, how to sustain the culture. It is clear that partnerships with patients at the clinical and organizational levels have developed slowly, and more educational preparation for both patients and providers is needed to improve results. Many leaders have employed an array of good ideas but lack the ability to foster a true culture change that integrates P&FCC into the strategic work of the hospital. What are the hallmarks of how nurses and other health professionals can help create the organizational culture, manage their own preparation, and include patients and families for an active role in their care? Transformation involves understanding the new mind-set about patient and family partnerships in care as well as reorienting organizational philosophy and operations, patient and family engagement in care, and changes in provider approaches.

Realigning Organizational Philosophy and Operations

Patient-centered care is a long-term commitment that drives organizational culture change by aligning an organization's values, strategies, and structures and engaging healthcare providers and patients in building and sustaining the culture. This shift in thinking may challenge long-held beliefs and practices providers hold about the intersection of patients and families with the healthcare delivery system and may require reflection on values clarification (Walton & Barnsteiner, 2012). Focus groups and surveys about hospital operations and philosophies are a first step to determine patient and provider priorities that address the needs of the communities served. Although the impetus for change sometimes arises in units or departments, achieving institutional culture change requires the support of organizational leadership to incorporate broad support to redesign physical environments, align institutional policies, and reinforce quality-improvement cycles that assess gaps so patients have a consistent experience across the system (Frampton & Guastello, 2010).

Patient and family inclusion in care planning involves a fundamental shift in corporate thinking about policies, procedures, and environmental design. Transformation to meet patient-centered goals means hospital administrators must understand the role of families in supporting the patient. Families bring personal knowledge of the patient, and their presence is often reassuring during the anxious, uncertain, vulnerable illness experience (Abraham & Moretz, 2012). Traditional hospital policies have restricted family presence and not fully included family in admission or discharge planning, even though their inclusion can ensure continuity in care for preexisting conditions or care for recovery from the current illness circumstance.

To build and operationalize a sustainable culture of patient-centered healthcare, hospitals must change traditional approaches and economic emphases that patients have come to expect and sometimes dread (Frampton, 2009). The Joint Commission (TJC, 2010) issued a roadmap for transforming organizations. *Advancing Effective Communication, Cultural Competence, and Patient and Family Centered Care: A Roadmap for Hospitals* describes ways hospitals can change specific operations, such as admission, assessment, end-of-life care, discharge, transfers, and organizational readiness. TJC further issued accreditation standards that ensure patients will be able to have a support person present throughout their hospital stay.

The Institute for Healthcare Improvement (IHI) has identified three core concepts required to develop the infrastructure needed to create partnerships between patients and providers and transform the patient and family experience (Balik, Conway, Zipperer, & Watson, 2011):

- Patients and families are treated with dignity and respect to honor patient and family perspectives, choices, knowledge, values, beliefs, and cultural backgrounds in care planning and delivery.

- Transparent, timely, complete, and accurate communication provides information to patients and families in affirming and helpful ways.

- Patients and families are invited and encouraged to participate in care and decision-making and are included in developing policy, facility design, education, and care delivery.

P&FCC philosophy and preparation come from organizational leaders who are themselves educated and committed to patient-centered philosophies to create the foundation and in turn lead physicians, nurses, and other caregivers to invite patient engagement. For instance, effective leadership engages the hearts and minds of staff and providers, which in turn provides a foundation for respectful team communication and partnerships with patients and families, which in turn reinforce staff and provider engagement. P&FCC improves transitions of care, increases patient and provider satisfaction, and reduces readmissions (Coulmont, Roy, & Dumas, 2013).

P&FCC is at the heart of providing an exceptional patient experience and is both integral and intertwined for improving quality and safety outcomes. Partnerships with patients contribute to safer care; patients and families must be included as active members of the care team to contribute to goals, help identify potential errors, and participate in improving care (Walton & Barnsteiner, 2012). The culture of P&FCC is not a set of isolated activities but is an integration of the philosophy that permeates the organization from executive leadership through all components of the system; it is a reinforcing philosophy lived out in how patients and families are treated and how the care experience is managed and continuously improved. Patients and families see the care experience as a synthesis of expert clinical care and coordination, teamwork and relationships with providers at all levels, and the impact of the overall hospital environment (Conway et al., 2006).

In providing P&FCC, providers shift from "doing to" to "doing with" patients and families. This shift in thinking across the organization influences how patients and families are facilitated and encouraged to actively engage in their care (Sofaer & Schumann, 2013). First and foremost is communicating effectively with patients and families so that care is personalized to accommodate personal preferences and circumstances in a way that empowers families to engage in care. Health institutions reflect the communities they serve, which are increasingly diverse; cultural beliefs and backgrounds are important considerations in planning quality, safe care, such as having places to worship and follow religious practices, food and nutrition that matches cultural preferences, and opportunities to follow daily hygiene routines (TJC, 2010).

Some who have resisted implementing P&FCC have argued that patients will have unrealistic demands or families will interfere with care, leading to delays, errors, and infections. Providers have expressed concerns that having patients and families participate in team meetings will inhibit staff from being open about patient concerns. Yet no evidence has emerged to support these arguments.

Education and Commitment of Providers

Moretz and Abraham (2012) identify three overall needs to successfully implement P&FCC: provider education, the preparation of team members for working together, and leadership involvement in creating the infrastructure to sustain and grow the new philosophy. Education is a critical starting point for changing long-held attitudes. Nurses and other providers may have been educated with P&FCC philosophies but lacked experiences in how to establish policies and organizational changes that are patient- and family-centered and in how to implement strategies to encourage active patient engagement (Sofaer & Schumann, 2013). To fill this gap, Walton and Barnsteiner (2012) have developed teaching strategies to prepare nurses to work in a patient- and family-centered culture, coordinate care across providers, and develop leadership skills.

Fully engaged providers are at the heart of P&FCC; patients' overall experience is linked to how providers interact with patients in conveying a sense of "I know you" (Balik et al., 2011). P&FCC cannot simply be mandated; providers must feel support from the organization. Providers must also bring clinical competence; competence inspires confidence through reliable care, communication, and teamwork. Provider interactions based on respect, addressing the patient's and family's emotional needs, actions that engender trust, and efforts to meet the patient's emotional needs convey the provider engagement and understanding of the P&FCC philosophy. Respectful, empathic relationships in combination with clinical quality are essential to achieving exceptional experiences.

Staff and providers are more effective in their work, provide safer care, and can achieve a better patient and family experience when they work in an organization whose values match their own, when they are supported by effective systems, and when they are recognized for the work they do (Conway et al., 2006). Organizations that are recognized as best employers and achieve outstanding patient and family experiences hire for fit with values; leaders recruit, select, develop, and retain people who share the commitment to outstanding patient and family experience. Finding the right talent and offering appropriate education and support are critical for implementing P&FCC.

Patient Engagement: Active Agents in the Hospital Experience

Consumers are increasingly involved in healthcare, in part because of the focus on quality and safety, and are driving public policy for adopting patient-centered approaches in care delivery. Data from public reporting in the United States of Hospital Consumer Assessment of Healthcare Providers and Systems (HCAHPS) allow the public to compare performance results from multiple hospitals and are fueling consumer interest in how patients and families are treated. Patient-centered healthcare is accountable care, focusing on value, quality, and patient satisfaction, but from the consumers' perspectives (IOM, 2001). For more information on HCAHPS, visit www.hcahpsonline.org.

Consumers themselves must be educated about seeking involvement, taking an active role, and managing their healthcare goals. It is a challenge to reverse the passive role patients have had in a paternalistic healthcare system and to reorient providers to include patients and families. Simply providing information and education will not be sufficient to motivate patients to participate in their care. They must see the connection between engagement and outcomes to help change the culture (Sofaer & Schumann, 2013). To accomplish a culture shift for P&FCC, patients and families need preparation to develop health confidence, viewed in some models as a sixth vital sign.

Health confidence is built through offering access to information, sharing decision-making, and involving family as care team members. It develops as the organization empowers patients to own their health through a patient-centered approach. Many patient-centered hospitals have developed patient and family partnership councils as an ongoing mechanism to solicit meaningful input and reactions from patients, families, and the community to better understand how to increase health confidence, promote engagement, and include the patient and family as team members (Michalak et al., 2010).

We can see an example of consumer-driven change in the dramatic shifts in obstetrics and delivery. Changes in care for childbearing women and families date to the 1960s and 1970s, when fathers and family members pushed to have a more active role in prenatal, perinatal, and postnatal care (Association of Women's Health, Obstetric, and Neonatal Nurses [AWHONN], 2012). Later, families with special-needs children who were technology dependent also sought a more active partnership and collaboration in caring for these children so that home care and even school participation were possible.

Today, maternity units routinely define patient-centered care as the acceptance by healthcare providers and systems of the values, culture, choices, and preferences of a woman and her family as relevant for promoting optimal healthcare (AWHONN, 2012; Katz, 2012). Balancing maternal-child safety and well-being with the woman's needs and desires, patient-centered care requires treating all childbearing women with kindness, respect, dignity, and cultural sensitivity and includes supportive resources, such as education and skilled attendants.

There are four main principles (AWHONN, 2012) to accomplish patient- and family-centered maternity care, which can be replicated throughout the organization in other service areas:

- **Communication:** Effective communication between and among all healthcare team members and with the patient provides information exchange in a language understandable to all.

- **Shared decision-making:** Patient and families participate in decision-making; providers recognize the knowledge the patient and family bring about patient health, unique situation, culture, and preferences in making decisions about care, ensuring informed choice, thus reducing risk and improving satisfaction and outcomes.

- **Teamwork:** Effective teamwork includes effective communication, shared goals and philosophy, monitoring performance, and avoiding hierarchy.

- **Quality improvement:** Process and outcome data are tracked with strategies for closing any gaps in care.

Exemplar Models of Care

Several models and resources are available to guide organizational design to achieve the hallmarks of P&FCC based on organizational change and active patient engagement in their care. Although the organizations briefly described here have independently supported P&FCC, the synergy that has developed among them has become a primary driver for P&FCC.

Institute for Healthcare Improvement

IHI has been a leader in promoting P&FCC through provision of resources and education to help organizations accomplish the culture shift (Balik et al., 2011). To promote P&FCC, IHI first collected an evidence base through interviews with experts, critical analysis of related research, and examination of organizations achieving exemplary outcomes.

From this in-depth review, a driver diagram was created to identify exceptional patient and family inpatient hospital experiences using the premise from the 2003 IOM report—care is patient-centered, safe, effective, timely, efficient, and equitable (Greiner & Knebel, 2003). A driver diagram was used to demonstrate a model for systematically collecting theories and concepts to achieve essential actions or primary drivers that will accomplish a specific goal or outcome, thus an improvement. Five primary drivers of exceptional patient and family inpatient hospital experience of care are leadership; staff hearts and minds; respectful partnership; reliable care; and evidence-based care (see Table 9.1).

TABLE 9.1 Primary Drivers for Patient- and Family-Centered Care

DRIVER	DESCRIPTION
Leadership	All elements of the organization are focused on P&FCC throughout the hospital and are demonstrated at the individual patient level, at the microsystem level, and in the governance structure and executive level.
Hearts and Minds	All members of the organization must be fully engaged through their hearts and minds to share respectful partnerships to demonstrate commitment to shared values of P&FCC.
Respectful Partnership	Every care interaction is anchored in a respectful partnership to address patient and family priorities for physical comfort and emotional, informational, cultural, spiritual, and learning needs.
Reliable Care	All patients receive reliable, quality care every hour of every day.
Evidenced-Based Care	Collaborative care is based on best practices from current evidence.

Sources: Balik et al., 2011; IHI, 2011

Institute for Patient- and Family-Centered Care

The primary aim of the Institute for Patient- and Family-Centered Care (IPFCC) is to promote patient and family care. The IPFCC has identified the following characteristics as hallmarks of P&FCC (IPFCC, 2010):

- People are treated with dignity and respect.
- Healthcare providers communicate and share complete and unbiased information with patients and families in ways that are affirming and useful.
- Patients and family members build on their strengths by participating in experiences that enhance control and independence.
- Collaboration among patients, family members, and providers occurs in policy and program development and professional education as well as in the delivery of care.

For more information, visit www.ipfcc.org.

The Picker Institute

The Picker Commonwealth Program for Patient-Centered Care and the Picker Institute initiated a research focus on patient-centered care in 1988 (Picker Institute, n.d.). Subsequently the group was renamed the Picker Institute, Inc., as an independent nonprofit organization dedicated to promoting the advancement of patient-centered care and the improvement of the patient's experience and interaction with healthcare providers. The organization ceased operations in March 2013, but in its 27 years of operation, the Picker Institute was a pioneer in providing evidence-based patient-centered care to prepare physicians and hospital staff for improving patient services from a patient's perspective and providing a standard metric for measuring performance used routinely by healthcare organizations worldwide.

The Picker Institute supported the principle that all patients deserve high-quality healthcare and that patients' active involvement is fundamental to improving care outcomes. Based on a definition of P&FCC as "improving health care through the eyes of the patient," eight essential dimensions of patient-centered care were identified (Picker Institute, n.d.):

- Effective treatment delivered by staff whom patients can trust
- Involvement in decisions and respect for patients' preferences
- Fast access to reliable healthcare advice
- Clear, comprehensible information and support for self-care
- Physical comfort and a clean, safe environment
- Empathy and emotional support
- Involvement of family and friends
- Continuity of care and smooth transitions

Education and research have been two main objectives of the Picker Institute. The Picker Institute promoted the advancement of patient-centered care through education programs, research grants, annual awards recognizing best practices, publications on patient-centered care topics, scientifically valid survey instruments, and the maintenance of research databanks. The Picker Institute sponsored research to identify patients' needs and preferences in order to understand patients' definition of high-quality care and design new models of care. Qualitative data from focus groups and interviews with patients and their families described their view of quality of care and were used to develop survey instruments to measure patients' experience of care. The Picker Awards for Excellence in the Advancement of Patient-Centered Care were established in 2003 to honor people and organizations as role models for advancing patient-centered care.

For more information, visit www.pickerinstitute.org.

The Planetree Model

Planetree, Inc., provides the most comprehensive model of P&FCC. Planetree is a not-for-profit organization established in 1978 to partner with hospitals and other healthcare organizations to transform organizational cultures and improve the patient experience (Planetree, n.d.a).

Planetree was first conceived by Angelica Thieriot, a former patient herself. The name comes from the type of tree Hippocrates, the father of medicine, sat under to work with his students in ancient Greece. The Planetree philosophy began as a new approach to hospital philosophy to enable patients to receive quality care in a healing environment with access to the information needed to become active participants in their own care. In developing the Planetree model, thousands of patients, family members, and hospital staff members participated in focus groups to define the main areas for improvement and strategies to create a patient-centered approach (Frampton, Chamel, & Planetree, 2008). An active patient voice has been and remains a critical part of how Planetree has integrated personalized healthcare practices. Staff, patients, and families are included in organizational assessments and focus groups to help design how P&FCC is implemented. The Planetree model is not prescriptive; each organization applies the philosophy to suit the needs of the unique population served.

Today Planetree has a global member network of more than 500 acute-care hospitals, continuing care facilities, ambulatory centers, community health centers, and health libraries in 32 U.S. states, Canada, and the Netherlands (Planetree, n.d.a). Planetree Designation recognizes achievement in patient-centered care based on evidence and standards; it is the only such program to formally recognize excellence in patient-centered care. Healthcare organizations of all types may apply for membership. Organizations first complete an organizational assessment, including focus groups with patients, families, and staff to identify community needs and ensure they agree with the Planetree belief model (see Table 9.2) and meet the standards for care based on the domains in Table 9.3.

TABLE 9.2   Planetree Core Beliefs

We are human beings, caring for other human beings.

We are all caregivers.

Caregiving is best achieved through kindness and compassion.

Safe, accessible, high-quality care is fundamental to patient-centered care.

A holistic approach meets needs of body, mind, and spirit.

Families, friends, and loved ones are vital to the healing process.

Access to understandable health information can empower individuals to participate in their health.

The opportunity for individuals to make personal choices related to their care is essential.

Physical environments can enhance healing, health, and well-being for patients and caregivers.

Illness can be a transformational experience for patients, families, and caregivers.

Source: Planetree, n.d.a

TABLE 9.3   Components of the Planetree Model

COMPONENT	EVIDENCED BY
I. Human Interactions/Independence, Dignity, and Choice	A healing environment includes personalized care, organizational cultures that support and nurture staff, and a continuing care community.
II. Importance of Family, Friends, and Social Support	Family and friends are encouraged to be active in patient care through patient-directed visiting, optional family presence during procedures and resuscitation, pet therapy, and overnight resources.
III. Patient/Resident Education and Community Access to Information	Patient records are open and available for family to read and add their own comments. Collaborative care conferences, patient information and education, Internet access, and health libraries provide the information patients and families need to be active in their care.
IV. Healing Environment: Architecture and Interior Design	The physical environment is part of well-being and is designed to be like a home environment, with a kitchen, library, lounges, activity rooms, green spaces, and space for overnights for families.
V. Nutritional and Nurturing Aspects of Food	Recognizing the role of nutrition in healing, dining options are flexible to suit patient preferences yet model healthy eating. Families may bring food from home and use kitchens provided.
VI. Arts Program/Meaningful Activities and Entertainment	The environment balances serenity and playfulness with careful attention to artwork. Patients may select art from carts; enjoy musicians, poets, and storytellers; and participate in activities to build fellowship.
VII. Spirituality and Diversity	Chapels, gardens, labyrinths, and meditation rooms provide opportunities for reflection and prayer. Chaplains are vital healthcare team members.
VIII. Importance of Human Touch	Touch reduces anxiety, pain, and stress benefiting patients, residents, families, and caregivers.

continues

TABLE 9.3 *continued*

COMPONENT	EVIDENCED BY
IX. Integrative Therapies/Paths to Well-Being	Patients may access resources other than Western medicine, such as aromatherapy, acupuncture and Reiki, heart-disease reversal programs, guided imagery, tai chi, and yoga.
X. Healthy Communities/Enhancement of Life's Journey	Hospitals are including efforts to improve the health of the larger community; environmentally friendly cleaning products, activities for children, walking clubs, and community gardens expand the role of hospitals from treating illness to promoting wellness. Life-stories programs capture patient stories.

Source: Planetree, n.d.a

Further details are on the website (www.planetree.org), but criteria based on a structured, operational framework are used to evaluate organizational systems and processes to measure organizational culture change (see Table 9.2). As such, these criteria collectively represent the hallmarks of what is required to implement and maintain a patient-centered culture, particularly the satisfaction of all stakeholders, patients, family members, frontline staff, leadership teams, the medical staff, patient and family advisors, and board members (DerGurahian, 2008). According to data on the Planetree website, as a group, Planetree member organizations exceed the national averages in each publicly reported HCAHPS category and outperform national benchmarks on the Centers for Medicare & Medicaid Services (CMS) process of care core measures and have lower readmission rates (Planetree, n.d.a).

Planetree's philosophy states that care should be organized around patient needs and desires to create a more personalized, humanized, and demystified healthcare experience. Implementing P&FCC changes the hospital culture so that daily operations are changed to match the goal of patient and family engagement and transform institutional culture.

Planetree provides resources to allow staff members to develop the expertise, tools, and support for transforming healthcare experiences for patients and caregivers. Resources are available on Planetree's extensive website and include an organizational assessment tool, educational materials, training sessions, webinars, conferences, consultations, idea sharing across institutions, and assistance with physical design. Educational resources are also available for patients and their families to learn how to become actively engaged as partners in managing their healthcare needs.

In becoming a Planetree member, hospitals implement processes and structures that inspire and enable caregivers to transform the healthcare experience. Caregivers and staff across the continuum must have the expertise, tools, and support to participate in continuous process improvement; develop an infrastructure to support sustainable culture change; and personalize the patient experience. The goal for Planetree facilities is to enhance the experience for patients, staff, and visitors by creating efficient and effective operations in the healthcare facility.

The resources extend to helping with physical design. Planetree also offers environmental design certification of architectural and design firms that have been vetted for their ability to match physical design and function with the Planetree philosophy. These firms focus on improving the patient and family experience through physical layout, with attention to respect for privacy, quieter environments, welcoming visitors, valuing human beings more than technology, and enabling patients to fully participate as care partners—all components of a patient-centered healing environment.

Planetree members focus on research and quality improvement by promoting translational research and evaluating patient-centered care and quality across the continuum of care settings. These opportunities include the development and testing of patient-centered measures of care, the identification of best patient-centered care practices, and individual and aggregate analyses of quantitative and qualitative data on healthcare provider performance.

Changing the Culture: Patient-Centered Approaches to Encourage Patient and Family Engagement

P&FCC is no longer a radical concept but a core component of healthcare quality in the IOM (Greiner & Knebel, 2003) framework. Acceptance in part stems from the popularity of the HCAHPS survey developed to measure exceptional patient care and patient and family inpatient hospital experience, defined by the IOM as care that is patient-centered, safe, effective, timely, efficient, and equitable (2001).

HCAHPS is a nationally standardized, publicly reported survey for evaluating the patient experience. There are three broad goals for the survey (CMS, 2013):

- Produce comparable data from the patient's perspective of care to be able to compare across hospitals in areas important to consumers.
- Create incentives for hospitals to improve quality of care.
- Promote public accountability through transparency of hospital data.

These publicly reported survey results indicate consumers' willingness to recommend a particular hospital by providing performance data on hospital performance. For more information, visit http://www.hcahpsonline.org.

Reframing Hospital Processes to Establish a Culture of P&FCC

Still, organizations have difficulty knowing how to actualize the concept, align policies and procedures with the philosophy, and prepare the workforce as well as patients and families. Decades of paternalistic healthcare have conditioned patients and families to have a passive role. Now both providers and patients need additional education to change mind-sets. Each organization will have a different starting point based on existing philosophies and practices.

Accurate assessment is a key place to begin. *Strategies for Leadership: Patient- and Family-Centered Care, a Hospital Self-Assessment Inventory* (American Hospital Association, 2011) is one self-assessment tool, in addition to the Planetree survey tool already mentioned, used to examine strengths and opportunities for the organization in establishing a patient-centered culture (Moretz & Abraham, 2012). This survey was a collaboration of the IHI, the National Initiative of Children's Healthcare Quality (NICHQ), and the IPFCC. Questions ask about family visitation, whether the environment supports family participation, and what advisory roles families may have. Another survey resource is the Planetree organizational survey previously discussed. From this information, organizations can have a starting point to begin provider and consumer discussions on priorities and needs for the communities served.

Resources to Help Change the Culture

The *Patient-Centered Care Improvement Guide* (Frampton et al., 2008), developed by Planetree, describes more than 150 practices that represent hallmarks for changing the culture to implement P&FCC and are incorporated within the 10 domains of care described earlier in Table 9.3. To create the guide, patients and families provided input in redesigning routine hospital processes, such as admission, patient care rounds, handoffs, diagnostic testing and ancillary departments, discharge planning, the overall environment, information resources, and family advisors or case managers to encourage active participation.

Another resource is the guide to Same Page Transitional Care provided by Planetree (n.d.c). It is difficult to coordinate complex care when patients transition from one care setting to another and interact with numerous providers. Each transition or handover is a high-risk time with potential for error. This guide to transitional care was created to facilitate common understanding among all members of the healthcare team before, during, and after transitions to ensure accurate communication and understanding of the patient's healthcare history, needs, priorities, and health goals. A toolkit (Planetree, n.d.b) can be accessed from http://planetree.org/online-tools-and-resources/.

Putting It Together: Hallmarks of P&FCC

Isolated strategies do not constitute a culture of P&FCC, but they are important ways that the philosophy is lived each day as providers interact with patients and their families (Frampton & Guastello, 2010). There are five aims that undergird the theoretical basis for planning patient-centered interventions:

- Building trust
- Providing positive orientation

- Promoting perceived control
- Promoting strengths
- Setting mutual health-directed goals

Providers build trust by demonstrating respect. Inviting the patient and family to engage in setting goals for the daily care plan integrates their priorities and preferences (Ahman & Dokken, 2012). The goals of the following are suggestions or starting points in considering how nurses and other providers must rethink traditional hospital practices.

Admission

Admission procedures must be more than a checklist; open-ended questions are ways to elicit particular information to help inform P&FCC. Family caregivers are often a valuable source of information about the patient's history, routines, symptoms, and other aspects of the healthcare situation. Because many are in ongoing caregiving roles before and after the patient's hospitalization, their inclusion is an important step in continuity of care. An accurate and personalized admission assessment is critical for providing safe quality care.

Exemplars detailed in Benner and Wrubel's 1989 work include personal assessment as part of expert nurses' work, evidenced in how nurses immediately notice signs and symptoms in the way the patient and family present for care. These clues represent patterns that can be followed in questioning. Tanner's model of clinical judgment (noticing, interpreting, responding, and reflecting) applied to the admission assessment can be employed in the initial assessment (Tanner, 2006). The well-known story of Lewis Blackman is a case of missed assessment (QSEN, 2008) in which providers fail to ask questions, assess critical signs and symptoms, and recognize patterns in the cues presented throughout the weekend as the patient deteriorated. For more information, see www.QSEN.org.

Patients need to be oriented on the role of P&FCC and encouraged to speak up when they are unsure what is happening, information is missing or confusing, and their preferences and priorities are ignored. Patients and families can be provided a small notebook to keep a healthcare journal of significant events during hospitalization and upon discharge to track their healthcare journey. They also need orienting on how to be active partners and encouraged to join the conversation by using the whiteboard in patient rooms, asking questions, and joining daily rounds. TJC (2010) identifies specific areas to cover in an assessment:

- Communicate in a way that conveys respect.
- Make introductions to begin to establish the relationship.
- Support patients for their level of understanding of health information and ability to act.
- Assess mobility needs.
- Understand cultural, religious, or spiritual beliefs and practices that affect care.

- Learn of dietary needs or restrictions affecting care.

- Identify a support person.

- Communicate unique needs to the healthcare team.

These eight bullets are key aspects of P&FCC to convey a welcoming, personalized approach. They are built on an accurate, personalized assessment that helps identify patient and family priorities, goals, and an understanding of the patient's healthcare needs.

Interprofessional Patient Rounds

The QSEN competencies (Cronenwett et al., 2007) based on the IOM framework (Greiner & Knebel, 2003) define teamwork and collaboration as including the patient and family as active team members. Interprofessional rounds at the patient's bedside engage the patient and family and provide care coordination across disciplines. Working with the patient and family to set a goal of the day helps personalize evidence-based care by incorporating the patient's desires and goals. Often written on a whiteboard in the patient's room so all disciplines see it, daily goals acknowledge family and patient contributions of information and insights.

Family Meetings

Family meetings are another way to engage the family in care (Weaver, Bradley, & Brasel, 2012). The family is likely the primary support system during illness, particularly for critically ill patients. Scheduled meetings are an effective strategy to improve communication about all aspects of care and increase the likelihood for successful discussion about goal-directed care (Weaver et al., 2012). Clear, thorough documentation of the meeting is a critical part of communication to ensure that the family and all healthcare providers understand important discussions, and it provides a record, whether written or on a voice recorder.

Flexible Schedules

Hospitals have traditionally followed set schedules for patients for meals, visiting hours, and other business. In responding to patient and family needs, where can schedules be flexible for the working spouse to be involved in care, or to honor cultural or personal preferences? Patients need autonomy, dignity, inclusion, explanations and information, and respect. Respect means taking someone's needs and preferences into account and acknowledging that person as an individual. Patients want to control their routines, to keep them much like they were, as a means of comfort and lessened anxiety. Allowing flexible schedules encourages active patient participation in managing their health. Rather than simply following a schedule set by the hospital staff, patients may want to get out of bed on their own schedule, manage their usual hygiene routines, and follow dietary habits.

Patient-Directed Visitation

Patient-directed visitation is defined as an unrestricted visiting environment in which the patient or the designated healthcare proxy determines what visitation parameters best suit the individual circumstances (IPFCC, 2010). The goal is to meet the psychological and emotional needs of the patient and family. Patients determine upon admission those persons whose presence would enhance their hospitalization (Bishop, Walker, & Spivak, 2013).

Berwick and Kotagal (2004) report that 88% of families surveyed found unrestricted patient visitation had a positive effect on their overall experience, and anxiety was reduced by 65%. Despite clear evidence that patient-directed visitation is what patients and families prefer, hospitals continue to struggle with the transition from traditionally restrictive visiting policies to patient-directed visitation. Concerns range from spread of infection and family members posing as impediments to clinicians' ability to provide care to concerns that open visiting hours may keep family members from getting a much-needed break from the bedside (Berwick & Kotagal, 2004). Patient-centered hospitals have addressed and successfully overcome these barriers in order to implement patient-directed visitation. Education helps all appreciate the need to balance visitation with patient rest periods and informs visitors about their responsibility to maintain a quiet, healing environment along with proper infection-control procedures. The following outline can also be applied to any quality-improvement strategy to improve P&FCC.

Steps for Implementing Patient-Controlled Visitation (or Other P&FCC Protocols)

1. *Begin with education for providers, hospital board members, and the community and share best-practice evidence from related studies.*

2. *Assess the organization, perhaps using* Strategies for Leadership: Patient and Family Centered Care, a Hospital Self-Assessment *(www.IHI.org), to examine strengths and opportunities for the organization to transform the culture and share results.*

3. *Identify physician and nursing champions who can work with departments for implementation.*

4. *Conduct a pilot study.*

    a. *Use a quality-improvement tool, such as Plan, Do, Study, Act.*

    b. *Share results to refine implementation plans.*

    c. *Spread to other units or departments.*

    d. *Interview patients, families, and staff for feedback.*

5. *Set a time frame for institutional implementation.*

6. *Finalize policies.*

7. *Establish liaisons across departments to maintain momentum and consistency.*

8. *Communicate to patients and families through newsletters, communication boards, electronic means, and brochures.*

9. *Recognize key adopters for being pilot starters.*

Source: Planetree, n.d.b

Patient/Family-Initiated Rapid Response Teams

Patients and families often feel powerless during hospitalization. Many hospitals have staff-initiated rapid-response teams to signal care when they see signs indicating that a patient's condition is deteriorating, such as difficulty breathing or a change in heart rate or rhythm; more recently, patients and families have the right to activate an alert. Patient/family–initiated rapid-response teams take this quality initiative one step further, encouraging patients and their families to alert care teams to noticeable clinical changes in patients' conditions. Patients and families are informed upon admission, signs are posted in patient rooms, and brochures are available describing when and how to activate a rapid response.

Spiritual Care

Providing emotional and spiritual care is based on patient and family preferences learned through admission and ongoing assessment (TJC, 2010). Providers need to know how to help patients access care for special needs, such as chaplains, priests, or other spiritual leaders, and how to locate places of worship for their religious preferences.

Respectful Partnerships

Every care interaction is anchored in a respectful partnership, anticipating and responding to patient and family needs for physical and emotional comfort and for information and education needs. It is a new realization for some providers that they are the ones who are guests in the patient's life, not the other way around in which patients are viewed as guests in the hospital (Johnson et al., 2008). People choose to participate in their care at different levels, with different preferences, and they bring different levels of education and understanding about their healthcare. Respecting and responding to each individual is an important part of the patient experience.

Nurse-to-Nurse Handoffs (Handovers)

Any change in provider or setting presents the possibility of miscommunication and error. Both *handoff* and *handover* generally mean the same thing—a change in provider—and this is a highly critical time for monitoring safety. Including the patient and family in information sharing can help transmit accurate information, includes them in discussions, and treats them as allies. Always maintain eye contact to communicate inclusion, use the first person, and include them in the conversation as meaningful partners.

Coordinating Care in Ancillary Departments

Patients have often been kept waiting on gurneys for hours, separated from family while waiting for x-rays and other diagnostic procedures, while in the perioperative area, and during other points of care transition. With available technology, it is now possible and desirable to reduce wait times with real-time notices for patients to be transferred only when their appointment times are available. Moving to patient-centered rather than provider-centered schedules and operations increases patient satisfaction and lessens fatigue.

Discharge Planning

Discharge planning begins at admission, with assessment in learning about the patient's background, available resources, goals for recovery, and family-support mechanisms. Continuing care coordination requires an important partnership between microsystems in the hospital and outpatient referral clinics or transitional care centers. Keeping a health journal is one strategy patients and families can use to assist care coordination between providers. They can use the journal to maintain a medication record, treatments and outcomes, and recovery goals.

Healing Environment

The importance of the environment has been emphasized throughout this chapter in consideration of family preferences as well as overall facility design to accommodate families. Healthcare environments can easily cause undue stress or offer a sense of calm, hope, and healing (Montague, Blietz, & Kachur, 2009). Paying attention to environmental details sends the message that *we are here to care for you* (DerGurahian, 2008; Frampton et al., 2008). Room design can be modified to accommodate family with caregiver zones and family zones, including Wi-Fi provision to remain connected. Safety features, such as handrails to guide the patient moving from the bed to the bathroom, can prevent falls. Colors, artwork, linens, and aromas are part of the healing environment. Noise, lighting, ease of finding your way (and staff who offer help), cleanliness, orderliness, comfortable settings, and staff appearance send both positive and negative messages to patients about the value of their experience.

Access to Nutrition Resources

Consideration of how family members access such simple provisions as water, coffee, and tea are important satisfiers. When parents or family members cannot leave the bedside, what resources can be provided to access food?

Information Resources

Access to a health library or health-information resource center in languages of the population served is an essential component to encourage patient engagement (TJC, 2010). Access to such a space guides patients and families toward trusted sources of information and motivates their engagement in care.

Working With Patient and Family Advisors

Many organizations have recruited patient and family advisors to help in reframing operations and procedures. Patients and families also fill vital roles on advisory boards for specialty units as well as for the organization to help guide and maintain transformation. In Chapter 23, Schlucter describes considerations for setting up patient/family advisory councils.

Conclusion

Recall the example of Lindy and her father from the beginning of this chapter. Presented here is an alternative situation that we would hope they could experience as the principles of this chapter are implemented.

> Ten-month-old Lindy had serious surgery on Wednesday at 8 a.m. in a large teaching hospital. Her young parents had been well prepared for the procedure with educational material provided both by the surgeon and his staff, but they also had come to the hospital for a preadmission orientation, during which they completed an assessment of dietary needs and preferences, their spiritual and religious practice, family constellation allowed to visit, their own plans for remaining overnight with Lindy post-operatively, expectations for post-op care, and plans for their participation in interdisciplinary rounds.
>
> On Thursday, the first full post-op day, the father had awakened after a calm night when the nurse came for the morning assessment. He then had time to shower, have coffee from the unit's family resource center, and hold Lindy to feed her with instructions from the nurse. Lindy's mother arrived prior to the interdisciplinary team including the surgeon, primary nurse, respiratory therapist, and dietitian arriving at Lindy's bed on schedule. They introduced each team member and their role in her care, discussed the previous night's care and progress, identified goals for the day and what would be required to meet them, asked the parents what they would like to see accomplished that day, recorded the goals on the whiteboard, asked for and answered questions from the parents, and suggested ways the parents could assist Lindy in recovery. The parents consulted their health journal to share their observations and concerns. They were informed of expectations for what complications they should watch for and how to inform staff of any concerns and told to expect swelling around the face from the surgery and how to best assist in providing for Lindy's comfort.

The parents participated in the discussion, shared concerns they felt, and commented on how they felt a part of the team. They knew what they had to do to help Lindy heal and were prepared to do their part.

How different is this experience from the first one? What were key interventions that helped?

P&FCC is recognized as a core component in safe, quality care. Education for providers, patients, and organizational leaders contributes to the capacity to implement and sustain P&FCC to replace traditional patriarchal operations and practices. P&FCC is based on entire organizational approaches, not isolated care practices, so that providers, consumers, and organizational leaders participate together to design the system based on needs and priorities of the communities served.

Several key points and implications for practice must be highlighted:

- Reconceptualizing the hospital experience based on P&FCC contributes to quality, safe care; reduces readmissions; and improves patient satisfaction.

- P&FCC creates a synergistic partnership to increase patient activism in their care, thus taking charge of their health.

- Both the physical environment and philosophical approaches must fundamentally change to help patients and their families achieve their health goals.

References

Abraham, M., & Moretz, J. G. (2012). Implementing patient- and family-centered care: Part I—Understanding the challenges. *Pediatric Nursing, 38*(1), 44–47.

Ahman, E., & Dokken, D. (2012). Strategies for encouraging patient/family member partnerships with the health care team. *Pediatric Nursing, 38*(4), 232-235.

American Hospital Association (AHA). (2011). *Strategies for leadership: Patient- and family-centered care. A hospital self-assessment inventory.* Retrieved from http://www.aha.org/content/00-10/assessment.pdf

Association of Women's Health, Obstetric, and Neonatal Nurses (AWHONN). (2012). Quality patient care in labor and delivery: A call to action. *Journal of Obstetric, Gynecologic, and Neonatal Nursing, 41*(1), 151-153.

Balik, B., Conway, J., Zipperer, L., & Watson, J. (2011). *Achieving an exceptional patient and family experience of inpatient hospital care.* IHI Innovation Series white paper. Cambridge, MA: Institute for Healthcare Improvement. Retrieved from http://www.ihi.org/resources/Pages/IHIWhitePapers/AchievingExceptionalPatientFamilyExperienceInpatientHospitalCareWhitePaper.aspx

Benner, P., & Wrubel, J. (1989). *The primacy of caring: Stress and coping in health and illness.* Menlo Park, CA: Addison Wesley.

Berwick, D., & Kotagal, M. (2004). Restricted visiting hours in ICUs: Time to change. *Journal of the American Medical Association, 292,* 736-737.

Bishop, S., Walker, M., & Spivak, M. (2013). Family presence in the adult burn intensive care unit during dressing changes. *Critical Care Nurse, 33*(1), 14-22.

Centers for Medicare & Medicaid Services (CMS). (2013). HCAHPS: Patients' perspectives of care survey. Retrieved from http://www.cms.gov/Medicare/Quality-Initiatives-Patient-Assessment-Instruments/HospitalQualityInits/HospitalHCAHPS.html

Conway, J., Johnson, B., Edgman-Levitan, S., Schlucter, J., Ford, D., Sodomka, P., & Simmons, L. (2006). *Partnering with patients and families to design a patient- and family-centered health care system: A roadmap for the future.* Institute for Family-Centered Care and Institute for Healthcare Improvement. Retrieved from http://www.ipfcc.org/pdf/Roadmap.pdf

Coulmont, M., Roy, C., & Dumas, L. (2013). Does the Planetree patient-centered approach to care pay off? A cost-benefit analysis. *Health Care Manager, 32*(1), 87-95.

Cronenwett, L., Sherwood, G., Barnsteiner, J., Disch, J., Johnson, J., Mitchell, P.,…Warren, J. (2007). Quality and safety education for nurses. *Nursing Outlook, 55*(3), 122-131.

DerGurahian, J. (2008). Focusing on the patient: Planetree guide touts patient-centered care model. *Modern Healthcare, 38*(43), 7.

Frampton, S. B. (2009). Creating a patient-centered system. *American Journal of Nursing, 109*(3), 30-33.

Frampton, S. B., Chamel, P. A., & Planetree (2008). *Putting patients first: Best practices in patient-centered care* (2nd ed.). Ames, IA: Wiley & Sons.

Frampton, S. B., & Guastello, S. (2010). Putting patients first: Patient-centered care: More than the sum of its parts. *American Journal of Nursing, 110*(9), 49-53.

Frampton, S. B., Guastello, S., Brady, C., Hale, M., Horowitz, S., Bennett Smith, S., & Stone, S. (2008). *Patient-Centered Care Improvement Guide.* Derby, CT: Planetree. Retrieved from http://planetree.org/wp-content/uploads/2012/01/Patient-Centered-Care-Improvement-Guide-10-28-09-Final.pdf

Frampton, S. B., Horowitz, S., & Stumpo, B. J. (2009). Patients first. Open medical records: Allowing patients access to their records increases their satisfaction. So why are hospitals resistant? *American Journal of Nursing, 109*(8), 59-63.

Greiner, A. C., & Knebel, E. (Eds.). (2003). *Health professions education: A bridge to quality.* Institute of Medicine. Washington, DC: The National Academies Press.

Institute of Medicine (IOM). (2001). *Crossing the quality chasm: A new health system for the 21st century.* Washington, DC: The National Academies Press.

Institute for Patient- and Family-Centered Care (IPFCC). (2010). *Changing hospital "visiting" policies and practices: Supporting family presence and participation.* Retrieved from http://www.ipfcc.org/visiting.pdf

Johnson, B., Abraham, M., Conway, J., Simmons, L., Edgman-Levitan, S., Sodomka, J. S., & Ford, D. (2008). Partnering with patients and families to design a patient and family-centered health care system. Retrieved from http://www.ipfcc.org/pdf/PartneringwithPatientsandFamilies.pdf

The Joint Commission (TJC). (2010). *Advancing effective communication, cultural competence, and patient- and family-centered care: A roadmap for hospitals.* Oakbrook Terrace, IL: Author.

Katz, B. (2012). New focus on family centered maternity care. *International Journal of Childbirth Education, 27*(3), 99-102.

Michalak, J., Schreiner, N. J., Tennis, W., Szekely, L., Hale, M., & Guastello S. (2010). "The patient will see you now." *American Journal of Nursing, 110*(1), 61-63.

Montague, K. N., Blietz, C. M., & Kachur, M. (2009). Ensuring quieter hospital environments. *American Journal of Nursing, 109*(9), 65-67.

Moretz, J. G., & Abraham, M. (2012). Implementing patient and family centered care: Part II, strategies and resources for success. *Pediatric Nursing, 38*(2), 106-109, 71.

Picker Institute. (n.d.). About Picker Institute. Retrieved from http://pickerinstitute.org/about/

Planetree. (n.d.a). About us. Retrieved from http://planetree.org/about-planetree/

Planetree. (n.d.b). Same page care tools and resources. Retrieved from http://planetree.org/online-tools-and-resources/

Planetree. (n.d.c). Same page transitional care. Retrieved from http://planetree.org/search-planetree/same-page-transitional-care/

Quality and Safety Education for Nurses (QSEN). (2008). The story of Lewis Blackman. Retrieved from http://qsen.org/videos/the-lewis-blackman-story/

Sofaer, S., & Schumann, M. J. (2013). Fostering successful patient and family engagement: Nursing's critical role [White paper]. Retrieved from https://naqc.nursing.gwu.edu/sites/naqc.nursing.gwu.edu/files/downloads/NAQC_PatientEngagementWhitePaper.pdf

Tanner, C. (2006). Thinking like a nurse: A research-based model of clinical judgment in nursing. *Journal of Nursing Education, 45*(6), 204-211.

Walton, M. K., & Barnsteiner, J. (2012). Patient centered care. In G. Sherwood & J. Barnsteiner (Eds.), *Quality and safety in nursing: A competency approach to improving outcomes* (pp. 67-90). Hoboken, NJ: Wiley-Blackwell.

Weaver, J., Bradley, C., & Brasel, K. (2012). Family engagement regarding the critically ill patient. *Surgical Clinics of North America, 92*(6), 1637-1647.

Chapter 10
Family Systems Theory

Jane H. Barnsteiner, PhD, RN, FAAN

Mavis was a 71-year-old admitted to the hospital for endoscopic surgery for an abdominal aneurysm. Her 80-year-old-husband, Tony, had multiple chronic illnesses, including severe osteoarthritis, which limited his mobility. Mavis also had multiple chronic illnesses and a long history of alcoholism and smoking (2 packs of cigarettes daily for 40 years, 80 pack years). Her 45-year-old daughter, Susan, often assisted her mother, taking her to various appointments when her father was not up to it.

Following an uncomplicated surgical procedure, Mavis showed symptoms of delirium tremens and developed a bowel obstruction that required a permanent colostomy. Susan, who was listed as the alternate decision-maker after her father, visited for long periods daily and often drove her father back and forth to the hospital to visit her mother.

Their 49-year-old physician son, Jeff, flew in from California. Normally he visited them annually when he returned home for the Christmas holidays, and they spoke by phone a few times a month. Jeff requested an immediate update from the ICU intensivist, queried the nursing staff on how and why his mother had developed a stage 3 pressure ulcer, and wanted to know why the nursing and medical staff had not anticipated the alcohol withdrawal. He rarely consulted with his father or sister for background information, automatically assuming the role of family spokesperson and healthcare expert. Neither Tony nor Susan intervened when Jeff was questioning the staff and seemed willing to let their son/brother, "the doctor," handle things. Mavis, who had developed a positive rapport with the nursing staff, noticed the nurses and medical residents were now coming into the room only when they had to carry out some procedure.

In the current healthcare environment, clinical nurses not only have to learn the latest technologies, procedures, and treatments for those in their care, but they also are expected to form helpful, caring relationships within a short amount of time. The American Nurses Association, in its *Nursing: Scope and Standards of Practice*, 2nd ed. (2010), asserts that nurses are patient advocates and must maintain a therapeutic and professional nurse-patient relationship with appropriate professional role boundaries.

Person- and family-centered care (P&FCC), an important framework for conceptualizing healthcare, is founded upon four principles (Cooper, Beach, Johnson, & Inui, 2006):

- Relationships in healthcare ought to include the personhood of all participants.
- Emotions and their expression are important components of these relationships.
- All relationships occur in the context of reciprocal influence.
- The formation and maintenance of authentic relationships in healthcare is morally valuable.

Although P&FCC considers the unique experiences, values, and perspectives of patients, clinicians, and all other participants in the healthcare process, it also focuses on the relationships between and among these participants at several levels: clinician with person and family, clinician with community, clinician with clinician, and clinician with self-awareness of one's own attitudes and experiences and their impact on interactions with others in the context of healthcare (Cooper et al., 2006).

Family systems theory (FST) was initially introduced to mental-health clinicians as a way to understand family dynamics and emotions (Bowen, 1978). As a theory of human behavior, its premise is that the family is a small group of interrelated and interdependent individual elements and also an emotional unit, or system. FST addresses interactions among members of a family and between the family and other systems. Furthermore, it proposes that a change in one family member will influence the entire system (Mehta, Cohen, & Chan, 2009). It has been demonstrated to be helpful in an array of settings and situations, such as teaching family practice residents (Yeheskel, Biderman, Borkan, & Herman, 2000), pediatrics (Barnsteiner & Gillis-Donovan, 1990), critical care (Leon & Knapp, 2008), ambulatory surgery (Mottram, 2009), and heart failure (Clancy, 2009).

This chapter reviews the principles and key concepts of FST and provides applications of the theory to the work of nurses and other healthcare professionals in their interactions with patients and families and in their interactions with colleagues. The concepts of systems thinking and therapeutic relationships are examined. In addition, recommendations are offered for ways in which nurses can use the principles of FST to enhance P&FCC.

Systems Theory

According to general systems theory, a *system* is defined as a whole with interrelated parts wherein the whole is more than the sum of its parts (Nichols & Schwartz, 2001). The system can be thought of as a set of interacting elements that are constantly changing; separating the parts from the whole reduces the overall effectiveness of the entity. A system can exist at the microlevel, such as a patient care unit, or at the macrolevel, such as a health system. As systems evolve over time, their natural tendency is to become increasingly more complex.

Clancy (2007a) notes that the complex system is characterized by multiple entities "interacting in a rich social network that is highly connected to both the internal and external environment" (p. 436). Complex systems are increasingly prevalent today and, as noted earlier, have been studied in many disciplines and for many situations. The field of systems theory seeks to understand man and his environment in the context of interacting systems.

Some of the most complex systems are found within healthcare. At one level, the healthcare industry is a mega-system, comprising healthcare providers, payers, pharmaceutical companies, professional societies, and consumer organizations, to name just a few of the moving parts. At another level, the integration of healthcare delivery and health professionals' education offers another complex system, the parts of which are complex in themselves and, when taken together, yield tremendous complexity. Developing plans to assess changes in the external environment and their impact on a hospital is one example of how managers apply the principles of systems thinking to the planning process in their organizations (Clancy, 2008). Accurately analyzing the current status of the organization draws from a wide array of resources, such as sociology, psychology, economics, engineering, medicine, and nursing, among others.

A special variation of complex systems is called complex adaptive systems (CAS). A CAS is a collection of individual agents who are free to act in ways that are not totally predictable and whose actions are interconnected. The component parts possess fuzzy boundaries, and membership of any one unit can change. Additionally, members can be part of several systems. Systems are embedded within other systems and co-evolve. Interaction leads to continually unfolding behavior, and there is an element of nonlinearity—that is, small differences in inputs can lead to huge differences in outcomes. One cannot fully understand one agent or system without considering others (Clancy, 2009).

Studies about social networks demonstrate that an organization is better equipped to handle environmental threats if there are a greater number of communications links among individuals in the system (Clancy, 2007b). This makes sense when realizing that no one person has all the information needed to solve a problem in a CAS. The reality is that most people have pieces of information that, when brought together, facilitate problem solving and decision-making. In this way, the whole truly is greater than the sum of the parts.

Family Systems Theory

Bowen's FST is derived from the broader framework of general systems theory (Bowen, 1978). It is a theory of human behavior that views the family as an emotional unit and uses systems thinking to describe the complex interactions within the family unit. In systems theory, people are viewed as part of their environment rather than separate from it. Bowen views the family as a system characterized by patterns of emotional interactions carried from generation to generation. He suggests that each member of a family plays a part in the way in which family members relate to each other, in the way in which the family's problems surface, and in the way that family members may deal with issues in other situations.

In FST, behaviors and concerns are translated into concepts about relationships. Key concepts in Bowen's model include:

- Boundaries
- Differentiation of self
- Balance
- Caretaker/person
- Overfunctioning and underfunctioning
- Triangles

The following sections describe each of these concepts in more detail.

Boundary

Boundary refers to where the self leaves off and the other person begins. Individual boundaries define a person's unique individuality. A family boundary delineates a unit apart from others.

Interactions between individuals within a group and between groups occur at the point where they meet or merge. Family members generally have characteristic ways that they relate to one another and to people outside the family, which stems from one's family of origin. Family of origin refers to the significant caretakers and siblings whom a person grows up with. Our early experiences provide a blueprint that forms our understanding of the world. Our family of origin has a major influence on how we see ourselves, others, and the world, and how we cope with and function in our daily lives.

Boundaries may be rigid, diffuse, or clear. Clear, well-defined boundaries indicate a balance of separateness and relatedness. In families with clear, well-defined boundaries, members are able to be separate and autonomous while simultaneously being related to each other. Family members thrive on each other's diversity, and individuals from such families have clear boundaries between themselves and others. They are able to be emotionally available and empathetic and relatively free of anxiety, bringing a calm perspective to emotionally upsetting or highly charged situations. They can serve as a helpful resource to each other.

Diffuse boundaries within families usually indicate too much relatedness, with members very involved with each other's lives and individuality and autonomy sacrificed. In families with rigid internal boundaries, members tend to be remote and underinvolved, or even uninvolved, with each other. Privacy, autonomy, and separateness are highly valued. Emotional styles exist on a continuum, and most people operate somewhere between rigid and diffuse boundaries.

Each system can be defined and understood by its boundaries. The boundary essentially defines the family unit or system and highlights the extent and type of contact between the system and other systems, including subsystems (Boss, Doherty, LaRossa, Schumm, & Steinmetz, 1993). It is the understanding of the family's boundaries and the degree to which they are permeable that allow healthcare professionals to gauge their ability to make an impact on the family unit. For example, if a family has extremely rigid boundaries that prevent exchange with other systems, the family members remain enclosed in the comfort or discomfort of their personal system and may have a difficult time interacting with individuals outside their system. Because families operate as a system, how one member behaves emotionally affects the behaviors and emotions of the other members of the family.

Differentiation

People who are well differentiated understand their selves well, including strengths and weaknesses, and accepts these as part of who they are, neither denying them or overstating them. People who are not well differentiated derive a great deal of their sense of self from someone else, perhaps someone who is stronger, or comparably weak (Gilbert, 1992). The ideal, according to FST, is a person who is fully differentiated and does not need another person to be complete but chooses to be in a relationship with another self-aware, differentiated person.

Families who share feelings and remain rigidly dependent may have members with low differentiation of self, oftentimes known as enmeshment (Bluestein & Bach, 2007). *Enmeshment* is a state characterized by poor individualization, amorphous interpersonal boundaries, reduced autonomy, and high emotional reactivity. Enmeshed families may be overprotective and overinvolved in care. Severely enmeshed families may be closed to outside influence from nursing staff or other clinicians, have unrealistic expectations, or insist on overly aggressive care. Clinicians may improve communication with enmeshed families by providing them with frequent updates and finding ways in which the family can participate in care.

Disengagement is described as a pattern manifested by family members who are emotionally distant or unresponsive. They may use denial or diversion in response to efforts to discuss care plans, may be unwilling to discuss advance directives, or be inclined to limit care prematurely.

Balance

Within the framework of FST, the concept of balance is one of the predictable tensions that exist. Balance must be sought and maintained between the needs of the individual and those of the family, and among members of the family. An example of the former could exist when a family's resources, whether they be financial or investments of time, are totally devoted toward the care of a family member who has a chronic illness. An example of the latter could exist when one child is supported in attending school, with full financial support, and another is forced to take on part-time jobs to pay tuition and expenses. Another example from an organizational perspective is if one department constantly receives a disproportionate share of the resources available; over time, unless the imbalance is explained and/or addressed, resentment can evolve among the system parts. An interesting application at the individual level occurs when one is spending an inordinate amount of time contributing to the pursuit of work goals to the detriment of personal goals; this also can lead to resentment. However, underinvestment can lead to feelings of guilt. Obviously, in all these situations, the goal is an acceptable balance among the component parts. Achieving this, in itself, can be a major pursuit.

Overfunctioning/Underfunctioning

Traditionally, common wisdom was that overfunctioners step in because the other person in a relationship is underfunctioning. However, a widely accepted premise in mental health is that overfunctioning in one person leads to, or creates, underfunctioning in another (Bowen, 1978). According to FST, the overfunctioner gains self-esteem by being in charge and in control and, therefore, is doing more than is required or than should be done to maintain balance. The underfunctioner may lack enough sense of self and does not make decisions, deferring to the other partner. In some situations, the relative underfunctioner can be a very competent individual who has fewer control issues, for whatever reason. Gilbert (1992) refers to this as inappropriate intrusion into another individual's space. Eventually the underfunctioner may become resentful of this dependent role and feel that a violation of personal integrity is occurring (Gilbert, 1992).

Triangles

A *triangle* is a three-part behavioral system that is automatic and has an unconscious relationship pattern. Bowen identifies the following in the triangulation process: When heightened anxiety is shared by two individuals and the heightened anxiety reaches a certain level of intensity, the two individuals tend to control their anxiety by diverting the attention to the third party or object. A problem with a triangular structure is that one side is usually closer to one side than the other. In this instance, tension forms and spreads through the members of the triangle in an attempt to find a new equilibrium (Gilbert, 1992). Obviously within family systems and larger organizational systems, there are multiple, overlapping triangles that need recognition, monitoring, and attention.

Individuals in the initial dyad of the triangle experience a comfortable relationship, and the third person is in a less comfortable position as the focus of the anxiety. Even though the third individual is experiencing discomfort, a crucial aspect of Bowen's theory (1978) is that this person allows triangulation to occur. By contrast, when anxiety is low, a two-person system can operate calmly without pulling in a third party. All individuals experience triangulation in various relationships and at various times in their lives. A common triangle occurs in many families where a child has two parents/care providers. Each person sits in a corner of the triangle. If the child is denied a request from one parent, she may seek out the other for permission, creating a two-against-one situation. These interactions can develop into problematic behavior patterns in the unwitting participants in the triangle.

The beginning patient vignette in Chapter 15 of the daughters' requesting a one-to-one for their mother is an example of a triangle in a patient situation when the nurse said no, and they then went to the resident physician, who ordered the one-to-one coverage. Left unaddressed, this creates tension and distancing or emotionally fraught relationships. In this case, the nurse addressed the situation with the daughters and closed the loop with the resident. Triangular relationships emerge wherever there are more than two people present—in families, among friends, and in work relationships.

Families of Origin

The *family of origin* is the group of caretakers and siblings with whom a person grows up. The family system remains a context in which individuals' beliefs and behaviors are sustained in the day-to-day life of adulthood (Fingerman & Berman, 2000). Adult family members describe a sense that they have gone back in time when they reunite with their families of origin (Fingerman & Berman, 2000). The larger family system rekindles old emotional patterns, behaviors, and roles, despite the fact that years have gone by and/or individual family members may have developed other patterns with their own life partners, children, coworkers, or friends. At the same time, families may provide a sense of reassurance. The rituals and customs of a given family lend comfort to individual members as they incur health problems, go through divorce, experience geographic moves, or even die.

Integrating the Concepts of Family Systems Theory Into Care Strategies

FST helps explain why family members behave as they do toward one another. They focus on what goes on in the context of the family level rather than merely examine individual family members. In order to understand family behavior, FST addresses communication, transactional patterns, conflict, separateness and connectedness, cohesion, and adaptation to stress. Between-family and within-family differences may be particularly evident at moments when families are forced to deal with issues that disrupt their homeostasis, such as an illness of a family member.

The family systems perspective provides a useful model for examining the association between familial characteristics and risk communication. The family systems perspective has been proposed by King and Quill (2006) as a framework for understanding how families may communicate with each other. It accounts for the reciprocal nature of family relationships, the broader social context in which families exist, and the multiple dimensions that comprise family functioning (King & Quill, 2006). An understanding of FST and its central concepts helps guide interventions that are aimed at stabilizing and supporting subsystems and addressing all parts of a family system.

In most instances, we are working with a person who is within a family, although the concept of family can be broadly defined. Stress levels of family members may lead to distortions of the situation or self-blame and, in complex situations, may approach clinical thresholds for anxiety or depression. Hence, we need to understand the backstory, anxiety, stress levels, and need for support of family members and their need for information, self-care, and guidance.

How families function affects caregiving and its outcomes. Some families handle crises by pulling together, while other families drift apart under the stress of the situation. As in other aspects of family life, insights into how adults react to crises that they encounter may be understood at the level of the larger family system rather than by merely examining individuals (Fingerman &

Berman, 2000; Quinn et al., 2012). Quinn and colleagues, in their study of end-of-life decision-making in adult intensive care units, identify multiple informal family member roles reflecting diverse responses to requests for family decision-making (2012). Clinician understanding of the formal and informal roles of family members is important to developing strategies and supporting family discussions and decision-making.

There are several specific applications of FST in providing P&FCC:

- Create a communication link for information exchange.
- Develop an appropriate communication care plan.
- Initiate family meetings.
- Understand sources of family anger and other strong emotions.
- Identify sources of collateral and historical information.
- Define family opinions and expectations.

Each of these applications is described in more detail in the following sections.

A Communication Link for Information Exchange

The family provides an important communication link for information exchange and support about family history and for the adoption of family-wide healthcare-related strategies (Harris et al., 2010). Individuals view and interpret health information through the lens of their family and disseminate that information within the family as well. For example, a health diagnosis in one family member often has implications for other family members, such as in a genetic predisposition to a disease. Thus, when one individual gets diagnosed with a healthcare condition, sharing this information can be crucial in leading to early screening or prevention activities to reduce morbidity and mortality.

> **NOTE**
>
> Because under Health Insurance Portability and Accountability Act (HIPAA) regulations healthcare professionals may be constrained not to share health information directly with relatives without the person's consent, it is vital to understand the properties of families that may aid or hinder this information from reaching appropriate family members. If the patient is communicative, check with the patient regarding who are the key communicators. Quinn et al. (2012) have found that many families have more than one spokesperson, and there may even be a spokesgroup.

Maintaining clear, open communication by frequently renegotiating a person's plan of care and updating information helps maintain a therapeutic relationship (Levine, 2011). Behaviors that assist in communicating with the person, family, and other healthcare providers to improve care include the following:

- Periodically assess the person and family to determine their current feelings, attitudes, responses, wishes, etc. and communicate these to professional colleagues, and update the healthcare record.

- Ask questions if the family is not participating in care. Look for anxiety, fear, feelings of intimidation, worry about making a mistake, or a perception of lack of competence.

- Keep communication channels open among self, family, and physicians and other care providers.

- Resolve conflicts and misunderstanding directly with those who are involved.

A comprehensive family assessment at the initiation of a relationship with a patient and the patient's family may be helpful for a person with whom there will be a long-term hospitalization or repeated occurrences, such as with cancer therapy. This provides valuable information on the family's functioning as a system and its boundary relationship style. The assessment should include a description of the family when family members believe everything is going well and what they do to restore balance in their family when members are upset (Walton, 2011).

An Appropriate Communication Care Plan

Another important nursing intervention is developing an appropriate communication care plan. Knapp and DelCampo (1995) stress the importance of using a family systems perspective in developing family care plans to provide a framework that will help healthcare professionals understand the complexity and diversity of family responses in the palliative-care population. Used as a communication tool, a plan should outline who are the members of the family system, what roles they play, and what they have identified as beneficial to them in terms of delivering care.

For example, if a family has an identified spokesperson(s), this information would be included in the care plan. The nurse would then know whom the family prefers having information passed to. Similarly, if the family has identified that receiving information about procedures decreases their anxiety level and helps restore the family's equilibrium, then nurses will know to provide clear explanations prior to any procedure.

This same communication plan should be used for transition in care planning rather than speaking to whoever happens to be with the patient at any point in time.

Family Meetings

Another intervention helpful in the care of complex patients is to organize and conduct a family meeting, allowing the family to participate, be heard, and be understood (Boyle, 2005; King & Quill, 2006). It is helpful to have each family- and clinician-participant think through and articulate their goals for the meeting in advance so they have time to plan for their participation. A family meeting provides an opportunity for the family members to voice questions and concerns, identify where all the "parts" are included, and it allows for some observations of relationships between the different parts of the family. A family meeting also provides a forum to acknowledge feelings and reactions other family members may be having. It helps the nurse identify the family's strengths and plan for further interventions. A family meeting is also an opportunity to observe the interrelatedness among the various parts of the family. Table 10.1 presents a scenario of a family meeting for the purpose of understanding family dynamics and family rules.

TABLE 10.1 Family Meeting Scenario to Understand Family Systems

Take time for introductions.

Thank attendees for coming to the meeting.

Review the purpose of meeting and ask if there are any other reasons why individuals are there. Family members should be able to prepare their goals for the meeting in advance so they can communicate among themselves, just as the clinical team should communicate their goals to the family. In this way, the clinical team can be prepared with information to respond to the family goals.

Open the meeting with a comment such as "Before we start, please tell me what your understanding is of _____'s condition." (This will reveal family perceptions and questions and information that may be important to participants.)

Demonstrate empathy by asking open-ended questions related to how the family has been managing the physical and emotional demands of care of the person, and whether there are other stresses or changes in the family at this time.

Elicit how the family has managed difficult situations (such as previous illnesses, loss of job, or deaths in the family) in the past.

Elicit information about any previous positive and/or negative past experiences with healthcare providers.

Ask for observations on helpful behaviors that staff can use to create a welcoming environment in which the family members can participate as they choose.

Sources of Family Anger and Other Strong Emotions

Understanding of FST can help clinicians understand possible sources of family anger and other strong emotions and thus respond less personally. Empathetic engagement, problem solving, and avoidance of defensiveness and personalization are more possible. Understanding FST can assist nurses in avoiding labeling people as "difficult" when they may actually be asserting their autonomy according to a long-established life pattern or "helpful" when they are people who stay in the background, have few requests and questions, and are actually "underfunctioners" who lack self-esteem and always defer to others. FST can also highlight other patterns of interaction among family members in order to avoid inadvertent triangulating and to most appropriately frame communication.

Sources of Collateral and Historical Information

The family becomes an important source of collateral and historical information. Observation can be extended to the family itself, through unobtrusive observation, noting who is there and who is not, who seems to be the most agitated or suffering the most, who sits near whom, body language, who talks and who does not, who is the leader, and who argues or agrees with whom. These data can help the clinician identify patterns suggested by FST and assist the nurse in selecting the most helpful communication strategies.

Family Opinions and Expectations

Eliciting family perspectives calls for defining family opinions and expectations and clarifying family member roles. This process is of particular importance in situations where people have complex chronic illnesses, are transitioning to long-term care, or are entering palliative or hospice care, because families may have received varied messages about prognosis and care recommendations across sites of care and different providers. Different family members may have different perceptions. Observing how family members interact with each other, and who takes the lead, is helpful.

Questions to ask might include:

- Who is considered part of the family?
- What role do family members play in healthcare?
- Who is the decision-maker in major decisions?
- What is the role of the adults in the family? Are there differences between the roles that men and women play?
- What is the role of children?
- What is the meaning of illness to the family?
- What communication patterns are used?
- Who speaks in important matters?

Family rules govern the degree of closeness and distance and who has the decision-making power in a family. Family rules dictate how conflict and differences are handled and shape each family's view of reality. The hierarchical family is one with a family leader or health expert who may see suggestions from the clinician as a challenge to the leader's authority. The clinician would do well to form a partnership with the family leader to the extent possible and to call on objective data to support healthcare-related recommendations when there is disagreement. Questions such as how each family member has reacted to the person's health or illness will provide a view into the family dynamics. Has the concern or challenge been communicated to family members?

> **NOTE**
>
> In Chapter 12 of this book, Dexheimer Pharris discusses approaches to use with the individualistic versus collectivist family.

Applying Family Systems Theory to Foster a Healthy Work Environment

A parallel of FST can be made to the work setting, i.e., each member of the work environment influences the group function and manifestation of work problems. The same patterns that exist in families may be present in work relationships. Members of a work group spend a significant portion of time together and build emotional relationship systems similar to those of a family. For instance, a behavioral change affecting the output of one healthcare team member's work affects all members of the unit and may affect overall patient care offered by the unit. The focus of systems theory is on understanding the interaction among the various parts of a system rather than on describing the function of each part.

Workplaces have their own rules, power structures, and communication patterns. FST can help us understand the complexity of relationship patterns among those with whom we work and how they can have an impact on efficiency and effectiveness. For example, just as families have family rules, family myths, family secrets, power structures, and communication patterns, so do workplaces. For example, in some settings, a common workplace rule is that personal problems should be left at the door when you come to work and should not interfere with job performance. Some workplaces still have a hierarchy structure where attending physician orders are never questioned. How such rules may or may not play out in our work areas will tell us something about our work relationships and systems and may well affect the delivery of P&FCC.

Understanding how individual staff members function is based on understanding the emotional process in organizations. FST also provides us with a way to understand the organization or unit as a human relationship system (Fox, 1990). The anxiety level of an individual influences the degree to which behavior is intellectually or emotionally driven. Higher anxiety results in more emotionally driven behavior. High anxiety–provoking factors among work groups lead to over- and underfunctioning, scapegoating, gossiping, and absenteeism. Such anxiety can be transferred to others in the workplace. Calmness, like anxiety, also is contagious, and anxiety can be reduced by thoughtful nonreactive behavior. Thus the organization and work group can benefit from leaders and nursing staff who are aware of and can manage their own anxiety.

Each nurse brings personal family experience to practice, as does each coworker and those in their care. Their families of origin will reflect the range of boundaries seen within family systems. Nurses from families with diffuse boundaries may have a tendency to get overinvolved with patients and families or may have reacted to such closeness and remoteness in their adult style, in which case they may lean toward underinvolvement. Alternatively, some nurses may tend toward overinvolvement to compensate for the isolation they felt from their family of origin. Nurses who have experienced clear boundaries in their lives appreciate the diversity of the team and its members. As with FST, they are able to be emotionally available and empathetic and relatively free of anxiety. They are able to bring a calm perspective to emotionally upsetting or highly charged situations with both people and families and their coworkers. For example, we have all worked with a colleague who is able to stay calm and decisive in an emotionally charged situation.

As FST suggests, in any relationship, boundaries differentiate us from others and give us a sense of who we are, what we think, and how we feel. Our personal boundaries determine how much we take responsibility for others and the degree to which we allow others to control us. In families with clear yet related boundaries, there is room for disagreement and recognition of what is and is not any individual's personal business. Nurses coming from families with clear internal boundaries allow themselves to engage in the helping process without becoming engulfed by the patients they care for and their family's problems.

Anxiety is often managed by distancing, conflict, over- and underfunctioning, and triangles. If avoiding certain individuals makes one feel calmer, then one might distance one's self from them by calling in sick when scheduled to work the same shift or by switching assignments. Some people feel better after having a direct confrontation. Others manage their anxiety by doing things themselves and overfunctioning for colleagues or people in their care and their families, leaving them in an underfunctioning situation. Lastly, we may relieve ourselves of relationship anxiety by bringing in a third party, creating a triangle. These behaviors are the way people manage anxiety and, in and of themselves, are neither good nor bad.

Therapeutic Relationships

Therapeutic relationships are described in the literature as a mixture of personal characteristics and caregiving skills. These qualities and skills include skilled communication, respect for patient autonomy and diversity, mutually agreed-upon goals and shared decision-making, empathy, and awareness of one's own skills and limitations (Canning, Rosenberg, & Yates 2007; Mottram, 2009).

A therapeutic relationship is one that is an interactive, clear, caring, boundaried relationship that is both positive and professional and that promotes people's control over their healthcare (Barnsteiner & Gillis-Donovan, 1990; Barnsteiner, Gillis-Donovan, Knox-Fischer, & McKlindon, 1994; Canning et al., 2007; O'Connell, 2008). It is an intentional relationship that is not aloof and is not a friendship. Professional nursing, regardless of setting, is emotionally complicated. It requires an ability to be meaningfully related to a person and their family yet separate enough to distinguish one's own feeling and needs. To be separate and related is challenging. One's caretaking style includes varying degrees of a need to be needed, which makes one susceptible to being caught in intense relationships. Day-to-day contact with patients and families makes it difficult to achieve a meaningfully related yet professionally separate balance. Being able to balance both simultaneously requires a level of professional objectivity and preservation of the self while caring for others.

Each of us enters nursing with personal motivations, values, and beliefs, along with unresolved family-of-origin challenges that can influence therapeutic relationships. A wish to help may reflect our need to be needed. Often, we do not understand how these needs may have led to our choice of profession. Understanding ourselves within a family systems framework assists us in understanding our motivations and in keeping our own goals clear. It requires an ability to relate meaningfully to a person and family yet remain separate. For example, a nurse assigned to care for a patient with alcoholism admitted for a liver transplant may respond to the person on the basis of his or her own family experience. If the nurse had a family member with this condition who ruined every holiday, he or she may react negatively to the patient for receiving a transplant organ that is in short supply. An understanding of self and what may cause heightened anxiety is important in developing therapeutic relationships.

Behaviors that help nurses become increasingly competent, confident, knowledgeable, calm, and in control include:

- Learning about one's own emotional responses to different people and situations
- Seeking to understand how one's own family-of-origin experiences influence reactions to individuals and families, especially as they affect tendencies toward overinvolvement or underinvolvement
- Working to have a calming influence and not one that will amplify emotionality
- Developing relational skills in addition to technical skills

Self-awareness and skill development related to therapeutic relationships and FST enable a healthcare professional to set appropriate boundaries and prevent excessive emotional vulnerability. These behaviors assist in facilitating a balanced relationship with patients and families and avoiding professional overfunctioning or underfunctioning.

Overfunctioning and Underfunctioning in One's Professional Role

A person's illness may create intense anxiety within a family and in those who serve them. Healthcare providers, and nurses particularly, are willing caretakers by professional choice and emotional style and are suited for most of the associated responsibilities. One's caretaking style includes varying degrees of a need to be needed, which increases one's susceptibility to get caught in intense relationships. Nurses who comes from families of origin with diffuse boundaries, where there was little privacy and everyone was in everyone's personal business, may be unclear about their own professional boundaries. They may then be susceptible to overinvolvement in their responsibilities. Coming from a family of origin with rigid boundaries where autonomy and separateness were highly valued may result in family members who are remote and uninvolved. Nurses from such families may carry out their professional relationships in an underinvolved manner, being unable to empathize or relate to a person with multiple illnesses and unable to loosen their personal boundaries to appropriately use the self to provide care. Underinvolved behavior is evidenced when the nurse may attempt to restrict family access by saying the unit is too busy or being consumed with the technical aspects of care and being aloof to the person and family.

The nature of the nurse-person relationship is dependent on the context in which nursing care is delivered. In areas with long-term relationships with patients and families, such as transplant, dialysis, and oncology units, day-to-day contact may make difficult a meaningfully related but professionally separate balance. Showing favoritism toward certain people or families and/or competing with other staff members for the favor of certain people and families are examples of overinvolved behavior. In situations such as these, more emotional energy is usually invested than is helpful to either the nurse or the patient. For example, the nurse may develop strong personal opinions on what is the appropriate course of action and attempt to influence the decisions of the patient or family rather than facilitate informed decision-making.

Possible reasons for the perceived threat to the formation of therapeutic relationships include time pressures on healthcare delivery and the increased use of technology (Beals, 2002; Foster & Hawkins, 2005). In today's healthcare environment, with short hospital stays and brief ambulatory visits, nurses may be consumed with the technical aspects of care and lose sight of the personhood of the patient they are working with and be underinvolved with the person and family. In critical care nursing, where technology can act as a barrier and compromise nurse-patient communication, it can be difficult to develop therapeutic relationships. O'Connell (2008) warns that without therapeutic relationships, nurses are reduced to objective technologists, while patients become objects to be examined and evaluated.

The short-stay surgery unit is an area where nurse and patient interaction is compressed into a very short time frame. In a study of short-stay surgery patients, Mottram (2009) details how nurses can develop therapeutic relationships even with short encounters. They can do this with the use of kind words, supportive touch, and engagement with the patient on a personal level, which all contribute to feelings of safety and comfort. Gestures such as these, although not prolonged or time-consuming, are remembered by patients for a long time afterward.

Appreciating that patients and their families have multiple and diverse needs is a fundamental principle for nursing practice. What may be less recognized or acknowledged is the role that the nurse's needs play in the care relationship. In optimal situations, the nurse is able to establish and maintain a therapeutic relationship with the individual and family, focusing on the goals of care that have been mutually established. In this relationship, the nurse employs compassion, which is an "investment of positive caring energy," separate from emotional entanglement (Schenck & Churchill, 2012, p. 14) and achieves a sense of pride and satisfaction in a meaningful care encounter.

However, if there is imbalance in this relationship, and either the nurse's need to be needed is inappropriate, or the nurse's need interferes with the plan of care for the patient or family, this is a problem. With P&FCC, nurses with clear boundaries grant rather than "allow" the person and family a level of control that balances the person's and family's needs for control, considering their stress level and capabilities, with their needs as nurses to organize the work environment and complete their work.

Self-Monitoring

The capacity for concurrent self-monitoring, ongoing moment-to-moment self-assessment, is an important component of the professional competence of all healthcare clinicians. *Self-monitoring* refers to the ability to notice our own actions, curiosity to examine the effects of those actions, and willingness to use those observations to improve behavior and thinking in the future (Epstein, Siegel, & Silberman, 2008). Self-monitoring allows for the early recognition of cognitive biases, technical errors, and emotional reactions and may facilitate self-correction and development of therapeutic relationships (Aronson, 2013). Self-monitoring requires cultivating an "observing self" within an otherwise chaotic and distracting environment in which clinicians work (Epstein et al., 2008, p. 5). The following are lessons for self-monitoring (adapted from Epstein et al., 2008):

- Self-monitoring is an aspect of self-assessment that may contribute to the quality of care and reduction in errors.

- Self-monitoring depends on the ability to regulate attention, maintain curiosity, and be flexible during daily work, especially when under stress and multitasking.

- Self-monitoring can be improved by cultivating an "observing self."

- Self-monitoring involves seeing "facts" as conditional, considering multiple perspectives, suspending categorization and judgment, and developing habits of self-questioning.

Conclusion

FST addresses interactions among members of a family and between the family and other systems, such as healthcare. Each member of a family plays a part in the way family members relate to each other, in the way in which the family's problems surface, and in the way that family members respond to situations. Application of the concepts of family systems thinking, which include therapeutic relationships, provides ways in which nurses may enhance P&FCC. Use of FST enables clinicians to develop helpful, caring relationships within a short amount of time. Understanding how families function and getting to know the informal roles of family members enable the healthcare team to develop effective strategies and support family decision-making. Ultimately it enables the provision of effective care for achieving mutually agreed-upon clinical outcomes.

References

American Nurses Association. (2010). *Nursing: Scope and standards of practice* (2nd ed.). Washington, DC: Author.

Aronson, L. (2013). "Good" patients and "difficult" patients—Rethinking our definitions. *New England Journal of Medicine, 369*(9), 796-797.

Barnsteiner, J. H., & Gillis-Donovan, J. (1990). Being related and separate: A standard for therapeutic relationships. *American Journal of Maternal Child Nursing, 15*(4), 223-228.

Barnsteiner, J., Gillis-Donovan, J., Knox-Fischer, C., & McKlindon, D. (1994). Defining and implementing a standard for therapeutic relationships. *Journal of Holistic Nursing, 12*(1), 35-49.

Beals, D. A. (2002). Does minimal access mean minimal relationship? Defining the physician-patient relationship in postmodern culture. *Seminars in Laparoscopic Surgery, 9*(4), 218-221.

Bluestein, D., & Bach, P. L. (2007). Working with families in long-term care. *Journal of the American Medical Directors Association, 8*(4), 265-270.

Boss, P. G., Doherty, W. J., LaRossa, R., Schumm, W. R., & Steinmetz, S. K. (1993). *Source book of family theories: A contextual approach.* New York, NY: Plenum Press.

Bowen, M. (1978). *Family therapy in clinical practice.* New York, NY: Jacob Aronson.

Boyle, D. K. (2005). Communication and end-of-life care in the intensive care unit: Patient, family and clinician outcomes. *Critical Care Nursing Quarterly, 28*(4), 302-316.

Canning, D., Rosenberg, J., & Yates, P. (2007). Therapeutic relationships for specialist palliative care practice. *International Journal of Palliative Care Nursing, 13*(5), 222-229.

Clancy, T. R. (2007a). Organizing: New ways to harness complexity. *Journal of Nursing Administration, 37*(12), 534-536.

Clancy, T. R. (2007b). Planning: What we can learn from complex systems science. *Journal of Nursing Administration, 37*(10), 436-469.

Clancy, T. R. (2008). Control: What we can learn from complex systems science. *Journal of Nursing Administration, 38*(6), 272-274.

Clancy, T. R. (2009). Putting it altogether: Improving performance in heart failure outcomes, Part 2. *Journal of Nursing Administration, 39*(9), 364-367.

Cooper, L. A., Beach, M. C., Johnson, R. L., & Inui, T. (2006). Delving below the surface: Understanding how race and ethnicity influence relationships in health care. *Journal of General Internal Medicine, 21*, S21-S27.

Epstein, R. M., Siegel, D. J., & Silberman, J. (2008). Self-monitoring in clinical practice: A challenge for medical educators. *Journal of Continuing Education in the Health, 28*(1), 5-13.

Fingerman, K. L., & Berman, E. (2000). Application of family systems theory to the study of adulthood. *International Journal of Aging and Human Development, 51*(1), 5-29.

Foster, J., & Hawkins, J. (2005). The therapeutic relationship: Dead or merely impeded by technology? *British Journal of Nursing, 14*(13), 698-702.

Fox, L. A. (1990). Fitting in, standing out: Leading effectively within your organization. *Journal of American Health Information Management, 76*(1), 24-28.

Gilbert, R. M. (1992). *Extraordinary relationships: A new way of thinking about human interactions.* Hoboken, NJ: Wiley-Blackwell.

Harris, J. N., Hay, J., Kuniyuki, A., Asgari, M. M., Press, N., & Bowen, D. J. (2010). Using a family systems approach to investigate cancer risk communication within melanoma families. *Journal of the Psychological, Social and Behavioral Dimensions of Cancer, 19*(10), 1102-1111.

King, D. A., & Quill, T. (2006). Working with families in palliative care: One size does not fit all. *Journal of Palliative Medicine, 9*(3), 704-715.

Knapp, E. R., & DelCampo, R. L. (1995). Developing family care plans: A systems perspective for helping hospice families. *American Journal of Hospice and Palliative Care, 12*(6), 39-47.

Leon, A. M., & Knapp, S. (2008). Involving family systems in critical care nursing challenges and opportunities. *Dimensions of Critical Care Nursing, 27*(6), 255-262.

Levine, C. (2011). The hospital nurse's assessment of family caregiver needs. *American Journal of Nursing, 111*(10), 1047-1051.

Mehta, A., Cohen, R., & Chan, L. S. (2009). Palliative care: A need for a family systems approach. *Palliative and Supportive Care, 7*(2), 235-243.

Mottram, A. (2009). Therapeutic relationships in day surgery: A grounded theory study. *Journal of Clinical Nursing, 18*(20), 2830-2837.

Nichols, M. P., & Schwartz, R. C. (2001). *The essentials of family therapy.* Boston, MA: Allyn and Bacon.

O'Connell, E. (2008). Therapeutic relationships in critical care nursing: A reflection on practice. *Nursing in Critical Care, 13*(3), 138-143.

Quinn, J. R., Schmitt, M., Baggs, J. G., Norton, S. A., Dombeck, M. T., & Sellers, C. R. (2012). Family members' informal roles in end-of-life decision making in adult intensive care units. *American Journal of Critical Care, 21*(1), 43-51.

Schenck, D., & Churchill, L. (2012). *Healers: Extraordinary clinicians at work.* New York, NY: Oxford University Press.

Walton, M. K. (2011). Supporting family caregivers: Communicating with family caregivers. *American Journal of Nursing, 111*(12), 47-53.

Yeheskel, A., Biderman, A., Borkan, J. M., & Herman, J. (2000). A course for teaching patient-centered medicine to family medicine residents. *Academic Medicine, 75*(5), 494-497.

Chapter 11

Ethical Dilemmas in Person- and Family-Centered Care

Mary K. Walton, MSN, MBE, RN

Katharine approaches the bedside of her patient, who is dying with cancer, with mixed feelings. It is evening, and it is immediately evident that her patient is suffering. Mr. Lefkakia, now enrolled in a Phase I chemotherapy trial, will, Katharine believes, die in a matter of days. She reflects on the past 2 weeks and the many days she has struggled with witnessing his deterioration. Two weeks ago, Katharine called the family meeting that brought Mr. Lefkakia and his three adult children together with the oncology team. One daughter is an oncologist, and his two sons are successful businessmen. Katharine could see the love and pain in their faces as they heard Dr. Siemans review the various treatment courses and their failure to bring the cancer into remission. Mr. Lefkakia trusted Dr. Siemans and shared that he understood, thanking him for keeping him so well informed of all treatment options as well as the progression of cancer over the past few years. Mr. Lefkakia stated that he knew about hospice from his wife's final months and would like to move from aggressive care to hospice care now. Katharine remembers how startled his daughter, Athena, looked when her father spoke the words of accepting hospice—she appeared to have been physically hit. An oncologist herself, although her practice was halfway across the country, she told her father, "You must continue to fight. I know there are Phase I trials—I will never forgive you if you give up now." At that point in the meeting, Mr. Lefkakia looked lovingly at his daughter and said to Dr. Siemans, "Let me tell you tomorrow if I want to enroll in that trial and go for another round of chemo."

So now it was 2 weeks later. Katharine still has a negative visceral reaction every time she hangs the chemo, knowing it will not benefit her patient and, in fact, will produce symptoms that cause physical suffering. Mr. Lefkakia accepts the treatment, and last week when she was sitting quietly with him, he shared how proud he was of his daughter's career. He well recognized that he was dying but wondered whether others would benefit from knowledge gained from his participation in a clinical trial; in fact, maybe one of his daughter's future patients might benefit. Although Katharine still regrets that her patient has consented to more chemotherapy, she has some understanding of the meaning of his choice for his end-of-life story.

Nursing takes us into the world of those for whom we care. As Diers so eloquently wrote, "Nursing puts us in touch with being human. Without even asking, we are invited into the inner spaces of other people's existence" (1982, p. 460). Entering another's world requires reflection on our own deeply held values and meaningful life experiences as we seek to honor the values and preferences of another person. Given the complexity of healthcare today, along with the diversity of human experience, patient needs and preferences will likely create dilemmas for clinical nurses. When these dilemmas are ethical in nature, nurses must consider both facts *and* values in order to determine the morally justifiable options. Providing person-centered care while also maintaining one's own personal and professional integrity is challenging. This chapter details ways of identifying and thinking through ethical dilemmas that clinical nurses may experience when they seek to let patient values guide clinical decisions. Organizational resources to assist nurses with morally distressing situations are identified and discussed.

Nursing and Ethics

Ethical practice has always been a concern of professional nursing. Discussion relating to the development of a code of ethics is evident as far back as 1896. Many of the ethical beliefs embedded within the current American Nurses Association (ANA) *Code of Ethics* can be traced back to the values found in the writings of Florence Nightingale. For well over a century, nurses have identified ethical concerns and developed strategies to address the ethical dilemmas that arise in practice (Badzek, 2008). More recently, attention is being given to the phenomenon of *moral distress*, the psychological impact of constraints to ethical practice.

Nursing

"Definitions of nursing have evolved to reflect these essential features of professional nursing:

- Provision of a caring relationship that facilitates health and healing
- Attention to the range of human experiences and responses to health and illness within the physical and social environments
- Integration of assessment data with knowledge gained from an appreciation of the patient or group
- Application of scientific knowledge to the processes of diagnosis and treatment through the use of judgment and critical thinking
- Advancement of professional nursing knowledge through scholarly inquiry

- Influence on social and public policy to promote social justice
- Assurance of safe, quality, and evidence-based practice" (ANA, 2010, p. 9).

Examining these essential features gives evidence of the importance of the nurse-patient relationship in concert with the individuality and experiences of the person for whom the nurse cares. Although the medical profession has adopted a strong preference for an evidence base for practice, at times to the exclusion of the values of the individual patient, nursing has sustained its focus on the caring aspects of the relationship and respect for the uniqueness of the individual along with rigor for the science supporting nursing practice (Altamirano-Bustamante et al., 2013).

Nursing Ethics

Within the field of ethics, the category of nursing ethics is recognized by many as a legitimate subcategory of biomedical ethics (or bioethics) with a focus on the study of the moral problems that nurses face in the healthcare setting (Fry, Veatch, & Taylor, 2011). *Nursing ethics* is the formal study of nurses' professional obligations to the individuals who require nursing care—how nurses make decisions and act in light of their professional identities as caregivers committed to the health and well-being of their patients.

Although concern with ethical practice is as old as the professions, bioethics as a field of study emerged as a result of scandals in research and the uncertainties that arose with advances in science and technology. It has quickly become very much a part of healthcare, given the prominence of some of the cases that have been covered in the public media. A major focus of bioethics is the study of the quandaries arising from life-sustaining therapies and limited resources. The focus of clinical bioethics on hospitalized patients is primarily concerned with questions relating to identifying the appropriate decision-maker, identifying the criteria to use to determine what treatment modalities should be used, and addressing conflicts that may arise with these decisions (Taylor, 1993). These issues usually relate to quandaries and the dramatic decisions related to technological modalities that can extend life.

Nurses were members of the early hospital-based ethics committee, and today nurses continue not only as members but often as leaders of committees and clinical ethics consultation services. Clinical nurses at the bedside are most often the frontline implementers of the decisions that save and extend life. The rapid advancement in care strategies over the past half century has proceeded without sufficient ethical reflection upon the effect of this care on the bedside nurse. While caring for the patients, particularly critically ill patients, nurses are the major communicators with family members seeking to grasp their loved ones' conditions. Given the complexity and importance of the ethical considerations in clinical practice, the new role of nurse ethicist is emerging to support not only nurses but the interprofessional teams and patients and families as well (Wocial, Bledsoe, Helft, & Everett, 2010).

Less well publicized, but equally important, are the troubling questions that arise for nurses at the bedside as they actually implement care reflecting the advances in knowledge and technology and work with the patient, family, and interprofessional team. For example, life-sustaining technology offered in intensive care units (ICUs) tends to foster the view of the patient as a body composed of organ systems, tissues, cells, and so forth. Often little attention is given to the body as a whole representing the personhood of the individual. Nurses, while giving intimate care and in close proximity to both the body and the patient's loved ones, may experience moral concerns when care is deemed to be overly aggressive or the burden of care is not seen as worthy of the potential benefit. Thus, there is increasing recognition of the need to also focus on the everyday issues that present moral concerns for clinical nurses. These daily challenges include "the role of relationships and gender in decision-making processes, the distribution of decisional power, and the mechanisms of empowerment and disempowerment of patient, relatives and health care workers because nursing is highly influenced by the caring approach as a normative theory of ethics" (Monteverde, 2009, p. 614). "Competence in ethics demands first that nurses reflect on and articulate their everyday ethical concerns and not limit their understanding to ethical breakdown and dilemmas. Genuine awareness of ethics unfolds in the concrete reality of what nurses live every day, not in the philosophical contemplation of right and wrong" (Wocial, 2012, p. 37)

Moral Distress

Moral distress, first identified by Jameton in 1984, is increasingly recognized as a significant issue for nurses and, more recently, other members of the clinical team (Bell & Breslin, 2008; Jameton, 1984; Ulrich, Hamric, & Grady, 2010). This phenomenon of moral distress occurs when one knows the right thing to do, but institutional constraints make it impossible to pursue the right course of action. Research on moral distress consistently reveals that the highest levels of distress relate to the provision of aggressive care to terminally ill patients (Hamric & Blackhall, 2007). Which aspects of this care create moral problems or concerns and the subsequent distress? What are the moral considerations that arise for the bedside nurse who recognizes physiological futility when the family and/or clinical team remain committed to continue aggressive care? These moral concerns might include the deterioration of the body, the isolation of the patient, the infliction of pain without benefit, and the nurse's perceived position of powerlessness.

A full discussion of the concept of moral distress is beyond the focus of this chapter. Rather, the purpose here is to consider the dilemmas arising in practice through the lens of person-centered care, where the values of the patient rather than the values of the nurse are guiding clinical decisions. How can clinical nurses move from their personal and clinical views when they experience dissonance with the wishes of a patient or family to both see and explore the situation through the life story of the patient? Once having this patient's view, how can nurses proceed to work in partnership with the patient and patient's loved ones to achieve their goals?

In the vignette at the opening of the chapter, the value that the nurse places on relieving suffering along with respect for patient autonomy must be considered in light of the patient's life history and relationships with family members. Initially this nurse might experience what is defined as moral distress—she believes moving from curative to comfort care is the right thing to do based on her professional values. Her thought process might include recognizing the patient as an autonomous individual with the right to self-determination; the patient, after understanding the medical facts, has the authority to reject further curative therapy and consent to hospice care. Yet

Katharine learns more about her patient and his values over time. Does Mr. Lefkakia's decision to honor his daughter's heartfelt plea to continue care reflect the value he places on his relationship and his long years of parenting a daughter who chose oncology as her life's work? Clinicians can never fully know their patients' life stories and all that influences their care decisions, yet some exploration of the patients' life stories may mitigate or prevent ethical stress when there is a deeper understanding of another's values. Furthermore, clinical nurses may find over time that, if they honor the patient's position and continue to be open and present, working in partnership, they might find opportunities to help the patient and family explore their own values in the context of the specific health crisis and move toward a common goal. Families need more time to process these unique experiences in contrast to nurses, who have gained experience working through many illness experiences.

Clinical nurses who continue to administer the chemotherapy, inducing symptoms and suffering, need to reflect not only on their role and their patient but on the family relationships and values informing the patient's decision-making. The existential suffering of the daughter should be recognized and of concern along with the physical suffering of the patient.

If the clinical nurses gave voice to the daughter's suffering, would it prompt a deeper discussion among the family members? An initial negative reaction based on seeing the daughter's prioritizing her own needs over her father's could be followed by considering what is unknown about the previous experiences with life, suffering, and death. The family's previous experiences, although invisible to the nurse, are at play in the current crisis. Could the daughter's previous experience with hospice be informing her reaction, perhaps even more so than her oncology expertise?

The traditional focus of clinical ethics' work has been on the four principles of bioethics set forth by Beauchamp and Childress in their *Principles of Biomedical Ethics* textbook, now in its seventh edition: respect for autonomy, nonmaleficence, beneficence, and justice (Beauchamp & Childress, 2012). Although these principles frame important moral considerations, attention to these moral considerations is only an important first step in seeing the myriad of ethical obligations and issues that arise in the biomedical context (Churchill, Fanning, & Schenck, 2013; Fiester, 2007; Taylor, 1993). When clinicians limit their moral considerations to a simplistic understanding of these four principles, they exclude important aspects of an individual's caring relationships as well as the nurse's professional obligations that are relevant to ethical decision-making.

Theories of Bioethics

Although nurses may not think they work through ethical dilemmas using theories, in actuality they do. These theories offer a framework to help us focus our concerns and discuss them with others. Consider four discrete theories and the questions they pose:

1. **Virtue ethics or character ethics** emphasizes the individual who makes choices and acts with the question *What sort of person/nurse ought I to be?* Nurses consider the following virtues, among many, to be important aspects of ethical practice: compassion, trustworthiness, and respectfulness.

2. **Principle-based or obligation-based ethics** asks, *What should I do to be ethical in a given situation?* Nurses use the principles of autonomy and nonmaleficence, or do no harm, to organize thinking through a situation relating to consent, as one example.

3. **An ethics of care** focuses on the traits valued in intimate personal relationships and privileges kindness, attentiveness, sympathy, and love. *How do I care for this person as an individual within his or her constellation of loving relationships?* Nurses working from this perspective would broaden their area of concern to include the patient's loved ones, who would be recognized as important recipients for nursing care.

4. **Feminist ethics** asks about the political and power bases in the clinical arena and who is advantaged or disadvantaged by them. Nurses ask, *Who has the power in a given situation? Where does that power originate? Who should have the power in a particular situation?* The sources of power within the hospital hierarchy as well as the patient's family system are all important considerations for nurses seeking to address ethical concerns.

Although presented as separate and exclusive theories, nurse ethicists Davis, Fowler, and Aroskar maintain that nurses use a combination of these ethical theories to explore and reason through different aspects of the ethical dilemmas clinical nurses face in practice (Davis, Fowler, & Aroskar, 2010, pp. 2–3).

Person-Centered Care

The concept of person-centered care, when examined using several well-established ethical theories, comes out as "just the right thing to do" (Duggan, Geller, Cooper, & Beach, 2006).

"The nurse-patient relationship is central to *care ethics* which directs attention to the specific situations of individual patients viewed within the context of their life narrative" (Fry et al., 2011, p. xxvii). Nurse ethicist Taylor's examination of the characteristics of the care perspective serves to illustrate the moral nature of person-centered care:

- The centrality of the caring relationship
- The promotion of the dignity and respect of patients as people
- The acceptance of particular patient and healthcare professional variables (beliefs, values, relationships) as morally relevant factors in ethical decision-making
- Redefinition of the fundamental moral skills to expand beyond principle-based ethics and controversy resolution to include moral skills, such as kindness, compassion, attentiveness, and reliability (Taylor, 1993)

Despite the nursing profession's espoused focus on caring, there is evidence to support that nurses, when faced with ethical dilemmas, tend to reason in a conformist way and are guided by workplace rules and norms rather than by critical reflection and creative problem solving

(Dierckx de Casterle, Izumi, Godfrey, & Denhaerynck, 2008; Goethals, Gastmans, & Dierckx de Casterle, 2010). Furthermore, in challenging situations, nurses do not necessarily move to a more patient-centered practice where the personal needs and well-being of the patient are paramount, but rather to one that tends to favor the nurses' moral perspective (Pavlish, Brown-Saltzman, Hersh, Shirk, & Rounkle, 2011). Clinical nurses struggle when family preferences in end-of-life care are honored over those of the patient; promoting patient autonomy is frequently expressed as the ethical priority. However, without clear and intimate knowledge of the patient, nurses' view of the best interest of the patient may in fact be rather paternalistic (Pavlish et al., 2011).

Gadow emphasizes this concern with her concept of existential advocacy—"the effort to help persons *become clear about what they want* to do, by helping them discern and clarify their values in the situation, and on the basis of that self-examination, to reach decisions which express their reaffirmed, perhaps recreated, complex of values" (1980, p. 85).

In this context, advocacy should not be based on the nurse's values grounded in clinical expertise or the belief that the nurse, rather than the patient, is in the position to determine what is in the patient's best interest. One can think of existential advocacy as the opposite of paternalism as well as a more comprehensive (developed) advocacy than just protecting the individual's rights to do what he or she wants.

What Makes a Dilemma Ethical in Nature?

Whether the term used is *ethical dilemma*, *problem*, *issue*, or *incident*, nurses face situations that require "value clarification, reflection on these values, and possibly actions of an ethical nature" (Davis et al., 2010, p. 9). The clinical practice of nursing includes systematic problem solving with nursing interventions and advocacy to meet patient care needs. When nurses attend to the range of human experiences and responses to health and illness, they make countless decisions in the provision of care. Decisions are made frequently and comfortably without reflection on the personal or professional values that inform their decision-making. Yet at times the clinical decisions or care options that nurses face will trouble them as they determine their course of action. Some situations will prompt reflection and questions—*What is the right thing to do in light of my professional identity? How do my personal values and beliefs influence my professional life? Whose values are privileged in care situations—the patient, the patient's loved ones, or the person providing care?*

Ethical issues can be recognized when one moves from the idea that one can do something to the position that one *ought* to do something involving a set of norms or judgments of values, rights, duties, and responsibilities. Judging the "right" thing to do is not a matter of personal preference.

Actions or decisions are considered ethical in nature when they are determined by our obligations, duties, and commitments, grounded in the caring relationship rather than a personal preference.

What Is a Dilemma?

By definition, a *dilemma* is a situation presenting a choice between what seems to be two equally desirable or undesirable alternatives. A dilemma can also be defined as a difficult problem seemingly incapable of a satisfactory solution or, alternately, a situation that presents two choices between equally unsatisfactory alternatives (Davis et al., 2010). Not all dilemmas that arise in nursing practice are ethical in nature. Many choices in daily life are simple choices among options without ethical implications. Raines found in a nationwide sample of more than 200 oncology nurses that they reported experiencing an average of 31.7 different types of ethical dilemmas within the previous year (2000). Other studies also report nurses experience frequent ethical concerns in practice (Pavlish, Brown-Saltzman, Hersh, Shirk, & Nudelman, 2011; Ulrich et al., 2007).

Examples of Ethical Dilemmas

Clinical nurses confront many ethical dilemmas in practice. Examples of dilemmas that may arise in the provision of person-centered care include:

- Whether and in what way to care for the patient characterized as "difficult" or "noncompliant"

- Nursing care of a dying patient receiving aggressive care based on directives from family in conflict with a patient's expressed wish

- Whether to maintain confidential information that a patient specifically expressed should not be shared with the family after the patient's deterioration, when family members are serving as surrogate decision-makers

- Willingness to care for a patient based on that person's lifestyle, behavior, or espoused beliefs that conflict with those of the nurse

- Whether to participate in procedures that conflict with the nurse's personal or spiritual values when there is an emergent care need

In these and many other examples, nurses must consider their obligations as professional nurses and the nature of the caring relationship. The intimacy and proximity of the nurse to the individual and the patient's loved ones during these health-related crises present complex situations for nurses to understand and respond to.

> **NOTE**
>
> Nurses will sometimes identify situations as being ethical in nature when they are disagreements without an ethical foundation. Examples of these include short-staffing, nurse-to-nurse conflicts, some disagreements over the plan of care, and resource shortages. Each of these situations is difficult, creates significant stress, and must be thoughtfully addressed. On occasion, they may have an ethical dimension, but it is incorrect to say that, by definition, one of these situations (such as a short-staffing situation) poses an ethical dilemma.

The Role of Values in Ethical Dilemmas

Values are deeply held beliefs that inform and guide our actions. As individuals, we hold personal values, and as clinicians, we adopt professional values. Clinicians are so well socialized into the culture of biomedical science that they may not recognize the extent and depth of the values integral to the practice of nursing and medicine. These powerful values, shaped through professional socialization about health, illness, healing, and the nature of a good death, are not universal and fuel the dilemmas that arise in the acute-care setting (Glen, 1999). We may believe that the values we hold are universal, but individuals are strikingly diverse in the values they hold.

Diversity—Discipline and Specialty Values

If we give attention to some of the professional and clinical subspecialty cultures that inform healthcare, there are many hurdles to overcome. Hospital-based acute care, where most nurses practice, is situated within many subcultures, including that of the organization, nursing unit, medical subspecialty, and the distinct professional culture of the provider. Culture is never static. For example, the medical standard of disclosure of bad news to patients has changed dramatically in the past 50 years from a norm of withholding (Veatch & Tai, 1980) to disclosing. Berger challenges the 1998 *American College of Physicians Ethics Manual* imperative that "however uncomfortable to the clinician or patient, information that is essential to the patient must be disclosed" (2001, p. 376). He notes that given varying cultural norms for disclosure, patients should define for the physician their personal requirements for disclosure.

I myself can remember using numerical codes on hospital paperwork to prevent a patient from seeing the diagnosis of cancer on hospital admission forms. Thus, the normative practice and culture of medicine have evolved from the therapeutic privilege of withholding information for the benefit of the patient to full disclosure, and now to consideration of patient preferences and values about what information should be shared and with whom (Barclay, Blackhall, & Tulsky, 2007; Ngo-Metzger, August, Srinivasan, Liao, & Meyskens, 2008). Another example of values evolving in the United States relatively recently is with the presence of a women's partner participating in childbirth or family presence during resuscitation efforts. Values are not static.

Findings from examinations of ICU cultures reveal another layer of specialty culture. Although the units are governed by the same institutional policies and procedures, with common formal rules, there are profound differences in interpretation and implementation. Surgical and medical ICUs handle the decision-making process about consent for tracheostomy and gastrostomy tube placement differently; value placed on Do Not Resuscitate orders ranges from being considered meaningless paperwork by surgeons to alternately being seen as a tool to promote communication and end-of-life care planning by medical practitioners (Baggs et al., 2007). Oncology, characterized as a moral world permeated by hope and optimism, fosters patient participation in aggressive research regimens until death (del Vecchio Good, Good, Schaffer, & Lind, 1990). Values differ; science is not neutral; and expert clinicians are not merely repositories of facts and technical skills (Kukla, 2007).

Nurse ethicist Fry believes there to be remarkable agreement among nurses around the world on the moral values of nursing and identifies these values as "honesty (or truthfulness), compassion, respect for others, doing good for others, competence, and keeping commitments" (2008, p. 51). The ANA *Code of Ethics* articulates these values along with others (2008). The International Council of Nurses (ICN) *Code of Ethics for Nurses* identifies these professional values: respectfulness, responsiveness, compassion, trustworthiness, and integrity (2012). A literature review of articles published in English and Persian language to identify and define nursing values offers examples of ethical values generally shared within the global community; however, the influences of socioeconomic, cultural, and religious beliefs result in varying definitions of these shared values (Shahriari, Mohammadi, Abbaszadeh, & Bahrami, 2013). Furthermore, even within the nursing profession in one country, there can be significant differences among values related to the sanctity of life, abortion rights, self-efficacy, and "acceptable" lifestyles. Although nurses may share a common bond, within and across countries, societal pressures and priorities will influence the individual nurse's values.

Identifying and Reflecting on Personal Values

Creating and supporting a culture of person-centered care demands that clinicians reflect on their own deeply held beliefs and values. Once these values are recognized, they can move to elicit and appreciate the values of patients and their families. Although there are universal and widely held values, such as do not kill, lie, or cheat, many values are context-specific. If values are what we believe are important and what we focus our attention on, consider the range of disciplines and the variation in attention. Specialty practices vary in their areas of concern. Does the clinical nutritionist focus on appetite and caloric intake differently than the physical therapist or medical resident? Consider how the social worker for a transplant service might focus on health-care insurance in contrast to the geriatric social worker. Roles will shape our focus. A clinical nurse serving as the charge nurse will differ in focus from the clinical nurse assigned to specific patients. Finally, our personal life experiences shape where we pay attention and what we believe to be important in our professional work. Consider the pregnant nurse caring for a critically ill newborn versus the nurse who is a new grandparent. How might their practice convey their values founded in their immediate life experiences or previous experiences?

Reflecting on your own values, whether they originated from your early family life or later in your professional socialization, is an important prerequisite for working with your patients' values:

- What are the situations or ethical risk factors in your practice world? Stated another way, what situations trouble you? What keeps you up when you should be sleeping? What clinical situations do you try to avoid?

- What are the values of your organization? Read and reflect on its mission and value statements. Do they shape your practice? If so, how? Or are these statements invisible? Are the statements visible, but not demonstrated? Do you practice in an academic setting? If so, how are the tripartite missions of education and research balanced with the commitment to patient care?

- What values are evident in the routine practices of your work unit or team? If you asked three colleagues what the primary values are in your group, would there be similarities or differences among their answers?

- What can you do, as a practicing clinician, to give voice to the ethical values that shape your practice? What about the values that foster concerns or conflict?

- Do you know the values of your local community or specific populations you serve? Have you ever been surprised by a value or belief of a patient or family? I remember how startled I felt when a family member shared her belief that a child's genetic condition was God's punishment for the parents' bitter divorce. How might this belief have influenced their caring relations?

- What are ways to promote interprofessional conversations about the values that raise ethical concerns?

When deeply held beliefs and values are recognized, they can be examined and discussed to promote understanding. When hidden, they surely influence behaviors, and specifically decisions about health and caregiving (Kleinman, 2011). Now consider if a colleague or patient understood your values and told you they were wrong. How would you feel? What would you say? Yet is this not what health professionals often do when seeking to influence patients into accepting our recommendations? Would rejection of your values promote trust and cooperation or create distance and silence?

Giving voice to values can serve to promote comfort with discussing and understanding the rich diversity of life experiences and the values they inform. Gaining comfort with recognizing the values embedded in practice is an important precursor for person-centered care. A simple statement that a patient or family member is asking too many questions conveys values of the speaker—values about time, curiosity, and meaning.

Value-Laden Conflict

The values espoused both in our domestic lives and professional practice reveal a very personal spectrum, reflecting the varied influences and emphases of cultural background, education, training, and experience. Badcott posits that it is "important for the individual that there is little or no dissonance between personal values in private life and professional values in healthcare practice" and that our genuine values should not be disposed of when we put on a uniform or white coat (2011, p. 186). However, if clinicians are to provide care based on the values of their patients, some dissonance is to be expected. How is this potential for conflict in values handled? One resource is the ethics consultation services developed to address value-laden conflicts that arise in healthcare and are driven by legal cases and regulatory mandates. And yet, because the diversity of values is to be expected, can the toll of conflict for all be prevented through a culture of person-centered care and a more proactive approach to recognizing and honoring the diversity of values? Many believe so (Pavlish, Brown-Saltzman, Fine, & Jakel, 2013; Schlairet, Kiser, & Norris, 2012).

> **NOTE**
>
> Refer to Chapter 16 for more details about ethics consultation.

Enablers for Voicing Values

What makes it easier to speak and act on our values? Some things are within our control; for others, we need help from colleagues and the organizations within which we work.

> **NOTE**
>
> The lists of the following factors are adapted from Appendix C of M. C. Gentile's *Giving Voice to Values: How to Speak Your Mind When You Know What's Right* (2010).

Things Within Our Own Control

- Enlisting allies: Who else shares our concern?
- Selecting and sequencing of audiences: Share your value conflict and invite a response (critique/alternate perspective, immediate response to how we present our value conflict).
- Gaining greater confidence in your viewpoint by securing more information: Family or clinician narrative/context/history
- Starting with questions rather than assertions
- Gaining greater understanding of others' motivations, needs, fears
- Lowering the stress by taking the conversation with dissenters or key supporters off-line, one-on-one, at a mutually convenient time, and in a quiet place
- Working through incremental steps
- Changing the frame of the problem: Position it as an opportunity to learn about another's perspective or as a "learning dialogue" rather than a reproach.
- Questioning assumptions, professional rationalizations, and seeming truisms/facts
- Appealing to shared purpose, values
- Normalizing (managing this kind of conflict is just part of doing the job): Value conflicts are expected.

Within the Organizational Context

- Having explicit organizational policies and values in place

- Seeing an organizational value placed on open debate, discussion

- Structuring explicit mechanisms for open debate and discussion within the organization

- Instituting systems for raising questions and gathering responses, having healthy disagreements

- Achieving a consistent and visible organizational track record of values-based leadership and an inclusive and respectful practice of correcting problems

Resources to Assist With Morally Distressing Situations

Clinical nurses who have recognized the importance of addressing ethical concerns can assess where there are opportunities for assistance. Consider that there are three levels of intervention:

1. **For an individual patient:** Organize team discussions and family meetings.

2. **For issues related to the unit or team culture:** Be proactive and look for and employ ideas that give voice to the group values and norms; engage leadership perspective on the concerns.

3. **At the organizational level:** Institute policies, procedures, and system resources.

When needs are identified, demonstrate a willingness to work with colleagues to create solutions to address values issues, remembering to bring the perspective of the patient and family forward, and acknowledge the impact on direct care providers.

Table 11.1 lists examples of resources that exist in many healthcare organizations to assist with clinical issues that present ethical concerns. Work with organizational leaders to access these services according to existing policies or to see whether these services can be put in place to support caregivers while improving patient care.

TABLE 11.1 Organizational Resources for Assistance in Addressing Ethical Concerns

RESOURCE	DESCRIPTION
Ethics Consult Service	Provides services in response to calls from patients, families, surrogates, and healthcare professionals who seek to clarify or resolve morally and/or ethically challenging situations arising in patient care. Identifies morally/ethically justifiable options in cases of value conflict. Provides full consults upon request or serves as a resource.

continues

TABLE 11.1   *continued*

RESOURCE	DESCRIPTION
Social Work Department	Assesses immediate and ongoing needs of patients, families, and staff; offers short-term counseling and support; links patients and families to community programs and resources; facilitates support groups for patients, families, and staff related to specific situations; assists with completing applications for benefits/financial assistance.
Pastoral Care/Chaplain	Assists families in distress; counsels patients and families; assists in preparing advance directives; offers spiritual support to patients and families as well as staff.
Caregiver Support Programs Related to Stressful or Traumatic Events	Assists staff to work through intensely stressful situations, such as the death of a long-term patient or staff member. Assists with debriefing staff when very traumatic situations have occurred.
Physician and Employee Assistance Programs	Provides confidential individual counseling, group consulting, and stress and conflict management for staff.
Patient and Guest Relations	Provides a judgment-free environment where patients and families can communicate concerns and connect with the appropriate staff/departments for resolution.
Office of General Counsel	Represents organization in legal matters generated by the work of the organization; initiates action to forestall problems and manage risks; interprets legal, regulatory, and policy mandates relevant to healthcare.
Risk Management	Addresses adverse incidents related to patient care; risk treatment; reduction opportunities; potential liabilities and injuries of patients, visitors, or employees; or events that may cause damage and/or loss to institutional or personal property.
Acute Pain Service	Specialty consultation service for recommendations for pain control.
Palliative Care Service	A multidisciplinary team to assist in care of patients/families affected by serious illness, including pain and symptom management, goals of care discussion, end-of-life issues, psychosocial or spiritual distress.
Professionalism Committee of the Medical Board	Provides intervention for disruptive or unprofessional behavior by staff.
External (Patients' Own) Clergy	Hospital chaplains can assist, especially for patients from out of town, who may wish a visit from a local imam, rabbi, minister or priest, or representative of other religious/spiritual traditions.

Conclusion

The Institute of Medicine (IOM) in its landmark book *Crossing the Quality Chasm* (2001, p. 40) defines patient-centered as "providing care that is respectful of and responsive to individual patient preferences, needs, and values and ensuring that patient values guide all clinical decisions." Recognition of the diversity of human beliefs and experiences—shaping an infinite range of beliefs about health and the illness experience—is fundamental.

"Nursing care aims to maximize the values that the patient has treasured in life and extends supportive care to the family and significant others" (ANA, 2008, p. 147). When patient and family values trouble us or even conflict with personal or professional values, we must make decisions to honor patient values while preserving our integrity as individuals and professionals. Reflection on our own life experiences, and the values and beliefs they inform, is the groundwork necessary for eliciting and subsequently honoring patient values, beliefs, and goals.

Clinical nurses who sincerely value the diversity of beliefs about health, illness, and the important role of family in the care experience will help achieve the needed cultural transformation toward person-centered care.

References

Altamirano-Bustamante, M., Altamirano-Bustamante, N. F., Lifshitz, A., Mora-Magana, I., de Hoyos, A., Avila-Osorio, M. T.,…Reyes-Fuentes, A. (2013). Promoting networks between evidence-based medicine and values-based medicine in continuing medical education. *BMC Medicine, 11*(39). Retrieved from www.biomedcentral.com/1741-7015/11/39

American Nurses Association (ANA). (2008). *Guide to the code of ethics for nurses: Interpretation and application.* M. D. M. Fowler (Ed.). Silver Spring, MD: Author.

American Nurses Association (ANA). (2010). *Nursing's social policy statement: The essence of the profession.* Silver Spring, MD: Author.

Badcott, D. (2011). Professional values: Introduction to a theme. *Medical Health Care and Philosophy, 14*(2), 185-186.

Badzek, L. (2008). Legacy and vision: The perspective of the American Nurses Association on Nursing and Health Care Ethics. In W. J. Ellenchild Pinch & A.M. Haddad (Eds.), *Nursing and health care ethics* (p. 8). Silver Spring, MD: American Nurses Association.

Baggs, J. G., Norton, S. A., Schmitt, M. H., Dombeck, M. T., Sellers, C. R., & Quinn, J. R. (2007). Intensive care unit cultures and end-of-life decision making. *Journal of Critical Care, 22*(2), 159-168.

Barclay, J. S., Blackhall, L. J., & Tulsky, J. A. (2007). Communication strategies and cultural issues in the delivery of bad news. *Journal of Palliative Medicine, 10*(4), 958-977.

Beauchamp, T. L., & Childress, J. F. (2012). *Principles of biomedical ethics* (7th ed.). New York, NY: Oxford University Press.

Bell, J., & Breslin, J. M. (2008). Healthcare provider moral distress as a leadership challenge. *JONA's Healthcare Law, Ethics, and Regulation, 10*(4), 94-97.

Berger, J. T. (2001). Multi-cultural considerations and the American College of Physicians Ethics Manual. *Journal of Clinical Ethics, 12*(4), 375-381.

Churchill, L. R., Fanning, J. B., & Schenck, D. (2013). *What patients teach—The everyday ethics of healthcare.* New York, NY: Oxford University Press.

Davis, A. J., Fowler, M. D., & Aroskar, M. A. (2010). *Ethical dilemmas and nursing practice* (5th ed.). Upper Saddle River, NJ: Pearson Health Science.

del Vecchio Good, M-J., Good, B. J., Schaffer, C., & Lind, S. E. (1990). American oncology and the discourse on hope. *Culture, Medicine and Psychiatry, 14*(1), 59-79.

Dierckx de Casterle, B., Izumi, S., Godfrey, N. S., & Denhaerynck, K. (2008) Nurses' responses to ethical dilemmas in nursing practice: Meta-analysis. *Journal of Advanced Nursing, 63*(6), 540-549.

Diers, D. (1982). Nursing reclaims its role. *Nursing Outlook, 30*(8), 459-463.

Duggan, P. S., Geller, G., Cooper, L. A., & Beach, M. C. (2006). The moral nature of patient-centeredness: Is it "just the right thing to do"? *Patient and Education and Counseling, 62*(2), 271-276.

Fiester, A. (2007). Why the clinical ethics we teach fails patients. *Academic Medicine, 82*(7), 684-688.

Fry, S. T. (2008). Philosophical and theoretical issues in nursing ethics. In W. J. Ellenchild Pinch & A. M. Haddad (Eds.), *Nursing and health care ethics* (pp. 45-55). Silver Spring, MD: American Nurses Association.

Fry, S. T., Veatch, R. M., & Taylor, C. R. (2011). *Case studies in nursing ethics*. Sudbury, MA: Jones and Bartlett Learning.

Gadow, S. (1980). Existential advocacy: Philosophical foundations of nursing. In S. F. Spicker & S. Gadow (Eds.), *Nursing images and ideals: Opening dialogue with the humanities* (pp. 79-101). New York, NY: Springer.

Gentile, M. C. (2010). *Giving voice to values: How to speak your mind when you know what's right*. New Haven, CT: Yale University Press.

Glen, S. (1999). Educating for interprofessional collaboration: Teaching about values. *Nursing Ethics, 6*(3), 202-213.

Goethals, S., Gastmans, C., & Dierckx de Casterle, B. (2010). Nurses' ethical reasoning and behaviour: A literature review. *International Journal of Nursing Studies, 47*(5), 635-650.

Hamric, A. B., & Blackhall, L. J. (2007). Nurse-physician perspectives on the care of dying patients in intensive care units: Collaboration, moral distress and ethical climate. *Critical Care Medicine, 35*(2), 422-429.

Institute of Medicine (IOM). (2001). *Crossing the quality chasm: A new health care system for the 21st century*. Washington, DC: National Academies Press.

International Council of Nurses (ICN). (2012). *The ICN code of ethics for nurses*. Geneva, Switzerland. Retrieved from www.icn.org

Jameton, A. (1984). *Nursing practice: The ethical issues*. Englewood Cliffs, NJ: Prentice Hall.

Kleinman, A. (2011). The divided self, hidden values, and moral sensibility in medicine. *The Lancet, 377*(9768): 804-805.

Kukla, R. (2007). How do patients know? *Hastings Center Report, 37*(5), 27-35. doi:10.1353/hcr.2007.0074

Monteverde, S. (2009). The importance of time in ethical decision making. *Nursing Ethics, 16*(5), 613-624.

Ngo-Metzger, Q., August, K. J., Srinivasan, M., Liao, S., & Meyskens, F. L. (2008). End-of-life care: Guidelines for patient-centered communication. *American Family Physician, 77*(2), 167-174.

Pavlish, C., Brown-Saltzman, K., Fine, A., & Jakel, P. (2013). Making the call: A proactive ethics framework. *HEC Forum, 25*(3), 269-283.

Pavlish, C., Brown-Saltzman, K., Hersh, M., Shirk, M., & Nudelman, O. (2011). Early indicators and risk factors for ethical issues in clinical practice. *Journal of Nursing Scholarship, 43*(1), 13-21.

Pavlish, C., Brown-Saltzman, K., Hersh, M., Shirk, M., & Rounkle, A. M. (2011). Nursing priorities, actions, and regrets for ethical situations in clinical practice. *Journal of Nursing Scholarship, 43*(4), 385-395.

Raines, M. L. (2000). Ethical decision making in nurses: Relationships among moral reasoning, coping style, and ethics stress. *JONA's Healthcare Law, Ethics, and Regulation, 2*(1), 29-41.

Schlairet, M. C., Kiser, K., & Norris, S. (2012). Clinical ethics support services: An evolving model. *Nursing Outlook, 60*(5), 309-315.

Shahriari, M., Mohammadi, E., Abbaszadeh, A., & Bahrami, M. (2013). Nursing ethical values and definitions: A literature review. *Iranian Journal of Nursing Midwifery Research, 18*(1), 1-8.

Taylor, C. (1993). Nursing ethics: The role of caring. *Association of Women's Health, Obstetrics, and Neonatal Nurses' Clinical Issues in Perinatal and Women's Health Nursing, 4*(4), 552-560.

Ulrich, C. M., Hamric, A. B., & Grady, C. (2010). Moral distress: A growing problem in the health professions? *Hastings Center Report, 40*(1), 20-22.

Ulrich, C., O'Donnell, P., Taylor, C., Farrar, A., Danis, M., & Grady, C. (2007). Ethical climate, ethics stress, and the job satisfaction of nurses and social workers in the United States. *Social Science & Medicine, 65*(8), 1708-1719.

Veatch, R. M., & Tai, E. (1980). Talking about death: Patterns of lay and professional change. *Annals of the American Academy of Political and Social Science, 447*(1), 29-45.

Wocial, L. D. (2012). Finding a voice in ethics: Everyday ethical behavior in nursing. In C. Ulrich (Ed.), *Nursing ethics in everyday practice* (pp. 37-48). Indianapolis, IN: Sigma Theta Tau International.

Wocial, L. D., Bledsoe, P., Helft, P. R., & Everett, L. Q. (2010). Nurse ethicist: Innovative resource for nurses. *Journal of Professional Nursing, 26*(5), 287-292.

Chapter 12

Patient-Centered Care in the Face of Cultural Conflict

Margaret Dexheimer Pharris, PhD, MPH, RN, FAAN

It was an especially hot, sweltering August day in the Deep South of the United States of America. The nurses on the intensive care unit were stretched thin, emotionally and physically, as they responded to the demands of caring for critically ill patients. They were an all–African-American nursing staff who partnered with the rest of the health-care team—environmental service workers, chaplains, physicians, nursing assistants, respiratory therapists, health unit coordinators, nurse managers, social workers, and physical therapists—in caring for the state's most vulnerable patients. They prided themselves on the high quality of patient- and family-centered care they provided as a cohesive team.

But this morning the nurses were weighted down by the heavy, humid air that made every movement an effort and by the intense suffering of several patients and families in their care. Just when it seemed like quick lunch breaks might be possible, the phone rang. The emergency department was sending a 38-year-old man, Ricky, who was comatose and on the verge of death after a suicide attempt. Three nurses converged in the room when the patient arrived to settle him in, do an assessment, and determine who would be most able to fit him into their already demanding schedule. As they transferred the patient to the bed, the eyes of the nurses simultaneously converged on the left side of Ricky's pale white chest, which prominently displayed a large tattoo of a Black man hanging from a tree with a noose around his neck. Terror rose up from the depths of their souls. They looked at one another and, together, heavily sighed, thinking, "Oh no, dear Lord, we do not have energy for this today!" The collective memory of each of their families contained sorrowful images of losing cherished loved ones to the violence of White hatred and disregard for Black life. A colleague had just shown them the Without Sanctuary *website, which displays lynching postcards, including images of smiling White families with their children in their best Sunday clothes, gathered around charred Black bodies hanging from trees (Allen & Littlefield, 2005). The reminder of this violent disregard for the sanctity of Black life on the chest of this new patient made them sick to their stomachs. Which of them had the emotional strength to best care for this patient, to nurture and protect his life?*

The Backbone of Patient-Centered Care in the Face of Cultural Conflict

For nurses, patient-centered care in the face of cultural conflict is rooted in the ethical standards of the profession, which form the framework for the culture of nursing around the world. The International Council of Nurses (ICN) *Code of Ethics for Nurses* (2012) states, "The nurse maintains a standard of personal health such that the ability to provide care is not compromised" (p. 4). Angeleen stepped forward to be Ricky's primary nurse and remained in that role until he left the unit. She stepped forward out of concern and respect for her colleagues, knowing that they will do the same for her someday in the future when her emotional reserve is low. And she stepped forward on behalf of her profession, which calls her to respect the human dignity of each individual in her care and states that she has the fundamental responsibility to promote health, prevent illness, restore health, and alleviate suffering (ICN, 2012, p. 2). She recalled her first fundamentals nursing course that stressed the importance of adhering to nursing codes of ethics, which called her to provide high-quality nursing care to all patients. The preamble of the ICN *Code of Ethics for Nurses* (2012) states:

> Inherent in nursing is a respect for human rights, including cultural rights, the right to life and choice, to dignity and to be treated with respect. Nursing care is respectful of and unrestricted by considerations of age, colour, creed, culture, disability or illness, gender, sexual orientation, nationality, politics, race or social status. (p. 1)

For Angeleen, personal health went far beyond making sure she was well rested and that she exercised adequately, ate nutritious foods, maintained emotional balance, and immersed herself in that which nourished her spirit. She also needed to do the mental and spiritual work that involved an analysis of the social structures that set up and maintain racism in her country, which is necessary core content in schools of nursing so that nurses understand the historical roots of racial conflict. Through this analysis, Angeleen knew that racism took root by pitting poor White people against poor Black people to make poor White people think that they were in some way superior. Even though poor Whites were working as sharecroppers and indentured servants, they did not experience the violence of being torn from their homeland, objectified, beaten, and having their families broken apart as loved ones were sold away by plantation owners, which was the experience of enslaved Black people in the Western hemisphere. Poor Whites were also much less likely to be victims of rape and lynching.

After slavery legally ended, from the 1880s to the 1960s, Jim Crow laws legally separated Blacks and Whites. For example, pertaining to the practice of nursing, the state of Alabama had a law stating, "No person or corporation shall require any white female nurse to nurse in wards or rooms in hospitals, either public or private, in which negro men are placed" (National Park Service, n.d.). These laws shaped and formed the structural violence perpetrated upon African Americans and portrayed on Ricky's chest. Angeleen understood that this violence oppressed both the perpetrator and the victim and that her professional code of ethics called her to uphold the human dignity of each person (American Nurses Association [ANA], 2010). Through her healing presence as a nurse, she could construct a new story, although it would not be easy. In their work on caring for "not so picture-perfect patients," Turkel and Ray (2009) draw on the work of Roach (2002) to propose that ethics in nursing implies a relational responsibility to care for the patient without discrimination related to who the person is, what the person has done, or what behaviors the person exhibits.

Employing great energy and moral fortitude, Angeleen concentrated on her nursing presence and responsibility so that she could attend to what it was that Ricky, from his perspective, needed to heal. She knew that when he woke up, she would have only seconds to reassure him with her words and her mannerisms that he was safe in her highly professional care. Yet the fear that Ricky might experience was miniscule compared to what Black patients often feel when they are in the care of White healthcare providers they do not know, given the enduring pattern of White violence and terror perpetrated against Black people in the United States. To adequately and sensitively provide patient-centered care to Black patients, all healthcare providers in the United States, but particularly those from the dominant White culture, should read Harriet Washington's (2006) *Medical Apartheid: The Dark History of Medical Experimentation on Black Americans from Colonial Times to the Present*. Patient-centered care is rooted in nursing codes of ethics and begins with an understanding of and sensitivity to the historical and sociocultural experience of patients.

Patient-Centered Care Calls for a Dual Focus on Systems and Individuals

Shim (2010) proposes a theory of Cultural Health Capital (CHC), which employs a "double vision" to simultaneously focus on biography and social structures—on the histories and cultures patients and healthcare providers bring into the healthcare interaction—as well as on the macro-level structures that profoundly shape the nature of the interaction (p. 4). Nurses know that many patients come into the healthcare system unable to advocate for themselves, and oftentimes they present in a manner that is confrontational and makes providing care a challenge. Or, patients simply do not have the energy or strength to clearly communicate what they need. Patient-centered care involves intense emotional and spiritual work so that the nurse is able to sort through the patient's pain, broken relationships, emotional trauma, and social differences to discern what healing means for *this* person in *this* situation and to collaborate with the patient's significant others and other members of the healthcare team to create the potential for healing and health. Active listening with one's whole being is essential—with eyes, ears, heart, and spirit wide open. In many healthcare environments, systemic forces place an undue burden on patients to act in a certain way in order to receive adequate care.

Studies demonstrate that patients need to fit a certain profile in order to be the easy recipients of quality care. Shim (2010) draws on the work of Malat, van Ryn, and Purcell (2006) to propose that in the U.S. healthcare system, patients do better—have more cultural health capital—when they:

- Possess knowledge and vocabulary of medical topics
- Know what information is relevant to healthcare personnel
- Can communicate health-related information succinctly and clearly to healthcare personnel
- Are proactive in taking charge of their own health
- Have an instrumental attitude toward their own bodies
- Value self-discipline and have the resources to carry it out
- Demonstrate future orientation in goals and actions
- Possess knowledge of interpersonal dynamics
- Can adapt their own interactional styles to the situation at hand
- Have "the ability to communicate social privilege and resources that can act as cues of favorable social and economic status and consumer savvy" (Shim, 2010, p. 3)

As a nurse reading this text, you know that these impression management strategies come at a cost, are difficult to maintain in stressful healthcare encounters, and are out of the reach of many patients, particularly those with limited resources, those who have been traumatized, and/or those who are not represented in the cultural makeup of the healthcare provider community.

Internationally, there is a trend away from this healthcare provider–centric practice toward patient- and family-centered care (P&FCC). Upon coming into the care of a nurse, patients should be able to bring their whole selves with them; they should be able to be themselves and not have to put on a mask and figure out how to act in a way that is more acceptable to the healthcare establishment just to ensure that they get adequate care. Figuring out how to act in such a way that health can optimally flourish is the responsibility of nurses. Cultural conflict is more likely to arise when patients fear that they will not be understood, valued, known, or respected for who they are. Nurses must work to understand the context of patients' lives so that they can receive each patient with positive regard and without judgment. The ANA (2010) refers to this ability as *moral imagination*—having insight into the experiences of those affected by injustices and other forms of suffering. Moral imagination is "the ability of individuals and communities to empathize with others" (ANA, 2010, p. 6) and involves understanding the life circumstances that shape the current health predicament and their responses to it.

Addressing the rapidly increasing disproportionate burden of diabetes on the poor, Shim (2010) points out that social status is strongly and persistently related to health status and that "health benefits tend to rebound to the resource-rich, and health risks to the resource-poor" (p. 5).

Patient-centered care, at its heart, calls nurses to analyze who is benefiting and who is suffering in the healthcare environment and in each encounter. We must conduct a systematic analysis of the flow of healthcare dollars and quality of care in order to discern whether certain populations are being saturated with healthy lifestyle chances and healthcare benefits while others are being deprived of health chances, discriminated against, bombarded with societal factors that threaten their health, and treated poorly by the very people who are being paid to care for them. The role of the nurse in these situations is to rebalance the flow of resources to ensure adequate quality care for all, but particularly for those most in need. This happens through taking leadership in systems change, education of the healthcare team, and coaching patients so that they are poised to receive the best possible care as they navigate the healthcare system.

Averting Cultural Conflict Through Caring Connection

Self-reflective and well-informed nurses foresee interactions that might result in cultural conflict, and they avert conflict by creating a healthy environment where caring connection can flourish. Pelletier and Stichler (2013) propose that relationship-based care in the context of a healthy work environment in an "accessible, well organized, accountable, supportive healthcare system" leads the way to patient and family engagement, patient activation, and improved healthcare outcomes (p. 53). Both interpersonal and system-level attentive and accessible support are essential for optimal health outcomes.

To weave a caring connection with patients, the first step is educating oneself on the historical and current social experiences of the populations in the community you serve. This knowledge will enable you to be sensitive to what *might be* the experience of a culture other than your own without making assumptions about this individual patient. With each new patient interaction, the nurse begins by coming to know the patient's world through active listening. Even in time-constrained situations, this can be done by simply asking, "What is of greatest concern to you right now?" and then sitting down at the patient's side and attentively listening so that a plan to maximize the patient's health can be mutually developed.

It is also helpful to ask who the important people are in the patient's life and how they might react to what the patient is going through. I remember coming into an emergency department to care for a woman who had been brutally assaulted. The woman, by physical appearance, looked to me to be African American; my priority was treating her with utmost respect and upholding her dignity and sense of safety, as I would with all patients, but in a more explicit manner. When I asked her about who was most important to her, she explained that her father was from eastern Costa Rica and was an African immigrant, and her mother was Native American, which presented two distinct cultural patterns I might need to be sensitive to. The patient went on to explain that her parents were no longer a part of her life and that when her mother abandoned her, she was raised by a Norwegian couple who had adopted her mother when she was young. This patient had grown up in a predominantly White rural community, eating lutefisk and lefse. Cultural care involves a graceful dance between what we know of a person's cultural background so that we can be sensitive and alert to potential health concerns and preferences and then listening carefully to who this unique person before us is and what is meaningful to this individual in this particular circumstance. It involves holding open a space where assumptions are suspended so that the patient can bring the whole self into a caring relationship where he or she is honored and respected for whomever and however he or she is. Cultural care involves a shift from focusing on differences to honoring our common humanity.

Fiester (2012) gives the example of a Persian couple coming into the hospital with a gynecological emergency. The couple adheres to Purdah—a custom in which women's bodies must be covered from the view of men. The husband refuses to allow a male healthcare provider to examine his wife. An uninformed staff member who is not Muslim or Hindi might find this request inconvenient and challenging or may see it as discriminatory. Fiester (2012) proposes the "obligations of hospitality" (p. 20) and calls healthcare providers to move from seeing mainly *otherness* to a focus on *commonality*, which leads healthcare providers to view the situation from the patient's and family's perspective, to respect their values, and to safeguard the woman's health. If no qualified female healthcare provider is available to examine the woman, the dialogue would focus on identifying common concern for the woman's safety and clearly explaining the treatment options and possible outcomes so that the couple can make an informed decision on whether to stay or seek care elsewhere. If the couple decides to stay, the manner in which the woman will be examined can be mutually determined. At the systems level, if this is not a novel situation at this particular hospital, then patient-centered care also requires a policy accommodation so that healthcare providers of both sexes are available at all times. Culturally sensitive patient-centered care involves accommodation at the interpersonal and systems levels to create the context for patient engagement and health.

In addition to the quality of the healthcare encounter, the extent to which patients and families engage in their own health and healthcare is shaped by their cultural beliefs, individual circumstances, and other factors in their lives (Sofaer & Schumann, 2013). These factors are of central concern for nurses as they plan their presence with and care for patients. Socioeconomic status, environmental exposures, transgenerational trauma, social isolation, discrimination, and inequities in health dissemination and healthcare delivery adversely affect people's health and hamper their engagement in the healthcare system. The Nursing Alliance for Quality Care (Sofaer & Schumann, 2013) has put forth guidelines for nursing engagement of patients and their families. These authors define patient engagement as "the involvement in their own care by individuals (and others they designate to engage on their behalf), with the goal that they make competent, well-informed decisions about their health and health care and take action to support those decisions" (p. 5). Patient engagement differs from adherence or compliance, which are driven by the dictates of the medical model. Patient engagement involves an active partnership and patient-defined confidentiality and rights as well as mutuality and consensus in decision-making. Nurses engage in advocacy when necessary but focus on building patients' skills and capacity to manage and optimize their own health as possible. Use of the Patient Activation Measure helps nurses to target engagement strategies resulting in increased patient satisfaction, decreased costs, and improved patient health outcomes (Hibbard & Greene, 2013). Acknowledgement and appreciation of diverse cultural, racial, and ethnic backgrounds are essential to the success of the engagement process, as are healthcare literacy and linguistically appropriate interactions (Sofaer & Schumann, 2013).

The Patient Activation Measure

The Patient Activation Measure (PAM) was developed by Judith Hibbard and colleagues at the University of Oregon to assess patients' knowledge, skills, and confidence in managing their own health and healthcare. The PAM has been widely tested to establish its validity and reliability (Hibbard, Stockard, Mahoney, & Tusler, 2004) to determine which stage patients are at in managing their own health. Four stages of activation have been identified with accompanying measures:

Stage 1: Believes an Active Role Is Important

- *When all is said and done, I am the person who is responsible for managing my health condition.*

- *Taking an active role in my own healthcare is the most important factor in determining my health and ability to function.*

Stage 2: Confidence and Knowledge to Take Action

- *I am confident that I can take actions that will help prevent or minimize some symptoms or problems associated with my health condition.*

- *I know what each of my prescribed medications does.*

- *I am confident that I can tell when I need to go get medical care and when I can handle a health problem myself.*

- *I am confident that I can tell my healthcare provider concerns I have even when he or she does not ask.*

- *I am confident that I can follow through on medical treatments I need to do at home.*

- *I understand the nature and causes of my health condition(s).*

Stage 3: Taking Action

- *I know the different medical treatment options available for my health condition.*

- *I have been able to maintain the lifestyle changes for my health that I have made.*

- *I know how to prevent further problems with my health condition.*

Stage 4: Staying the Course Under Stress

- *I am confident that I can figure out solutions when new situations or problems arise with my health conditions.*

- *I am confident that I can maintain lifestyle changes, such as diet and exercise, even during times of stress. (Hibbard, Mahoney, Stockard, & Tusler, 2005, p. 1923)*

The PAM is available from its authors. Its use helps nurses enter into the world of the patient in order to effectively engage with the patient to generate ideas for maximizing the patient's health.

Unconscious Bias

A significant body of literature addresses healthcare provider bias and its untoward effects on patients' health (Burgess, van Ryn, Crowley-Matoka, & Malat, 2006; Hall & Fields, 2013; Malat & Hamilton, 2006; Malat et al., 2006; Smedley, Stith, & Nelson, 2003; van Ryn & Burke, 2000; van Ryn & Fu, 2003; Williams, Neighbors, & Jackson, 2003). Not all of this bias is overt or intentional. Bias comes from employing stereotypes. Healthcare providers must be adept at organizing vast amounts of incoming data into categories of how things work based on previous experience so that they can make decisions regarding how to proceed in any given situation. In this process, stereotypes are automatically activated without conscious knowledge of how they influence emotions, perceptions, behaviors, and outcomes. Stereotype-linked bias is an automatic and unconscious process that occurs even among people who are not prejudiced. The situational factors that increase stereotype usage are time pressure, need for quick judgments, high cognitive demand, task complexities, resource constraint, and the presence of anger or anxiety—many of which are common in healthcare encounters. The activation of negative stereotypes results in discrimination against people who fall into that stereotyped group (van Ryn & Fu, 2003). Deep self-reflection and analysis are necessary to untether negative stereotypes and thus remove discrimination from healthcare practice. Analysis of stereotype activation is essential as we deepen our knowledge and appreciation of the variations between and within cultural groups.

Patient-Centered Care Across Cultural Care Belief Systems

In order to provide effective, high-quality, patient-centered care for people whose culture(s) are different from yours, it is essential that you understand the cultures in which you grew up and currently affiliate with and examine how your cultural beliefs affect your responses, particularly in high-stress situations. Take a moment and envision the people you spend most of your non-work hours with—the people who gather with you for celebrations, the people in the social organizations you belong to, the people you vacation with, the people who come to memorial services when someone close to you has died. If the people who are around your table or at your side in good times and bad do not reflect the cultures and appearance of your patients, you likely have a considerable amount of work to do to provide patient-centered care, particularly to be effective when cultural conflicts arise. Campinha-Bacote (2002, 2011) presents a model for nurses to engage in the ongoing process of becoming more and more culturally competent; the process moves from cultural awareness to cultural knowledge, cultural skill, cultural encounters, and cultural desire. When nurses sense a disconnect with patients from a culture different from their own, the first step is to critically analyze the differences and similarities between the two cultures and reflect on any strong emotions or thoughts that arise when caring for patients from that culture. The next step is researching the culture and discerning ways to sensitively provide care within the culture. It behooves nurses to spend time within the new culture—going to restaurants, cultural events, and community gatherings with an open spirit and desire to learn. However, self-awareness is the critical first step.

For example, to begin the process of cultural awareness and move students through the process of becoming culturally competent, my nurse educator colleagues and I have used racial-moment journaling with nursing students to help them become aware of how issues of "race" and racism play out in their personal and professional lives. [The word "race" is placed in quotation marks to remind the reader that it is a sociological construct.] This process may be of help to you. Using a "racial moments" awareness process developed by Karis (2008), we instruct students to keep a journal for a few weeks in which they record every time the concept of "race" comes to mind. We instruct students to pay attention to and record what they were thinking and feeling at the time and then later, when they have more time to think and reflect, to analyze the situation and their response to it.

Self-Awareness Through Racial-Moment Journaling

A White graduate student, who prided herself for her cross-cultural competence in her multicultural, multilingual work environment, was shocked to suddenly realize that she held some deep-seated racial prejudices. She described coming out of a grocery store after an evening class, heavily laden with bags. She dropped her purse and one bag. A young Black man quickly and kindly came to her rescue and helped pick up her fallen belongings from the street. Her immediate response was to grab her purse. She was both shocked and horrified by her response of fearing he was trying to steal her purse, which she realized she might not have noticed had it not been for the racial-moment journaling exercise. She pondered whether she was seeing the full potential of the young Black men she worked with.

She became even more alarmed as the journaling continued and she realized that everything she did outside work was in a totally "White world." Her church was all White, as were her children's sports teams, neighbors, and friends. She realized that she had significant lifestyle changes to make if she was going to see her patients for who they fully are and regard them as she would her mother, father, sister, brother, son, daughter, or beloved friend.

The journaling process recommended by Karis can be adapted to gain insight into other areas of unconscious bias, such as heterosexism, ableism, or classism. Being aware of our deep-seated cultural beliefs and biases is the first step in patient-centered care, particularly in the face of serious cultural conflicts. Karis (2008) terms this *compassionate awareness,* which helps us recognize that we have been socialized into a racially stratified society and creates the fertile ground for exploring our racial misperceptions and thus knowing ourselves and our patients more deeply and fully. Hall and Fields (2013) propose that by raising consciousness about the ways in which we "propagate subtle racism, nursing can progress faster in eliminating health disparities" (p. 164). These authors describe how even more damaging the effects of subtle racism are than overt racism, because subtle or aversive racism is more difficult to confront and more likely to be internalized, thus resulting in increased hypertension, prolonged anger, headaches, and generalized tension.

Nursing in the Midst of Serious Cultural Conflict

Ting-Toomey and Oetzel (2001) make the case that culture provides the primary imprint in our habitual responses to conflict (p. xii). These intercultural conflict theorists assert that conflict is a testing ground for the resilience of our everyday relationships and, if managed well, that conflict can bring about positive changes and set the stage for deeper dialogue and understanding in the face of crisis. The Chinese character for crisis is two symbols joined together; the first signifies danger, end times, or something horrible about to happen, but the second stands for opportunity—the possibility for a new beginning. When realizing that there is an opportunity for deeper meaning and understanding in the face of crisis and conflict, nurses are able to be mindful of their commitment to patients and move into collaborative dialogue to find a resolution that points toward health and well-being for the patient. When conflict is not well managed, the result is defensiveness, verbal criticism, suppression of anger, or anger explosion—all of which have negative physiological and emotional consequences. Good conflict management is a life skill that buffers emotional strain. As a nurse, it is imperative that you recognize and understand that patients' behavior may have a different and often contradictory meaning than what the same behavior would have within your own culture. For example, a smile in most cultures indicates pleasure and receptivity, but in some cultures it also represents nervousness, embarrassment, and discomfort.

An understanding of the broad cultural beliefs, values, and norms of the patient populations you work with provides a helpful map for navigating cultural differences. These loose stereotypes, or broad generalizations about a culture, can help decrease unpredictable guesswork and shed light on possible sources of conflict or misunderstanding; however, generalizations about cultural beliefs and norms need to be verified for each individual patient and family. Negative stereotypes can perpetuate and deepen destructive cycles of conflict and produce tremendous pressure and threats to self-identity. As previously pointed out, these negative stereotypes can be internalized and operate without conscious employment; therefore, self-awareness of negative stereotypes is an important, ongoing reflective process for every nurse if conflict is going to be managed. Ting-Toomey and Oetzel (2001) propose 10 constructive conflict-management skills that can be employed when serious cultural conflict arises (see sidebar).

Constructive Cultural Conflict-Management Skills

1. *Mindful observation (observing, describing, interpreting, and suspending evaluation)*

2. *Mindful listening (attending delicately and intently with eyes, ears, and focused heart)*

3. *Mindful reframing (creating a new context to understand the behavior/conflict event)*

4. *Identity validation (respecting desired identities and confirming other's self-worth)*

5. *Face work management (understanding power difference and collectivist concerns from the patient's cultural perspective to maintain face or restore face loss)*

6. *Productive power balancing (being mindful of your power currency to focus on enhancing patient's power and self-agency)*

7. *Collaborative dialogue (employing an ethnorelative lens to focus on patient's perspective of health, listening and sharing knowledge on how to collaboratively achieve health)*

8. *Problem-solving skills (differentiating approaches, describing the problem in mutually understandable terms, and integrating a mutually agreed-upon plan for health)*

9. *Transcendent discourse (discovering healthy and creative ways in which moral differences and underlying assumptions can be expressed and understood)*

10. *Interaction adaptability (avoiding interventionist and prescriptive approaches; opening your thinking pattern to be flexible and adaptable as you meet the specific needs in the situation)*

Source: Adapted from Ting-Toomey & Oetzel, 2001, pp. 179–195

In order for you to be successful in recognizing and managing cultural conflict, it is important to first understand your own cultural norms, values, and beliefs:

- Cultural norms are the collective expectations related to what constitutes proper behavior in any given situation. Norms are readily inferred and observed. They are the manifestation of deep-seated and invisible cultural values and beliefs.

- Cultural values and beliefs are the priorities and motivational base that guide desirable or undesirable behaviors. They mold and shape cultural attitudes and behaviors and drive how we respond to conflict when it arises.

The greater the cultural difference, the more likely it is that assessments or judgments will be polarized and misconstrued (Ting-Toomey, 2007). One of the most important cultural values differences to understand in yourself and others is the collectivist-individualistic cultural value orientation. Collectivist cultures emphasize group harmony, fitting in, and relational interdependence—they focus on harmony and communal well-being in the face of crisis. Individualistic cultures stress the importance of pursuing personal goals, autonomy, and independence—they focus on equity during conflict situations. Conflict styles are shaped by where a person is on the individualistic-collectivist values continuum. People with low concern for self and low concern for others will usually employ an avoiding style. Those with low concern for self and high concern for others will use an obliging or accommodating style. People with low concern for others but high concern for self will use a dominating or competing style. Those with moderate concern for self and moderate concern for others are more apt to compromise in the face of conflict. High concern for self and high concern for others promotes an integrating, collaborative style of resolving conflict (Ting-Toomey & Oetzel, 2001).

A second important cultural values difference relates to power distance. Small power difference cultures emphasize individual credibility and expertise, democratic decision-making, and equitable rewards, punishments, rights, and relationships. In small power difference cultures, it is common for children to contradict parents and for professional relationships to be collaborative without regard to title, age, rank, or seniority. Large power distance cultures place emphasis on status, hierarchical decision-making, and rewards based on age, rank, status, title, and seniority. In these cultures, children are expected to obey their elders, and subordinates carry out and defer to the demands of those in charge or those who hold a title (Ting-Toomey & Oetzel, 2001).

Another important concept in cross-cultural conflict is face-negotiation, which is shaped by individualistic-collectivist and power distance values. Ting-Toomey (2007) proposes a conflict face-negotiation theory, stressing that "intercultural conflict often involves different face losing and face saving behaviors," with "face" referring to a person's desired social self-image (p. 256). Face-loss involves identity claims' being ignored or challenged and is more serious in emotionally threatening or vulnerable situations (as exemplified in the story of the Gutierrez family, which follows).

Saving Face and Optimizing Health for the Gutierrez Family

The Gutierrez family is from a small town in Chiapas, Mexico, but has lived in the United States for more than 30 years. The family consists of Don Francisco; his wife, Doña Josefa; 8 eight children; and 18 grandchildren. Don Francisco and Doña Josefa go back and forth between their two countries a few times a year. They transition between their two cultures several times a week—mostly during medical interactions at the university health center. They have dozens of close relatives and friends who move in and out of their house for celebrations or to stay for extended periods of time. Their social and religious communities are 100% Mexican. Their business interactions are predominantly with people who are also from Mexico. Both Don Francisco and

Doña Josefa receive medical care from the university hospital system because of their complex physical health challenges. Back in their hometown in Chiapas, Doña Josefa was a curandera—*a traditional healer who uses plants and traditional methods of healing sicknesses and restoring health. She is known in her current community as a source of health information and healing treatments. Her knowledge is well respected in the community, which gives her great pride.*

The university health center, known for its high-quality care, is always bustling with activity. Both Mr. and Mrs. Gutierrez have heart disease and diabetes and receive their care from a highly competent adult nurse practitioner (NP), Donna Johnson, whom they respect for her intelligence and medical knowledge. In spite of Dr. Johnson's good care, Mr. Gutierrez's blood pressure and blood sugars have been increasingly high, and he is showing signs of renal failure. A series of medication adjustments do not help. Mr. Gutierrez goes on dialysis and experiences large fluctuations in his blood pressure and blood sugars; his condition is worsening. Dr. Johnson asks Mrs. Gutierrez whether they are following the medication regime, and she replies, "Yes, yes, we are doing everything you have told us to do," firmly nodding her head and looking directly into Dr. Johnson's eyes.

There are often children present at the clinic visits, and although there seem to be varying opinions about Mr. Gutierrez's care, the children always defer to their mother. Perplexed and realizing that Mr. Gutierrez's life is in danger, Dr. Johnson asks the Gutierrezes whether they would accept a home health nurse coming to their home to help them learn how to manage Mr. Gutierrez's medications and treatments. They reluctantly agree.

The home health nurse, Anna James, comes to the Gutierrez home. She walks in and shakes hands with everyone, warmly greeting each and inquiring about their names. Even though Mr. and Mrs. Gutierrez provide their first names, she refers to them as Don Francisco and Doña Josefa to denote the respect she has for them as elders. In her position, Anna is able to be less medico-centric than if she were working within a medical center. She is able to hold open the space for multiple healing modalities and thus provide more culturally congruent care, beginning with essential "social chit-chat," which is often impossible in overscheduled clinics but essential for establishing a trusting relationship within the Mexican culture (Huerta & Sánchez, 2009). Anna is able to spend 2 hours getting to know the Gutierrezes, their family story, and what is important to them. She asks about all the healing practices they draw upon, leaving an opening for Doña Josefa to talk about her practice as a curandera, *which traditional treatments she has been giving Don Francisco, and how he feels well at home but then goes to the hospital and receives the strong medications and gets even sicker and more unstable. Doña Josefa believes she has to do whatever is possible to save her husband's life.*

Anna understands that the Gutierrez family comes from a culture that is both collectivist and has a high power difference, so they would probably make decisions based on what is best for the family and community and they would be unlikely to challenge their NP, Dr. Johnson, or the nurses and physicians in the hospital. Doña Josefa confides that when she talks to people in the hospital and clinic, she feels like they may think she is stupid and does not care about her husband, which makes her feel horrible, so she just says, "yes, yes" to everything they say and ask. Don Francisco trusts his wife's decisions and the long-standing traditions from his community but also looks to the university health system for a possible cure so that he can get back to caring for his family. Anna realizes that she needs to help both Don Francisco and Doña Josefa save face, stay connected to their community and its traditions, and negotiate how they will draw on the expertise of the university health system. She collaborates with the Gutierrez family to carefully develop a plan to help them learn and be aware of the benefits of and interactions between traditional and Western medications and treatments so that they can choose wisely the healing modalities they want to draw upon. The entire family feels good about the plan they have developed and are excited that there are concrete things they can all do to restore health to Don Francisco and relieve the burden on Doña Josefa. Anna realizes that she can help them all learn about how to restore the healthy diet and lifestyle their ancestors had in Chiapas as a path to healing for the entire family. In doing so, she will help Don Francisco, Doña Josefa, and their children and grandchildren make healthier choices while claiming pride in themselves and their heritage.

Sharing the knowledge she has gained about the health practices and beliefs of the Gutierrez family with the primary care NP could serve to improve the family's health and well-being through coordinated, culturally consistent care while in the clinic and hospital setting. Anna obtains Don Francisco and Doña Josefa's consent to coach their NP, Dr. Johnson, on how to best care for them. Anna and Dr. Johnson also strategize on how to best obtain information from patients on their health practices and beliefs, drawing in the recommendations of The Joint Commission (TJC; 2010) roadmap Advancing Effective Communication, Cultural Competence, and Patient- and Family-Centered Care, *particularly Kleinman's questions (p. 15). Anna suggests that Dr. Johnson add a question, such as, "What traditional Mexican treatments have you found to be helpful?" following up with a question about which treatments they have tried. This would normalize the use of indigenous healing practices and open the door for Doña Josefa to talk freely about her practice and beliefs. Depending upon the warmth and spirit with which that door is opened, Doña Josefa may or may not choose to enter.*

Engaging Patient Perspectives to Create Systems of Cultural Care

Ideally, healthcare systems have patient and family voices on their advisory boards so that optimal systems of care can be designed and cultural conflict can be minimized. TJC (2011) has established guidelines for care of the lesbian, gay, bisexual, and transgender community. These guidelines include:

- A leadership checklist to ensure adequate policies are in place; a care, treatment, and services checklist detailing best practices

- A workforce checklist aimed at ensuring equitable and inclusive employment practices for LGBT employees

- A data-collection checklist to ensure that comprehensive data are collected and maintained in a sensitive and respectful manner

- And finally, a patient, family, and community engagement checklist to ensure that LGBT patients and families have input into policies related to the provision of care to the LGBT community through the use of surveys, focus groups, and advisory councils

This engagement process helps collect data related to satisfaction and staff responsiveness, shape policies, create sensitive assessment tools, illuminate acceptable practices, redesign printed materials and website messages, and promote community outreach. Including marginalized populations in an action research process helps shape systems of care in which cultural conflict and misunderstandings are minimized and health flourishes (Pavlish & Pharris, 2012).

Implications for Practice

As a nurse committed to patient-centered care, you will be able to minimize cultural conflict in your practice by:

- Rooting your practice in the nursing codes of ethics, which call you to uphold the human dignity, worth, and uniqueness of all people (ANA, 2010; ICN, 2012)

- Being aware of your deep-seated cultural beliefs and biases through intentional self-reflection and analysis

- Understanding that what appears to be difficult or oppositional behavior is likely springing forth from fear of not being known, valued, understood, or respected (Aim to understand, value, respect, and know who your patients are.)

- Educating yourself on the cultural norms and sociohistorical backgrounds of the patient populations you serve and ways in which to best interact in a culturally sensitive manner

- Preparing yourself for the intense emotional and spiritual work of sorting through your patient's pain, broken relationships, emotional trauma, and social differences to discern what healing means for *this* person in *this* situation and to collaborate with the patient's significant others and other members of the healthcare team to create the potential for healing and health

- Realizing that at its heart, culturally sensitive patient-centered care calls nurses to analyze who is benefiting and who is suffering in the healthcare environment and in each encounter (You have the potential not only to advocate for your patients but to take steps to rebalance the flow of resources and to ensure adequate quality care for all, but particularly for those most in need.)

- Embracing the cultural diversity and unique differences of patients, communities, and members of the healthcare team (Diversity of backgrounds and cultures within your interprofessional team is a valuable resource to enhance your ability to best serve patients and their families [Interprofessional Education Collaborative Expert Panel, 2011].)

- Engaging in relational presence and mindful practice (for example, the mindfulness program developed by nurse educators Constance Green and Colleen Prunier, available at http://qsen.org/eight-week-mindfulness-program-for-nursing-students/, or Margaret Newman's 2008 book *Transforming Presence: The Difference Nursing Makes*)

- Delving more deeply into the principles of patient engagement, as outlined by the Nursing Alliance for Quality Care (Sofaer & Schumann, 2013)

Conclusion

Patient-centered care flourishes when nurses possess cultural knowledge and skill but also requires system-level accommodations to avert cultural conflict. Patient-centered care in the face of serious cultural conflict takes time and calls upon relational presence, cultural knowledge, and mindful practice. It is firmly rooted in the commitments expressed in nursing codes of ethics. NP Donna Johnson understood this when she recognized that her patient needed more than what the clinic visit environment offered, and she made the home health nurse referral. Anna James understood this as she artfully wove her caring and collaborative relationship with the Gutierrez family to chart a new path toward health that incorporated traditional Mexican as well as Western healing practices.

And finally, going back to the opening story of this chapter, Angeleen understood this as she nurtured Ricky back to health in the ICU—that relationship was particularly difficult to negotiate due to the power difference and loss of face. Angeleen's mindful presence, highly competent care, and direct and caring communication—along with the collective knowledge and spirit of the ICU healthcare team—provided a healing environment for Ricky on many levels. Ricky was cared for by nurses who rose above their personal pain to embody their professional code of ethics and uphold his human dignity, which not only saved his life but transformed his spirit. This was evident in this true story when, a few months after his discharge, Ricky came back to the ICU to thank the healthcare team. He pulled Angeleen aside and unbuttoned his shirt to reveal the healing space where a tattoo once had been.

References

Allen, J., & Littlefield, J. (2005). *Without sanctuary: Photographs and postcards of lynchings in America.* Retrieved from http://withoutsanctuary.org/main.html

American Nurses Association (ANA). (2010). *Position statement: The nurse's role in ethics and human rights: Protecting and promoting individual worth, dignity, and human rights in practice settings.* Retrieved from http://www.nursingworld.org/MainMenuCategories/Policy-Advocacy/Positions-and-Resolutions/ANAPositionStatements/Position-Statements-Alphabetically/Nursess-Role-in-Ethics-and-Human-Rights.pdf

Burgess, D., van Ryn, M., Crowley-Matoka, M., & Malat, J. (2006). Understanding the provider contribution to Race/Ethnicity disparities in pain treatment: Insights from dual process models of stereotyping. *Pain Medicine, 7*(2), 119-134.

Campinha-Bacote, J. (2002). The process of cultural competence in the delivery of health services: A model of care. *Journal of Transcultural Nursing, 13*(3), 181-184.

Campinha-Bacote, J. (2011). Coming to know cultural competence: An evolutionary process. *International Journal for Human Caring, 15*(3), 42-48.

Fiester, A. (2012). What "patient-centered care" requires in serious cultural conflict. *Academic Medicine, 87*(1), 20-24.

Hall, J., & Fields, B. (2013). Continuing the conversation in nursing on race and racism. *Nursing Outlook, 61*(3), 164-173.

Hibbard, J. H., & Greene, J. (2013). What the evidence shows about patient activation: Better health outcomes and care experiences: Few data on costs. *Health Affairs, 32*(2), 207-214.

Hibbard, J. H., Mahoney, E. R., Stockard, J., & Tusler, M. (2005). Development and testing of a short form of the patient activation measure. *Health Research and Educational Trust, 40*(6), 1918-1930.

Hibbard, J. H., Stockard, J., Mahoney, E. R., & Tusler, M. (2004). Development of the patient activation measure (PAM): Conceptualizing and measuring activation in patients and consumers. *Health Service Research, 39*(4), 1005-1026.

Huerta, C., & Sánchez, M. S. (2009). Influence of culture on knowing persons. In R. C. Locsin & M. J. Purnell (Eds.), *A contemporary nursing process: The (un)bearable weight of knowing in nursing* (pp. 481-503). New York, NY: Springer.

International Council of Nurses (ICN). (2012). *The ICN code of ethics for nurses.* Geneva, Switzerland: Author.

Interprofessional Education Collaborative Expert Panel. (2011, May). *Core competencies for interprofessional collaborative practice: Report of an expert panel.* Washington, DC: Interprofessional Education Collaborative.

The Joint Commission (TJC). (2010). *Advancing effective communication, cultural competence, and patient- and family-centered care: A roadmap for hospitals.* Retrieved from http://www.jointcommission.org/assets/1/6/aroadmapforhospitalsfinalversion727.pdf

The Joint Commission (TJC). (2011). *Advancing effective communication, cultural competence, and patient- and family-centered care for the lesbian, gay, bisexual, and transgender (LGBT) community: A field guide.* Oak Brook, IL: Author.

Karis, T. A. (2008). The psychology of whiteness: Moving beyond separation to connection. In R. Osborne & P. Kriese (Eds.), *Global community: Global security* (pp. 97-108). New York, NY: Rodopi.

Malat, J. R., & Hamilton, M. A. (2006). Preference for same-race health care providers and perceptions of interpersonal discrimination in health care. *Journal of Health and Social Behavior, 47*(2), 173-187.

Malat, J. R., van Ryn, M., & Purcell, D. (2006). Race, socioeconomic status, and the perceived importance of positive self-presentation in health care. *Social Science & Medicine, 62*(10), 2479-2488.

National Park Service. (n.d.). *Jim Crow laws.* Retrieved from http://www.nps.gov/malu/forteachers/jim_crow_laws.htm

Newman, M. A. (2008). *Transforming presence: The difference nursing makes.* Philadelphia, PA: F. A. Davis.

Pavlish, C., & Pharris, M. D. (2012). *Community-based collaborative action research: A nursing approach.* Sudbury, MA: Jones and Bartlett.

Pelletier, L. R., & Stichler, J. F. (2013). American Academy of Nursing action brief: Patient engagement and activation: A health reform imperative for improvement opportunity for nursing. *Nursing Outlook, 61*(1), 51-54.

Roach, M. (2002). *Caring, the human mode of being* (2nd rev. ed.). Ottawa, Canada: Canadian Hospital Association Press.

Shim, J. K. (2010). Cultural health capital: A theoretical approach to understanding health care interactions and the dynamics of unequal treatment. *Journal of Health and Social Behavior, 51*(1), 1-15.

Smedley, B. D., Stith, A. Y., & Nelson, A. R. (Eds.). (2003). *Unequal treatment: Confronting racial and ethnic disparities in health care.* Washington, DC: The National Academies Press.

Sofaer, S., & Schumann, M. J. (2013). *Fostering successful patient and family engagement: Nursing's critical role.* Retrieved from http://www.naqc.org/WhitePaper-PatientEngagement

Ting-Toomey, S. (2007). Intercultural conflict training: Theory-practice approaches and research challenges. *Journal of Intercultural Communication Research, 36*(5), 255-271.

Ting-Toomey, S., & Oetzel, J. G. (2001). *Managing intercultural conflict effectively.* Thousand Oaks, CA: Sage.

Turkel, M. C., & Ray, M. A. (2009). Caring for "not-so-picture-perfect patients": Ethical caring in the moral community of nursing. In R. C. Locsin & M. J. Purnell (Eds.), *A contemporary nursing process: The (un)bearable weight of knowing in nursing* (pp. 225-249). New York, NY: Springer.

van Ryn, M., & Burke, J. (2000). The effect of patient race and socio-economic status on physicians' perceptions of patients. *Social Science & Medicine, 50*(6), 813-828.

van Ryn, M., & Fu, S. S. (2003). Paved with good intentions: Do public health and human service providers contribute to racial/ethnic disparities in health? *American Journal of Public Health, 93*(2), 248-255.

Washington, H. A. (2006). *Medical apartheid: The dark history of medical experimentation on Black Americans from colonial times to the present.* New York, NY: Harlem Moon Broadway.

Williams, D. R., Neighbors, H. W., & Jackson, J. S. (2003). Racial/ethnic discrimination and health: Findings from community studies. *American Journal of Public Health, 93*(2), 200-208.

Chapter 13

Special Considerations of Person- and Family-Centered Care Related to Age

Tara A. Cortes, PhD, RN, FAAN

Cheristi Cognetta Rieke, DNP, RN

Abigail and John DiCarlo live in San Francisco with their daughter, Amy, 6 years old, and son, Ian, 2 years old. Their daughter was born with multiple disabilities. She is in a wheelchair, is deaf, and has the developmental level of a 2-year-old. Abigail, John, and their children have a routine and a lifestyle that works. Amy does have frequent stays in the hospital, as she tends to aspirate her food and develop upper respiratory problems and has a frequent occurrence of urinary tract infections. Abigail usually stays in the hospital with Amy when this happens, but John travels for business and Abigail always needs to find a neighbor to stay with Ian when John is away and Amy is hospitalized.

Abigail's mother is a widow who lives in Indiana. She has been living independently since her husband died 2 years ago. Abigail speaks to her mother every day. About 6 months ago, Abigail became concerned when her mother seemed to be repeating herself frequently in their conversations. This became worse, and 3 months ago Abigail asked her mother what she had for dinner that night. Her mother could not remember. Abigail flew to Indiana the next day and found her mother disheveled and confused about why Abigail was "not at school." Abigail took her mother to the primary care provider, who examined her, ordered tests, and 3 days later diagnosed her with Alzheimer's dementia. Abigail knew she could not leave her mother alone in Indiana, and Abigail was her only child. She called her husband and told him she had no choice but to bring her mother back to their home in California.

One month later, Abigail and John felt as if their orderly existence with a child who had multiple challenges was in a tailspin. They had an established routine, healthcare team, and support services that worked around the health needs of Amy. They did not have this system in place for Abigail's mother. They were exhausted, confused, and not sure what to do. Abigail's mother seemed happy to be with her daughter and family, and her confusion seemed to lessen. She did, however, seem somewhat depressed. And any disruption in the day or any setback in Amy's health seemed to set off agitation and anxiety in Abigail's mother. Abigail and John realized that their family and home life had suddenly become more complex, and they were at a loss for how to manage all of it.

This scenario is becoming more typical of many families across the country. Any acute or chronic illness in a child is a stressor to any family. And as the baby boomers age, more and more families are taking on the burden of caregiving for their parents. This chapter provides insights for the reader on unique ways to incorporate age-specific concepts into patient- and family-centered care (P&FCC). There has never been a more important time for the healthcare team to understand the impact these caregiving activities have on the patient and the family. Healthcare providers need to have the knowledge and skills to bring the patient and family on board as integral to the healthcare team and fully involve them in decision-making and planning care. In this chapter, we discuss strategies to engage and empower patients and families across the healthcare continuum to maximize their involvement.

P&FCC has become an integral part of the healthcare vocabulary, but perhaps the impact of P&FCC is most felt in the early years and later years of the life continuum, during which time patients may not be their own best advocates. It is the very young and the very old and those in between with chronic conditions and/or disabilities who are often dependent on families as caretakers, decision-makers, and surrogates. These families are affected by the illness, and their needs are often overlooked and forgotten. Unless patients and their families are recognized as members of the healthcare team and included in decision-making and care giving, these patients will become more burdensome on the healthcare system, utilize more resources, have a poorer quality of life, and have less than optimal outcomes. Today's paradigm of healthcare delivery must shift from hospital-centric to patient-centric. Coordination, collaboration, communication, and integration across all parts of the healthcare system must be done with the patient and family fully informed and participating as decision-makers. This chapter addresses some of the unique needs and characteristics of the children and older adults in the healthcare system and how we can best position them and their families as partners in the healthcare team.

Population Relevant Statistics

In 2011, nearly 5.2 million children 17 years and younger were receiving special education or special needs/disabilities services. This equates to 7% of all U.S. children (U.S. Department of Health and Human Services Centers for Disease Control and Prevention National Center for Health Statistics, 2012).

There is resounding evidence displaying the importance of capturing the psychosocial elements of a child's being admitted to an acute care hospital setting to help engage the child in decision-making and to direct individualized, patient-centered care. This includes effective communication, active assessment of competence, and a policy of inclusion (Kelsey, Abelson-Mitchell, & Skirton, 2006; Prilleltensky, 2010; Prilleltensky, Nelson, & Peirson, 2001; Reed, Smith, Fletcher, & Bradding, 2003; Sartain, Clarke, & Heyman, 2000). Despite the growing body of literature that emphasizes the need to talk directly to the child and stresses the importance of obtaining the child's view, this is rarely done in practice. Sadly, children are often silent consumers of healthcare; children's voices remain generally excluded from decision-making and care planning in acute care hospital settings (Coyne, 2006). Lack of consultation along with an imposed inferior role may negatively affect the physical and emotional well-being of the child (Coyne, 2006). Research suggests there is a relationship between self-esteem, self-worth, and medical outcomes. This reinforces the importance of seeking and including children's perceptions in the delivery of healthcare (Prilleltensky, 2010).

On the other end of the age continuum, patients 65 years and older represented 40% of hospitalized adults and nearly half of all healthcare dollars spent on hospitalization in 2008, but comprised less than 13% of the population in the United States (Agency for Healthcare Research and Quality, 2008). Furthermore, hospitalization-associated disability is the long-term loss of ability to perform daily living tasks associated with acute hospitalization (Covinsky, Pierluissi, & Johnston, 2011). Those people who experience this condition have lost abilities basic to everyday living—independent living—such as walking, getting themselves to and from the toilet, or dressing or bathing themselves. Hospitalization-associated disability occurs in approximately one-third of those over the age of 70 who are hospitalized. This percentage increases with the age of the patient (Covinsky et al., 2011). Older patients discharged with hospitalization-associated disability require more care either through a long-term care placement or a caregiver, who often is a family member. AARP defines P&FCC as "an orientation to the delivery of healthcare and supportive services that considers an older person's needs, goals, preferences, cultural traditions, family situation and values" (Feinberg, 2011, p. 1). It is estimated that of older people needing assistance and living at home, about 66% get that care from family caregivers, about 26% receive that care from a combination of family and paid caregivers, and 9% receive assistance from only paid caregivers (Doty, 2010). In 2009, 42 million family caregivers were providing 40.3 billion hours of unpaid care at an estimated economic value of $450 billion (Feinberg, Reinhard, Houser, & Choula, 2011). The caretaker burden is heavy but even heavier if that caretaker is not a full partner in the healthcare team.

Challenges

Acute illness, chronic illness, and disability create stress for patients and families. Events ranging from broken bones to the diagnoses of serious illness, chronic disease, and disability create life-changing situations for patients and their families. Whether these events are temporary, as with a broken bone, or persistent and will require extensive changes in the family, such as a chronic illness or loss of limb, stress is a factor. Children have more emotional needs and often have a limited understanding of what is happening to them. Older adults often have multiple comorbidities that need to be managed, and, as previously noted, they may lose significant function when hospitalized. The unique needs of the two populations require different types of patient and family engagement with the healthcare team.

Age-Specific Needs—Children

Anytime children or adolescents are interacting with healthcare professionals and/or the healthcare system, care providers need to understand the developmental milestones of the pediatric patient population. As healthcare providers, we can nurture, involve, and empower children within the healthcare setting by better understanding their world. Children absorb and understand the world around them through their senses: touch, sight, sound, smell, and feel. All children learn via observation and have highly developed nonverbal skills. Children experience stress, fear, and pain. How children manage these physiological symptoms is shaped by their personality, temperament, age, and life experiences. Play is a very important part of a child's world; it is considered their work. Children learn and experience their surroundings through play. It validates their understanding and allows for imaginative exploration. Children live in the present moment—in the "now." Each child has a unique personality and wants to be recognized as the individual that he or she is (Brazelton & Sparrow, 2001).

The parents and family of children who have chronic medical conditions and those who have special needs require true partnerships with the healthcare industry and healthcare providers to ensure that P&FCC and expected outcomes are achieved. The Federation for Children With Special Needs has a mission to provide "information, support and assistance to parents of children with disabilities, their professional partners, and their communities; and are committed to listening to and learning from families, and encouraging full participation in community life by all people, especially those with disabilities" (Federation for Children With Special Needs, 2013, para. 1). Often the care being provided to children who have special healthcare needs is multifaceted and provided by a variety of members from the immediate and extended family, the healthcare system, the school, and the community. Caregivers from across this vast continuum need to fully understand the significance of involving the child in the care being provided. It is imperative for the caregivers to have access to education regarding policy and advocacy, community and school programs, and resources and support for the role they have as a full-time or part-time caregiver.

Age-Specific Needs—Older Adults

Good care for older adults with complex, chronic needs and functional challenges requires a collaborative approach, which builds family caregivers into the team as partners and provides them with the information to understand what is happening to their loved ones and how to contact a health professional when they need to. The continuum of healthcare for older people with chronic diseases is variable, as many of these people live independently. These patients and their families need to be engaged in the management and monitoring of their chronic conditions and given the information to keep them at an optimum level of function.

On the other end of the continuum are those patients with multiple chronic diseases who have cognitive and/or physical disabilities that require full-time or at least part-time caregiving. Often these caregivers are family members, and sometimes there are direct caregivers supervised by the family who are providing at least some of the care. These people need to be able to assist with medications, provide treatments, monitor the diseases, ensure tests are carried out and results are communicated, make appointments, and transport the patient to appointments. They also need to know how to recognize changes in conditions; when to call the physician, nurse practitioner (NP), or visiting nurse; and how to communicate any observation about the patient. These skills and tasks are very difficult, but they are even more difficult if that caretaker is not an informed member of the team.

Clearly, when the patient is a child or older adult, P&FCC is particularly important, because the family is very often the caretaker. The concepts of communication, collaboration, and coordination are essential to the integration of the family caretaker as a member of the team.

Communication With and Integration of All Families

Effective communication includes assertiveness; trust; mutual respect; recognizing and valuing of diverse, complementary knowledge and skills; and humor.

Communication with the patient and families is essential to good P&FCC. Healthcare providers must be transparent in sharing information with the patient and family.

Ideally, healthcare providers would respect patient and family choices and incorporate their values into the care being delivered. Communication would be open and transparent, collaboration would be valued and fostered, and coordination would be a shared activity with jointly developed outcomes for care. If the patient is at the center of the system, then the patient's personal needs, goals, and preferences must be considered and integrated into the care. Again, this is so important for the very young and very old for whom the middle generation most often incurs the responsibility of caregiving, and without information and opportunities to make decisions, these caretakers become marginalized in their role.

The communication of timely, accurate, and complete information enables patients, families, and providers to make decisions and plan for care. Communication involves listening as well as speaking, and it is as necessary for providers to be giving and sharing information with the patient and family as it is for the patient and family to be giving and sharing information with the rest of the healthcare team. This is what empowers every member of the team to plan appropriately, make choices, and manage healthcare. This openness also reduces the caretaker burden, as caretakers are informed and confident in their care because they understand the needs and the behavior of the patient.

For example, a diagnosis of Alzheimer's dementia is often a shock to a patient and their family as they contemplate the future and what might happen. Sometime family members ask physicians not to tell the patient the diagnosis. Ethically, the provider is required to tell the patient; just as importantly, the patient needs to know in order to be part of the decision-making while still able to do so. A similar example could take place with a child as the patient; and the parents ask the physicians not to tell the patient of the diagnosis based on the assumption that the child is "too young to understand." As noted earlier in this chapter, children are able to actively participate in care planning and making care decisions as long as we share information with them and include them in the process.

Respecting the patient and family by acknowledging their ideas and values is essential if the healthcare and management of the patient is to be consistent and reliable. This is often seen in dietary restrictions, and we then blame patients for not following a regimen. Or we see families of patients with dementia struggling with changes in their behavior but not understanding what those changes mean, and we then blame them for hostile behaviors. Without involving the patient and family in planning that regimen and recognizing their values and behaviors, we will never get participation from them. It should be noted that often the caregivers of both very young patients and of older patients are the best resources to fully understand the individual patient preferences and norms in the home setting.

It is essential that the healthcare team and other support services communicate with the patient and the family in a way that is supportive, builds trust, and helps decision-making. Offering informational resources to the family to inform them about the patient's condition, where to find community resources, and what to expect in long-term outcomes is helpful.

Accommodations to consider for optimizing communication with both of these special patient populations, the pediatric patient and the older adult, would include the following:

- Use the patient's story to connect with the individual and to develop trust and rapport, a good ground for open communication to take place.

- Speak in terms that are familiar to the patient and the family; frame what you are trying to communicate in a way that will make sense to the younger or older patient.

- Be mindful of the tone, volume, and pace of communication. Children are receptive to softer volumes and higher pitches, while older adults may require louder volumes and lower pitches in order to hear well.

- Written communication should be in larger print for older adults and in a pictorial display with multiple colors for children.

- As a healthcare professional, understand the cognitive and developmental abilities of the patient you are caring for; stretch yourself to view the situation through a child's eyes or an older adult's eyes.

Collaboration and Integration With All Families

Collaboration is an interaction that requires both communicative and behavioral competencies. Hanson and Spross (2009) define *collaboration* as a "dynamic, interpersonal process in which two or more individuals make a commitment to each other to interact authentically and constructively to solve problems and to learn from each other to accomplish identified goals, purposes, or outcomes. The individuals recognize and articulate the shared values to make this commitment possible" (p. 285). This definition implies that individuals form a partnership; have shared values, commitment, and goals; and demonstrate mutual respect for differences in opinions and approaches to problem solving. Hanson and Spross (2009) identify essential characteristics of collaboration as clinical competence and accountability, common purpose, interpersonal competence, and effective communication.

Collaboration implies a circular relationship between the providers and the patient and family. This means that there is an exchange of information, and listening and learning are valued by both sides. Mutual respect and integration are necessary components of collaboration. This type of relationship actively engages patients to participate in decision-making and have better health outcomes. When the patient and family caregivers become part of the process through active collaboration and integration, fragmentation, lack of coordination, and poor quality often go by the wayside.

For children and adolescents to collaborate in their care, we need to be sure to address children and adolescents within the healthcare setting according to their developmental stage in life. Involving the patient and family in decisions empowers them to be part of the healthcare team. Children need to be empowered to make choices and to be involved in making decisions that will affect their own health and treatment. The literature has found that when children have a feeling of control over stressful situations, this aids in their individual coping with the stress of their illness and/or hospitalization (Kelsey et al., 2007). Further involving the child and encouraging active participation in care planning and decision-making affords the child a better understanding of the illness and allows the child to prepare for procedures (Coyne, 2006).

Very often, older adults move to sub-acute care from hospitalization before going home. These transitions are opportunities for miscommunication, medication duplication, and lack of coordination. Several transitional care models have been developed, and many of them incorporate P&FCC as a basic element. These models recognize the essential component of a collaborative relationship between the provider and the patient and family to reflect integration, increase coordination, enhance communication, and produce best outcomes. Patients with multiple chronic diseases are often taking multiple medications. If a family member is informed and takes charge of medication reconciliation as the patient moves from one level of care to another, there will be more effective medication management. Medication reconciliation is just one of the processes that is critical to safe discharges across the continuum and can be managed by family members or caretakers.

Both of these special patient populations, the young and the old, are dependent on others more than other patient populations, and this makes collaboration central to their care planning and wellness. The family and/or caretakers of patients from these special populations need to be expert in knowing the patient's needs, preferences, routines, and norms and, therefore, need to be knowledgeable about what to expect and fully involved in all aspects of the care planning, patient/family education, and implementation.

Coordination and Integration of All Families

A patient- and family-centered approach to care decreases fragmentation and enables quality, coordinated care. Families can assume responsibility for coordinating appointments and tests and ensuring that follow-up information is shared with the provider. Families need to know what information needs to be shared immediately and what can wait until the next appointment with the provider. As previously stated, if coordination is to be successful, the healthcare team regards the patient and family as an integral part and shares any new information with them as well. For coordination to really lead to better outcomes, all information must be transparent and shared. Healthcare is complex, and there are more and more demands on the health team. There are instances when a member of the healthcare team and/or a member of the family believes that there is something "wrong" or that there are "difficulties" with the patient or the plan of care. It is important for members of the healthcare team to employ an interprofessional approach and shared decision-making techniques directly with the patient and family to resolve these situations.

Patients and families want to be involved in the plan, and coordination is not a new activity for most people. People coordinate many activities during their lives. Coordination of their healthcare allows them to do what they can do as a full partner on the healthcare team. This robust care coordination may include many people and settings, including the patient's primary care providers, family, caregivers, community, school, child-care setting, adult day care, church, and community.

Exemplar of Person-Centered Care for the Special Patient Population

Today's paradigm of healthcare delivery must shift from hospital-centric to patient-centric. Coordination, collaboration, integration, and communication across all parts of the healthcare system must be done with the patient and family fully informed and participating as decision-makers. A visual diagram of this (Figure 13.1) depicts all the crucial elements (coordination, collaboration, integration, and communication) directly circling into the patient/family as the center of gravity for the decision-making, direction, and pace of the care. This would redefine the notion of patients and families receiving healthcare to a model where patients and families partner with healthcare providers to fully understand and play an active role in both health and care.

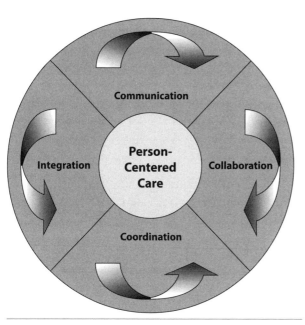

FIGURE 13.1

Integrated Model of Person-Centered Care for the Special Population.

Key Points and Practical Implications

This section provides specific strategies for both organizational structural changes to support P&FCC and strategies the professional can use to support persons and families as members of the healthcare team. The development and infusion of technology will enable patients and families to have more information to be meaningful and engaged partners with healthcare providers.

Communication, Coordination, and Collaboration Across the Care Continuum

Healthcare organizations today are complex and simultaneously manage multiple competing priorities. In order for these organizations to be successful in the dynamic industry of today, healthcare organizations need to be agile and innovative, and they must capitalize on collaboration. It is essential to identify elements that differentiate groups within and among organizations and understand the boundaries of those groups. Once these differences and boundaries are recognized and identified, leaders can employ specific strategies to transform them into opportunities that can be used to catapult the organization to new frontiers. P&FCC initiatives, much like most of the work within the healthcare setting, is highly dependent on interprofessional collaboration, cooperation, and accountability; ensuring that patient and family preferences are shared and honored across the care continuum requires many boundaries to be spanned. However, this is possible and necessary for the patients and families whom we are called to serve.

Strategies to Ensure Emphasis and Rigor Are Applied to P&FCC Initiative

P&FCC initiatives should be held to the same standards and have the same priority and esteem as all other quality and safety-outcome measures within the healthcare arena. Involving patients and families in care being delivered is invaluable in providing high-quality, safe, effective care. Some suggested strategies to ensure emphasis and rigor follow:

- Involve patients and families in the creation and implementation of P&FCC initiatives within the healthcare organization. Hospital and other healthcare system entities have established patient- and family-centered cultures through the participation of patients on advisory boards. It is important to have children from multiple age groups and older adults included on these advisory boards.

- P&FCC initiatives should have associated reliable metrics to show the value of the initiative and to make incremental updates/improvements as needed in a process-improvement approach. Patient representatives from these special patient populations could help guide how to measure values of the P&FCC initiative.

- P&FCC initiatives should be embedded into the fabric of the healthcare organization. This can be done by including age-specific measures of competence on annual per-formance evaluations and including P&FCC principles in organizational policies and procedures of practice.

- The Picker Institute's Always Events framework was developed specifically to elevate patient experience within the healthcare setting. This framework serves as a guide for organizations to develop and implement strategies to promote P&FCC. Age-specific strategies must be included to address the unique needs of the family caretakers in these special populations.

Age-Specific Strategies

1. *Establish organizational consumer boards to represent all ages in P&FCC.*

2. *Invite patients of all ages to comment on their perception of engagement qualitatively and quantitatively.*

3. *Assess the staff member's ability to personalize care (such as in the use of specific equipment or medication dosages) according to differences in the patient's age or size.*

4. *Develop a patient's Bill of Rights that is tailored to and co-created by children and adolescents.*

5. *Design a Patient Satisfaction Survey that uses pictures and cartoons for children under 5 years of age.*

Leveraging Technology to Provide and Embed P&FCC Within an Organizational Structure

Technology is a mainstay within the healthcare setting today. Technology can be a valuable tool for gathering, housing, transferring, and hard-wiring P&FCC within the healthcare setting. For example, the electronic health record (EHR) is widely used across the healthcare continuum today, and many EHR systems have functionality for patients and families to access their records or charts from home. This is an excellent place to record a patient's individual preferences and expressed needs for care where it can be seen and used to provide individualized centered care by all care professionals who interact with the patient. Innovation and optimization of the EHR has the potential to create high reliability and consistency of the patient's care experience across continuums of care. As we look into the future and realize the ability for patient access to their own EHRs, it will be imperative for pediatric and older patients that the design includes the ability to give proxy access to caregivers in situations where these patients cannot do it themselves. The monitoring of chronic conditions, so often part of the complex nature of caring for children or older adults, will move into e-mobile platforms. Families will need to know how to access these tools and resources and input data to inform providers of changes in a condition.

Conclusion

In order to transform the care that patients and families are receiving across the healthcare continuum today, it is imperative for leaders within the healthcare industry to continuously embed patient-centered care models and initiatives. This calls for leaders who understand and value P&FCC, are well versed in its philosophy, and can engage and inspire others to collaborate with patients and their families as full partners within an ever-changing environment. In addition, leaders need to understand that family caregivers for very young and very old patients have additional burdens, and caretaking often begins to rule their lives.

Several strategies are suggested for achieving P&FCC for vulnerable age groups:

- Use process improvement methodology to develop P&FCC initiatives and institute special patient population advisory boards to guide this work.

- Involve pediatric patients/families and older adults/caregivers in the creation and implementation of special patient population P&FCC initiatives.

- Deliver ongoing age-specific education to all interprofessional staff within the healthcare setting to ensure both confidence and competence of staff for caring for pediatric patients and the older adult patient population.

- Capitalize on technology to hardwire P&FCC initiatives at the point of care (for example, EHR).

- Embed P&FCC initiatives within the organization's fabric (mission, vision, policies, procedures, expected behaviors, and annual performance reviews).

- Use pediatric and/or older adult case studies and scenarios to demonstrate the value of P&FCC initiatives for these special patient populations.

Perhaps of most importance is to trust and use qualitative data—for example, the patient's story—to guide P&FCC work within the organization. That is the essence of person-centered care.

References

Agency for Healthcare Research and Quality. (2008). Statistics on hospital-based care in the United States. *Healthcare Cost and Utilization Project Facts and Figures 2008.* Retrieved from http://www.hcup-us.ahrq.gov/reports/factsandfigures/2008/section1_TOC.jsp

Brazelton, T. B., & Sparrow, J. D. (2001). *Touchpoints 3 to 6: Your child's emotional and behavioral development.* Cambridge, MA: Perseus Publishing.

Covinsky, K. E., Pierluissi, E., & Johnston, C. B. (2011). Hospitalization-associated disability: "She was probably able to ambulate, but I'm not sure." *Journal of the American Medical Association, 306*(16), 1782-1793.

Coyne, I. (2006). Consultation with children in hospitals: Children, parents' and nurses' perspectives. *Journal of Clinical Nursing, 15*(1), 61-71.

Doty, P. (2010). The evolving balance of formal and informal, institutional and non-institutional long-term care for older Americans: A thirty-year perspective. *Public Policy and Aging Report, 20*(1), 3-9.

Federation for Children with Special Needs. (2013). *Our mission.* Retrieved from fcsn.org/about_us.php

Feinberg, L. (2011). Moving toward person-centered care. *AARP Public Policy Institute. Insight on the Issues, 51,* 2011.

Feinberg, L., Reinhard, S. C., Houser, A., & Choula, R. (2011). Valuing the invaluable: 2011 update: The growing contributions and costs of caregiving. *AARP Public Policy Institute. Insight on the Issues, 51,* 2011.

Hanson, C. M., & Spross, J. A. (2009). Collaboration. In A. B. Hamric, J. A. Spross, & C. M. Hanscon (Eds.), *Advanced practice nursing: An integrative approach* (4th ed.) (pp. 283-314). St. Louis, MO: Saunders Elsevier.

Kelsey, J., Abelson-Mitchell, N., & Skirton, H. (2007). Perceptions of young people about decision making in the acute healthcare environment. *Pediatric Nursing, 19*(6), 14-18.

Prilleltensky, I. (2010). Child wellness and social inclusion: Values for action. *American Journal of Community Psychology, 46*(12), 238-249.

Prilleltensky, I., Nelson, G., & Peirson, L. (2001). The role of power and control in children's lives: An ecological analysis of pathways toward wellness, resilience and problems. *Journal of Community & Applied Social Psychology, 11*(2), 143-158.

Reed, P., Smith, P., Fletcher, M., & Bradding, A. (2003). Promoting the dignity of the child in hospital. *Nursing Ethics, 10*(1), 67-76.

Sartain, S. A., Clarke, C. L., & Heyman, R. (2000). Hearing the voices of children with chronic illness. *Journal of Advanced Nursing, 32*(4), 913-921.

U.S. Department of Health and Human Services Centers for Disease Control and Prevention National Center for Health Statistics. (2012). *Summary health statistics for the U.S. population: National health interview survey, 2011.* Retrieved from http://www.cdc.gov/nchs/data/series/sr_10/sr10_255.pdf

Chapter 14

Advocating for Patients and Families

Carol Taylor, PhD, RN
Sarah Vittone, MSN, MA, RN

Mrs. Esposita is an independent 96-year-old woman whose 71-year-old son accompanies her to her routine cardiologist appointment. She is in complete heart failure. Her heart rate is 30 bpm, but her son reports that she is asymptomatic unless active—which she rarely is. The cardiologist tries to get her to sign consent for a permanent pacemaker without adequate disclosure of anticipated risks and benefits and the option of non-pacemaker treatment. When the patient hesitates, asks questions, and seems incapable of signing the consent form, the cardiologist turns to the son. The physician tells him that this procedure would benefit his mother and instructs him to sign the consent for her.

A nursing instructor and two bachelor of science in nursing (BSN) students are present and observe this clinical encounter. The nursing instructor is immediately outraged, knowing that many patients in similar situations would elect not to get the pacemaker— a chance not being offered Mrs. Esposita. Should he advocate for Mrs. Esposita? Does he have a professional duty to advocate? What is the best practice for resolution in the case?

Increasingly, hospitalized patients are being cautioned to have a family member at the bedside 24/7, because there are no guarantees that the healthcare team will work collaboratively to promote and protect their interests. Sadly, even when family members are present, they may lack the knowledge and confidence to effectively advocate for loved ones, as shown in the preceding vignette. Those seeking healthcare services in the community have even fewer guarantees about getting the right care, from the right provider, in the right setting, and at the right cost.

This chapter examines the advocacy responsibilities of nurses and their collaboration with other professional caregivers in person- and family-centered care (P&FCC). We return to the opening case study before we conclude.

Defining Patient Advocacy

Every professional caregiver who designs and implements a plan of care for patients and families is obligated to advocate for their interests. As you will read in a moment, advocacy is central to nursing's essence.

The *What* of Patient Advocacy

Bu and Jezewski (2007) have published a middle-range theory of patient advocacy, which was completed through a concept analysis on the topic. They identify three broad core attributes for patient advocacy: (a) "safeguarding patient's autonomy," (b) "acting on behalf of patients," and (c) "championing social justice in the provision of health care" (p. 104). Autonomy is the capacity to be self-determining. When internal or external variables interfere with an individual's ability to act on healthcare preferences and choices, advocates can get involved to promote the patient's interests.

Patients can be individuals, families, or communities. A nurse can advocate for *a patient* whose plan of care is no longer addressing priority needs; for *families*, such as those struggling to cope with the complex needs of veterans returning home to months of rehabilitation made all the more challenging because of post-traumatic stress disorder (PTSD); and for *communities,* such as those that recently suffered weather-related disasters, tornadoes, hurricanes, or earthquakes. Generally, the more vulnerable patients are because of poverty, illiteracy, or disabilities, the greater the need will be for advocacy. In a country like the United States, where there is a growing divide between those with and those without financial and other resources, the need for nurses to pay attention to social justice issues to ensure a fair distribution of scarce health resources is critical.

> **NOTE**
>
> Ask yourself before reading further, what is reasonable for everyone to expect of U.S. healthcare? What difference should my socioeconomic status make if I arrive in the emergency department (ED) after a motor vehicle accident?

A group of Iranian nurses defined *advocacy* as informing and educating, valuing and respecting, supporting, protecting, and promoting quality of care for patients (Negarandeh, Oskouie, Ahmadi, & Nikravesh, 2008). Distinctive of the Iranian study is that its nurses also believed that advocacy could take place only if there was respect for patients' individuality and their inherent human dignity. This insight immediately raises the question about who gets our advocacy efforts. By referencing "inherent human dignity," the Iranian nurses are claiming that everyone, by virtue of being human, commands our respect and simultaneously our advocacy efforts as needed. In the world of healthcare, the disparities that characterize so much of society and the way we distribute human goods should not be present. Sadly, this is not so.

There are basically three models of healthcare decision-making: paternalism, patient sovereignty, and shared decision-making. See Table 14.1.

TABLE 14.1   Three Models of Healthcare Decision-Making

MODEL	DEFINITION	CONSIDERATIONS
Hippocratic (Paternalistic)	Physician/clinician decides what is in the best interests of the patient. Grounded in *beneficence* and *nonmaleficence (primum non nocere)*.	Because humans are more than biological machines, what physicians believed to be in the best medical interests of patients was not always what patients wanted. Abuses of paternalism were corrected by championing the autonomy of the patient (patient's right to be self-determining). Strong consensus now exists in the United States that (1) all patients with intact capacity have the right to say yea or nay to any and all indicated medical treatment; (2) loss of capacity does not entail loss of the right to be autonomous and to have one's preferences respected; (3) to the extent the preferences of the patient with diminished capacity are known, they should be honored.
Patient Sovereignty	The patient or the patient's surrogate decides what should be done and informs the physician/clinician. Instead of *giving orders to* the patient, the clinician *takes orders from* the patient or the patient's surrogate. Grounded in *non-interference model of respect for autonomy*.	Opposite end of the continuum—there is nothing to protect the patient from poor or ill-advised choices grounded on misperceptions, guilt, etc. The patient/surrogate's autonomous choice does not obligate clinicians to sacrifice their integrity or that of the profession. However, many clinicians today prefer to think of themselves as "technicians" who implement the wishes of patients and their surrogates "for a price"; some may have abdicated accountability for their actions.

continues

TABLE 14.1 *continued*

MODEL	DEFINITION	CONSIDERATIONS
Shared Decision-Making	The treating team works collaboratively with the patient/surrogate and family to secure the health and well-being or good dying of the patient in a manner that privileges the beliefs, values, and goals of the patient and the clinical knowledge and experience of clinicians.	The President's Commission in 1982 rejected both extreme models of decision-making and instead recommended a model of shared decision-making. Benefits of shared decision-making: It improves patient autonomy, which aids patients in two ways: (1) It satisfies their desire for more information; and (2) it improves their overall well-being. It provides clinicians with more insight into their patients' lives and their ability to tolerate the negative effects of certain treatment options—which improves a clinician's ability to advise patients about treatment options. Alert: Shared decision-making can easily slip back into either paternalism or patient sovereignty.

In the 1960s, the United States was just beginning to transition out of paternalistic medicine and to champion patient autonomy. Nurse philosopher Gadow (1980) has recognized that respecting autonomy means much more than not interfering with the choices patients make—and argues that nurses are uniquely positioned to promote real patient self-determination using existential advocacy. Gadow (1980) bases her concept of existential advocacy upon the principle that freedom of self-determination is the most fundamental and valuable human right. In negative terms, this implies that the right of self-determination ought not to be infringed upon, even in the interest of health.

Writing at a time when it was still common for clinicians to believe they knew what was good for patients better than patients ever could, Gadow states clearly that it is not the professional but the patient who determines what "best interest" shall mean:

> In positive terms, the ideal which existential advocacy expresses is this: that individuals be assisted by nurses to authentically exercise their freedom of self-determination. By authentic is meant a way of reaching decisions which are truly one's own—decisions that express all that one believes important about oneself and the world, the entire complexity of one's values. (p. 85)

Gadow asserts that advocacy is not based on an assumption about what individuals *should want* to do, nor does it consist of protecting individuals' *rights* to do what they want:

[Advocacy] is the effort to help persons become clear about what they want to do, by helping them discern and clarify their values in the situation, and on the basis of that self-examination, to reach decisions which express their reaffirmed, perhaps recreated, complex of values. Only in this way, when the valuing self is engaged and expressed in its entirety, can a person's decision be actually self-determined instead of being a decision which is not determined by others. (p. 85)

> **NOTE**
>
> What Gadow could not have foreseen in 1980 is the degree to which the pendulum would shift from paternalism to patient sovereignty. When patients were first characterized as clients to negate the passiveness associated with patient status, few realized that the next transition would be from client to customer—with the customer always being right.

What Gadow is advocating is shared decision-making in which nurses and other members of the team work in partnership with patients and families, providing the knowledge and support they need to make decisions that truly serve their best interests. Today, the need for advocacy to protect patients and their surrogates from poor or ill-advised health decisions is equal to the need to protect them from abuses of paternalism.

This chapter is based on the conviction that the object of all clinical decision-making is *first and primarily* to secure the health, well-being, or good dying of the patient and to simultaneously do this in a manner that respects the integrity of all participants in the decision-making process—the patient, the family, and healthcare professionals. This makes the dignity and autonomy of patients central and respects the integrity, expertise, and experience of clinicians. This is true shared decision-making. A final caveat: Shared decision-making plays out differently in every scenario, depending on the knowledge, experience, and ability and desire to be self-determining of the patient and family and similar characteristics of healthcare professionals.

If we return to the opening vignette, we see that Mrs. Esposita and her son are being pressured to authorize a permanent pacemaker without first finding out more about her goals at this point in her life and whether the pacemaker is compatible with these goals. The physician doing the pressuring may simply be paternalistically seeing a "problem" that needs to be "fixed"—or, worse, may be motivated by greed to secure approval for a costly intervention. In either scenario, the physician is failing to provide the information and support Mrs. Esposita and her son need to make a truly authentic decision.

However, let's imagine that Mrs. Esposita presents in the ED in crisis and her son demands that "everything—including a permanent pacemaker—be done." If healthcare professionals comply without first making sure that the son understands the request he is making and any reservations the team has about the appropriateness of his requests, they are failing to exercise existential advocacy. Gadow sets a high standard.

The *Who* of Patient Advocacy

Everyone who is part of designing and implementing a plan of care is responsible for patient advocacy. Ideally, the interprofessional team functions collaboratively to advocate for the patient according to their knowledge of the patient, professional role, and scope of practice. Whoever first realizes that something is interfering with a patient's receiving appropriate care should bring this to the attention of the team. Often, existential advocacy simply involves helping patients and families understand what is at stake with pending health decisions and evaluate options in light of their values and preferences.

Although nurses have long claimed that advocacy is essential to their professional role, they do not "own" advocacy. Those who viewed (or, worse, promoted) advocacy as the nurse's saving the patient from an indifferent physician contributed to unhelpful adversarial relationships between physicians and nurses. Again, the ideal is to foster collaborative advocacy. Nurses are often well positioned to lead advocacy efforts when their intimate knowledge of patients, families, and communities results in keen appreciation for the challenges patients encounter. Nurses are also well positioned to lead because of their expertise and experience with care coordination and their ability to relate to persons during difficult and challenging experiences.

The Urban Institute's Health Policy Center (2010) describes *vulnerable populations* as groups that are not well integrated into the healthcare system because of ethnic, cultural, economic, geographic, or health characteristics: "This isolation puts members of these groups at risk for not obtaining necessary medical care, and thus constitutes a potential threat to health" (para. 1). Vulnerable populations with special advocacy needs include cultural, racial, and ethnic minorities; the economically disadvantaged; low-income children; the elderly; the homeless; those with chronic health conditions, including severe mental illness; those with language illiteracy; and those living in rural areas. The Centers for Disease Control and Prevention (CDC; 2014) lists as other at-risk/vulnerable populations cancer survivors, immigrants and refugees, incarcerated men and women, persons who use drugs (PWUD), pregnant women, and veterans. To read more about vulnerable populations, see the Resources section at the end of the book for this chapter.

It is probably most important to remember that anyone can be rendered vulnerable by illness and require advocacy. A person can be wealthy, well educated, and otherwise resourceful, and yet when a new cancer diagnosis is made, the person can easily become confused and experience great difficulty navigating a complex healthcare arena. Individual characteristics that indicate a need for advocacy include:

- Limited or deficient ability to communicate
- Limited or absent capacity for decision-making
- Limited or deficient health literacy
- Deficient social support and resources
- Limited or lacking coping skills

Considering these characteristics, any individual has the potential to be vulnerable and to require the advocacy skills of nurses when experiencing a healthcare need.

The *How* of Patient Advocacy

Being an effective patient advocate means making the healthcare system "work" for those who need it—making the system responsive to the unique needs of individual patients, families, and communities. Sometimes this is as simple as discovering what these needs are and bringing them to the attention of the team. Sometimes it entails finding or creating the resources to address these needs. Often this entails helping the patient or family advocate for their own needs—explaining their rights, helping them navigate the healthcare system, or preparing them to speak up or request a family meeting. Sometimes it means fighting for the underdog to ensure that everyone has fair access to the team's time, attention, expertise, and resources. This can be especially challenging in climates that condone suboptimal treatment for the marginalized.

Consider for a moment the elderly nursing home resident who arrives in the ED with a fractured hip, cold, wet, and confused—and without family. Or consider the migrant worker appearing in the same ED with multiple injuries stemming from a farm accident—and no money to pay. Or imagine yourself as a new obstetrical nurse receiving an incarcerated pregnant woman in active labor—and being told that she is to remain handcuffed to the bed. In these instances, advocacy is about ensuring that these patients and families receive safe, respectful, evidence-based, individualized care that meets their physical, psychological, social, and spiritual needs. It may also entail challenging an institutional culture or policy or even national or local legislation that interferes with these needs' being met: Do we need to develop additional resources? Should the incarcerated woman remain in handcuffs? Are there safe alternatives? What treatment is reasonable for the migrant family to receive? Should public monies be used for non-U.S. citizens?

Exactly how advocacy is implemented is dependent on context and complexity. Advocacy interventions required for any situation range from simple to complex. It is the experience, competence, and empowerment of the nurse and the complexity of the situation that determines the extent and relevance of interventions to achieve positive outcomes for the patient. One strong example of an opportunity for nurses to advocate is during the discharge process, when the patient is particularly vulnerable. The discharge process is generally the last assessment the nurse makes with the patient, after which the patient is released from acute, urgent, or rehabilitative care to self-care or lower level of skilled care. The patient is in a highly vulnerable situation, and it is the nurse who must make that final agreement that a previously determined collaborative plan of care with the clinical team remains suitable for the patient.

A contextual example when a simple set of advocacy actions might be utilized would be during the discharge process of a capable adult with supportive family present after elective surgery. During the discharge discussion of self-care related to activities of daily living, dressing changes, and medication administration, the nurse may deem it best to use a simple set of interventions, including establishing a short-term therapeutic relationship, supportive listening, reactive problem solving, support for patient self-advocacy and due diligence toward disclosure, and collaborative decision-making, thereby assuring the success of the discharge and transition to home.

A more complex contextual example of discharge might be from an ED to home. Further adding to the intricacy of any discharge would be patients whose capacity by diagnosis, by disease progression, or by age (children) require more complex advocacy interventions. These more complex advocacy interventions include supportive and active listening, enhanced communication, reactive and proactive problem solving, establishing long-term therapeutic relationships either with self or other clinicians, enabling patient/surrogate self-advocacy in collaborative decision-making with due diligence to disclosure, and establishing patient wishes and/or best interest as outcome drivers.

In the most complex cases, many advocates from differing clinical perspectives will be helpful to achieve positive outcomes. The patient who refuses care and desires discharge against medical advice or the psychiatric patient who refuses medication are both examples of complex situations, when how the nurse advocates is of great importance.

> **NOTE**
>
> For the sake of continuity and consistency, all advocacy interventions must be documented in the medical record.

Advocacy requires intentionality; we have to value being effective advocates and work to develop these capacities. Periodically pausing to reflect on our individual capacity (knowledge, attitudes, and skills) for advocacy and the role our institutional culture plays in promoting or thwarting advocacy is essential. See Tables 14.2 and 14.3.

Advocacy Reflection

Advocacy does not just happen because we are good people and want to help others. If we are intentional about developing our capacity to advocate effectively, we can begin by evaluating whether we and our institutions have the prerequisite knowledge, attitudes, and skills. Review the following concepts and self-reflection questions (see Tables 14.2 and 14.3) to determine which areas you may want to focus on.

TABLE 14.2 Reflections for the Professional Caregiver/Nurse

CONCEPT	QUESTIONS FOR REFLECTION
Own advocacy as central to professional role/intentionality	Do I believe that advocacy is absolutely central to my professional identity—that I cannot be a good nurse unless I am an effective advocate?
	Do I value learning how to enhance my commitment to advocacy and my advocacy practice?

CONCEPT	QUESTIONS FOR REFLECTION
Motivation	Is my heart in the right place?
	Am I approaching each patient, family, and community with respect, open to their vulnerabilities, willing to commit my experience and expertise to securing their interests, even when this means sacrificing my comfort and well-being?
Primacy of the patient	Do I routinely pause to make sure that my commitment and loyalty to myself, my colleagues, my employer, or other entities do not compromise my primary commitment to the patient?
Openness	Do I harbor bias, discrimination, or worse that blinds me to the needs of some patients or makes me reluctant to get involved?
Empathy and compassion	Have I sufficiently "walked in my patients' shoes" to grasp relevant physical, mental, social, and spiritual needs?
	Do I resist thinking I know what is wrong and how to fix it before listening to the patient's narrative?
	Do I understand the barriers that are preventing the patient, family, or community from getting excellent care?
Engagement/trusting partnership with patients	Is my engagement with the patient such that we have formed a real, working partnership?
	Does the patient feel "heard" and understood and able to trust and confide in me?
	Does the patient have confidence in me?
Collaborative team partnerships	Have I established collaborative relationships with other members of the professional caregiving team in order to enhance our team's capacity for advocacy?
	Can I approach other team members with my concerns, confident that I will be heard and that collective effort will go toward addressing patient needs?
	Is my reputation that I am worth paying attention to?
Confidence and expertise	Am I confident in my ability to advocate effectively?
	Am I intentional about learning how to do this better from role models?
	Do I know how my institution works?
	Can I identify and access power players, and do I know where to direct my concerns?

continues

TABLE 14.2 *continued*

CONCEPT	QUESTIONS FOR REFLECTION
Courage and persistence	Do I have the courage to call attention to what is not working—especially in an efficiency-driven system?
	Am I willing to get involved?
	If my initial efforts to bring about change fail, am I willing to reflect on what happened to better understand the forces at work in order to try again?
Authenticity	If asked to describe examples of successful patient advocacy, would they come readily to mind—or would I have to "dig deep" to remember a situation where I made the critical difference for a patient or family?

TABLE 14.3 Reflections for the Agency/Institution

CONCEPT	QUESTIONS FOR REFLECTION
Advocacy central to mission	Have we clearly communicated to every employee that advocacy is absolutely central to our mission—that we expect every professional caregiver and staff member to advocate for the needs of patients, families, and communities?
Evaluating for advocacy	Do our annual performance reviews call out advocacy and highlight its importance to our mission?
	Are we holding frontline caregivers accountable for effective advocacy?
Supporting advocacy	Is leadership at all levels advocating for frontline caregivers—making sure that they have the time and resources to be effective advocates?
	If asked, would frontline caregivers confirm that this is the case?
Educating for advocacy	Are our educational efforts targeting populations within the agency or institution who pose the greatest advocacy challenges and suggesting workable strategies to meet these needs?
Troubleshooting for advocacy	If asked, to whom would they turn if initial efforts to advocate for patients met failure?
	What percentage of our frontline caregivers could name an individual within the agency or institution they trust to respond positively to their concerns?
Celebrating advocacy	Are there institutional strategies to celebrate successful advocacy?

Once we are intentional about cultivating the knowledge and attitudes that promote successful advocacy, it is time to begin practicing advocacy skills.

Advocacy as a Skill

Advocacy must be intentionally taught and learned as a skill. Opportunity to reflect during the student experience is valuable self-learning. Our experience during Ethics Rounds with undergraduate BSN students has been successful in this area. For example, one senior graduating student shared this reflection after Ethics Rounds:

> This case had a big impact for me in terms of what the nurse's responsibility is. When I am given a patient with a difficult case, I can do one of two things as a nurse: I can just get through the day and pass that patient on to the next nurse, or I can be the patient's advocate and find the problem and work to fix it.

Table 14.4 highlights examples of patient advocacy competencies and relevant knowledge, skills, and attitudes.

TABLE 14.4 Patient Advocacy Competencies

COMPETENCY	DESCRIPTION
Supporting autonomy	1. Determining and documenting the patient's decision-making capacity; ensuring that agency/institutional policies specify how this is to be done and identify responsible parties
	2. Protecting the right of patients with decision-making capacity to be self-determining
	a. Ensure that the patient understands the medical condition and pending diagnostic and treatment decisions.
	b. Facilitate communication and documentation of the patient's preferences.
	c. Anticipate the types of treatment decisions that will likely need to be made.
	d. Assist in the preparation of advance directives.

continues

TABLE 14.4 *continued*

COMPETENCY	DESCRIPTION
Supporting autonomy *(continued)*	3. Promoting authentic autonomy (authentic decisions reflect the individual's identity, decisional history, and moral norms)
	4. Identifying the morally as well as legally valid surrogate decision-maker for patients who lack decision-making capacity
	5. Supporting the surrogate decision-maker; clarifying the surrogate decision-maker's role
	6. Identifying limits to patient/surrogate autonomy and limits to caregiver autonomy
	7. Developing agency/institutional policies that identify the professional caregivers responsible for and the procedures to be used to identify and support the appropriate decision-makers
Promoting patient well-being	1. Clarifying the goal of therapy: cure and restoration; stabilization of functioning; preparation for a comfortable, dignified death
	2. Determining the medical effectiveness of therapy
	3. Weighing the benefits and burdens of therapy
	4. Ensuring that all interventions are consistent with the overall goal of therapy
	5. Ensuring that the patient's priority needs are addressed (bio-psycho-social-spiritual needs)
	6. Ensuring continuity of care as the patient is transferred among services and within and without the institution
	7. Weighing the moral relevance of third-party interests (family, caregiver, institution, society)
	8. Identifying and addressing forces within society and the healthcare system that compromise patients' well-being

COMPETENCY	DESCRIPTION
Preventing and resolving ethical conflict	1. Establishing that preventing and resolving ethical conflict falls within the authority of all healthcare professionals engaged in the care of a patient
	2. Developing awareness of and sensitivity to the conscious and unconscious sources of conflict
	3. Facilitating timely communication among those involved in decision-making: one-on-one meetings and periodic meetings of the patient, family, and interdisciplinary team to clarify goals and plan of care
	4. Documenting pertinent information on the patient record
	5. Referring unresolved ethical issues to the ethics consult team or the institutional ethics committee
	6. Identifying and addressing system variables that are contributing to recurrent ethical problems

Critiquing the Adequacy of One's Personal, Team, and Institutional Ability and Willingness to Advocate for Patients and Families

Presented in this section are three opportunities for you to assess your individual, team, and institutional advocacy capacities and familiarity with pertinent advocacy strategies. Read through the scenarios that follow and assess your ability and readiness to advocate for these patients. Feel free to substitute clinical scenarios more pertinent to your practice. Then review the suggested advocacy activities. Which might be appropriate in your setting? What other strategies might you try?

Scenario 1: "Staying the Course"

You believe that the plan of care for Ms. Jones is no longer helping to cure or even to sustain her. She has had two lengthy abdominal resections and is left with less than a foot of bowel, which is riddled with fistulas and seeping feces. Not surprisingly, she is septic. She has been ventilated in the surgical intensive care unit (ICU) for 3 months, and the team has treated complication after complication—seemingly without ever revisiting the overall goals of treatment. Her family is beginning to question whether medical therapies should be continued, but the surgeon is adamant about "staying the course." The daughter confides to you that she is sure that her mother would tell everyone "there are worse things than death" if only she were able to speak.

Consider now the following questions, circling your level of confidence for each:

How confident are you that *you* would step up to advocate for the team's meeting to revisit the goals of care—even if the surgeon dismisses the need to do so or pulls rank?				
Not very confident				Extremely confident
1	2	3	4	5

How confident are you that *your team* would appropriately address the need to revisit the goals of care—even if the surgeon initially dismisses the need to do so or pulls rank?				
Not very confident				Extremely confident
1	2	3	4	5

How confident are you that *your institutional culture* would support individuals' advocating for patients like Ms. Jones—in fact, would *actively promote everyone's doing so?*				
Not very confident				Extremely confident
1	2	3	4	5

Based on your answers to the preceding questions, what needs to change at the level of yourself, your team, or your institution to ensure that the needs of patients like Ms. Jones are met?

Here are some suggested key advocacy actions to undertake:

- Be an active and supportive listener.
- Establish who the decision-maker is.
- Provide information on the role, responsibilities, and rights of the surrogate decision-maker.
- Establish patient desires, wants, and wishes for treatment and/or outcome as described by the surrogate.
- Collaborate with the clinical team on medical care, all options, and directions.
- Facilitate a care conference with the surrogate, family, clinical team, and other stakeholders.
- Focus care on goals that benefit and meet the patient's wishes based on collaborative decision-making.

Scenario 2: "Don't Rock the Boat"

You are an experienced obstetrical nurse with 20 years of experience conducting prenatal classes and providing perinatal care and assisting with deliveries. You work closely with the women you coach, and they tend to be comforted when they find you when they arrive in the birthing center in labor. They trust you. Last year a new obstetrician, Dr. Kumar, was hired and quickly became popular with patients. She has two children, ages 4 and 6, and values being home at their dinner and bed times. You have begun to notice a pattern of increased Caesarean deliveries after 5 p.m. and suspect she is recommending Caesarean deliveries so that she can leave the hospital. You strongly believe that this is not in the best interests of the women and infants being delivered. When you report this to the center's nursing and medical leaders, they caution you not to "rock the boat." The medical director directly tells you that he noticed the same pattern, but because her patients seem happy, he is reluctant to challenge her. You believe her patients are happy because she tells them she needs to do Caesarean deliveries to save their babies' lives.

Consider now the following questions, circling your level of confidence for each:

How confident are you that *you* would persist in advocating for this obstetrician's patients—even in the face of initial counsel to "stand down"?				
Not very confident				Extremely confident
1	2	3	4	5

How confident are you that *your team* would share your concerns once alerted to what is happening and find a way to correct the problem?				
Not very confident				Extremely confident
1	2	3	4	5

How confident are you that *your institutional culture* would support everyone's advocating for these women—in fact, would *actively promote everyone's doing so?*				
Not very confident				Extremely confident
1	2	3	4	5

Here are some suggested key advocacy actions to undertake:

- Actively foster the collegial relationship between the nursing staff and Dr. Kumar.
- Identify respect and trust as key aspects.

- Identify key patient indicators for plan-of-care options and the associated disclosure elements.

- Establish an open communication channel among the staff and Dr. Kumar to ensure information is heard without fear of conflict or retaliation.

- Establish regular team meetings to review quality indicators set by the team and for respectful communication of acclaim and concern.

Scenario 3: Compassionate Use...Maybe?

Carlos is a 10-year-old with significant solid tumor growth 3 years after remission of osteosarcoma. His parents are knowledgeable about his disease but are hesitant to ask questions, leaving decisions to the doctor. They trust the doctors and the nurses without question. Carlos is clearly in acute pain, which has been managed up to this point with standard therapy. The clinical team has been very involved with the family and is hopeful that Carlos will be able to return home.

You are aware of various research protocols, including a Phase 3 study at your facility that Carlos might meet inclusion criteria for if he were 12 years old. Many children on the study have had good results—some lifesaving. You are aware that compassionate use of the therapies might even be available (although the cost must be absorbed by the facility). You know that last year, a 6-year-old was enrolled for compassionate use. Your nursing unit manager would not discuss this with you for fear of bringing more costs to the unit, and although you think it might be important for the family to know, you do not know how to reach the investigators and are hesitant to bring this possibility up to the team or the family.

Consider now the following questions, circling your level of confidence for each:

How confident are you that *you* would persist in advocating for patients like Carlos—even in the face of initial counsel to "stand down"?				
Not very confident				Extremely confident
1	2	3	4	5

How confident are you that *your team* would share your concerns once alerted to what is happening and find a way to correct the problem?				
Not very confident				Extremely confident
1	2	3	4	5

How confident are you that *your institutional culture* would support everyone's advocating for patients like Carlos—in fact, would *actively promote everyone's doing so?*

Not very confident				Extremely confident
1	2	3	4	5

Here are some suggested key advocacy actions to undertake:

- Engage the nurse manager in the discussion of patient care options and your role as an advocate for this child and family.
- Contact the study team for information about the enrollment and the study itself. Be informed.
- If information proves fruitful, discuss the option with the clinical team.
- If the clinical team disagrees with this option on grounds unrelated to potential benefit, disclose to the team your obligation to the child and family to reveal this disparity to them.

The *When* of Advocacy

Patient advocacy is called for whenever a patient, family, or community is finding it difficult to secure needed healthcare resources. In many of these situations, members of the healthcare team, the patient, and/or members of the family may be in conflict about what should be done. Not infrequently, patients are vulnerable to coercion from the family or team. The earlier efforts are made to address deficiencies, the more likely these efforts are to result in optimal patient outcomes. Advocacy is also indicated when interests other than the well-being of the patient are influencing medical decisions (e.g., when the desire to generate revenues motivates a clinician to promote a costly but suboptimal intervention).

The *Why* of Advocacy

Bu and Jezewski (2007) recognize that the antecedents to patient advocacy included, at the macro or organizational level, a complex hospital system (and we would add a dizzying array of diagnostic and treatment choices), and at the micro or work-unit level, issues of vulnerability, poverty, language barriers, patients who feel intimidated, severity of illness, and level of consciousness, among other factors.

Although we can continue to debate whether advocacy is an ethical ideal or nonnegotiable moral obligation for professional nurses, the profession is clear in its standards. The *primacy of the patient* is central to the ethics of all in healthcare professions and to the very notion of professionalism.

The American Nurses Association (ANA) *Code of Ethics for Nurses* reads:

> "The nurse's primary commitment is to the patient, whether an individual, family, group or community."

> "The nurse promotes, advocates for and strives to protect the health, safety and rights of the patient." (ANA, 2001, provisions 2 and 3)

The ANA's *Nursing's Social Policy Statement: The Essence of the Profession* identifies advocacy as an essential nursing action:

> The aims of nursing actions (also nursing interventions) are to protect, promote, and optimize health; to prevent illness and injury; to alleviate suffering; and to advocate for individuals, families, communities, and populations. Nursing actions are theoretically defined, evidence-based, and require developed intellectual competencies. (2010a, p. 11)

The ANA *Scope and Standards of Practice* (2010b) similarly identifies advocacy as essential to professional practice:

> The registered nurse "[a]dvocates for health care that is sensitive to the needs of healthcare consumers, with particular emphasis on the needs of the diverse." (Standard 5. Implementation, p. 38)

> The registered nurse "[a]dvocates for the delivery of dignified and humane care by the interprofessional team." (Standard 5A. Coordination of Care, p. 40)

Recently, the Nursing Alliance for Quality Care (Sofaer & Schumann, 2013), believing that (1) the active engagement of patients, families, and others is essential to improving quality and reducing medical errors and harm to patients and that (2) nurses at all levels of education and across all healthcare settings must play a central role in fostering successful patient and family engagement, included among its guidelines: "Advocacy for patients who are unable to participate fully is a fundamental nursing role. Patient advocacy is the demonstration of how all of the components of the relationship fit together" (p. 6).

The alliance recognizes that nurses' daily experience includes working with patients and families who have often fared poorly because patients' concerns, preferences, and knowledge have not been valued. The alliance also realizes that many factors reduce a nurse's willingness and effectiveness in advocacy. Its report promises to detail

> a set of strategies that will support every nurse as an advocate, will educate each nurse regarding techniques that foster well-informed decision-making by patients and

families, and will demand that the healthcare system stop, listen, translate effectively, and respond appropriately to keep patients safe from harm due to medical error or insufficiently responsive healthcare professionals. (p. 8)

The challenge the nursing profession faces, having clearly identified advocacy as central to the profession of nursing, is continuing to promote healthcare practice environments that make advocacy possible. A nurse should not have to be a hero to be an advocate. A great sadness for the authors is no longer hearing many nurses complain about the difficulties of trying to advocate for patients, because they have given up trying to advocate: "We're lucky to get the bare minimum for our patients accomplished during our shifts—everyone is so busy." Even worse is this sentiment: "You get paid the same whether you just show up and do the minimum or try to advocate for what needs to change." Clearly there is a gap between what the profession demands of nurses and what practice environments make possible.

One nurse who worked hard to change this was Denise Thornby. President of the American Association of Critical-Care Nurses (AACN), the world's largest specialty association for registered nurses (RNs) representing more than 500,000 critical care nurses, Thornby used her monthly newsletter to encourage senior nurses to mentor new nurses in the skills of effecting needed change. In her presidential speech to the AACN, aptly titled "Make Waves, the Courage to Influence Practice," Thornby called for action from her critical care colleagues:

> Every day, every moment, you make choices on how to act or respond. Through these acts, you have the power to positively influence. As John Quincy Adams sagely said, "The influence of each human being on others in this life is a kind of immortality." So I ask you: What will be your act of courage? How will you influence your environment? What will be your legacy? (Thornby, 2012)

Hopefully Thornby will challenge us all to reflect on the legacies we are creating. As we walk out of clinical encounters, what is in our wake—are people better for having experienced us?

Arguments Debating the Role of the Nurse Advocate

As many rights-based movements gained steam in the 1960s (e.g., civil rights, women's rights), changes were also happening in healthcare. Winslow (1984), writing in *The Hastings Center Report,* a prestigious bioethics journal, notes that nursing was transitioning out of its military metaphor phase, which valued loyalty and obedience, into a legal metaphor phase, valuing advocacy and rights. The transition was hardly a smooth one.

Bernal (1992), writing later in the same journal, questions the claim that nurses should be patient advocates, given all the constraints on their practice. She was one of the first to link successful advocacy with nurses' freedom to practice. She also was quick to see the dangers of nurses demonizing physicians to patients and the public and astutely recommended that a less combative, more cooperative model of the profession would serve nurses better.

Hewitt (2002) issues similar cautions, writing that nurses need to be empowered first if they are to empower patients: "There may, however, be more suitable candidates for the role of patient advocate and nurses should recognize that they do not have a monopoly on ethical decision making" (p. 440).

Common to these critiques is the need for nurses to embrace a collaborative stance toward advocacy, as this chapter recommends. Writing in 2006, MacDonald calls for more empirical studies related to the role of advocacy in nursing, arguing that because advocacy is universally considered a moral obligation in nursing practice, we need to advance our knowledge about its nature in nursing.

Advocating for Advocates

One group of nurse leaders spent a morning trying to define what constitutes a good nurse. The result was the following two-sentence definition:

> A good nurse is a competent, compassionate, collaborative advocate for patients and families. A good nurse is remembered for making the critical difference.

Immediately after affirming this definition, one nurse spoke up, saying, "But we cannot be this nurse unless someone advocates for us." Although each nurse has to advocate for her- or himself, there are larger initiatives now championing nursing.

> **NOTE**
>
> You may want to check the American Academy of Nursing website (http://www.aannet.org/advocacy-resources) and the American Nurses Association website (http://www.nursingworld.org), which list advocacy resources. Be sure to also read the Institute of Medicine (IOM) report *The Future of Nursing: Leading Change, Advancing Health* (2010).

Tomajan (2012) urges nurses in all settings to seize opportunities to make a positive impact on the profession through advocating daily for nurses and the nursing profession:

> Point-of-care nurses have an opportunity to build on their public image of being the most trusted profession by communicating and advocating for a more accurate view of their contributions to healthcare and society. Managers and administrators work daily, advocating to obtain adequate resources for their nursing staff and to promote positive work environments. Nurse educators play a critical role in preparing nurses to strengthen the profession through advocacy. (para. 39)

Constraining and Facilitating Forces for Advocacy

Before ending this chapter, we want to provide a quick look at some of the constraining and facilitating forces that influence how effectively nurses can fulfill their advocacy responsibilities. Being familiar with these forces can help nurses committed to becoming better advocates.

Constraining Forces

Although the evidence presented thus far is great with respect to expectations and support for nurses in their advocacy role, frequently nurses are observed failing to act as advocates or perhaps failing to be aware of their opportunity to promote change or impact outcomes. They fail in the professional advocacy role through a lack of education or a lack of personal motivation, investment, or understanding of the nursing role. They may be inexperienced, lacking in confidence in their own skills. They are unable to lead or are overly reliant on others to lead, transforming nurses to a dependent and powerless role. When the nurse does not actively perform the professional nursing role, quality, safety, and outcomes are affected negatively. The dependent role this nurse assumes eventually leads to reluctance to engage in conflict.

This reluctance to bring forward information as an advocate has been identified in two recent studies. According to a 2005 study by Maxfield, Grenny, McMillan, Patterson, and Switzler called *Silence Kills,* more than half of nurses and physicians studied witnessed behaviors negatively affecting patient care. Further, while observing risks to patients, the study showed that less than 10% of physicians, nurses, and others advocated for the patients.

In 2010, Maxfield, Grenny, Lavandero, and Groah in conjunction with the Association of peri-Operative Registered Nurses (AORN) performed a larger second study called *The Silent Treatment.* This second study confirmed the findings of the first study and further identified a category of communication breakdowns in which risks are known but not discussed. *The Silent Treatment* examines the decision-making and communication failures resulting from failed advocacy. The authors suggest that enhancing knowledge, individual skills, and personal motivation must be in conjunction with organizational and collegial elements that will support engagement and advocacy in the face of conflict and power discrepancies (Maxfield, Grenny, Lavandero, & Groah, 2010). Nurses need to feel comfortable and empowered in their advocacy role.

Negative power differentials stifle positive outcomes for patients. Positive organizational and collegial elements are key to resolve the noncommunication that comes from fear by those who feel powerless. Lack of empowerment by nurses to fulfill their professional obligations, communicate problems, and affect patient outcomes is commonly identified as a limiting factor to the advocacy role, patient safety, and, according to Gordon (2010), the rescue of patients. Nurses' failure to rescue patients due to of their lack of empowerment and lack of advocacy action, identified by Silber, Williams, Krakauer, and Schwartz (1992), is still enabled today through organizations and individuals who wield power specifically inhibiting the actions of nurses. Those in identified leadership positions, administrators, nurses, or physicians may use this capricious power to streamline processes without regard for individual differences either in patients or nurses. Further, those nurses who "rock the boat," who advocate assertively, may be viewed as "trouble-makers" both by leaders and by nurse peers.

Hanks (2010) conducted advocacy research to develop, determine the psychometric properties, and support the validity of the Protective Nursing Advocacy Scale (PNAS), which measures nursing advocacy beliefs and actions from a protective perspective. The PNAS has four subscales related to advocacy:

- Acting as an advocate
- Work status and advocacy actions
- Environment and education
- Supports and barriers to advocacy

Interestingly, this study validated previous work on the subject with regard to nurses' being risk takers who act as advocates, and that those who advocate are labeled as "disruptive."

Research has identified peer support or resistance as significant to the organizational environment's acceptance of the advocacy role. Peers may not reinforce advocacy efforts and may undermine the effects of an individual advocate through horizontal violence. The ANA statement on workplace violence (ANA, n.d.b) identifies lateral (horizontal) violence as a long-term issue for nursing, in which nurses inflict overt or covert psychological distress that affects them and their professional role, specifically deteriorating the quality of patient care. According to Black in her 2011 analysis of the Las Vegas Hepatitis-C outbreak of 2007 to 2008, fear of retaliation cannot be ignored. In this study, one in six nurses knew there was a significant problem but failed to speak up, resulting in poor outcomes for many.

Finally, to complicate this and due to the contextual nature of advocacy, if the nurse lacks a relationship with the patient, this too will limit the success of nursing advocacy for the patient. The relationship of the patient to the nurse has been severely affected over the last two decades through increasing complexity of care, lack of continuity in nursing care, and the relinquished collaborative role in shared decision-making. In this relinquished role, the nurse will "agree by default" with all the patient's requests for plan of care (or the physician's plans) without regard for professional obligations to evidence-based practice, clinical excellence, or collaborative care and decision-making.

Facilitating Forces

Facilitators for advocacy as a professional obligation for nurses may be described in three layers. Starting at the most macro layer, various professional organizations identify advocacy as a nursing responsibility, but it is most prominently highlighted by the ANA in its definition of nursing: "Nursing is the protection, promotion, and optimization of health and abilities, prevention of illness and injury, alleviation of suffering through the diagnosis and treatment of human response, and *advocacy* [emphasis added] in the care of individuals, families, communities, and populations" (ANA, n.d.a, para. 1).

Further, advocacy is a skill that must be taught and modeled. Nursing faculty whose role in the clinical setting is observed and replicated by students actively influence the future nursing practice of these students. The American Association of Colleges of Nursing (2008) identifies advocacy in four elements in the *Essentials of Baccalaureate Education* for nurses:

- **Essential I:** Liberal Education for Baccalaureate Generalist Nursing Practice (p. 12)
- **Essential II:** Basic Organizational and Systems Leadership for Quality Care and Patient Safety: Knowledge and skills in leadership, quality improvement, and patient safety are necessary to provide high-quality healthcare (p. 13)
- **Essential VI:** Interprofessional Communication and Collaboration for Improving Patient Health: Communication and collaboration among healthcare professionals are critical to delivering high-quality and safe patient care (p. 23)
- **Essential VIII:** Professionalism and Professional Values: "Ethics is an integral part of nursing practice and has always involved respect and advocacy" (p. 27)

The American Association of Colleges of Nursing (2011), in the *Essentials of Master's Education in Nursing,* also highlights advocacy. Specifically, in Essential VI: Health Policy and Advocacy, the association "[r]ecognizes that the master's-prepared nurse is able to intervene at the system level through the policy development process and to employ advocacy strategies to influence health and health care" (p. 20), and in Essential IX: Master's-Level Nursing Practice, in which advocacy is a key concept in the integration of master's prepared nursing practice (p. 26).

At the middle layer, healthcare organizations identify nursing advocacy as key to organizational mission, tied to patient outcomes and patient satisfaction. Strong organizational expectations for nursing leadership may be identified overtly, such as in the Magnet Recognition Program. The Forces of Magnetism, first identified in 1983, are attributes that currently exemplify nursing excellence (American Nurses Credentialing Center, 1983). In Force 1:

> Quality of Nursing Leadership: Knowledgeable, strong, risk-taking nurse leaders follow a well-articulated, strategic and visionary philosophy in the day-to-day operations of nursing services. Nursing leaders, at all organizational levels, convey a strong sense of advocacy and support for the staff and for the patient. The results of quality leadership are evident in nursing practice at the patient's side. (para. 3)

In Force 13:

> Interdisciplinary Relationships: Collaborative working relationships within and among the disciplines are valued. Mutual respect is based on the premise that all members of the health care team make essential and meaningful contributions in the achievement of clinical outcomes. Conflict management strategies are in place and are used effectively, when indicated. (para. 16)

At the micro layer, nurses find an obligation to advocacy tied to personal values attached to holistic care and human flourishing. The synergy model developed by the AACN embraces such values as caring in the active practice of nursing. The synergy model quantifies various nursing competencies, including advocacy. Table 14.5 describes the various levels of expertise, ranging from competent (1) to expert (5).

TABLE 14.5   Levels of Advocacy Expertise

Advocacy and Moral Agency

Works on another's behalf and represents the concerns of the patient/family and nursing staff; serves as a moral agent in identifying and helping resolve ethical and clinical concerns within and outside clinical setting.

Level 1

Works on behalf of patient; self-assesses personal values; is aware of ethical conflicts/issues that may surface in clinical setting; makes ethical/moral decisions based on rules; represents patient when patient cannot represent self; is aware of patients' rights.

Level 3

Works on behalf of patient and family; considers patient values and incorporates in care, even when differing from personal values; supports colleagues in ethical and clinical issues; believes that moral decision-making can deviate from rules; demonstrates give and take with patient's family, allowing them to speak/represent themselves when possible; is aware of patient and family rights.

Level 5

Works on behalf of patient, family, and community; advocates from patient/family perspective, whether similar to or different from personal values; advocates ethical conflict and issues from patient/family perspective; suspends rules—patient and family drive moral decision-making; empowers patient and family to speak for/represent themselves; achieves mutuality within patient/professional relationships.

Source: AACN, 2008

Nurses must recognize and be accountable for their power in creating change and driving outcomes for and with patients. The nurse is skilled in assessment, planning, providing evidence-based interventions, and evaluating care with continuing assessment. This continuing nursing process—along with knowledge and skills in communication, leadership, and collaboration—render advocacy for patients an obvious strength of the professional nurse's role in the team.

Conclusion

Our willingness to advocate for patients, families, and communities literally has the power to influence:

- How people are born, live, suffer, and die

- The peace or torment families experience as a result of their role in decision-making

- The personal and professional integrity of healthcare professionals and healthcare institutions

- The way scarce healthcare resources are utilized in the United States

Advocacy is an intentional leadership skill and an obligation that nurses embrace to support the autonomy of vulnerable persons in their professional practice. It is identified by professional organizations as a significant role for nursing. It is best applied through collaboration with patients, families, and the healthcare team.

The case of Mrs. Esposita at the beginning of the chapter highlights many elements that must be addressed through advocacy interventions both simple and complex. The assessment priorities begin with the patient. Is the patient capable? Does she make her own decisions? Does she have understanding, appreciation, and reasoning for the decision related to the procedure? Verify that she names a surrogate for the future. Is she vulnerable? Does she or her son speak English as a first language? What is their level of health literacy? Do they know family or friends who have pacemakers? Create a therapeutic relationship with the patient and son. Utilize active and passive listening.

If your assessment reveals that Mrs. Esposita does not meet the elements of a capable decision-maker, inform the physician for a collaborative assessment. Consider whether the son is the correct surrogate decision-maker. If there is a language barrier, how can we provide enhanced communication—through interpreter or other? Further, what is the physician's motivation for offering the procedure? What is the desired outcome? Speak with the physician to more fully understand the indications for treatment. Invite exploration of the physician's values and share your values and assessment of the patient and son.

As for Mrs. Eposita and her son, how can the patient make this decision voluntarily? How can the information elements be enhanced? Use teach-back when assessing understanding. Use due diligence and active problem solving to ensure transparency. Allow the patient to speak with you privately about any questions, concerns, and her own goals for care. Address questions and assist the patient and son in formulating their own questions; support them in their query with the physician mediating this discussion. In the larger sense, if the patient's heart failure is significant, is there urgency in this decision, and what is the outcome of not doing the procedure? Are there end-of-life concerns or plans in place? Ultimately, have a team meeting removed from the patient and family to resolve plan-of-care options, then meet with the patient and son. Support their goals and respect the stress and complexity of this decision.

Regarding the nursing instructor and students, yes, the nursing instructor is a key team member in this situation and must collaborate with the physician and the unit nurses. The obligations to the patient extend to all the nurses by their relationship or presence in context. As witnesses to the process, the faculty and students must ensure the elements of disclosure and consent are met. The faculty member must assume leadership and be responsible for the communication process. Engage the clinic nurse and clinic manager for transparency of process. Additionally, what impact does the action of the nursing instructor have on the BSN students or on the physician and clinic nurses?

The nursing instructor is a role model and has professional obligations to the BSN students to address and document the issues identified. Although he may not see this patient concern to resolution, he is obligated to identify and address to the team his assessment and suggestions for resolution and process improvement. If the nurse instructor chooses not to be involved and does not lead in this moment, the BSN students who observe this will learn to ignore their own advocacy role in future situations. This may lead to their feelings of powerlessness and failure to embrace one of the professional obligations of nursing. Finally, the nursing instructor owes a professional obligation to the physician and clinic nurses as a partner in collaborative care. As faculty in clinic, the nurse articulates the process and supports the team in evaluating their own process to support patient decision-making for the future. Rather than criticizing the process, the faculty must provide assessment and interventions to the clinic for a quality improvement outcome, with potential impact on all patients of the clinic.

References

American Association of Colleges of Nursing. (2008). *The essentials of baccalaureate education for professional nursing practice.* Washington, DC: Author.

American Association of Colleges of Nursing. (2011). *The essentials of master's education in nursing.* Washington, DC: Author.

American Association of Critical-Care Nurses (AACN). (2008). The AACN synergy model for patient care: Characteristics of patients, clinical units and systems of concern to nurses. Retrieved from http://www.aacn.org/wd/certifications/content/synmodel.pcms?menu=

American Nurses Association (ANA). (2001). *Code of ethics for nurses.* Washington, DC: Author.

American Nurses Association (ANA). (2010a). *Nursing's social policy statement: The essence of the profession.* Silver Spring, MD: Author.

American Nurses Association (ANA). (2010b). *Scope and standards of practice.* Silver Spring, MD: Author.

American Nurses Association (ANA). (n.d.a). What is nursing? Retrieved from http://nursingworld.org/EspeciallyForYou/What-is-Nursing

American Nurses Association (ANA). (n.d.b). *Workplace violence.* Retrieved from http://nursingworld.org/MainMenuCategories/Policy-Advocacy/State/Legislative-Agenda-Reports/State-WorkplaceViolence

American Nurses Credentialing Center. (1983). Task force on Nursing Practice in Hospitals. Forces of Magnetism. Characteristics that distinguish hospitals. Retrieved from http://www.nursecredentialing.org/Magnet/ProgramOverview/HistoryoftheMagnetProgram/ForcesofMagnetism

Bernal, E. (1992). The nurse as patient advocate. *Hastings Center Report, 22*(4), 18–23.

Black, L. M. (2011). Tragedy into policy: A quantitative study of nurses' attitudes toward patient advocacy activities. *American Journal of Nursing, 111*(6), 26–35.

Bu, X., & Jezewski, M. A. (2007) Developing a mid-range theory of patient advocacy through concept analysis. *Journal of Advanced Nursing, 57*(1), 101–10.

Centers for Disease Control and Prevention (CDC). (2014). Other at risk populations. http://www.cdc.gov/minorityhealth/populations/atrisk.html

Gadow, S. (1980). Existential advocacy: Philosophical foundation of nursing. In S. F. Spicker & S. Gadow (Eds.), *Nursing images and ideals: Opening dialogue with the humanities* (pp. 79–101). New York, NY: Springer Publishing Company.

Gordon, S. (2010) Nursing needs a new image. *International Nursing Review, 57*(4), 403–404.

Hanks, R. (2010). Development and testing of an instrument to measure protective nursing advocacy. *Nursing Ethics, 17*(2), 255–267.

Hewitt, J. (2002). A critical review of the arguments debating the role of the nurse advocate. *Journal of Advanced Nursing, 37*(5), 439–445.

Institute of Medicine (IOM). (2010). *The future of nursing: Leading change, advancing health.* Washington, DC: National Academies of Science. Retrieved from http://books.nap.edu/openbook.php?record_id=12956&page=R1

Maxfield, D., Grenny, J., McMillan, R., Patterson, K., & Switzler, A. (2005). *Silence kills.* Aliso Viejo, CA: AACN.

Maxfield, D., Grenny, J., Lavandero, R., and Groah, L. (2010). *The silent treatment.* Aliso Viejo, CA: AACN.

MacDonald, H. (2006). Relational ethics and advocacy in nursing: Literature review. *Journal of Advanced Ethics, 57*(2), 119–126.

Negarandeh, R., Oskouie, F., Ahmadi, F. & Nikravesh, M. (2008). The meaning of patient advocacy for Iranian nurses. *Nursing Ethics, 15*(4), 457–467.

President's Commission for the Study of Ethical Problems in Medicine and Biomedical and Behavioral Research. (1982). *Making health care decisions.* Washington, D.C.: U.S. Government Printing Office.

Silber, J. H., Williams, S. V., Krakauer, H., & Schwartz, J. S. (1992). Hospital and patient characteristics associated with death after surgery: A study of adverse occurrence and failure-to-rescue. *Medical Care, 30*(7), 615–629.

Sofaer, S., & Schumann, M. J. (2013). *Fostering successful patient and family engagement: Nursing's critical role.* Washington, DC: American Association of Colleges of Nursing. Retrieved from https://naqc.nursing.gwu.edu/sites/naqc.nursing.gwu.edu/files/downloads/NAQC_PatientEngagementWhitePaper.pdf

Thornby, D. (2012). Obituary. Retrieved from https://www.gonetoosoon.org/memorials/denise-thornby

Tomajan, K. (2012) Advocating for nurses and nursing. *OJIN: The Online Journal of Issues in Nursing, 17*(1), Manuscript 4. doi:10.3912/OJIN.Vol17No01Man04

Urban Institute Health Policy Center. (2010). Vulnerable populations. http://www.urban.org/health_policy/vulnerable_populations/index.cfm

Winslow, G. (1984). From loyalty to advocacy: A new metaphor for nursing. *The Hastings Center Report, 14*(3), 32–40.

Chapter 15

Using the Techniques of Mediation to Promote Person- and Family-Centered Care

Mary K. Walton, MSN, MBE, RN

Katharine Smith, an 82-year-old woman with significant dementia, suffers a fall in the assisted-living center where she has resided for 2 years. An ambulance transports her to the academic medical center, where she is diagnosed with several rib fractures and placed in a brace. Her two daughters arrive shortly after her admission to the inpatient neuroscience unit and immediately request that their mother receive one-to-one supervision.

An experienced clinical nurse orients Mrs. Smith's daughters to the unit and describes the expertise of the nursing staff with patients such as their mother. In addition, the nurse explains that, based on the nursing assessment, one-to-one supervision is not indicated, and she assures the daughters that their mother is now safe. Fall-reduction strategies, including the placement of a bed alarm, are implemented and explained to the family members. The nurse believes that the daughters have accepted her plan of care.

However, the daughters seek out the attending physician and express their belief that their mother requires one-to-one supervision, stating if she falls, "That will be on you." The attending physician immediately directs the physician trainee to place an order for one-to-one supervision. This resident physician informs the nurse. The nurse, now furious, vents to his colleagues that this is a waste of resources as he proceeds to find a staff member to provide the one-to-one supervision for the night shift.

Conflict, such as the one described in the preceding vignette, is no stranger to the professional nurse. The hierarchical structure of medicine; issues of race, gender, and class; and the nature of healthcare and demands of patient safety all contribute to the prevalence of conflict in clinical healthcare settings. In fact, "resolving conflict in the context of patient care" is an essential competency for registered nurses (American Nurses Association [ANA], 2010, p. 57). Because nurses anticipate, predict, mitigate, and manage conflict in the clinical setting on a daily basis, it is not surprising that nursing literature reflects the professional interest in alternative dispute resolution processes and, specifically, mediation (Gerardi, 2004; Philipsen, 2008; Saulo & Wagener, 2000; Schlairet, 2009; Ward-Collins, 1998).

In the acute-care setting, nurses are administratively responsible for managing patient care units, operating suites, and emergency departments as well as the allocation of scarce resources. Typically, nurses are the on-site administrators during nights and weekends; they run codes and handle crises dealing with disruptive physicians, employees, patients, and visitors. In addition, they handle organization-level conflicts that may arise with emergency situations, whether internal (floods, power outages) or external (weather-related access emergencies).

Nurse managers and leaders develop skill in navigating disputes that are both employee- and patient-related. Clinical nurses also develop significant skill in preventing or mitigating conflict with patients, their loved ones, and the interprofessional team when patients or family members perceive that care is not reflecting their wishes, preferences, and values. Nurses who are successful at working through conflict most likely employ some of the skills used by trained mediators in a well-defined formal process. It is invaluable to develop skills to effectively respond to concerns in a manner that respects the patient perspective. Conflict related to staff or room assignments, plans of care, or access to equipment or other hospital resources are everyday issues in the acute-care setting. Medical errors and end-of-life care may promote even higher-stakes conflicts and involve many team members and disciplines. In all these situations, clinical staff who develop and master mediation skills will be well prepared to address disputes at the bedside.

Mediation offers approaches and techniques that foster therapeutic relationships, promote effective communication, and prevent or mitigate conflict. The purpose of this chapter is to describe and illustrate selected techniques of the mediation process that, when integrated into the communication skills of nurses, prevent, mitigate, and resolve conflict and promote care that reflects the preferences, values, and needs of patients in the acute-care setting.

What Is Mediation?

Mediation is a form of assisted negotiation by which the parties can prevent or resolve conflict by reaching consensus. Formal mediation consists of using a neutral third party to facilitate a discussion between two opposing parties in an environment where the parties have the opportunity to discuss accusations and points of conflicts toward the goal of repairing the relationship and promoting healing (Meruelo, 2008). The process includes:

1. Eliciting both facts and emotions
2. Identifying a range of options for consideration
3. Developing a plan that both parties find acceptable for moving beyond the conflict

Fiester (2012) characterizes mediation as "a carefully monitored dialogue intended to help the stakeholders find a shared resolution that brings the cherished values and interests of those involved into clear focus" (p. 11).

Well recognized as an effective dispute resolution technique, the formal mediation process is based on three core principles: "party autonomy, informed decision-making, and confidentiality" (Dubler & Leibman, 2011, p. 11). These principles are essential because "being voiceless, powerless, marginalized, silenced, dominated are potential vulnerabilities or liabilities of anyone engaged in a dispute—of any kind" (Fiester, 2012, p. 10). Given the hierarchical nature embedded in healthcare and the vulnerability of an individual who is hospitalized, attention to these three principles is a fundamental responsibility of the nurse.

Mediation techniques foster understanding and help reveal the underlying issues, needs, and interests of all the participants. A hallmark of mediation is the uncovering of the underlying need or concern rather than the initial stated position or demand. With this knowledge, the mediator asks purposeful questions and tests options that address the needs and interest of both parties and moves the participants toward shaping a solution that honors all participants.

Multiple models of mediation have emerged as viable options for dealing with conflict in the clinical care setting (Fiester, 2007; Gibson, 1994). The American Society for Bioethics and Humanities (ASBH; 2011) recognizes mediation as one approach for clinical ethics consultation. Dubler and Liebman (2011) have developed a process called bioethics mediation, using ethical principles and the formal processes and techniques of mediation used in law to achieve what they call a "principled resolution" (p. 14). Schlairet (2009) outlines the role and importance of nursing advocacy with bioethics mediation. Bergman and Fiester (2009) posit that a more representative term is *health care mediation* given the recognition that many conflicts are grounded in communication issues rather than ethical dilemmas (p. 174).

Although a variety of mediation models is used in clinical ethics consultation, all models recognize the importance of communication that empathically addresses the emotion of the participants engaged in decision-making and conflict in the acute-care setting (Arnold, Aulisio, Begler, & Seltzer, 2007).

Using Mediation in Healthcare

Similarities between the nursing process and mediation have been identified in the literature (Ward-Collins, 1998). Furthermore, nurses are identified as excellent candidates to train for the role of a hospital-based bioethics mediator (Dubler & Liebman, 2011).

Saulo and Wagener (2000), in their study of health professionals who were formally trained in mediation techniques, found an increased comfort level with conflict among those professionals who had formal training. In addition to using the skills in a formal mediation process, they also found that the skills these professionals learned were transferable to their everyday interactions with patients, families, and coworkers. Gerardi (2004) has developed a framework for using four mediation techniques in the critical-care setting to create a healthy work environment:

- Listening for understanding
- Reframing
- Elevating the definition of the problem
- Creating clear agreements

Her premise is that these techniques, when learned, can be integrated into the communication skills of nurses with the result of avoiding the conflict—and, more importantly, without requiring a neutral third-party mediator. When nurses specifically employ selective mediation techniques, disagreements can be managed early and directly by those involved in the critical-care setting.

The Unique Position of the Clinical Nurse

Clinical nurses navigate among competing perspectives within the highly structured medical hierarchy and have long been characterized as "in the middle" position caught between physicians or between patients and families (Murphy, 1993, p. 3). Furthermore, clinical nurses describe enacting their moral agency within "a shifting moral context; working in-between their own identities and values and those of the organizations in which they worked; working in-between their own values and the values of others; and working in-between competing values and interests" (Varcoe et al., 2004, p. 319).

Hamric (2001), while acknowledging that this position may present moral challenges, points out that it also offers opportunity for patient advocacy. In this position, nurses "can better contend for the needed cooperation because they share the medical side of the decision with the physician, the hospital policy side with hospital administration, and the personal side with the patients" (p. 255). Thus, being positioned with exposure to the perspectives of all stakeholders should prime the clinical nurse to learn and integrate the techniques of mediation to avert or resolve conflict in the patient care setting.

Formal mediation requires a neutral third party to assist the parties in conflict find common ground and shape their (not the mediator's) shared solution. Mediators consider themselves neutral with regard to outcomes; the participants own the process and the solution (Gibson, 1999a). In healthcare, this concept of neutrality has been challenged as impossible in theory or practice. Moreover, some would say there is value in the nurses' process expertise and pursuit of the best possible outcome for patients as the goal (Gibson, 1999b).

Although a clinical nurse may not feel at all neutral or impartial in these situations and, in fact, may hold a position that represents the interests of one of the stakeholders, this recognition of the different perspectives of the clinical nurse and mediator help the clinical nurse clarify and play his or her role and move the process forward in a positive direction. The clinical nurse, in contrast to a neutral third-party mediator who needs to seek out and understand varied positions and interest, already has an appreciation of the perspectives that are setting up the conflict. Thus clinical nurses who use the techniques of mediation in their communication with patients, families, and colleagues are well positioned to efficiently and effectively manage situations that often provoke conflict or inhibit person- and family-centered care (P&FCC) in the inpatient setting.

Techniques to Promote Person- and Family-Centered Care

Clinical nurses are the professionals with patients for sustained time periods during an acute care hospitalization. This proximity—both physical proximity, nearness to the body, and narrative proximity, understanding the story—affects a nurse's ability to identify needs and seek solutions (Peter & Liaschenko, 2004). Nurses who incorporate the techniques of mediation as they care for patients (rather than as a separate skill to employ when conflict is emerging) will recognize the patients' expertise and values and form effective partnerships for person-centered care. Mediation techniques that can be integrated into routine nurse-patient communications include:

- Listening for understanding
- Preparing
- Summarizing
- Distinguishing between positions and interests
- Reframing
- Questioning

Listening for Understanding

Words can be harsh and hostile when individuals perceive a threat—or there may be no words readily found to express a fear, need, or vulnerability. Given the high stakes of care provided in the inpatient setting, the ability to listen for understanding is an essential skill for nurses and other care providers who must manage the potential for conflict inherent in the inpatient setting. Here the listener follows the lead of the speaker, taking in not only the words but also emotions and nonverbal cues. The goal is for the listener to hear the needs and concerns underlying the spoken words and for the speaker to feel heard and in control of the content.

Listening for understanding, a well-recognized and essential communication skill, demands that a clinician be fully present in the encounter with patients and families. Schenck & Churchill (2012), in their synthesis of interviews of physicians identified by their peers as extraordinary clinicians, highlight the importance of practicing presence that is "willing to be led and not feeling like you have to orchestrate" (p. 73). Listening for understanding requires using all our senses for what is unsaid—"listen with the third ear" (p. 13) that is, and use our eyes to follow not only the words—but also "voice tone, body language, facial expression, and gaze" (Koloroutis & Trout,

2012, p. 137). While listening may be portrayed as a simple thing to do, it actually takes energy and concentration; it is a way of focusing or giving attention and tells the patient, "You are worth my time. I think this interaction with you is important. I am willing and able to be with you rather than somewhere else" (Churchill, Fanning, & Schenck, 2013, p. 60).

Koloroutis and Trout (2012) describe the importance of "attunement (undivided attention) and a willingness to wonder (by inquiring), follow (by listening and acknowledging), and hold (by delivering the one thing that is most important to this individual patient)" to establish a human connection (p. 277). They ask the reader to consider how clinicians might respond if anger were assessed as the emotional equivalent of bleeding, prompting not judging or disconnecting but moving in to respond to the anger as a symptom needing attention. For busy clinicians comfortable with being in control and directing the flow of information, this requires not only skill but also a sincere interest in understanding the experience of the other.

Listening for understanding requires openness and an ability to suspend judgment and refrain from conclusions based on first impressions or previous experiences. To do this:

- Be curious and wonder how this individual or family sees the situation from their unique perspective.

- Do not evaluate the validity of their stated position or demand.

- Do not interrupt, ask for clarification, or correct their story.

- Seek to understand rather than respond. The listener who understands the speaker's story as it reflects the individual's experience may find the underlying needs and concerns revealed.

> **NOTE**
>
> See Chapter 12 for an in-depth discussion of listening for understanding as it relates to cultural difference and conflict. See Chapter 19 for an in-depth discussion of narrative approaches to understand patient and family perspectives.

Koloroutis and Trout (2012, pp. 148–150) identify seven obstacles to what they term "conscious" or "therapeutic" listening and attribute them to a drive for self-protection when the possibility of conflict is apparent:

- **Fixing:** Listening with a fixed ear for problems that can decisively be solved, thus closing off access to the full range of valuable information.

- **Advising:** Offering recommendations or giving directions that may prematurely shut down the ability or willingness of the other to express thoughts.

- **Educating:** Instructing or coaching; if initiated before the speaker is ready to learn, it will likely be unsuccessful.

- **Storytelling:** Offering to tell one's own similar story. Although it may be intended to create connection, it interrupts the focus of the speaker and redirects attention back to the clinician.

- **Distancing and shutting down:** Responding to intense emotions and behaviors, such as anger and criticism, by becoming emotionally unavailable.

- **Explaining or correcting:** Taking control of the situation, potentially leaving the other party feeling unseen, unheard, and misunderstood.

- **Excessive responding:** Too many or repetitive expressions of support, such as "Oh my!", "I know what you mean", "That is awful." When overdone, interferes with the speaker's ability to express and stay on track.

Preparing

Helping resolve conflict requires preparation, not only by gathering information but also by identifying where the work can be best accomplished. The environment in an active clinical setting may not be conducive to listening for understanding. Whenever possible, select or prepare a location that will support or enhance communication. The amount of activity and noise level surrounding a patient will influence the ability of participants to give their full attention to the conversation.

Consider also the need for confidentiality; for example, does the patient or family member need to speak in private? Does the physician trainee want to share her perspective out of the earshot of an attending physician? Might the new-to-practice nurse feel overwhelmed sharing frustrations in the main nurses' station?

Finally, consider the need for privacy, quiet, and comfort; ensure that all participants can sit down. Patient rooms and hospital corridors are familiar places for clinicians to have important conversations, yet not so for patients and families, who may find it harder to tune out the surrounding individuals and activity. Is there a family caregiver center away from the inpatient unit that is more tranquil for a challenging conversation to unfold? Taking the time to identify a space and moving participants there may actually save time as well as signal the importance of the conversation.

Summarizing

Once a patient, family member, or colleague has shared his or her perspective and conveyed his or her emotions—whether they are expressed as a concern, demand, or threat—summarizing, often repetitively, is a valuable technique to promote understanding. Synthesizing and reflecting back what has been heard and understood serve a number of key purposes in addressing conflict (Dubler & Liebman, 2011):

- It lets the participants know the listener has really been listening.

- It lets listeners test their current understanding of what has been said.

- It helps all the participants organize their thoughts.
- It helps the participants hear what others are saying.
- It shows the parties areas of common interest.
- It brings order to the discussion.
- It reminds parties of any progress being made in the process.

When mediating conflict, summarizing is not merely repeating back what was said after an exchange of information or request or demand. Rather, the summary should begin the process of identifying the issues, interests, and feelings of the participants and offer the participants the opportunity to clarify or confirm the content in the summary. Here is an example based on the vignette at the beginning of this chapter:

> *If I understand what is most important to you at this time, it is that your mother is very vulnerable given her pain, dementia, and admission to a completely new and unfamiliar environment, and that you believe only direct supervision at this point in time will assure you that she will be safe here. Did I capture your thoughts and feelings well enough? Is there any other information you want me to understand?*

Distinguishing Between Positions and Interests

In working through conflict, it is essential to distinguish between positions and interests. A *position* is what the individual wants, in contrast to the individual's *interests,* or what really matters most. An initial position may not address all the issues or more concrete things that relate to solving the problem. For example, in the introductory vignette at the beginning of this chapter, one issue needing consideration is the availability of an individual to provide one-to-one supervision.

Fisher, Ury, and Patton (1991) describe interests as desires and concerns that are "the silent movers behind the hubbub of positions" (p. 41). Interests are the needs and concerns that are threatened by failure to resolve the issues and must be satisfied if solutions are to be workable. In mediation language, interests can be multifaceted, and it may be helpful to think about the various categories when trying to understand the underlying concerns in an emerging conflict. For example, does the patient or family want resources, such as nursing care hours, equipment, different space (substantive interests), or respect and face-saving (psychological interests), and/or a different experience or feeling of being heard in the decision-making process (procedural interests) (Dubler & Leibman, 2011)?

Conflict often is recognized or gets attention when someone states a position or demand that prompts a negative reaction or push back from the receiver of the demand. Think about a patient, family member, or colleague's demand as a position that does not convey or reveal what the individual really wants or cares about—the issues and interests that lead the person to take a certain position. Consider the vignette at the beginning of this chapter where the daughters present what seems to be a clear demand to the physician. Now try to imagine what might really be important to them as they address nurses and physicians.

Position: *This is what we want.*

- One-to-one supervision of our mother

Interest: *This is what really matters to us.*

- To keep our mother safe
- To be good daughters
- To learn about and evaluate the quality of care in this hospital
- To assert our authority over our mother's care—perhaps based on a failure to do so in other situations
- And other interests

The ability to work from a stated demand or position to then uncover what really matters most to a patient or family member is invaluable and promotes therapeutic relationships in the intense acute-care setting. Patients and families are vulnerable; responding to their expressed emotions in contrast to using demanding words or threats will support effective communication and help with problem solving.

Reframing

Reframing is an extremely valuable communication technique and essential in the summarization process. Here the problem or issue is restated without any hostile or inflammatory language while still acknowledging the emotions. Reframing helps move the conversation from hostile and confrontational language to more positive and problem-solving language. Reframing creates the opportunity for validation. Positions are restated as interests, stories about the past are posed as questions about the future, and individual concerns are offered as shared concerns (Dubler & Leibman, 2011).

Gerardi (2004) highlights four steps for reframing a statement:

1. Acknowledge emotion.
2. Remove inflammatory language.
3. Restate the problem or issue.
4. Request or wait for clarification or validation from the speaker.

Consider a patient or family member who presents a concern or demand in a loud voice with a hostile tone. Clinicians who respond with a directive, whether to promote a conversation or defend oneself, might respond with, "I can see you are angry about this, but you must lower your voice," or "Don't talk to me that way." Restating the concern and neutralizing the language might include a response that identifies the feelings yet may be less likely to escalate the emotions: "I can see you have a lot of energy about this issue. This really matters to you, and I want to understand more." This statement serves to convey that the emotion has been heard and the listener wants to hear more about the problem or learn more of the details. The word *energy* in contrast to the word *anger* has a more positive and inviting connotation. Think of it as responding to the emotion in a caring, inquisitive, positive way rather than responding to the facts in a defensive manner. For example, if the accusation is unfounded, rather than offer contradictory information, respond to the feelings.

Consider this statement: "No one has been in to examine my mother since we have been here." A clinical nurse might want to respond defensively: "Both the admitting physician and I were in with your mother for more than 30 minutes immediately before your arrival." An alternative response that reframes and neutralizes the language might be: "I hear your concern for your mother. Let me share the information I have about her since she arrived here."

Here's another example from one of the daughters from the opening vignette, addressing the nurse assigned to their mother—in a loud tone of voice:

> No one gets the care they need in any healthcare facility these days. Look what happened to our mother in a place that was supposed to keep her safe. No one here is to be trusted. Nurses do not understand the needs of the patients. I guess we have to deal with the head physician to get care for our mother. I am not going to waste any more time talking to nurses.

Reframed, the response might sound like the following:

1. **Acknowledge the emotion:** "You sound upset about your mother's fall and injuries."

2. **Remove the inflammatory language:** "I understand that you have just learned of your mother's injuries and have just met us. I know that you do not trust us yet. We will work hard to hear your concerns and plan care together. We want your mother to be well cared for and to keep her safe."

3. **Restate the problem or issue:** "Let's talk about a plan to keep your mother safe. We need to learn more about your mother so we can meet her needs. I would like to talk with you now, but would you feel more comfortable if I asked your mother's attending physician to join us?"

4. **Request or wait for validation or clarification:** "Of course I am upset about the fall. This is devastating. We have to protect our mother."

If these reframing steps seem awkward or artificial, try one or two of them out at first and see how they work. For example, accepting and acknowledging the emotion of an angry patient or family member will likely get the person's attention. The individual may be relieved to really be heard and more willing to move forward with you as you gather more information.

Questioning

Asking questions can serve many purposes. Effective questioning can advance the understanding of the situation, clarify the issues to be addressed, and uncover viable options and creative solutions. An anthropologic approach, known as *Kleinman's Questions*, is well recognized as an effective strategy for understanding a patient's health-related beliefs and practices (Kleinman, Eisenberg, & Good, 1978). Although published more than 30 years ago, these eight questions continue to be recognized in the literature to support P&FCC (The Joint Commission, 2010; Walton, 2011).

Think about the information needed when forming questions; in general it is best to ask one question at a time. How the question is asked will shape the content and quality of the response (see Table 15.1).

TABLE 15.1   Types of Questions and Examples of Answers They Might Produce

QUESTION TYPE	EXAMPLE
Open-ended questions give the speaker the opportunity to offer what is most important or relevant from his or her perspective. This can provide unexpected information and valuable insight relating to needs and interests.	"Please tell me about your mother." "Tell me more about your experience with previous hospitalizations."
Narrow questions focus the speaker on a specific topic.	"I understand your mother has fallen before. Can you tell me the details of that fall as you understand them?" "What information was given to you when you were notified that your mother had fallen in her residence?"
Closed questions typically generate limited yes or no answers.	"Has your mother fallen before in her current residence?" "Has your mother fallen before during a hospitalization?"
Clarifying questions help all participants develop insight into the meaning of statements, demands, and positions.	"I understand that you believe one-to-one direct supervision will keep your mother safe. Has that been successful before?"

Source for types of questions: Dubler & Leibman, 2011, p. 80.

Reflect on the various types of questions and how they will guide the listener's response. In tense or high-conflict scenarios, be selective about the information needed and how to best elicit it. The right questions will help identify what really matters and make the values and interests of patients and families visible so they can be addressed. Answering questions serves to help the responders to gather their thoughts and organize their needs for the questioner.

Elevating the Definition of the Problem

Gerardi (2004) defines this technique as offering a statement or response that combines multiple opposing or disparate positions by reflecting back on an issue that is common to everyone involved. The goal is to establish some common ground and start to build or rebuild trust. Finding common ground also "enables people to begin to see the whole person again rather than just a symbol of one's angst" (p. 190).

Using this technique, a nurse might respond to the daughters described in the vignette like this:

> *I understand that you are very concerned that your mother be kept safe here in the hospital, especially given her fractures and inability to fully understand directions. The physicians and nurses share this concern and consider your mother's safety of great importance as we evaluate and treat these injuries. There are many ways to promote safety, especially to prevent falls for patients such as your mother—you already know about one-to-one observations, and along with that intervention, we have numerous others to consider. You know your mother best, and the clinical staff is familiar with assessing and providing safety measures. Together we must plan which measures will best provide for your mother's safety over the next 24 hours.*

Here the nurse specifically invites the daughters to share their expertise about their mother's history and needs as well as their assessment of what is needed. If their demand for direct observation by the staff reflected their need to be involved and protect their mother, this opens up the opportunity for nurses to learn more about the patient as well as elicit the daughters' needs and interests. Recognition that the daughters bring their expertise to the encounter is essential. The nurse in the opening vignette, with all good intentions, sought to impress the daughters with nursing expertise but missed the opportunity to invite the daughters to share their knowledge of their mother for the clinicians to incorporate into the plan of care. Patient-centered care requires partnership—bringing together clinical expertise and patient and family expertise.

What matters most to individuals is often hidden and unspoken. Nurses and physicians are very familiar with the hierarchy and norms embedded in healthcare. Patients and family members may at times hesitate to express themselves for fear it will create problems with clinicians or upset the balance in the family constellation (Kleinman, 2011). Over time, concerns held back may eventually erupt and be expressed in nonconstructive ways. Eliciting the underlying interests, making them visible, and framing them in a way that invites all stakeholders to work toward a shared solution will fuel conflict resolution in the acute-care setting.

Eliciting the Medical Facts

Often a linguistic, cultural, and professional gulf separates patients and families from the clinical staff. What medical facts have been shared? More importantly, how have they been understood? How do patients and family members appreciate the meaning of the facts? In academic medical centers with multiple trainee programs, patients and families may have heard a variety of opinions based on the same facts.

When there is conflict, it is essential to elicit the patient's and family's understanding of the healthcare information presented; appreciate the basic tenet of communication that what is said may not be what is heard. To understand the underlying interests of patients and family members, clinicians must seek to view the information as the patient sees it and the patient's experience with the illness—in contrast to viewing the information as clinical facts about disease pathology. Asking more than once and requesting a patient to "Tell me more" is one approach based on the principle that one must build on the knowledge and understanding an individual already holds before one can teach or clarify miscommunication (Back, Arnold, Baile, Tulsky, & Fryer-Edwards, 2005).

Think about how a clinical nurse moves among patient, family, and clinician discussions. The same medical facts might be characterized in dramatically divergent viewpoints. Consider the critical care nurse who successfully discharged a patient home on a ventilator versus another nurse whose patient had a different and very disastrous discharge process. One can imagine they might discuss a subsequent planned discharge to home differently based on their previous experiences.

Just as previous clinical/professional experiences shape how nurses view a current situation, the same is true for family members. Imagine that the daughters in the opening vignette had previous experience with their mother in another hospital. How might their relationship with nurses and previous caregivers shape how they perceive their mother's current needs? If the conflict is driven by inaccurate information or past experience, uncovering these facts is essential to moving forward. How might the nurse appreciate the daughters' demand if he learned that their mother had fallen in several previous hospital stays, despite nursing expertise and fall precautions? Did the nurse elicit any history from the daughters about previous care when explaining why one-to-one supervision was not indicated? Did he know what was informing the daughters' request?

Caucusing

The term *caucus* refers to a private meeting between the mediator and one of the parties in dispute. When one of the participants appears "intimidated or disempowered, a caucus can provide the emotional, intellectual, and sometimes physical space for quiet contemplation, perhaps allowing him or her to regain emotional composure to better understand the facts, implications and options" (Dubler & Leibman, 2011, p. 88). When tension is palpable or open conflict is emerging, offering or directing one of the participants the opportunity to move to another space that perhaps affords privacy and/or separation from an instigating situation can be helpful. The intensity of a clinical setting or the appearance of a sick loved one can overwhelm an individual and contribute to losing composure. Also consider that sitting quietly and silently with individuals after a tense or hostile outburst can convey caring and commitment and is a therapeutic intervention.

The purpose of a private meeting may be to help the individuals articulate their questions, explore their needs and interests, or outline their values and preferences. The goal is to help one of the parties prepare to move forward with the next step in planning.

Developing Options and Packaging Proposals

Creating plans of care and presenting them to others for input or authorization is a standard practice for clinical nurses. Shaping and presenting proposals that reflect a solution acceptable to all stakeholders is key to mediating conflict. If the daughters from the vignette at the beginning of this chapter accept the offer to discuss their mother's care, and together a plan is shaped and agreed upon, the nurse will need to present the plan to another stakeholder in this scenario—the physician colleague. When planning how to present a proposal, think about the recipients. What are their issues and concerns? If the physician ordered the one-to-one supervision in response to a threat of litigation by family members, that needs to be addressed in packaging the proposal for acceptance.

The discussion might start like the following:

> *I know you talked with the daughters of our patient about the need for safety and the initial plan was for one-to-one observation. As you probably recognized, they had just learned about their mother's injury and were quite upset. I understand they demanded continuous direct observation. We have talked in detail about their mother and their specific concerns about her care, including her dementia and her past history of falling. Together we have created a plan for the next 24 hours that we all believe will keep her safe. The plan includes one of her daughters staying overnight at the bedside, placement of a bed alarm, and 30-minute rounds to check for comfort and toileting. I believe, based on the information shared in my meeting with the daughters and the current nursing assessment, one-to-one observation is not necessary. If you do not have any other information that I am missing, I believe the order for one-to-one supervision can be discontinued. Tomorrow morning, I will reassess together with the daughters and the night-shift staff.*

Shaping and presenting proposals that reflect a solution acceptable to all stakeholders is key to mediating conflict.

Establishing a Clear Agreement

Once the parties have stated their positions and the content has been summarized and reframed, the goal is to develop a plan that is specific and reflects the needs and interests of the participants. An agreed-upon plan for reassessment should be part of the care plan. This plan should be captured and communicated.

Conclusion

Clinical nurses, uniquely positioned at the bedside, readily identify the potential for the early signs of conflict. Conflict can occur due to many reasons, but what is relevant here is when care is not centered on the values, needs, and preferences of patients and their families. Using the techniques of mediation, clinical nurses can avert or mitigate conflict among patients, families, and clinical care providers. These techniques are developed as an alternative to litigation and are successfully used in addressing ethical issues by clinical ethics consultants. Because many conflicts arise from communication problems rather than ethical dilemmas, the approaches and strategies used in mediation can be used to prevent or mitigate conflict in daily bedside issues. Becoming skillful in working from a stated position or demand, attending to emotions, and uncovering underlying interests will empower clinical nurses to effectively and therapeutically work with patients and their families. If they are adept at listening for understanding, at reframing demands as needs and interests, and at assisting stakeholders in shaping a shared solution, they can also contribute toward moving an organizational culture to one that consistently responds to the values, needs, concerns, and preferences of patients and families.

References

American Nurses Association (ANA). (2010). *Nursing scope and standards of practice* (2nd ed.). Silver Spring, MD: Author.

American Society for Bioethics and Humanities (ASBH). (2011). *Core competencies for healthcare ethics consultation* (2nd ed.). Glenview, IL: Author.

Arnold, R., Aulisio, M., Begler, A., & Seltzer, D. (2007). A commentary on Caplan and Bergman: Ethics mediation—Questions for the future. *Journal of Clinical Ethics, 18*(4), 350-354.

Back, A. L., Arnold, R. M., Baile, W. F., Tulsky, J. A., & Fryer-Edwards, K. (2005). Approaching difficult communication tasks in oncology. *CA: A Cancer Journal for Clinicians, 55*(3), 164-177.

Bergman, E. J., & Fiester, A. (2009). Mediation and health care. In V. Ravitsky, A. Fiester, & A. L. Caplan (Eds.), *The Penn Center guide to bioethics* (pp. 171-180). New York, NY: Springer.

Churchill, L. R., Fanning, J. B., & Schenck, D. (2013). *What patients teach: The everyday ethics of health care.* New York, NY: Oxford University Press.

Dubler, N. N., & Liebman, C. B. (2011). *Bioethics mediation: A guide to shaping shared solutions.* Nashville, TN: Vanderbilt University Press.

Fiester, A. (2007). The failure of the consult model: Why "mediation" should replace "consultation." *American Journal of Bioethics, 7*(2), 31-32.

Fiester, A. (2012). Mediation and advocacy. *American Journal of Bioethics, 12*(8), 10-11.

Fisher, R., Ury, W., & Patton, B. (1991). *Getting to yes: Negotiating agreement without giving in* (2nd ed.). New York, NY: Penguin Books.

Gerardi, D. (2004). Using mediation techniques to manage conflict and create healthy work environments. *AACN Clinical Issues, 15*(2), 182-195.

Gibson, J. M. (1994). Mediation for ethics committees: A promising process. *Generations, 18*(4), 58-60.

Gibson, K. (1999a). Mediator attitude toward outcomes: A philosophical view. *Mediation Quarterly, 17*(2), 197-211.

Gibson, K. (1999b). Mediation in the medical field: Is neutral intervention possible? *Hastings Center Report, 29*(5), 6-13.

Hamric, A. B. (2001). Reflections on being in the middle. *Nursing Outlook, 49*(6), 254-257.

The Joint Commission (TJC). (2010). *Advancing effective communication, cultural competency, and patient-and family-centered care: A roadmap for hospitals.* Oakbrook Terrace, IL: Author.

Kleinman, A. (2011). The divided self, hidden values, and moral sensibility in medicine. *Lancet, 377*(9768), 804-805. doi:10.1016/S0140-6736(11)60295-X

Kleinman, A., Eisenberg, L., & Good, B. (1978). Culture, illness, and care: Clinical lessons from anthropologic and cross-cultural research. *Annuals of Internal Medicine, 88*(2), 251-258.

Koloroutis, M., & Trout, M. (2012). *See me as a person: Creating therapeutic relationships with patients and their families.* Minneapolis, MN: Creative Health Care Management.

Meruelo, N. C. (2008). Mediation and medical malpractice: The need to understand why patients sue and a proposal for a specific model of mediation. *Journal of Legal Medicine, 29*(3), 285-306.

Murphy, P. (1993). Clinical ethics: Must nurses be forever in the middle? *Bioethics Forum, 9*(4), 3-4.

Peter, E., & Liaschenko, J. (2004). Perils of proximity: a spatiotemporal analysis of moral distress and moral ambiguity. *Nursing Inquiry, 11*(4), 218-225

Philipsen, N. C. (2008). Resolving conflict: A primer for nurse practitioners on alternatives to litigation. *Journal for Nurse Practitioners, 4*(10), 766-772.

Saulo, M., & Wagener, R. J. (2000). Mediation training enhances conflict management by healthcare personnel. *American Journal of Managed Care, 6*(4), 473-483.

Schenck, D., & Churchill, L. R. (2012). *Healers: Extraordinary clinicians at work.* New York, NY: Oxford University Press.

Schlairet, M. C. (2009). Bioethics mediation: The role and importance of nursing advocacy. *Nursing Outlook, 57*(4), 185-193.

Varcoe, C., Doane, G., Pauly, B., Rodney, P., Storch, J. L., Mahoney, K.,…Starzomski, R. (2004). Ethical practice in nursing: Working the in-betweens. *Journal of Advanced Nursing, 45*(30), 316-325.

Walton, M. K. (2011). Communicating with family caregivers. *American Journal of Nursing, 111*(12), 47-53.

Ward-Collins, D. (1998). Alternative dispute resolution: A mediation process for conflict resolution of healthcare issues. *Journal of Legal Nurse Consulting, 9*(3), 2-7.

Chapter 16

Ethics Consultation

Mary K. Walton, MSN, MBE, RN

Ms. Georgia, exhausted and frustrated, asked her daughter's nurse how she could have an ethical concern addressed. Directed to the office of the hospital ethics committee nurse co-chair, she found an empathic and listening ear as she shared her daughter's story. Her daughter, Mena, now 35 years old, suffered with liver disease among other comorbidities for more than 20 years. A liver transplant 7 years ago brought only a few years of relative well-being. With full knowledge that her transplant had failed and that she was not a candidate for a second transplant, Mena continued to want all aggressive care to sustain her life. Despite multiple admissions to the medical intensive care unit (ICU) over the past year, her overall health continued to deteriorate. A few brief discharges to home only prompted another readmission for complications, and Mena continued to agree to, or even request, transfer to the ICU when sepsis or respiratory distress developed. Many physician trainees recommended referral to hospice over the past year to Mena, recommendations that she adamantly rejected. Ms. Georgia reported that this last episode infuriated her daughter and that her daughter felt "bullied" by these repeated, and at times strident, recommendations for referral to hospice rather than aggressive care and transfer to the ICU. She noted that the nurses witnessed these discussions yet did not weigh in with their perspective. Ms. Georgia shared that she did not understand how her daughter had the strength to continue; if it were she, she would have refused life-sustaining therapy months ago. As her mother, she felt she needed to support her daughter's wishes, values, and preferences. Thus Ms. Georgia initiated a formal ethics consultation for her daughter with the question to the consultant: "Can you make these physicians stop pushing hospice referral?"

Patient-centeredness is defined by the Institute of Medicine (IOM) as "providing care that is respectful of and responsive to individual patient preferences, needs and values and ensuring that patient values guide all clinical decisions" (IOM, 2001, p. 40), and by Quality and Safety Education for Nurses (QSEN) as "the patient is the source of control and full partner" (Cronenwett et al., 2007, p. 123). These definitions are well aligned with the purpose and goals of clinical ethics consultation. Ethics consultation, a well-established formal process in most U.S. hospitals, offers a resource to patients, families, and staff to achieve patient-centered care (Fox, Myers, & Pearlman,

2007). This consultative process encompasses a variety of services provided in response to questions from patients, families, surrogates, and healthcare professionals "who seek to resolve uncertainly or conflict regarding value-laden concerns that emerge in health care" (American Society for Bioethics and Humanities [ASBH], 2011, p. 2). Stated another way, ethics consultation can be seen as a remedy for care that is not based on patient values, needs, and preferences—care that is provider- or organization-centered rather than patient-centered.

However, because ethics consultation responds to issues that relate to values, and values differ among individuals, the concerns of the staff must also be addressed. Because practitioners represent many disparate professions and clinical specialties and because complex healthcare systems are too often organized around the preferences, needs, and values of the organization, ethics consultations are helpful in sorting out the issues and developing a plan that acknowledges and reconciles the different points of view. Supporting the rights of staff to honor their values, enact their moral agency, and hopefully mitigate any developing moral distress must be considered in concert with ensuring that patient values guide all clinical decisions. This chapter reviews how ethics consultation supports patient-centered care as well as the professional and individual moral values of staff members. Examples are offered to illustrate the role of the clinical nurse using the ethics consultation as a strategy to ensure that care reflects the values and care preferences of patients and their families.

Origins of Ethics Consultation Services

Hospital-based ethics committees and consultation services emerged during the patient rights movement in the 1970s to recognize the ethical values of self-determination, well-being, and equity. The President's Commission for the Study of Ethical Problems in Medicine and Biomedical and Behavioral Research supported the value of self-determination as "the capacity to form, revise, and pursue his or her own plans for life" (President's Commission, 1983, p. 26). As advances in knowledge and technology introduced myriad treatment options along with multiple decision points in the acute-care setting, patients were often unprepared or physically incapable of participating in care decisions. In fact, ethics committees and consultation services can be traced back to the recognition of the rights of individuals and their implications for patient care from the highly publicized legal cases of Karen Ann Quinlan (1976), Baby Doe (1980s), and Nancy Cruzan (1990). Each of these cases involved families who sought to bring their values into the clinical decision-making equation (Aulisio & Arnold, 2008).

With emerging recognition that the care setting rather than the courts was the better place to address these value-laden decisions, The Joint Commission (TJC) initiated a requirement for a formal process to address ethical issues and protect patients' rights in 1992 (Joint Commission on Accreditation of Healthcare Organizations, 1992). Today, along with hospital accreditation standards (TJC, 2014), additional quality standards, such as Magnet designation and the Beacon Award for Excellence, specifically require that nurses have a resource to identify and address care-related ethical issues (American Association of Critical-Care Nurses [AACN], 2011; American Nurses Credentialing Center [ANCC], 2008). Thus, ethics committees providing a clinical consultation service emerged as an essential organizational structure, recognizing and honoring patient rights in the hospital setting.

What Is Healthcare Ethics Consultation?

Ethics consultation is a "set of services provided by an individual or group in response to questions from patients, families, surrogates, healthcare professionals, or other involved parties who seek to resolve uncertainty or conflict regarding value-laden concerns that emerge in health care" (ASBH, 2011, p. 2). The goal of this set of services is to improve the quality of healthcare through the identification, analysis, and resolution of ethical questions and concerns. Consultants assist in analyzing the nature of the value uncertainty or conflict and facilitate resolution within a respectful atmosphere, giving attention to the interests, rights, and responsibilities of all those involved (ASBH, 2011).

Literature Regarding Ethics Consultation

Although this definition reflects the great variability in consultation practice, the importance of the service in providing a safe moral space to address ethical concerns is well recognized and widely endorsed (Aulisio & Arnold, 2008; Dubler et al., 2009; Fox et al., 2007; Walker, 1993). There is increasing evidence that these services offer a safe venue to raise ethical questions for healthcare providers (Danis et al., 2008). However, there is little empirical evidence about how patients and families value ethics consultations (Nilson, Acres, Tamerin, & Fins, 2008). Two early single-institution studies found varying perceptions of the value of the consultation process from the patient and family perspective (McClung, Kamer, DeLuca, & Barber, 1996; Orr, Morton, deLeon, & Fals, 1996). Today, the healthcare hierarchy continues to be complex in the acute-care setting, and the need for early recognition of ethical concerns to prevent or mitigate ethical conflicts about care is receiving increasing attention (Pavlish, Brown-Saltzman, Fine, & Jakel, 2013). Although legally the authority for care decisions remains with the patient or the patient's legally authorized surrogate, both perception and reality at times indicate that providers assume consent or even usurp patient authority at times.

Although the provision of patient-centered care is recognized as the goal of interprofessional teamwork, the challenges are great given the diversity of values among team members (Interprofessional Education Collaborative Expert Panel, 2011, p. 20). Professions, specialty practices, and individual patient care units develop and hold a wide range of values that inform the work of healthcare professionals and staff (Baggs et al., 2007). Individual preferences, values, and cultural differences within families also present challenges to clinicians (Quinn et al., 2012). Power imbalances are inherent despite the continued recognition of patient self-determination as a goal. Although consulting specialty experts is routine in the acute-care setting, initiating an ethics consult may unfortunately be seen as implying unethical practice on the part of a colleague or, alternately, a strategy to coerce a patient to accept medical recommendations.

Today, despite decades of formal support for seeking assistance with ethical issues, there is evidence that nurses may lack knowledge or experience with this resource or be hindered from accessing the resource by the organizational processes or power gradients (Danis et al., 2008; Gaudine, Lamb, LeFort, & Thorne, 2011; Gordon & Hamric, 2006; Pavlish, Hellyer, Brown-Saltzman, Miers, & Squire, 2013). However, one study revealed that nurses pursued consultation with less concern for repercussions when the patient's family sought the request (Gordon & Hamric, 2006). Alternately, interacting with a "difficult" patient or family member was cited as a common reason for ethics consultation by internal medicine physicians who practice in critical care and oncology (DuVal, Sartorius, Clarridge, Gensler, & Danis, 2001). Ethics consultation, by definition, is a service that supports patient-centered care and should serve as a valued resource providing a safe moral space for patients, families, and professionals to address the complex issues that arise today in healthcare.

How Does Ethics Consultation Promote P&FCC?

Qualified clinical ethics consultants bring specific knowledge and skills to the bedside. Their goals include helping to clarify and articulate the patients' preferences, bridging gaps between these preferences and reality (if there is a discrepancy) while promoting and ensuring respect for not only the requester's values but those of all stakeholders, including patient, family, and providers (Craig & May, 2006). These goals all serve to promote the values, needs, and preferences of patients within the context of what is actually feasible given the skill and resources available in the patient's current healthcare setting.

Quality in Ethics Consultation

Responding to an ethical concern in the practice setting is increasingly recognized as a high-stakes endeavor with the potential to benefit patients or, alternately, put patients at risk, if not handled correctly (Kodish et al., 2013; Tarzian & ASBH Core Competencies Update Task Force, 2013). Thus, a national movement is well underway to ensure that ethics consultants are qualified to provide this service and to ensure that the focus is maintained on the values of the patient or family (Dubler et al., 2009; Kodish et al., 2013; Magill, 2013). Although a variety of approaches, such as credentialing or certification, are under consideration, the ASBH Core Competencies, which are the nationally established standards, offer a patient-centered approach (Dubler et al., 2009; Silverman, Bellavance, & Childs, 2013). Although there may be some variability in qualifications, ethics consultants who possess the requisite competencies will bring specific knowledge and skills that support patient- and family-centered care (P&FCC) to the requester seeking assistance as well as other stakeholders in the care constellation.

Core skills for ethics consultation identified by ASBH (2011) include ethical assessment and analysis skills, process skills, the ability to facilitate formal meetings, and a range of interpersonal skills. Consider the components of the interpersonal skills. An ethics consultant with these abilities will support care that is centered on the values, needs, and preferences of the patient when an ethical concern or conflict emerges:

- "[L]isten well and to communicate interest, respect, support, and empathy to all involved parties
- [R]ecognize and attend to various relational barriers to communication present among those involved in a consultation—in particular, suffering, moral distress, and strong emotions
- [E]ducate involved parties regarding the ethical dimensions of the consultation
- [E]licit the moral views of involved parties
- [R]epresent the views of involved parties to others
- [E]nable involved parties to communicate effectively and be heard by other parties" (ASBH, 2011, p. 24)

Core knowledge areas delineated by ASBH for ethics consultants include moral reasoning and ethical theory, bioethical issues and concepts (such as patients' rights, informed consent, surrogate decision-making, substituted judgment, and best interest standard), the clinical context and knowledge of the important health and spiritual beliefs of the local communities that influence healthcare (ASBH, 2011, pp. 26–31).

Bringing the Patient Voice Forward

Many of the fundamental elements of a clinical ethics consultation bring the perspective and voice of the patient and family forward in a meaningful way. Below are selected examples of the interventions a trained clinical ethics professional will employ:

- Respond to the request from the patient or family member without requiring authorization by a professional.
- Visit the patient and family specifically to seek their perspective and elicit their values and preferences.
- Involve the patient and family with the clinical care providers toward the goal of promoting communication, exploring options, and seeking consensus.
- Employ expert discussion of bioethical principles, practices, and norms supporting respect for the individual.
- Use reason, facilitation, negotiation, or mediation to seek agreement about the plan of care going forward.
- Attend to the social, psychological, and spiritual issues that are at play in disagreements (Dubler et al., 2009, p. 25).

Thus, patients and families who believe their values, preferences, and needs are not being either recognized or honored by the professional care team should expect expert assistance in navigating treatment and care decisions. Clinical nurses can recommend this resource to patients and families when ethical concerns are raised. Alternately, clinical nurses should initiate the consult process if they assess that the patient's values are not being respected in a given care situation.

Although patients and family members may initiate a consult, the literature primarily reflects consults requested by physicians, nurses, and other members of the clinical care team, although the request may in fact be prompted by the patient or family member. No matter who initiates the consult, the consultant will directly engage the patient. If the patient is unable to participate, the consultant will actively seek out the surrogate decision-maker and other family and friends who can speak to the patient's values and preferences as previously expressed. This attention to understanding and bringing the patient's values and preferences forward is fundamental to the ethics-consultation process. Clinical teams who may have inadvertently lost the patient perspective, especially given the technological imperative so pervasive in U.S. hospitals, should find this specific attention on identifying and working with the patient's perspective invaluable.

Recognition of the Important Role of the Family

The bioethics principle of respect for autonomy with emphasis on the individual in isolation from the family constellation has not served the patient well in the acute-care setting. Respecting the personhood of a patient demands respecting this person's relationships and supporting the patient's ability to draw on these relationships during health crises (Berlinger, Jennings, & Wolf, 2013). The routine of visiting hours and restrictions on family presence at a patient's bedside is a classic example of provider or organization-centric care. From the inpatient's perspective, the need for comfort, solace, or assistance with myriad treatment decisions provided by friends and family at the bedside is evident. Yet the value placed on efficiency and expedience for routine tasks, such as rounds and informed-consent documentation, eliminates the opportunity for patients to have the support of family. Now, federal regulation requires hospitals to respect the patient's right to the continual presence of a support person even in the ICU (Centers for Medicare & Medicaid Services [CMS], 2010). Increasingly, families are supporting patients through involvement in care routines, such as interdisciplinary rounds and patient handoffs (see accompanying sidebar).

P&FCC and Patient Handoffs

The Institute for Healthcare Improvement (IHI) has resources regarding its ISHAPED patient-centered approach to nurse shift change bedside report at http://www.ihi.org/resources/Pages/Tools/ISHAPEDPatientCenteredNurseShiftChangeBedsideReport.aspx

The Agency for Healthcare Research and Quality (AHRQ) published an implementation handbook for Nurse Bedside Shift Report as part of a Guide to Patient and Family Engagement in Hospital Quality and Safety. See http://www.ahrq.gov/professionals/systems/hospital/engagingfamilies/index.html for more detail.

The goal of these particular strategies is to ensure a safe handoff of care between nurses by involving the patient and family in the process. Ideally, a patient and family member at the bedside could expect the nurses going off and coming on duty to do the following:

- *Introduce the nurse coming on duty.*

- *Be invited to take part in the report process.*

- *Talk about the details of care over the past time interval and the plans for the starting shift.*

- *Check medications that are currently being given.*

- *Follow up on any tests or procedures done or planned for.*

- *Elicit the patient's and, if the patient directs, the family members' assessment of care and hopes/personal goals for the starting shift.*

- *Encourage the expression of questions and concerns for the nurse to discuss with colleagues.*

If a patient welcomes a family member to participate in bedside support, the family member will gain an understanding of the goals and plans of care and how the patient is progressing. Questions can be answered in real time, as they are developing, and a family member may become comfortable with the care team members and express fears, needs, and concerns.

The landmark Quinlan case served to recognize the role of the family in healthcare decision-making when the highest court in New Jersey established the patient's father's right to make healthcare decisions. Twenty years after the Quinlan family ordeal, her parents wrote of their "deep desire to do the right thing for Karen and to respect her wishes. We had to fight for what we believed in" (Quinlan & Quinlan, 1996). Today the role of family members as surrogate decision-makers is well established by the courts, yet the movement for patient-centered care indicates there is still progress to be made if the personhood of the individual within the context of family is to be fully honored.

Ethics consultants are expected to be skilled in family dynamics and often work with family members around care issues in the critical-care setting when patients are unable to give consent for care. Managing the complexity of surrogate decision-making, particularly relating to end-of-life care, is sensitive and challenging work. Consultants work to bring the "patient's voice into the decision-making" and help family members reflect on the patient's previously stated values as they wrestle with the burden of decision-making (Lehmann, 2012, p. 67). Family members fulfill many informal and essential roles when a patient is unable to direct care decisions (Lehmann, 2012; Quinn et al., 2012). Family members who need to serve as surrogate decision-makers may benefit from working with an ethics consultant as they understand treatment options and translate their loved one's values into decisions for care. In bioethics, the concepts of substituted judgment and best interest standard are well defined as standards, but for loved ones they are a formidable and typically novel responsibility. An advance directive or living will, although informative and helpful, may not mitigate the stress. Ethics consultants offering expert guidance and support can help family members as they navigate through end-of-life decision-making.

When Patients Can't Speak for Themselves

There are three established standards of healthcare decision-making when the patient's voice is either temporarily or permanently unavailable to direct care. Family and friends may be essential to answering questions to bring forth the patient's values and preferences when a particular decision needs to be made.

- *Previous expressions: "What do we know about this person's wishes based on what she has said or written in the past?"*

- *Substituted judgment: "Knowing what we know about this person's behavior, values, and prior decisions, what do we think she would want done in these particular circumstances?"*

- *Best interest standard: "What do we believe would best promote this person's well-being in these particular circumstances?"*

Source: Post, Blustein, & Dubler, 2007, p. 31

Identifying the Value-Laden Concerns

Ethics consultation is a service responding to value-laden concerns. Identifying the values informing or driving the concerns is an essential part of the consultation process. Furthermore, the values of all the participants are relevant: the patient and the patient's family and all members of the caregiving team.

What Are Values?

Simply defined, *values* are what we pay attention to—what we believe to be important. Values can be identified in the everyday lives of individuals, whether expressed through behaviors or verbalized in conversation. Values can also be hidden and unexpressed, thereby undermining both personal and clinical interactions (Kleinman, 2011).

Sources of values include early family life, professional socialization, and organizational goals. These strongly held beliefs, ideals, principles, and standards inform practice and ethical decision-making. Values may be individually held or grounded in professional codes or culture. The

American Nurses Association (ANA) *Code of Ethics* is one expression of the values of professional nursing. In essence, "the relationship between the nurse and patient occurs within the context of the values and beliefs of the patient and the nurse" (ANA, 2010, p. 6).

Recognition of the diversity of values among professional groups who practice as members of interprofessional teams is essential and a prerequisite to providing care that centers on the values of the patient (Glen, 1999). Healthcare itself is not a value-neutral science, because, as clinicians develop expertise, their behavior is governed by particular values related to such things as "the badness of pain, a picture of human flourishing and wellness, the nature of dignity, and more" and there is "no extractable core of value-neutral knowledge that forms the essence of the clinician's skilled expertise" (Kukla, 2007, p. 32). Consider various clinical specialties and reflect on how practitioners focus on aspects of care. Are there differences between internal medicine, transplant services, oncology services, and surgical services? Consider advance directives and how they are encouraged, recognized, or invisible. What are the underlying values expressed in routine protocols and practices? How do individual, familial, and cultural values influence patient-directed advance-care planning?

Family members serving as surrogate decision-makers for critically ill loved ones may struggle with identifying and translating values into care decisions. Scheunemann, Arnold, and White (2012) offer a framework for clinicians to help surrogates identify and explore specific values and value conflicts in the context of critical illness. Using questions to elicit a narrative about the patient's life experience and to explore such values as longevity, maintenance of physical or cognitive function, and adherence to spiritual beliefs is an approach that can help a family during this difficult time.

Consider the vignette at the beginning of the chapter—how does the physician trainees' behavior serve to express their values? Did they value the relief of suffering over the patient's expressed desire to live as long as possible? What value was given to the limited resource of an ICU bed, and how may it have influenced the recommendation to forego another ICU transfer? Did the physicians' behavior relate to a professional orientation of an objective focus on the patient's body and treatment of disease pathology rather than "the new subjective medicine" that explicitly incorporates the patient's assessment of individual healthcare needs (Sullivan, 2003)? Although the ethical principle of respect for autonomy is well recognized in Western medicine, why would physicians continue to push for hospice over the aggressive treatment that was consistently successful in stabilizing the patient and extending her life?

Also consider the mother's values as she expressed them in her request for ethics consultation. Here the mother shared that her daughter's value of living as long as possible should trump her own values of minimizing her daughter's suffering. And what of the patient's values? An individual who has experienced an intensive care admission in the past can be considered well informed about a request for such care again. Is this informed consent? How is the patient's value to live another day even with significant illness requiring inpatient care honored? How might the physician trainees and the patient differ in assessing her quality of life? Does each party understand the other's perspective? Are there facts that need to be clarified?

And what might be the values of the clinical nurses? How did they value their obligation to advocate for what their patient wanted? Did the nurses fear speaking up? A group of nurses who may hold core nursing values can also be expected to have varying personal values and beliefs that will inform their professional practice. Did they discuss their values among themselves? Did they support ongoing aggressive care? Were they troubled by transferring the patient to the ICU or did they breathe a sigh of relief? Did the nurse who directed Mena's mother to the nurse ethicist's office silently support her? Was she relieved a consult was being called? What are the values of the clinical nurses who reportedly were consistently silent when witnessing the repetitive discussion that upset the patient? Is avoiding conflict a value? How did they view their obligation to the patient in contrast to their obligations to their physician colleagues when Mena expressed distress in the repetitive discussions about the goals of care?

Did anyone ask the patient to prepare an advance directive as a useful tool to communicate her preferences for care, especially given so many providers? Do health professionals value advance directives for patients, for themselves, for their own loved ones? How are cultural and spiritual perspectives that do not value advance-care planning represented with the regulatory requirement/organizational value placed on advance directives?

Recognizing and exploring the values informing ethical concerns are essential to the consultation process. What are the values embedded in the care? Whose values are they? What role are they playing in the emerging conflict or moral distress? The above queries represent questions that the ethics consultant might ask while gathering information about the values at play in the situation. Prompting reflection by questioning helps bring the values forward so they can be identified and discussed.

Identifying the values in conflict helps all the participants begin to see the ethical concern driving the conflict. In the vignette, Mena values every day of her life, despite being hospital-bound and quite ill. We can speculate that the physicians value curing or mitigating acute illnesses. Furthermore, they may place a value on an ICU bed for reversal of illness to support a "quality of life" not dependent upon continued acute care. The physicians may also value protecting themselves from witnessing the suffering of a patient who in their estimation did not have a long-term benefit from transplantation. The values of the clinical nurses are less clear, yet we can speculate that they did not value their advocacy role over the value of avoiding conflict or clinical team cohesion. Prompting reflection on the thoughts and feelings engendered at the bedside helps reveal the values involved.

Formulating an Ethics Question

Identifying the ethical concern and the embedded values is an important early step in the consultation process. When the consultant hears the presenting concern as described by the requester, ethical issues will be recognized. What makes something an ethical issue in contrast to a personal preference is the movement from the idea that one *can* do something to the position that one *ought* to do something based on norms or judgments about values, rights, duties, and responsibilities. *What is the right thing to do, and what makes it so?*

When an ethics consultant receives a request, a well-recognized approach is to formulate the initial information into a question so the uncertainty and/or conflict can be highlighted (see accompanying sidebar). Organizing initial information into a question helps both the requester and the consultant focus on the values at play and plan the subsequent steps.

Template for Framing an Ethics Question

- *Given (uncertainty or conflict about values), what decisions or actions are ethically justifiable?*

- *Given (uncertainly or conflict about values), is it ethically justifiable to (decisions or action)?*

Source: Fox, Berkowitz, Chanko, & Powell, 2006

Assuming direct confirmation of the information by the patient, here are examples of some initial formulations of the ethics question for the introductory scenario:

- Given the patient's expressed request for continued aggressive care so that she may live as long as possible and the medical team's recommendation for hospice care, what decisions or actions are ethically justifiable?

- Given the patient's specific request for all life-sustaining treatment and the medical team's recommendation for hospice care, is it ethically justifiable for the medical team to continue to recommend referral to hospice?

- Given the patient's specific request for intensive care to treat her life-threatening complications and the medical team's belief that this treatment is no longer warranted or medically futile, is it ethically justifiable to deny transfer to the medical ICU?

The details and context shape the formulation of questions. The ethics question may be formed in a variety of ways and will change as more information is gathered and discussed.

For example, although the patient's mother has initiated the consult, because the patient has decision-making capacity, she must be interviewed so she can directly present her concerns. If the patient were unable to communicate her concerns, the consult from the family member would be accepted. In the opening vignette, it would be important to know whether the patient and the mother were unified in the ethical concern. The possibility exists that a family member would frame the ethical concern differently. In addition to the patient and her mother, the consultant will need to gather information from other key stakeholders on the care team, most notably the physicians and nurses. The consultant is obligated to seek first-person information and should not assume that one professional can or should represent another's position or ethical concern. In fact, "an effective consultation process creates deliberate opportunities to seek the perspective of all the involved parties, anticipating and even expecting that they may frame the issues and questions differently and may have different and competing perspectives" (ASBH Clinical Ethics Task Force, 2009, p. 63). In this vignette, the physician trainees and clinical nurses might very well characterize their behavior and ethical concerns differently from the patient and her mother. The patient may also identify other family members who are troubled and/or have information to be shared in the process.

Transparency

"Nothing about me without me" is one way to summarize or conceptualize person-centered care (Delbanco et al., 2001). Whether patients or providers initiate an ethics consult, the standard is that patients should be informed of the consultation request and the reason for the consult, given explanations about the process, and invited to participate if they so choose. Reasonable exceptions to this standard relate to conflict between professionals only (ASBH, 2011, p. 16). It could be argued, however, that any differences in opinions among professionals should be shared with patients in the spirit of informed consent and given the goals of full disclosure and transparency. The standard is also that the attending physician should be notified of a consult involving one of her or his patients, because the attending physician is ultimately responsible for the care of the patient.

The opening vignette offers the perspective of the adult patient's mother, who presents as representing the patient's voice. One of the first questions to be asked by an ethics consultant is, *"Does your daughter know you are bringing this concern to the hospital ethics consultation service?"* The consultant needs to know this in order to frame the question being asked and to determine the next step. Family members might bring an issue forward that represents their own concern rather than a direct concern of the patient. Certainly there are times when the patient and family members have a disparate view of the ethical question and/or hoped for resolution. All perspectives are important to the consultant. Furthermore, it was not that long ago that the standard professional practice norm was to disclose bad news to the family rather than to the patient (Veatch & Tai, 1980).

Talking directly to the patient is essential to gain a deeper understanding of the individual's values and needs. A patient who may be weak, in pain, frustrated, or fearful is clearly vulnerable and may not be in a position of strength. An ethics consultant with knowledge of the organizational system and how to strategically bring concerns forward can take the patient's voice further and perhaps more effectively—framing and articulating the patient's perspective and/or working through a complex hospital system to meet the patient's goals. For example, in the opening vignette, physician trainees are key stakeholders. We can anticipate that this consultation will include communication with medical leadership to implement a plan in response to this patient's request to honor her authority to consent to life-sustaining care. Addressing this ethical concern with only the individuals currently on service would solely be a short-term intervention. Additionally, the consultant can follow up with education and emotional support as necessary for the physician trainees.

The Nursing Role in Using Ethics Consultation to Promote P&FCC

The need for nurses to have a resource to address ethical concerns is well established in both regulatory and quality standards. All hospitals accredited by TJC will have a policy outlining the process for initiating an ethics consultation. Nurses, given their time at the bedside, may be the clinicians who have the most informed perspective on the patient and family values that are guiding them during an acute-care hospitalization. Observing patient behaviors around self-care, ambulation, information seeking, response to pain, family involvement, spiritual rituals, and communication patterns with friends, work colleagues, or community connections provides evidence of individual values. Attention to these behaviors, in concert with seeking the patient or family "story" as it relates to the patient's life rather than more narrowly to the patient's illness, will enable a nurse to identify and bring the values of concern to the team and/or the ethics consultant. See Chapter 19 for a detailed discussion of narrative approaches to elicit the patient's illness experience and identify the patient's values and beliefs.

Initiating an Ethics Consultation

Because the nurse at the bedside has a particular relationship with the patient and family, nurses are often in a position to recognize the need for a consultation and to take steps to initiate one (see Table 16.1). One variable that serves to empower clinical nurses is the support of the nurse manager or clinical nurse specialists in raising ethical concerns and initiating ethics consultation (DeWolf Bosek, 2009; Gaudine et al., 2011; Gordon & Hamric, 2006). Unit- or program-based leaders influence the ethical climate of the work group and how difficult care situations are addressed (Bell & Breslin, 2008).

TABLE 16.1   Clinical Nurses: Preparing to Initiate an Ethics Consultation

1. **Know the organizational policy for initiating an ethics consultation.**

   Does the attending physician or nurse manager need to be informed first? Consider whether it would be helpful even if not required by policy.

2. **Explore your ethical concern with a trusted colleague and sincerely seek that individual's perspective on the situation. Invite or even probe for a different perspective on the issues.**

   I am troubled by continuing to provide aggressive care to one of my patients. Could I share my concerns and thoughts with you? I am especially interested in seeing whether you might think about this differently.

continues

TABLE 16.1   *continued*

3. **Reflect on the values of all stakeholders.**

Seek the perspective of at least one person with a non-nursing lens. Ask the patient, resident, social worker, or clinical nutritionist to spend a few minutes with you to share his or her thoughts on the issue that is troubling, or less specifically on the goals of care. What does this person see as the likely outcome? Whose values are reflected in this perspective? Do they differ from yours? How does this person frame the issue—from a patient or provider perspective?

I know I am looking at this patient's care as a nurse and carrying with me some previous similar clinical experiences. I am wondering how you look at this based on your role and past experience. Could you share some of your thoughts with me?

4. **When ready to initiate the consult, present your concern as an ethical one rather than an emotional or power-based issue; frame it in values and patient-centered goals rather than in emotions or roles.**

The patient has expressed how much she values every day of her life despite being hospital-bound. Although the ICU stays are burdensome, her goal is to live as long as possible. Hospice referral is raised with every service change—I see how upset she becomes every time the recommendation is encouraged. I am concerned we are not respecting her values.

5. **Frame the presentation as a professional obligation rather than personal opinion or objection to the plan of care.**

Dr. Young, I know you may be very familiar with our patient's treatment course and consistent refusal of a referral to hospice. It is my obligation as Mena's nurse to share my concern about the repeated recommendations for hospice by the physician trainees. During my time at the bedside, it is evident to me that this refusal to accept her position is stressful to her as well as to her family. I believe we need a team meeting to discuss the differing values and perspectives that are creating some tension at the bedside. We are all working so hard to do the right thing for Mena. Could we pick some times that would work from our schedules so I can coordinate with other team members?

6. **Invite and actively listen to the perspectives of others to identify the values of importance to them.**

Be curious and wonder when a perspective divergent from yours is offered. Seek to understand and encourage the person to share—*Tell me more*. The primary goal is to understand other perspectives before explaining your perspective.

Gaining knowledge of diverse, multiple perspectives will help address the value-laden conflicts that typically prompt clinical ethics consultations.

I know you are the chaplain whom Mena asks to talk with occasionally. Could you spend a few minutes talking with me? How do you feel about her repeated admissions to the ICU? How does her suffering affect you?

I know you have cared for Mena during the last two ICU admissions. What do you think about her goals of care and request for ICU admissions? Have you cared for other patients who have been hospitalized so long without any clear hope of discharge to home? What do you think about your work with her?

7. **Frame positively.**

> *Given the diversity of values involved, I believe we need assistance sorting through the ethical concerns—our ethics consultation service is the resource that can help us. I will start the process by calling in the request.*

Assisting in the Ethics Consultation Process

Once the consultation has been initiated, clinical nurses can play a key role in assisting in the process (Walton, 2012). Although a variety of approaches to ethics consultation has evolved over the past decades, generally every consult should have two distinguishable stages: gathering all the necessary information to facilitate a sound recommendation and formulating a written report with analysis and recommendations for the chart (Spike, 2012, p. 42). One useful characterization of ethics consultation is *slow the process down.* Although participants may seek a quick answer, gathering relevant and accurate information takes time and thoughtful discourse among the stakeholders. Bedside nurses are essential stakeholders in the consultation process given their consistent position at the bedside. Furthermore, they have knowledge of patient and family engagement, have observed response to treatment, and often are the care providers who enact the plan of care.

Identify the Key Stakeholders

The clinical nurse might recognize stakeholders whom the consultant should involve in the process. A question to ask to identify potential stakeholders is *Who else cares about this patient or, alternatively, this particular ethical concern?* For example, a clinician on a previous rotation might have established an effective working relationship with the patient and family during a care crisis or alternately was involved with an encounter of good news or successful treatment. A permanent night-shift nurse or respiratory therapist or the patient's neighbor might bring an important perspective to the consultation. Identifying key stakeholders is especially valuable when the patient is unable to speak or when there is conflict among family members in identifying the patient's values and preferences.

> **Identifying Stakeholders**
>
> *To identify stakeholders:*
>
> - **Ask the patient:** *Who shares your concern? Who could help you (or us) work through this important decision? Prompt the identification of individuals beyond family, such as community supports: Is the patient a member of a support group related to a chronic health condition, a faith community, or a resident in a veterans facility?*

- *Ask the representatives of clinical departments: Who is invested in this patient's care and/or might have relevant information or perspectives to share? Examples include medicine, surgery, clinical nutrition, pastoral care, social work, physical therapy, occupational therapy, and speech/language clinicians.*

Given the patterns of clinical nurses' care as well as work schedules, it may be important to ensure that clinical nurses who know the patient's care well are invited to participate in the process. In addition to hospital staff, there may be home-care nurses who have relevant information to offer.

Illustrate the Patient's Daily Life

Concerns about the patient's quality of life often arise in ethical discussions. Only the patient can self-evaluate the quality of life despite the oft-heard clinicians' expression, whether in sadness or frustration: "*This patient has no quality of life.*" Illustrating the patient's daily life can serve to give insight into the patient's experience while recognizing that we can never fully appreciate another individual's life experience. In the hospital setting, a description of the patient's experience of care can inform other stakeholders who do not have the benefit of proximity and intimacy that patients and clinical nurses share. Consider painful and extensive nursing care procedures, for example. Family members and physicians may not appreciate the extensive physical pain, bodily deformity, or functional impairment that the nurse witnesses during the provision of nursing care. This is of particular relevance when a patient cannot represent this experience to others. Alternately, a nurse's knowledge of how a patient tolerates and accepts limitations and suffering might be very relevant to assessment of care benefits and burdens. The nurse may be able to bring forward the experiences bringing pleasure or solace to the patient—making visible what may be invisible to others.

Support the Patient and Family

As unfamiliar as ethics consultation might be to clinical nurses, it may be even more so to the patient and the patient's family. This is most likely a once-in-a-lifetime experience at a critical time in a family's life. Illness or trauma requiring hospitalization is a major life disruption. Patients and families are also burdened as they struggle to determine "what is the right thing to do." We can imagine the burden of Mena's mother as she brought her daughter's concern forward. Attention to emotional and spiritual needs is important, and consulting other organizational resources to assist may be warranted.

Participate in Consult Meetings

Any ethics consultation meeting concerning an inpatient should have a representative of the nursing staff involved in the process. If a nurse initiated the consult, it is expected that the requesting nurse would participate fully in the process. Additionally, the nursing perspective on the experience and burden of care is essential. Also, as various treatment options are discussed, the nurse can provide reality testing. Proposed clinical interventions might not be feasible, or alternatively, nurses' creativity in developing work-around solutions may be invaluable. Nurses can speak to the organization's resources and their ability to access them. Any clinical nurse's ethical concerns should be made visible to the ethics consultant, even if these concerns represent a singular or minority perspective. Professional integrity should not be compromised, and, in fact, the ethics consultation process should address this. Clinicians who explore the perspectives of others and reflect on all the values in play may successfully refocus on their obligation to honor the patient's values and thereby recognize they are not compromising their own values or professional obligations.

Learning From the Consultation Process

Although a variety of methodologies exist for clinical ethics consultation, if the consultant engages in ethical analysis and facilitates moral deliberation among all stakeholders, the experience should be a learning one for clinical nurses. The outcomes of the process will vary and might include identifying the ethically appropriate decision-maker, distinguishing the benefits and burdens of possible treatment options that can be ethically justifiable, or supporting a patient's right to reject or receive life-sustaining therapies. Consultants also give attention to moral distress on the part of clinical staff. Many organizations consider staff support an essential role for ethics consultants, with follow-up discussions, ethics rounds, debriefings, or facilitated ethics conversations to promote a healthy ethical climate and mitigate any moral distress (Helft, Bledsoe, Hancock, & Wocial, 2009; Nelson, 2009; Wocial, Hancock, Bledsoe, Chamness, & Helft, 2010). Consultants often include in their medical record entry references and background literature to facilitate understanding of the ethical dimensions of the case. After the consultation is documented, some consultants continue to follow the patient's care.

Conclusion

Technological advancements have changed the nature of illness by increasing the degree and duration of sickness and rendering near invisibility to the line between extending a life and extending a death as well as constantly changing the probabilities of therapeutic outcomes (Callahan, 2000). The ever-changing landscape of treatment options, and the decisions they present for patients and those who care for them, create challenges and uncertainties for all involved. Ethics consultation services are a resource to support patients, their families, and the clinical care team to navigate the many values and beliefs that both inspire and trouble all involved in healthcare. Bringing the knowledge and skill of the ethics consultant to the bedside represents sensitivity to the complexity of ethical issues embedded in healthcare. Clinical nurses are key stakeholders in care and are strategically positioned to recognize potential or emerging value conflicts. Requesting ethical advice is a professional obligation and should not be seen as a critique or indictment of others when values and beliefs are fueling uncertainty or conflict about what is the right thing to do. Nurses and physicians who reflect on their own values in contrast to those for whom they care will promote a culture of P&FCC—both at the bedside and within the organizations where they practice.

References

Agency for Healthcare Research and Quality (AHRQ). (n.d.). *Guide to patient and family engagement in hospital quality and safety.* Retrieved from http://www.ahrq.gov/professionals/systems/hospital/engagingfamilies/index.html

American Association of Critical-Care Nurses (AACN). (2011). *Beacon award for excellence application handbook.* Retrieved from http://www.aacn.org/wd/beaconapps/content/mainpage.pcms?menu=beaconapps

American Nurses Association (ANA). (2001). *Code of ethics for nurses.* Washington, DC: Author.

American Nurses Association (ANA). (2010). *Nursing's social policy statement: The essence of the profession.* Silver Spring, MA: Author.

American Nurses Credentialing Center (ANCC). (2008). *Magnet recognition program: Application manual 2008.* Silver Spring, MD: Author.

American Society for Bioethics and Humanities (ASBH). (2011). *Core competencies for healthcare ethics consultation* (2nd ed.). Glenview, IL: Author.

American Society for Bioethics and Humanities (ASBH) Clinical Ethics Task Force. (2009). *Improving competence in clinical ethics consultations: An education guide.* Glenview, IL: American Society for Bioethics and Humanities.

Aulisio, M. P., & Arnold, R. M. (2008). Role of the ethics committee: Helping to address value conflicts or uncertainties. *Chest, 134*(2), 417-424.

Baggs, J. G., Norton, S. A., Schmitt, M. H., Dombeck, M. T., Sellers, C. R., & Quinn, J. R. (2007). Intensive care unit cultures and end-of-life decision making. *Journal of Critical Care, 22*(2), 159-168.

Bell, J., & Breslin, J. M. (2008). Healthcare provider moral distress as a leadership challenge. *JONA's Healthcare Law, Ethics, and Regulation, 10*(4), 94-97.

Berlinger, N., Jennings, B., & Wolf, S. M. (2013). *The Hastings Center guidelines for decisions on life-sustaining treatment and care near the end of life* (2nd ed.). Oxford, UK: Oxford University Press.

Callahan, D. (2000). *The troubled dream of life: In search of a peaceful death.* Washington, DC: Georgetown University Press.

Centers for Medicare and Medicaid Services (CMS). (2010). Medicare and Medicaid programs: Changes to the hospital and critical access hospital conditions of participation to ensure visitation rights for all patients. *Federal Register, 75*(223), 70831-70844.

Craig, J. M., & May, T. (2006). Evaluating the outcomes of ethics consultation. *The Journal of Clinical Ethics, 17*(2), 168-180.

Cronenwett, L., Sherwood, G., Barnsteiner, J., Disch, J., Johnson, J., Mitchell, P., … Warren, J. (2007). Quality and safety education for nurses. *Nursing Outlook, 55*(3), 122-131.

Danis, M., Farrar, A., Grady, C., Taylor, C., O'Donnell, P., Soekem, K., & Ulrich, C. (2008). Does fear of retaliation deter request for ethics consultation? *Medicine, Health Care, and Philosophy, 11*(1), 27-34.

Delbanco, T., Berwick, D. M., Boufford, J. I., Edgman-Levitan, S., Ollenschläger, G., Plamping, D., & Rockefeller, R. G. (2001). Healthcare in a land called PeoplePower: Nothing about me without me. *Health Expectations, 4*(3), 144-150.

DeWolf Bosek, M. S. (2009). Identifying ethical issues from the perspective of the registered nurse. *JONA's Healthcare Law, Ethics, & Regulation, 11*(3), 91-99. doi:10.1097/NHL.0b013e3181b7a010

Dubler, N. N., Webber, M. P., Swiderski, D. M., & the Faculty and the National Working Group for the Clinical Ethics Credentialing Project. (2009). Charting the future: Credentialing, privileging, quality, and evaluation in clinical ethics consultation. *Hastings Center Report, 39*(6), 23-33.

DuVal, G., Sartorius, L., Clarridge, B., Gensler, G., & Danis, M. (2001). What triggers requests for ethics consultations? *Journal of Medical Ethics, 27*(Suppl 1), i24-i29.

Fox, E., Berkowitz, K. A., Chanko, B. L., & Powell, T. (2006). *Ethics consultation: Responding to ethics question in health care.* Washington, DC: Veterans Health Administration. Retrieved from http//:www.ethics.va.gov/docs/integratedethics/Ethics_Consultation_Responding_to_Ethics_Questions_in_Health_Care_20070808.pdf

Fox, E., Myers, S., & Pearlman, R. A. (2007). Ethics consultation in United States hospitals: A national survey. *American Journal of Bioethics, 7*(2), 13-25.

Gaudine, A., Lamb, M., LeFort, S. M., & Thorne, L. (2011). Barriers and facilitators to consulting hospital clinical ethics committees. *Nursing Ethics, 18*(6), 767-780.

Glen, S. (1999). Educating for interprofessional collaboration: Teaching about values. *Nursing Ethics, 6*(3), 202-213.

Gordon, E. J., & Hamric, A. B. (2006). The courage to stand up: The cultural politics of nurses' access to ethics consultation. *Journal of Clinical Ethics, 17*(3), 231-254.

Helft, P. R., Bledsoe, P. D., Hancock, M., & Wocial, L. D. (2009). Facilitated ethics conversations: A novel program for managing moral distress in bedside nursing staff. *JONA's Healthcare Law, Ethics, and Regulation, 11*(1), 27-33.

Institute for Healthcare Improvement (IHI). (n.d.). ISHAPED patient-centered approach to nurse shift change bedside report. Retrieved at http://www.ihi.org/resources/Pages/Tools/ISHAPEDPatientCenteredNurseShift ChangeBedsideReport.aspx

Institute of Medicine (IOM) Committee on Quality of Health Care in America. (2001). *Crossing the quality chasm: A new health system for the 21st century.* Washington, DC: National Academy Press.

Interprofessional Education Collaborative Expert Panel. (2011). *Core competencies for interprofessional collaborative practice: Report of an expert panel.* Washington, DC: Interprofessional Education Collaborative.

The Joint Commission (TJC). (2014). *Comprehensive accreditation and certification manual for hospitals.* (L.D.04.02.03, EP 1, EP 2). Author.

The Joint Commission on Accreditation of Healthcare Organizations. (1992). *Hospital accreditation manual* (Sections RI1 and R12). Chicago, IL: Author.

Kleinman, A. (2011). The divided self, hidden values, and moral sensibility in medicine. *Lancet, 377*(9768), 804-805.

Kodish, E., Fins, J. Braddock III, C., Cohn, F., Dubler, N. N., Danis, M.,…Kuczewski, M. G. (2013).Quality attestation for clinical ethics consultants: A two-step model from the American Society for Bioethics and Humanities. *Hastings Center Report, 43*(5) 26-36.

Kukla, R. (2007). How do patients know? *Hastings Center Report, 37*(5), 27-35.

Lehmann, L. S. (2012). Family dynamics and surrogate decision-making. In D. M. Hester & T. Schonfeld (Eds.), *Guidance for healthcare ethics committees* (pp. 63-70). New York, NY: Cambridge University Press.

Magill, G. (2013). Quality in ethics consultation. *Medicine, Health Care, and Philosophy, 16*(4), 761-774. doi:10.1007/s11019-013-9489-x

McClung, J. A., Kamer, R. S., DeLuca, M., & Barber, H. J. (1996). Evaluation of a medical ethics consultation service: Opinions of patients and health care providers. *American Journal of Medicine, 100*(4), 456-460.

Nelson, W. A. (2009). Ethical uncertainty and staff stress. *Healthcare Executive, 24*(4), 38-39.

Nilson, E. G., Acres, C. A., Tamerin, N. G., & Fins, J. J. (2008). Clinical ethics and the quality initiative: a pilot study for the empirical evaluation of ethics case consultation. *American Journal of Medical Quality, 23*(5), 356-364.

Orr, R. D., Morton, K. R., deLeon, D. M., & Fals, J. C. (1996). Evaluation of an ethics consultation service: Patient and family perspective. *American Journal of Medicine, 101*(2), 135-141.

Pavlish, C., Brown-Saltzman, K., Fine, A., & Jakel, P. (2013). Making the call: A proactive ethics framework. *HEC Forum, 25*(3), 269-283. doi:10.1007/s10730-013-9213-5

Pavlish, C., Hellyer, J. H., Brown-Saltzman, K., Miers, A. G., & Squire, K. (2013). Barriers to innovation: Nurses' risk appraisal in using a new ethics screening and early intervention tool. *Advances in Nursing Science, 36*(4), 304-319.

Post, L. F., Blustein, J., & Dubler, N. N. (2007). *Handbook for health care ethics committees.* Baltimore, MD: The Johns Hopkins University Press.

President's Commission for the Study of Ethical Problems in Medicine and Biomedical and Behavioral Research. (1983). *Deciding to forego life-sustaining treatment: A report on the ethical, medical, and legal issues in treatment decisions.* Washington, DC: U.S. Government Printing Office.

Quinlan, J., & Quinlan, J. (1996, April 12-13). Commemorative essay. *Conference proceedings: Quinlan: A twenty-year retrospective.* Princeton, NJ: Princeton University.

Quinn, J. R., Schmitt, M., Gedney Baggs, J., Norton, S. A., Dombeck, M. T., & Sellers, C. R. (2012). "The problem often is that we do not have a family spokesperson but a spokesperson group": Family member informal roles in end-of-life decision-making in adult ICUs. *American Journal of Critical Care, 21*(1), 43-51. doi:10.4037/ajcc2012520.

Scheunemann, L. P., Arnold, R. M., & White, D. B. (2012). The facilitated values history: Helping surrogates make authentic decisions for incapacitated patients with advanced illness. *American Journal of Critical Care Medicine, 186*(6), 480-486.

Silverman, H. J., Bellavance, E., & Childs, B. H. (2013). Ensuring quality in clinical ethics consultations: Perspectives of ethicists regarding process and prior training of consultants. *American Journal of Bioethics, 13*(2), 29-31. doi:10.1080/15265161.2012.75039

Spike, J. (2012). Ethics consultation process. In D. H. Hester & T. Schonfeld (Eds.), *Guidance for healthcare ethics committees* (pp. 42-47). New York: Cambridge University Press.

Sullivan, M. (2003). The new subjective medicine: Taking the patient's point of view on health care and health. *Social Science and Medicine, 56*(7), 1595-1604.

Tarzian, A. J., & ASBH Core Competencies Update Task Force. (2013). Health care ethics consultation: An update on core competencies and emerging standards from the American Society for Bioethics and Humanities' Core Competencies Update Task Force. *American Journal of Bioethics, 13*(2), 3-13.

Veatch, R. M, & Tai, E. (1980). Talking about death: Patterns of lay and professional change. *Annals of the American Academy of Political and Social Science, 447*(1), 29-45.

Walker, M. U. (1993). Keeping moral space open: New images of ethics consulting. *Hastings Center Report, 23*(2), 33-40.

Walton, M. K. (2012). Ethics consultation. In C. Ulrich, (Ed.), *Nursing ethics in everyday practice* (pp. 67-84). Indianapolis, IN: Sigma Theta Tau International.

Wocial, L. C., Hancock, M., Bledsoe, P. D., Chamness, A. R., & Helft, P. R. (2010). An evaluation of unit-based ethics conversations. *JONA's Healthcare Law, Ethics, and Regulation, 12*(2), 48-54.

Chapter 17

High-Intensity Situations That Provoke Conflict

Victoria L. Rich, PhD, RN, FAAN
Rita K. Adeniran, DrNP, RN, NEA-BC

Tamika is a 24-year-old, new-to-practice registered nurse (RN) who has completed 6 months of orientation as an operating room (OR) nurse at Packer Community Hospital (PCH) on the day shift and is now scheduled for the 3–11 p.m. shift. She is apprehensive because she has heard many stories about the attitudes of a number of nurses on that shift and is concerned that they may not help her if she asks. Her first shift went well, but her second shift takes a drastic turn. The unit is very busy and short-staffed, and the nurse manager approaches Tamika: "Tamika, we are in a bind and if there are any emergencies, I need you to circulate. You will be fine. Just remember everything you were taught. The other staff will help you." Later that evening, a bus overturns, and seven patients are sent to PCH. Tamika is assigned to circulate with Dr. Chen, a new general surgeon to Packer. As the case proceeds, the patient starts to hemorrhage; Dr. Chen demands instruments that Tamika has never heard of. Tamika breaks scrub and tries to find someone to help her. Everyone is busy and harshly tells her to ask someone else. Tamika finally finds the instruments, scrubs, and returns to the OR. As she proudly rushes into the room and says, "Dr. Chen, I found what you need!" Dr. Chen peers over his mask and yells: "You are too late! I don't need it now. You are totally incompetent, and I will see to it that you NEVER work with me again!"

Put yourself in this situation as a new nurse. How do you feel? What should you do next?

Conflict is an inescapable human phenomenon affecting all forms of social relationships. In healthcare, conflict is inevitable because of the high stakes of events and emotions involved (Gerardi, 2004). Forces of conflict in healthcare include poor communication; lack of alignment of values and preferences among patients, families, and healthcare providers; the unprecedented pace of change in an evolving healthcare system; and heightened consumerism. Conflict is embedded in the continuous shift in the roles and responsibilities of the interprofessional healthcare team, who may have divergent training philosophies, backgrounds, and personal values (Marshall & Robson, 2005). Healthcare providers' intense pressures to balance competing priorities of patient care, data gathering and integration, resource management, and care coordination with members of the interdisciplinary care team create the perfect environment for high-intensity conflict situations. When conflict, especially emotionally charged, high-intensity conflict, is handled in a positive manner, improved interpersonal relationships, productivity, and patient safety can be achieved. Moreover, when it is handled negatively and unprofessionally, fear, retaliation, turnover, and anger can occur, and patient safety can be jeopardized (Cox, 2006).

This chapter presents a high-intensity situation vignette to generate a starting point for thought, discussion, and constructive approaches among nurses and other healthcare providers. This particular situation involves intra-personal conflict among peers, but the principles can apply to other kinds of conflict, such as between staff and the family (as seen in Chapter 18 of this book), or among family members (Chapter 10). This chapter then attempts to equip healthcare providers with evidence-based wisdom to be readily and skillfully prepared to handle high-risk, emotionally charged situations. As is discussed later, conflict is inevitable within healthcare and sometimes can be helpful; what this chapter focuses on, however, is the high-intensity nature of healthcare that sets up so many situations for conflict, some avoidable, some not.

Defining Conflict

There is no universally accepted definition for conflict; however, there is agreement that conflict is rooted in miscommunication, perception of incompatible interests, tension, and divergent views between involved parties with potential for constructive or destructive effects (Brinkert, 2011). For the purpose of this chapter, *conflict* is defined as "the interaction of interdependent people who perceive incompatibility and the possibility of interference from others as a result of this incompatibility" (Folger, Poole, & Stutman, 2009, p. 4).

Prevalence of Conflict in Healthcare

Despite agreement on the destructive potential of unresolved, damaging, or toxic conflict, no broad-based epidemiological data are readily available regarding the prevalence of conflict in healthcare (Azoulay et al., 2009). However, some specialty studies provide indication of the pervasiveness of conflict. Breen, Abernethy, Abbott, and Tulsky (2001) report that healthcare providers perceived conflict in 78% of cases of critically ill patients who required decision-making. They also reported the presence of tension in the form of definite disagreement between staff and the patient's family in 33% of cases requiring recommendation to either limit or not limit life-sustaining treatments. Congruent with observations made by Breen et al. (2001), in a study of 656 ICU patients, Studdert et al. (2003) found that conflict occurred between the care team and patient/family in at least one out of every three patients with a prolonged stay. Causes of team-family conflict in the ICU included incongruent life-sustaining treatments, poor communication, uncertainty in patient wishes, and coping problems (e.g., uncertainty, fear, and anger).

Both studies reported three types of conflict in healthcare. They are:

1. Conflict between patients and/or their families and the healthcare team (team and patient/family conflict)
2. Conflict among members of the interdisciplinary care team (team conflict)
3. Conflict within families (intrafamily conflict)

Conflict between patients and/or their families and the healthcare team (team and patient/family conflict) was the most commonly reported form of conflict cited. Two landmark studies from the Institute of Medicine reports *Crossing the Quality Chasm* (2001) and *Unequal Treatment* (2003) underscore the imperative of effectively managing and resolving conflict in healthcare so that conflict does not impede quality and safety. Unresolved conflict can decrease patient safety and lead to poorer health outcomes and lower quality of care.

In 2009, The Joint Commission (TJC) recognized the changing cultural landscapes and the accompanying opportunities and challenges in healthcare. A new hospital accreditation standard, Leadership Standard LD.02.04.01, was implemented: Hospitals need to manage such conflict so that healthcare safety and quality is protected (Schyve, 2009). LD.02.04.01 requires hospitals to manage conflict between leadership groups to protect the quality and safety of care and also stipulates that hospitals establish a conflict-management process. Also, in July 2008, TJC issued a sentinel event alert that underscores the responsibilities of both the organization and individual members of the interdisciplinary care team in eliminating intimidating destructive behaviors or conflicts that have potential to undermine safe, quality healthcare (TJC, 2008). However, conflict can have positive effects. According to Dinkin, Filner, and Maxwell (2013) in the book *The Exchange Strategy for Managing Conflict in Health Care,* conflict is a necessary element and is unavoidable if people are working together: "Conflict is not about professional proficiency or training, it is about the reality of being human" (p. 11). Keys to keep in mind: Healthy conflict can (1) diffuse more serious conflicts, (2) stimulate a search for new facts or resolutions, and (3) increase group cohesion and performance.

Causes and Sources of High-Intensity Conflict in Healthcare

A hospital is a classic example of a work environment that is susceptible to misunderstandings and disputes (Marshall & Robson, 2005). Conflicts may arise from hospital policies; disagreements between providers and patients; providers' trying to balance competing priorities of research, education, and practice; and power struggles among members of the interdisciplinary care team. Differing values of changing patient and provider demographics that include ethnic, sociocultural, and religious diversity can potentially escalate a situation quickly into a conflict. These factors, individually or collectively, heighten the propensity for high-intensity conflicts in healthcare environments.

To prevent or effectively manage intense conflict, one must first understand its source. Sources of intense conflict in healthcare have been extensively discussed in the literature (Marshall &

Robson, 2005; Moore, 2003; Moore & Kordick, 2006). Moore (2003) provides a useful framework for understanding sources of conflict. According to Moore, conflicts may be categorized into five main types:

1. Data source of conflict
2. Interest source of conflict
3. Structural source of conflict
4. Relationship source of conflict
5. Value source of conflict (2003)

Data Source of Conflict

Data source of conflict occurs when there is divergence in healthcare information sharing and interpretation. These situations are likely to occur when professional nurses or other healthcare providers consciously or unconsciously withhold health information; provide inadequate information; or when information is late, error-ridden, and poorly interpreted by patients and/or their families (Gold, Philip, McIver, & Komesaroff, 2009; Moore & Kordick, 2006). For example, advanced practice providers and physicians sometimes withhold or fail to provide full disclosure of adverse events to their patients in the name of therapeutic privilege (Reichman, 2006). Therapeutic privilege undermines the patient-provider trust relationship and often provokes conflict. Information transparency is important to prevent data-source conflict in healthcare (Tang & Lansky, 2005; Weiss & Miranda, 2008).

Interest Source of Conflict

Interest source of conflict results from bureaucratic issues that frustrate patients and families. A hospital's policies, processes, and protocols may prompt interest source of conflict (Moore & Kordick, 2006). Emotionally charged interest-source tensions can produce high-intensity conflict between patients and families with staff, among staff, and among family members. Policies that restrict family visiting time for their loved ones during hospitalization are known to often cause unpleasant worries for families and tension in hospitals (Hardin, Bernhardt-Tindal, Hart, Stepp, & Henson, 2011; Lee et al., 2007; Whitton & Pittiglio, 2011).

Other interest-based conflicts may occur when professional nurses and other providers are not responsive to family requests—for example, refusing to have team conferences at a time that is compatible with the family's schedule, or not adapting hospital routines to a patient's routine (such as bathing in the evening rather than the early-morning hours, or not allowing patients to take their medications on their home schedules).

Relationship Source of Conflict

Relationship source of conflict arises from misperceptions and/or poor communication that generates strong emotions of disrespect, such as from uncaring attitudes or stereotyping or discriminatory comments. Relationship sources of conflict are likely to occur when professional nurses and other providers are more concerned with the need to complete tasks for the patients than giving emotional attention (McCabe, 2004; Moore & Kordick, 2006). In Tamika's situation described at the beginning of the chapter, her future relationship with Dr. Chen and her peer nurses will certainly affect her self-esteem and her professional demeanor not only to healthcare colleagues but possibly also to patients and families.

Structural Source of Conflict

Structural source of conflict arises from differing care goals or lack of clarity around goals, differing experience and power levels, and/or tension around the status of stakeholders involved in conflict (Brinkert, 2010). An example of a structural source of conflict is the physician-nurse power imbalance, in which some physicians feel privileged or may use aggressive tactics and behaviors to get their way. The high-intensity situation at the beginning of the chapter embodies this issue. Structural conflict is well documented in the OR and is labeled "surgical personality." This is when surgeons utilize intimidating behaviors to maintain control over the other members of the interdisciplinary care team whom they perceive to be of lower rank (Katz, 2007; Rogers et al., 2013). Structural conflict also occurs between patients and professional nurses and other providers when they are perceived as dictating treatment (medical paternalism) that the patient may refuse (Ho, 2009). Many nurses and other healthcare providers have difficulty adapting to the growth of patient and family engagement and consumerism. Walton and Barnsteiner (2012) describe *patient- and family-centered care* (P&FCC) as a healthcare service approach where the patient or designee is recognized as the main source of control and equal partner in providing compassionate and coordinated services that honor the patient's and family's preferences, values, and needs.

Structural conflict tends to be more common with patients who suffer from chronic and serious illnesses, causing some form of resource dependence and a long-term relationship with the medical care team (Moore & Kordick, 2006). The tension may come from the patient's request for more resources from the provider, who may be unable to provide these resources due to structural constraints, such as insurance limits or the patient's/family's attempt to participate in decision-making.

Value Source of Conflict

Value source of conflict occurs when involved parties utilize different criteria for evaluating the situation at hand. It occurs when deeply held beliefs and values drive the tension (Moore & Kordick, 2006). In situations where family or patients and staff hold different views, a value-based conflict occurs.

In addition to the five sources of conflict provided by Moore (2003), fear is a major source of conflict in healthcare that requires some discussion. Marshall and Robson (2005) state: "A culture of fear is a culture of conflict" (p. 39). Nurses' and other healthcare providers' and administrators' fear of litigation, professional discipline, increased insurance premiums, bad publicity, and/or the fear of simply being viewed as incompetent create anxiety and mistrust, posing barriers to effective communication, collaboration, and teamwork, ultimately causing conflict (Spears, 2005). In an attempt to be perfect, do no harm, be in charge, and protect one's self-esteem, the culture of fear has become entrenched in healthcare providers and has been termed the "stress strap of professionalism" (Nelson, 2012, p. 183). *Stress strap of professionalism* is a condition where an individual tries to defend healthcare decisions even when they are wrong (Waddington & Fletcher, 2005; Welch, 2011). Despite the current drive to manage medical errors with transparency and full disclosure in a just manner for all involved, fear and mistrust continue to be a source of tension for healthcare providers, patients, and families.

Conflict may also be categorized by intensity or duration. The intensity of conflict ranges from minor disagreements and differences of opinion and personality clashes to blatant hostility and violence. Duration of conflict can be expressed in time frames of occurrence, such as acute, subacute, chronic, and interminable (Katz, 2007). The outcome of any conflict situation is highly dependent on the source, intensity, duration, task at hand, and the conflict-resolution skills of those involved in the conflict.

Preventing, Resolving, and Managing High-Intensity Conflict

Because the sources of conflict in healthcare are numerous and multilayered, a comprehensive and multipronged approach is required to address it. Strategies must include techniques to prevent, manage, and eliminate destructive conflict, while promoting constructive outcomes (Way, Black, & Curtis, 2002). Often the source of conflict itself is less of a challenge than ineffective management when conflict escalates (Ting-Toomey et al., 2000). Utilizing the most appropriate conflict management or resolution strategy is critical to success. Early recognition of potential conflict situations and an ability to deal with conflict proactively and/or resolve conflict early in the process is an essential and important goal (Vivar, 2006).

Once a high-intensity conflict is identified, the goal is to work through opposing views or tension to reach a common goal of mutuality for best health outcomes. Constructively resolving high-intensity conflicts requires effective communication and problem-solving skills that are often lacking in the professional nurse and other providers' educational and training curriculum (Lee et al., 2008; Slaikeu, 1989, 1992; Walczak & Absolon, 2001). Constructive conflict-resolution skills can enhance relationships, provide freedom for decision-making, empower parties to innovate, solve problems, and bring about creative solutions to strengthen the patient/family-provider relationship as well as the relationships within and among members of the interdisciplinary care team (Smith, Tutor, & Phillips, 2001).

Researchers propose principles of gracious space, effective communication, and principled negotiation as systematic and effective tools to reduce, prevent, and constructively resolve conflict (Gerardi, 2004; Hughes, 2004; Marshall & Robson, 2003). These strategies can be employed individually or in combination to address any conflict.

Gracious Space

Gracious Space is a spirit and a setting where we "invite the stranger" and "embrace learning in public" (Hughes, 2004, p. 11). *Inviting the stranger* means we are open to diverse perspectives in order to gain clarity. *Learning in public* means that we truly listen to new thoughts or conflicting ideas and we are open to changing our minds (Hughes, 2004). Gracious Space can help create a safe place for authentic dialogue, fostering understanding and acceptance. The Gracious Space principles direct individuals or groups to give opinions without fear of criticism; have deep respect for differences in spite of disagreements or conflicting ideas; hold off judging based on diverse perspectives or culture; step back and reflect on assumptions, especially in conflicting situations; be curious, willing to learn and be influenced; and slow down and actively listen. When members of the interdisciplinary care team commit to using Gracious Space principles as a guide to their interactions, they appreciate the fact that multiple truths may exist in a particular situation and do not assume their own truth to be the only solution in dealing with each other or treating patients. They are more likely to show empathy when they attempt to feel something the "other" feels and to be more compassionate. Compassion gives rise to conviction of possibility, whereby conflict situations can be authentically discussed and potentially resolved.

Effective Communication

Communication is the process of exchanging information and feelings. It provides an opportunity to express viewpoints, share assumptions, and inquire about other ways of thinking. It involves the process of utilizing active listening skills to arrive at a shared understanding and a course of action (Bub, 2004; Saulo & Wagener, 2000). Effective communication skills are essential in resolving conflict because they reduce misconceptions and increase understanding through active listening.

Active Listening

Active listening involves being open, temporarily putting aside individual or group feelings, making a conscientious attempt to listen and to understand, to be truly curious about the other's experience. Examples of behaviors that demonstrate active listening include nodding the head, summarizing and/or restating the other person's or group's concerns in one's own words, and allowing the other person to finish speaking without interruption. These behaviors demonstrate empathy and acknowledgment of the information provided by the opponent. Other active-listening tactics involve using "I" instead of "you" when sending messages (Dusenbury, Falco, Lake, Brannigan, & Bosworth, 1997) and carefully and appropriately planning the time and setting for communicating certain information (Baile et al., 2000).

Using "I" Instead of "You" in Sending a Message

Using "I" to express your own feelings is a much more effective way to communicate, which conveys accountability for your own perspective. The "you" message may connote blame and accusation, with a tendency to label the other. The "I" message is less likely to put the other person on the defense than the "you" message. For example, when discussing options of transfer to an alternate level of care with a husband who disagrees with the idea, a possible response might be, *"I know this must be difficult for you. What are you most concerned about regarding your wife's transfer?"* The dialogue can progress onto a more positive path with this response, illustrating the goal of effective communication.

Appropriate Timing and Setting

The timing and setting of communication can have a great impact on the effectiveness of information exchange. It is important to assess yourself as well as the opposing party for readiness to engage in the issue that led to the conflict. A setting is optimal when the parties involved in conflict are alone in a private area and have ample time to discuss the issue. In the chapter's opening scenario, it is clear that the situation cannot be resolved in the middle of the OR during a surgery. The surgeon's response was inappropriate—but responding angrily in return is not helpful either. Rather, Tamika could seek the counsel of a valued colleague, talk over the situation, and discuss how to approach Dr. Chen in a neutral setting. If necessary, depending on his communication patterns, a charge nurse or the nurse manager might be invited to join the conversation to help achieve a respectful interaction.

Principled Negotiation

According to Fisher and Ury (1983), principled negotiation is an effective strategy for reaching good agreement in contentious situations. *Good agreement* is a wise, fair, and efficient approach to improving opposing parties' relationships by satisfying their divergent interests. Usually during negotiations, each party opens the discussion with his or her position, a strategy termed *positional bargaining*. Positional bargaining tends to neglect the other parties' interests, a tactic that perpetuates conflict and promotes insolvability. Principled negotiation provides a better way of reaching good agreements (Fisher, Ury, & Patton, 1991). Fisher and Ury (1983) have established four fundamental guidelines for principled negotiation as a process that can be effectively used to resolve conflict in almost any type of dispute. The four strategies are:

1. Separate the people and issues
2. Focus on interests, not positions
3. Generate options for mutual gains
4. Use objective criteria

Table 17.1 explains in detail the four principles of principled negotiation. We developed the tactics to operationalize the principles toward conflict resolution in 2012.

TABLE 17.1   Four Principles of Principled Negotiation (Fisher & Ury, 1983)

PRINCIPLES	EXPLANATION OF PRINCIPLE	TACTICS TO OPERATIONALIZE PRINCIPLES TOWARD CONFLICT RESOLUTION
Separate people and issues	This principle underscores the importance of recognizing that all conflicts involve two problems: (1) Relationship (2) Substance or content The two problems tend to be intertwined, so it is imperative to separate them in order to resolve the conflict situation. Separating people, self, and/or ego problems from the content helps reduce feeling personally attacked by the opposing party. Further, this principle directs the parties in conflict to be mindful of the following three types of relationship concepts: **Emotions:** Be emotionally aware by recognizing your own and others' emotions. **Perception:** Everyone has his or her own version of reality; be careful not to misinterpret other's intentions. Intentions do not always equal impact. **Communication:** Parties may not be speaking to each other; rather, they may be grandstanding for their respective constituencies. The parties may not be listening to each other but may instead be planning their own responses.	• Make a conscientious effort to understand the opponents' viewpoint and not misinterpret their intentions. • Openly acknowledge your feelings about the situation and encourage others to do the same. This will help acknowledge the legitimacy of emotions. The goal is to channel emotions to productive vision of conflict resolution. • Parties should not assume that their worst fears will become the actions of the other party. • Use active-listening skills to understand, appreciating the fact that understanding does not constitute agreement.

continues

TABLE 17.1 *continued*

PRINCIPLES	EXPLANATION OF PRINCIPLE	TACTICS TO OPERATIONALIZE PRINCIPLES TOWARD CONFLICT RESOLUTION
Focus on interests, not position	Position is something one has already decided, while interests are the purpose for the decision. Defining a problem in terms of positions means that at least one party will lose. Alternatively, problems defined in terms of interests can find shared and compatible solutions behind the contentions. It is easier to find a common ground that often leads to a win-win outcome when discussions are focused on interest.	• Identify the parties' interests in the polarizing issue. • Ask why the parties hold the positions they do and why they do not hold some other possible positions to clarify interest. • Identify commonality in opposing parties' interests, such as economic, security, or safety interests, and leverage findings to frame a shared solution. • Remain open to discussing desired solutions rather than focusing on past events, and be ready to accommodate the interests of both parties.
Generate options for mutual gains	This principle accentuates the imperative of exploring all possibilities for a shared solution. Fisher, Ury, and Patton (1991) have identified four challenges to generating creative options for solving a problem. They are: (1) Deciding on an option prematurely, failing to consider other alternatives (2) Narrowing options to find a single solution or answer to the problem (3) Defining the problem in win-lose terms (4) Alluding that the opposing party must come up with the solution Parties in conflict should make conscientious efforts to mitigate these challenges.	• Brainstorm to generate a variety of possible solutions; propose solutions that can appeal to the opposing parties. • Search for mutual solutions, and merge different interests to be compatible and possibly complementary. • Identify party's decision-makers and design goals that appeal to them.

PRINCIPLES	EXPLANATION OF PRINCIPLE	TACTICS TO OPERATIONALIZE PRINCIPLES TOWARD CONFLICT RESOLUTION
Generate options for mutual gains *(continued)*	Fisher et al. (1991) also suggest four techniques for overcoming the obstacles of generating options for mutual gains: (1) Separate the process of inventing options from the act of judging them (2) Broaden the options and consider many ways to find solutions (3) Search for mutual gains (4) Invent ways of making decisions easy They concur that this principle is the hardest in using principled negotiation for conflict resolution.	• Reconcile different interests by identifying and conceding on items that are of low cost to one party but of high benefit to the other and vice versa. • Evaluate, refine, and improve solutions, starting with the most promising proposal.
Use objective criteria	The principle of objective criteria declares that solutions should be based on merits independent of the will of either side. Decisions based on merits (such as scientific findings, professional standards, or legal precedent) make agreement easier. Merit consideration should address partners' interest, not position; pushing hard on interest can stimulate partners to create innovative, mutually advantageous solutions.	• Establish which criteria are best for the situation. • Utilize legitimate and practical criteria. • Test objectivity of criteria, asking if both sides would agree to be bound by those standards • Use other parties' reasoning to support your own opinions when applicable. • All parties should commit to keeping an open mind. • Yield to principles; be reasonable and accommodative, but do not succumb to threats, pressures, or bribes. • When the other party stubbornly refuses to be reasonable, discussion may shift from a search for substantive criteria to a search for procedural criteria.

As seen in Table 17.1, principled negotiation offers useful, logical, and systematic options to effectively resolve conflict and strengthen relationships. It has potential to promote authentic dialogue, effective communication, and good agreement (Fisher et al., 1991). Healthcare providers can apply principled negotiation tactics to resolve or mitigate many of the inherent high-intensity situations that produce conflict in healthcare.

Conflict Management

Conflict management stems from the view that all conflicts cannot be avoided or perhaps even resolved, but all conflicts can be managed, minimized, or diffused to prevent escalation. Effectively managing conflicts can reduce unnecessary escalation and ultimately reduce the negative consequences of conflict. The literature has identified five main strategies to manage conflict. They are (1) avoiding, (2) compromising, (3) integrating, (4) accommodating, and (5) competing (Blake & Mouton, 1964; Rahim & Magner, 1995; Thomas, 1976). It is the responsibility of the individual or group involved in the conflict to identify the most suitable style to manage a specific conflict situation (Al-Hamdan, Shukri, & Anthony, 2011). Choosing the most effective and appropriate strategy to manage a particular circumstance can make the difference between constructive and destructive conflict management. Table 17.2 identifies and summarizes five styles of conflict management from the literature.

TABLE 17.2 Conflict Management Styles

CONFLICT MANAGEMENT STYLE	STYLE EXPLANATION	STYLE APPROPRIATE AND USEFUL WHEN
1 Avoiding	Avoidance is a conflict management style that seeks to evade conflict entirely. This style can be effective in very few situations, but overall, it is a weak and ineffective management style.	• Agreement is impossible • Tension is too trivial • There is someone in a better position to handle the conflict
2 Accommodating	Accommodation operates when one party is willing to meet the needs of the other at the expense of their own. The accommodator is not assertive and is highly cooperative and may stand to lose more.	• Issues matter more to the other • Peace is more valuable than winning • Expecting a greater benefit than the outcome of the conflict situation

CONFLICT MANAGEMENT STYLE	STYLE EXPLANATION	STYLE APPROPRIATE AND USEFUL WHEN
3 Collaborating	Collaboration works to meet the needs of involved parties. Opponents may be highly assertive, yet they are cooperative and able to acknowledge the importance of everyone involved.	• Leverage multiple viewpoints for best solution or innovation. • Interest is very important and cannot be met by few or any tradeoffs.
4 Competing	Competition is used when parties take a firm stand about their positions and will not budge. Competition as a strategy can escalate conflict, leaving opponents feeling bruised and resentful.	• There is an emergency. • Defend against someone who is trying to exploit a situation selfishly.
5 Compromising	Compromise seeks to find solutions that partially satisfy the parties involved in the conflict. Everyone is expected to give up something to reach a shared agreement or decision.	• The cost of conflict is greater than the cost of losing ground. • Equal-strength opponents are at a standstill. • There is a deadline looming.

Consequences of Unresolved Conflict in Healthcare

The consequences of conflict in healthcare can be serious, with physical and psychological manifestations in people as well as organizational effects (Almost, 2006; Walczak & Absolon, 2001). Conflicts threaten one's esteem and can elicit feelings of anger, disgust, and fear (McEwen, 1998). Conflict can cause providers to become angry, rigid, uncooperative, and dissatisfied with their work (Cox, 2003; Katz, 2007). Persistent conflict in healthcare organizations has been found to be associated with a lower level of job satisfaction, increased turnover, absenteeism, lower job commitment, and more reports of grievances (Almost, 2006; Danna & Griffin, 1999). Conflict distracts providers' focus on patients, causing harm that can jeopardize patient safety, quality care, and best outcomes (Katz, 2007). Pervasive conflict interferes with collaboration among members of interdisciplinary care teams and their departments and increases providers' error rates (Watson & Steiert, 2002). Unresolved conflict can be costly, serving as the instigator for malpractice claims (Levinson, Roter, Mullooly, Dull, & Frankel, 1997). As healthcare organizations strive to deliver excellence and improve quality of healthcare, there is no doubt that providers must continue to acquire the skills necessary to alleviate, manage, reduce, and avoid the negative consequences of conflict.

A Patient- and Family-Centered Approach to Preventing Conflict in Healthcare

Analysis of research and anecdotal evidence reveals that traditional provider-centered approaches (medical paternalism) to delivery of care contribute to inevitable conflict situations (Ho, 2009; Rodriguez-Osorio & Dominguez-Cherit, 2008). Disagreements may arise from medical paternalism, providers' dominance, and ethnocentrism in planning, delivering, and evaluating healthcare for patients (Ho, 2009; Putsch III & Joyce, 1990); poor provider communication skills; hospital policies and routines that limit the patient's and family's participation in care planning and delivery (Ågård & Lomborg, 2011; Berwick & Kotagal, 2004); and patient and family feelings of pressure to make certain healthcare decisions, including end-of-life decisions (Choong et al., 2010). Hospital policies can often create conflict, such as when a husband wants to stay with his wife at the hospital following admission but is asked to leave because hospital policy does not support family members' staying with patients. Such decisions go against the principles of P&FCC. A P&FCC approach of dignity and respect for the patient and family encourages patient and family engagement, which allows for the establishment and further development of a trusting relationship, which is needed to navigate the challenging situations that can ensue. Furthermore, family members can alert clinicians to change in the patient's status and can promote timely and effective communication of information, enhancing transparency, participation, collaboration, and trust building.

The concepts of P&FCC, including dignity and respect for patients and families, information sharing, and active participation of the patient and family in care planning, promote a positive patient-provider relationship that prevents and reduces conflict situations, along with laying the foundation to facilitate effective resolution of unavoidable conflicts (Abraham & Moretz, 2012; Choong et al., 2010). Indeed, it is logical to conclude that the P&FCC approach to healthcare delivery is a proactive strategy to prevent all types of conflict found in healthcare settings: (1) healthcare team and patient/family, (2) interdisciplinary healthcare team members, and (3) intra-family conflicts. Further, by appreciating, acknowledging, and responding to the patient's and family's unique circumstances, emotions, and health challenges, providers can alleviate and reduce conflict in healthcare, fostering a culture of graciousness, compassion, and excellence.

Ways to demonstrate graciousness and compassion involve a provider's skills to perceive and address impending conflict and to present treatment options, including end-of-life decisions and bad news. Nurses and other providers can also promote excellence in healthcare by their ability to understand and appreciate the patient/family perception of their health challenge or situation and cultural values or preferences, fully participating in care planning and goal establishment, timely and effective communication, and transparency. These concepts are the hallmarks of P&FCC.

Conclusion

Conflict is inherent in the healthcare environment and can occur between patients and their families and the healthcare team (team and patient/family conflict), within the members of the interdisciplinary care team (team conflict), and among family members (intra-family conflict) (Studdert et al., 2003; Walczak & Absolon, 2001). Some provider behaviors that cause conflict are avoidable. To alleviate avoidable conflict in healthcare, it is essential that providers acknowledge that conflict exists, analyze the causes and sources of conflict, and take action to prevent, reduce, and mitigate the causes of conflict in healthcare.

Providers should also be aware of and sensitive to how illness affects individual patients and their families and be ready to mediate the dissonance that may exist in the patient/family and providers' perspectives of the patient experience, care planning, and treatment decisions. When conflict does occur, providers should use the most appropriate strategy to resolve or manage conflict.

In pursuit of excellent, safe, and cost-effective healthcare, hospitals and other healthcare organizations are employing a P&FCC approach that is grounded in mutually beneficial partnerships among healthcare providers, patients, and families to mitigate the inherent burden of illness and disease, including alleviating conflict-provoking situations (Abraham & Moretz, 2012). Hospitals that utilize P&FCC welcome family members, not only lifting the many restrictions that have historically limited their involvement but also actively partnering with patients and families in care planning and decision-making. The P&FCC approach to care helps establish a firm relationship between patients/families and providers that ultimately helps reduce conflict occurrence and facilitate ease in conflict resolution if that becomes necessary.

References

Abraham, M., & Moretz, J. G. (2012). Implementing patient- and family-centered care: Part I—Understanding the challenges. *Pediatric Nursing, 38*(1), 44-47.

Ågård, A. S., & Lomborg, K. (2011). Flexible family visitation in the intensive care unit: Nurses' decision-making. *Journal of Clinical Nursing, 20*(7/8) 1106-1114. doi: 10.1111/j.1365-2702.2010.03360.x

Al-Hamdan, Z., Shukri, R., & Anthony, D. (2011). Conflict management styles used by nurse managers in the Sultanate of Oman. *Journal of Clinical Nursing, 20*(3/4), 571-580.

Almost, J. (2006). Conflict within nursing work environments: Concept analysis. *Journal of Advanced Nursing, 53*(4), 444-453.

Azoulay, É., Timsit, J. F., Sprung, C. L., Soares, M., Rusinová, K., Lafabrie, A.,...Schlemmer, B. (2009). Prevalence and factors of intensive care unit conflicts. *American Journal of Respiratory and Critical Care Medicine, 180*(9), 853-860.

Baile, W. F., Buckman, R., Lenzi, R., Glober, G., Beale, E. A., & Kudelka, A. P. (2000). SPIKES—A six-step protocol for delivering bad news: Application to the patient with cancer. *The Oncologist, 5*(4), 302-311. doi: 10.1634/theoncologist.5-4-302

Berwick, D. M., & Kotagal, M. (2004). Restricted visiting hours in ICUs: Time to change. *JAMA: Journal of the American Medical Association, 292*(6), 736-737.

Blake, R. R., & Mouton, J. S. (1964). *The managerial grid.* Houston, TX: Gulf.

Breen, C. M., Abernethy, A. P., Abbott, K. H., & Tulsky, J. A. (2001). Conflict associated with decisions to limit life-sustaining treatment in intensive care units. *JGIM: Journal of General Internal Medicine, 16*(5), 283-289.

Brinkert, R. (2010). A literature review of conflict communication causes, costs, benefits and interventions in nursing. *Journal of Nursing Management, 18*(2), 145-156.

Brinkert, R. (2011). Conflict coaching training for nurse managers: A case study of a two-hospital health system. *Journal of Nursing Management, 19*(1), 80-91.

Bub, B. (2004). The patient's lament: Hidden key to effective communication: How to recognize and transform. *Medical Humanities, 30*(2), 63-69.

Choong, K., Cupido, C., Nelson, E., Arnold, D. M., Burns, K., Cook, D., & Meade, M. (2010). A framework for resolving disagreement during end of life care in the critical care unit. *Clinical & Investigative Medicine, 33*(4), E240-E240.

Cox, K. B. (2003). The effects of intrapersonal, intragroup, and intergroup conflict on team performance effectiveness and work satisfaction. *Nursing Administration Quarterly, 27*(2), 153-163.

Cox, K. B. (2006). Power and conflict. In D. L. Huber (Ed.), *Leadership and nursing care management* (pp. 501-542). Philadelphia, PA: Saunders Elsevier.

Danna, K., & Griffin, R. W. (1999). Health and well-being in the workplace: A review and synthesis of the literature. *Journal of Management, 25*(3), 357-384.

Dinkin, S. P., Filner, B. A., & Maxwell, L. (2013). *The exchange strategy for managing conflict in healthcare: How to diffuse emotions and create solutions when stakes are high.* New York, NY: McGraw Hill.

Dusenbury, L., Falco, M., Lake, A., Brannigan, R., & Bosworth, K. (1997). Nine critical elements of promising violence prevention programs. *Journal of School Health, 67*(10), 409-414.

Fisher, R., & Ury, W. (1983). *Getting to yes: Negotiating agreement without giving in.* New York, NY: Penguin Books.

Fisher, R., Ury, W., & Patton, B. (1991). *Getting to yes: Negotiating agreement without giving in.* London, UK: Random House.

Folger, J. P., Poole, M. S., & Stutman, R. K. (2009). *Working through conflict: Strategies for relationships, groups, and organizations.* Boston, MA: Allyn and Bacon.

Gerardi, D. (2004). Using mediation techniques to manage conflict and create healthy work environments. *AACN Clinical Issues: Advanced Practice in Acute & Critical Care, 15*(2), 182-195.

Gold, M., Philip, J., McIver, S., & Komesaroff, P. A. (2009). Between a rock and a hard place: Exploring the conflict between respecting the privacy of patients and informing their carers. *Internal Medicine Journal, 39*(9), 582-587.

Hardin, S. R., Bernhardt-Tindal, K., Hart, A., Stepp, A., & Henson, A. (2011). Critical-care visitation: The patients' perspective. *Dimensions of Critical Care Nursing, 30*(1), 53-61.

Ho, A. (2009). "They just don't get it!" When family disagrees with expert opinion. *Journal of Medical Ethics, 35*(8), 497-501.

Hughes, P. (2004). *Gracious space: A practical guide for working better together.* Seattle, WA: Center for Ethical Leadership.

Institute of Medicine (IOM). (2001). *Crossing the quality chasm: A new health system for the 21st century.* Washington, DC: National Academy Press

Institute of Medicine (IOM). (2003). *Unequal treatment: Confronting racial and ethnic disparities in healthcare.* Washington, DC: National Academies Press.

The Joint Commission (TJC). (2008). Sentinel event alert: Behaviors that undermine a culture of safety. Retrieved from http://www.jointcommission.org/assets/1/18/SEA_40.PDF

Katz, J. D. (2007). Conflict and its resolution in the operating room. *Journal of Clinical Anesthesia, 19*(2), 152-158.

Lee, L., Berger, D. H., Awad, S. S., Brandt, M. L., Martinez, G., & Brunicardi, F. C. (2008). Conflict resolution: Practical principles for surgeons. *World Journal of Surgery, 32*(11), 2331-2335.

Lee, M. D., Friedenberg, A. S., Mukpo, D. H., Conray, K., Palmisciano, A., & Levy, M. M. (2007). Visiting hours policies in New England intensive care units: Strategies for improvement. *Critical Care Medicine, 35*(2), 497-501

Levinson, W., Roter, D. L., Mullooly, J. P., Dull, V. T., & Frankel, R. M. (1997). Physician-patient communication: The relationship with malpractice claims among primary care physicians and surgeons. *JAMA, 277*(7), 553-559.

Marshall, P., & Robson, R. (2003). Conflict resolution in healthcare: An overview. *Interaction, 16*(1/2), 1-7. Retrieved from http://www.mediatecalm.ca/pdfs/conflict_resolution_overview.pdf

Marshall, P., & Robson, R. (2005). Preventing and managing conflict: Vital pieces in the patient safety puzzle. *Healthcare Quarterly, 8*(Sp), 39-44.

McCabe, C. (2004). Nurse-patient communication: An exploration of patients' experiences. *Journal of Clinical Nursing, 13*(1), 41-49.

McEwen, B. S. (1998). Protective and damaging effects of stress mediators. *New England Journal of Medicine, 338*(3), 171-179.

Moore, C. W. (2003). *The mediation process: Practical strategies for resolving conflict.* San Francisco, CA: Jossey-Bass.

Moore, J. B., & Kordick, M. F. (2006). Sources of conflict between families and health care professionals. *Journal of Pediatric Oncology Nursing, 23*(2), 82-91.

Nelson, H. W. (2012). Dysfunctional health service conflict: Causes and accelerants. *Health Care Manager, 31*(2), 178-191.

Putsch III, R. W., & Joyce, M. (1990). Dealing with patients from other cultures. In H. K. Walker, W. D. Hall, & J. W. Hurst (Eds.), *Clinical methods: The history, physical, and laboratory examinations* (3rd ed.) (pp. 1050-1065). Boston, MA: Butterworths.

Rahim, M. A., & Magner, N. R. (1995). Confirmatory factor analysis of the styles of handling interpersonal conflict: First-order factor model and its invariance across groups. *Journal of Applied Psychology, 80*(1), 122-132.

Reichman, J. H. (2006). Withholding information from patients (Therapeutic privilege) (CEJA Report 2-A-06). Retrieved from http://www.ama-assn.org/resources/doc/code-medical-ethics/8082a.pdf

Rodriguez-Osorio, C. A., & Dominguez-Cherit, G. (2008). Medical decision making: Paternalism versus patient-centered (autonomous) care. *Current Opinion in Critical Care, 14*(6), 708-713

Rogers, D. A., Lingard, L., Boehler, M. L., Espin, S., Mellinger, J. D., Schindler, N., & Klingensmith, M. (2013). Surgeons managing conflict in the operating room: Defining the educational need and identifying effective behaviors. *The American Journal of Surgery, 205*(2), 125-130.

Saulo, M., & Wagener, R. J. (2000). Mediation training enhances conflict management by healthcare personnel. *American Journal of Managed Care, 6*(4), 473-483.

Schyve, P. M. (2009). *Leadership in healthcare organizations: A guide to Joint Commission leadership standards.* San Diego, CA: The Governance Institute.

Slaikeu, K. A. (1989). Designing dispute resolution systems in the health care industry. *Negotiation Journal, 5*(4), 395-400.

Slaikeu, K. A. (1992). Conflict management: Essential skills for healthcare managers. *Journal of Healthcare Materiel Management, 10*(10), 36-38.

Smith, S. B., Tutor, R. S., & Phillips, M. L. (2001). Resolving conflict realistically in today's health care environment. *Journal of Psychosocial Nursing & Mental Health Services, 39*(11), 36-45.

Spears, P. (2005). Managing patient care error: Nurse leaders' perspectives. *Journal of Nursing Administration, 35*(5), 223-224.

Studdert, D. M., Mello, M. M., Burns, J. P., Puopolo, A. L., Galper, B. Z., Truog, R. D., & Brennan, T. A. (2003). Conflict in the care of patients with prolonged stay in the ICU: Types, sources, and predictors. *Intensive Care Medicine, 29*(9), 1489-1497.

Tang, P. C., & Lansky, D. (2005). The missing link: Bridging the patient-provider health information gap. *Health Affairs, 24*(5), 1290-1295.

Thomas, K. W. (1976). Conflict and conflict management. In M. D. Dunnette (Ed.), *Handbook of industrial and organizational psychology* (pp. 889-935). Chicago, IL: Rand McNally.

Ting-Toomey, S., Yee-Jung, K. K., Shapiro, R. B., Garcia, W., Wright, T. J., & Oetzel, J. G. (2000). Ethnic/cultural identity salience and conflict styles in four U.S. ethnic groups. *International Journal of Intercultural Relations, 24*(1), 47-81.

Vivar, C. G. (2006). Putting conflict management into practice: A nursing case study. *Journal of Nursing Management, 14*(3), 201-206.

Waddington, K., & Fletcher, C. (2005). Gossip and emotion in nursing and health-care organizations. *Journal of Health Organization & Management, 19*(4/5), 378-394.

Walczak, M. B., & Absolon, P. L. (2001). Essentials for effective communication in oncology nursing: Assertiveness, conflict management, delegation, and motivation. *Journal for Nurses in Staff Development, 17*(3), 159-162.

Walton, M. K., & Barnsteiner, J. (2012). Patient-centered care. In J. G. Sherwood & J. Barnsteiner (Eds.), *Quality and safety in nursing: A competency approach to improving outcomes* (pp. 67-89). West Sussex, UK: Wiley Blackwell.

Watson, V., & Steiert, M. J. (2002). Verbal abuse and violence: The quest for harmony in the OR. *SSM, 8*(4), 16-22.

Way, J., Black A. L., & Curtis, J. R. (2002). Withdrawing life support and resolution of conflict with families. *British Medical Journal, 325*(7376), 1342-1345.

Weiss, P. M., & Miranda, F. (2008). Transparency, apology and disclosure of adverse outcomes. *Obstetrics and Gynecology Clinics of North America, 35*(1), 53-62.

Welch, S. (2011). Quality matters: Deny and defend: Apologizing hampered by physician culture, risk management. *Emergency Medicine News, 33*(3), 12, 24.

Whitton, S., & Pittiglio, L. I. (2011). Critical care open visiting hours. *Critical Care Nursing Quarterly, 34*(4), 361-366.

Chapter 18

Working With Abusive, Bullying, or Violent Patients and Families

Susan A. Phillips, MSN, RN, PMHCNS-BC

Marjorie, a registered nurse (RN), arrived early to work the night shift on the postpartum unit of a community hospital where she has been employed as a clinical staff nurse for 5 years. Marjorie found that she was assigned to care for a 19-year-old, married, female patient named Paula who had delivered a healthy baby girl earlier that day. The mother had experienced no physiological complications during the pregnancy or birth and the baby girl had a good APGAR score in the delivery room. The mother was resting comfortably in bed and breastfeeding was being initiated. Paula's husband Jay had been in and out of Paula's hospital room several times to make phone calls and to obtain food since Marjorie started work at 7:00 p.m. Marjorie noted the patient's husband was supportive and attentive in response to the new mother's needs. However, the situation changed abruptly later that evening at about 8:15 p.m. when another young male visitor arrived to visit Paula, whom Marjorie immediately recognized as being intoxicated with alcohol. This was evidenced by the odor of alcohol on his breath, slurred speech, and an unsteady gait. When he arrived in Paula's room, he announced quite loudly that he was the baby's father and told Jay to get out of the room. Paula recognized the young man and addressed him by name, but she was obviously frightened, humiliated, and shocked at this confrontational and dangerous situation taking place before her in her hospital room. Marjorie recognized that this stressful family situation was quickly getting out of control and she knew that help was needed right away. Marjorie was also aware that alcohol and/or drug abuse is a contributing factor to violence. Marjorie was afraid harm could come to the infant, the mother, herself, or either of the two men, and possibly other people in the vicinity of the patient's room, especially if a weapon had been brought into the hospital. Jay refused to leave and now a heated argument was taking place between the two young men. It looked like neither man was going to back down. Marjorie needed to act quickly.

Could this incident happen at your facility? Would you know how to respond? Fortunately, most family members that nurses encounter are grateful for the care and treatment provided to their loved ones in the healthcare setting. A small percentage of families are more challenging to interact with, and occasionally family members may exhibit behaviors that disrupt the flow of patient care and may become hostile or aggressive toward healthcare providers. For that reason, anger management is becoming increasingly important and relevant to nursing care. In 2004, among healthcare and social assistance workers, there were 11,790 workplace assaults; compared to American workers in other industries, healthcare has the highest rates of assault injuries in the workforce (American Nurses Association [ANA], 2006). This chapter will focus on working with abusive, bullying, or violent patients, family members, and visitors with strategies for individual nurses, organizations, and treatment teams to prevent and manage violent situations that may arise in healthcare.

What Is Workplace Violence?

The National Institute for Occupational Safety and Health (NIOSH) defines workplace violence as "violent acts, including physical assaults and threats of assault, directed toward persons at work or on duty" (NIOSH, 1996, para. 4). The Emergency Nurses Association (ENA, 2010) published a position statement which defines workplace violence as any physical assault, emotional or verbal abuse, threatening, harassing, or coercive behavior in the workplace that causes physical or emotional harm. The emergency department is particularly exposed and vulnerable to workplace violence because it is well known by drug seekers and gang members that emergency departments keep a lot of drugs and are easy to access (Allen, 2009). Weiss defines *disruptive behavior* as "any act by patients (or family members or visitors) that threatens the safety of staff, creates an intimidating environment, or interferes with the capacity of staff to provide safe and empathic care" (2012, p. 1).

Workplace Violence Statistics

Current statistics on workplace violence in healthcare organizations are alarming. Consider the following:

- Healthcare workers account for approximately two-thirds of non-fatal workplace violence injuries involving missed days from work, placing healthcare workers at five times the risk for workplace violence injuries than the overall workforce (National Institute for Occupational Safety and Health [NIOSH], 1996).

- In a survey conducted by the ENA in 2011, findings over a 7-day period demonstrated that 12.1% of respondents experienced physical violence and 42.5% of respondents experienced verbal abuse (ENA, 2011).

- Violence accounted for about 17% of all fatal work injuries in 2012 (Bureau of Labor Statistics, 2013).

- In a study of student nurses, 52% reported having been threatened or having experienced verbal abuse at work (Longo, 2007).

Violence can be exhibited in many forms, such as verbal abuse, sexual or racial harassment, bullying, threats, damage to property, physical assault, or homicide (Zuzelo, 2007). Workplace violence significantly affects nursing practice and contributes to physical injuries, psychological trauma, decreased productivity, and low morale among nurses. In addition to the physical and psychological effects on victims of workplace violence, negative effects incurred by healthcare organizations may include financial loss from insurance claims, lost productivity, legal expenses, property damage, and staff replacement costs (ANA, n. d.).

Why Patients and Families Exhibit Violent Behavior

Many patients and families come into the hospital with complex psychosocial issues and significant psychological issues. A patient's medical/surgical condition or traumatic injuries that are compounded by psychosocial issues may complicate hospitalization and generate conflict (Phillips, 2007). Families may be reacting to the stress of a loved one's illness or hospitalization and have exhausted the internal resources needed to enable them to cope. Patients may be experiencing pain, drug or nicotine cravings, discomfort, irritability, and distress. Often family members feel they must speak up on behalf of their loved ones and sometimes they may exhibit aggressive behavior in their efforts to advocate for their loved ones. Frustration can be exacerbated by poor interpersonal skills or cognitive impairment that limits emotional expression. When interpersonal stress and conflict occurs with patients and family members, the nurse's concerns for personal safety increases.

Factors That Contribute to Violence

Nurses work in close contact with patients and family members who may present to hospital nursing units in impaired, fatigued, or angry states (Zuzelo, 2007). Some individuals have learned to respond to stress with anger and may become violent when expectations are unmet or they encounter hospital rules and authority figures. Nurses must have an understanding of the complexity of workplace violence to be able to intervene appropriately.

There are numerous factors that may contribute to the onset of violence from a visitor, significant other, or family member that are beyond the nurse's control in the healthcare setting. There are both intrinsic and extrinsic factors that may contribute to violence. Intrinsic factors are experienced by the individual internally, whereas extrinsic factors are factors external to the individual in the environment.

TABLE 18.1 Intrinsic and Extrinsic Factors That Contribute to Violence

INTRINSIC FACTORS	EXTRINSIC FACTORS
Alcohol withdrawal	Long wait times
Confusion	Poor communication with medical staff
Delirium	Inexperienced practitioners
Pain	Misinformation
Anxiety	Rigid hospital policies and procedures
Irritability	Delayed access to care and treatment
Nicotine cravings	Temperatures too hot or too cold
Cognitive disorders (e.g., dementia, traumatic brain injury)	Overcrowded waiting rooms
An unfamiliar environment	Understaffing
Personality disorders (e.g., antisocial personality disorder)	Poor care coordination
Psychosis (e.g., hallucinations, delusions, paranoia)	
Frustration	
Emotions (e.g., fear, shame, humiliation)	
Impulsivity	
Poor interpersonal skills	
Fear of the unknown	
Feeling trapped	
Getting bad news	
Financial pressures	
A history of violence	

Sources: Crisis Prevention Institute, 2005; Gillespie, Gates, Miller, & Howard, 2010; NIOSH, 2002; Phillips, 2007

Substance Abuse

Substance abuse is a global issue affecting healthcare in both rural and urban areas of the country. Substance abuse includes addictive substances such as stimulants, opioids, cannabis, and hallucinogens, and recently bath salts have become problematic. Polysubstance abuse is common, especially when combined with alcohol. Patients may experience extreme withdrawal symptoms and cravings in the hospital that may or may not be adequately addressed, which often leads to premature discharges against medical advice, power struggles, and sometimes violence. Methamphetamine is an addictive central nervous system stimulant, and chronic use leads to depletion of the neurotransmitters dopamine and serotonin and structural brain alterations that have detrimental mental effects on the brain and results in cognitive impairment from drug-induced brain injury (Thompson et al., 2004). Unfortunately these changes may have a negative impact on the individual's interpersonal skills and limit their ability to resolve conflict in an adult manner. Bullying and intimidation are common behaviors that are influenced by drug and alcohol use (Zuzelo, 2007).

Although methamphetamine use is down by almost 50%, illicit drug use in America has been increasing, with an estimated 22.5 million Americans aged 12 or older (8.7% of the population) using an illicit drug or abusing a psychotherapeutic medication (such as a pain reliever, tranquilizer, or stimulant) within the past month (National Institute on Drug Abuse [NIDA], 2012). Use of hallucinogens and synthetic compounds is also down, but the rapid creation of new drugs poses problems in diagnosing their presence and identifying countermeasures for their effects. Rapid mood swings and wildly aberrant behavior are associated with a number of these drugs, which makes it difficult to anticipate violence or other disruptive acts.

Societal Influences

Societal and global violence is currently much more evident and problematic than in previous decades. News broadcasts on television, newspapers, movies, websites, video games, television crime shows, sports, and books all portray violence vividly and repeatedly expose countless people around the globe to violence on a daily basis. What is considered acceptable behavior in society today has significantly changed over previous decades. Disrespect and incivility toward healthcare professionals such as nurses and physicians has become more normal.

Why Are Nurses Vulnerable?

Unfortunately, nurses often become the targets of violence in healthcare settings. This may be for a variety of reasons, but mainly it is because nurses are the primary caregivers and providers of direct, hands-on patient care (Allen, 2009). The next section will explore the following: the nature of the nurse-patient and nurse-family relationship, education needs of nurses, nurses' perceptions of workplace violence, the phenomenon of underreporting, environmental influences, the negative impact of violence, and nurses' responses.

The Nature of the Relationship

Nurses often become the target of a patient or a family member's hostility and anger. There are a variety of reasons why nurses become potential targets for violence. Nurses manage the patient care setting and spend the most time with the patient and family members. Nurses are more available when compared to other healthcare disciplines because nurses are the frontline healthcare providers who provide direct, hands-on care to patients. Nurses also tend to be tolerant of inappropriate or disruptive behaviors that could lead to violence. Nurses may minimize and make excuses for disruptive behaviors. Nurses often put others' needs before their own. They may be fearful that addressing the behaviors or setting limits will exacerbate the behaviors. Nurses may be fearful that if they report the behaviors, they will be blamed for causing them, or feel inadequate that they are unable to stop them. Nurses also sometimes provide painful treatments to patients (such as IV insertion and wound care treatments), causing an increase in anxiety, stress, and pain.

A Lack of Skill

Many nurses lack the skills and training needed to manage aggressive patients and/or family members. When nurses work with patients and/or families who have the potential for violence, clinical knowledge and expertise, evidence-based practices, and tools are needed that will empower nurses and enhance clinical judgment, critical thinking, and decision-making (Phillips, 2007). Ideally, the nurse will have the knowledge and skills to be able to defuse escalating aggressive behaviors in the clinical setting, reducing the likelihood of violence occurring.

Nurses must set limits with patients and family members, which leads to patient frustration, resentment, and adversarial relationships. For example, hospital visitation policies for the intensive care unit (ICU) may restrict the number of visitors at one time, and the visitation hours may also be restricted to certain times of the day. Nurses may be put into a position of enforcing visitation policies they did not put into place.

An Assumption That It's Part of the Job

Violence may be expected as part of the job, but it should not be tolerated (Barthel, 2004). The importance of reporting violence may be minimized as nurses may fear reprisal from patients or family members. This may include fear of retaliation, job loss, negative reports to managers, or harm from patients or family members. Nurses may take personal responsibility for provoking a violent act or not preventing it. Nurses may also fear inadequate administrative support and may be reluctant to report incidents to avoid blame for providing what nurses may perceive as inadequate care.

Underreporting

Lack of data and reporting of violent incidents may inadvertently lead to the promotion of future violence. Hospitals need reporting mechanisms, and all staff should be encouraged to report all episodes of disruptive behavior. Administrators must be made aware of the violent episodes occurring within the healthcare facility. Tracking and trending workplace violence data will have a greater impact on making organizational change, developing a safer work environment, and improving the delivery of patient care. The decision to form a workplace violence committee is a proactive measure that organizations can take to address workplace violence incidents and focus on employee and environmental safety.

A nurse may fail to report violence, aggression, verbal abuse, or disruptive behaviors for a variety of reasons. The nurse may be too busy to complete the document or the nurse may believe the violence is insignificant (Zuzelo, 2007). It is possible that the nurse may empathize with the patient in their situation. The nurse may also not be aware of the law as it pertains to assaults on healthcare workers. Laws pertaining to assault and battery on healthcare workers vary from state to state (ENA, 2013).

Environmental Influences

The environment can have either a positive or negative effect on the behavior of patients and family members. A waiting room that is messy, with overflowing trash cans, few magazines or newspapers to read, no windows, and that is too hot or cold or too crowded is conducive to increased frustration, irritability, and hostility. A waiting room painted with calm, comforting colors, with coffee, tea, or water available, current reading materials, clean restrooms, and a clean, fresh smell is much more conducive to calm, rational behavior (Zuzelo, 2007).

Impact of Violence

Negative reactions in employees who are victims of workplace violence can include increased stress and fear of becoming victimized in the future; fear and anxiety at work; self-blame; lack of trust in others; and decreased job satisfaction and can lead employees to considering changing positions or leaving the profession (American Association of Occupational Health Nurses, 2012).

Healthcare Professional's Responses

Healthcare providers may also inadvertently contribute to conflict and unintentionally or unknowingly aggravate stressful situations (Hollinworth, Clark, Hartland, Johnson, & Partington, 2005). When clinical situations are emotionally charged, well-meaning healthcare providers may respond defensively, rudely, impatiently, or abruptly due to a variety of contributing factors including:

- Fatigue
- Burnout
- Highly stressful work environment
- Inadequate staffing patterns
- Feeling threatened and fearful
- Previous experiences of violence from patients or visitors

- Lack of support from management
- Lack of staff training and education
- Lack of experience in the healthcare workplace

What Would Be Marjorie's Best Course of Action?

I want to return to Marjorie, the RN from the beginning of the chapter, to see how she handled the situation with the new mother and baby. We all can learn many lessons from Marjorie's harrowing encounter that day. It was an experience that Marjorie will not forget anytime soon and demonstrates that violence can occur in a hospital anywhere and anytime.

Marjorie's first reaction was to remove the infant immediately to the nursery and call security for backup support. Marjorie had recently taken a course to assist her with developing verbal de-escalation skills, but she also understood her limitations. Marjorie's first goal was to maintain safety for everyone involved. While the two men were arguing, a nurse and a nursing assistant arrived in response to the shouting they overheard coming from the patient's room. At that time, Marjorie was able to successfully remove the infant to the safety of the nursery, call security, and have the unit secretary call the house supervisor STAT. The additional nursing staff assisted by getting the two men to momentarily stop arguing. Security staff arrived and they were able to intervene without any escalation of violence. Marjorie remembered from her class that it was necessary to keep a safe distance from any individual who was escalating toward violence. She attempted to remain calm and positioned herself so that she had an escape route out of the room. She kept her voice low and made no sudden movements. She explained to Paula that the best decision would be to take the infant out of the room to keep her safe and Paula agreed.

Marjorie's peers demonstrated excellent teamwork by intervening in a challenging situation. The nurse was able to set limits with the visitors by stating clear expectations and boundaries about their unacceptable behavior. They only needed to be reminded that there were other patients and visitors in the area that were feeling unsafe and insecure due to their inappropriate behavior. No clinician should be expected to deal with a potentially violent situation alone. Always utilize all available resources. When the house supervisor arrived, she commended all three of the nursing staff for defusing a potentially violent situation. She also encouraged Marjorie to take a break in the staff lounge for 30 minutes. Afterward, the house supervisor led a debriefing to make sure everyone involved was able to return to work. Later that evening, Marjorie completed an incident report so there would be a record of the occurrence.

Proactive Organizational Strategies to Counter Workplace Violence

Several studies have demonstrated that patients and families are confused by the visiting hour restrictions that are still in existence today in many hospitals and the inconsistency in enforcing these policies (Smith, Medves, Harrison, Tranmer, & Waytuck, 2009). Evidence suggests that open visitation policies can be beneficial to patients and family members (Smith et al., 2009). As hospitals begin to gradually expand their visiting hours, nursing staff must become more aware and better prepared to maintain safety on the nursing units. Hospitals have been slow to accept violence as an occupational hazard that affects healthcare providers. However, hospitals are microcosms of society, and our society is changing. Healthcare administrators must recognize the dangers and implement proactive strategies to keep patients and employees safe. Administrators are concerned with patient satisfaction and recognize that healthcare consumers feel entitled to receive quality service, yet quality service and safety are inseparable (Zuzelo, 2007).

Hospital administrators and nurse leaders must make a commitment to a violence-free environment. The commitment begins with the chief executive officer and the commitment must be communicated throughout all levels of the organization (Gulinello, 1998). Organizations that commit to developing a well-designed plan that embraces patient- and family-centered care and prevents workplace violence—thereby ensuring a safe and healthy work environment—will enhance nurse job satisfaction and retention, decrease staff turnover, improve patient satisfaction, and decrease assaults and injuries. We recommend that hospitals implement the proactive measures listed in the following sidebar.

Organization Strategies to Eliminate Violence in the Workplace

1. *Change the organizational culture and develop a zero tolerance policy for violence. No threatening or violent behavior is acceptable and no violence will be ignored (Zuzelo, 2007):*

   a. *Develop a workplace violence policy and procedure.*

   b. *Develop a protocol for an administrative discharge on the rare occasion this is needed.*

2. *Form a workplace violence committee:*

   a. *Address all violent incidents monthly.*

   b. *Analyze security data (e.g., codes for combative or aggressive individuals, violent behavior restraint situations, and disruptive behavior calls).*

   c. *Analyze occupational health data regarding missed days from work and light duty days related to employee assaults and injuries.*

   d. *Include security officers and risk management as committee members.*

3. *Provide interactive employee education to empower employees:*

    a. *Educate employees who work in the emergency department, behavioral health, and employees who may be assigned as companions or sitters (e.g., Crisis Prevention Institute).*

    b. *Develop a toolkit of available resources on workplace violence prevention accessible to all employees on the Intranet or Web.*

    c. *Utilize simulation activities for training staff whenever possible.*

4. *Implement security measures:*

    a. *Post signage to educate the public about state law.*

    b. *Install panic alarms in every department and nursing unit.*

    c. *Lock down entrances and exits to the facility when visiting hours end.*

    d. *Ensure adequate security officers and consider adding a K-9 unit to the security department personnel.*

    e. *Develop a collaborative relationship with the local police department to provide backup support when needed.*

    f. *Consider hiring off-duty police officers for key areas of the hospital on the night shift to increase visibility, especially on weekends (e.g., in the emergency department).*

    g. *Consider using security wands or installing metal detectors at entrances to identify weapons.*

    h. *Consider hiring detectives or off-duty deputy sheriff officers for surveillance outside patient rooms to keep the staff safe in the event a family member has been asked not to return for visitation.*

    i. *Develop a code for potentially violent or assaultive situations and a code for individuals who present with a weapon, accompanied by education on the two different types of employee responses.*

5. *Implement clinical interventions based on best practices:*

    a. *Research the current literature on workplace violence prevention.*

    b. *Introduce a flagging system for the electronic medical record (EMR) to use as a communication method for patients with a significant history of violence.*

    c. *Implement evidence-based treatment protocols (e.g., alcohol withdrawal protocol, nicotine replacement protocol).*

    d. *Provide unit-based debriefings by a trained facilitator following the occurrence of all critical incidents.*

    e. *Develop guidelines or flow diagrams to help nurses with clinical decision-making skills.*

  f. Survey nurses to determine the severity of concern about violence in your organization.

  g. Develop a process of evaluation for psychiatric intervention and care.

  h. Respond to potential or actual volatile family situations by de-escalating disruptive behavior and assisting in multidisciplinary family interventions.

 6. *Mobilize resources, disciplines, and departments:*

  a. Utilize hospital chaplains for employees (as well as patients and families) for spiritual and emotional support.

  b. Utilize patient relations to provide specialized advice, consultation, and intervention in challenging patient/family situations.

  c. Collaborate with social services to develop a treatment plan.

Working With Disruptive Family Members

Chapter 5 in this book offers a number of thoughts and strategies for differentiating "difficult" patients from those who are truly disruptive. Professional judgment must be exercised to determine the cause of behavior that, in some situations, may be seen as disruptive (e.g., frequent phone calls to the patient care unit) but may actually reflect an unmet need of the patient or family member.

However, if a family member is truly being disruptive by shouting, making verbal or physical threats, making unreasonable demands on the nursing staff, arriving intoxicated, or being verbally abusive, there are a number of interventions the nurse can implement. The nurse's initial response should always be to implement crisis intervention tools and techniques to de-escalate the family member's anger and hostility. These proactive intervention skills may include (Crisis Prevention Institute, 2005):

- Maintaining a safe distance
- Positioning oneself so the exit is not blocked
- Remaining calm and approachable
- Being mindful of non-verbal messages
- Maintaining a low tone of voice
- Breathing slowly and deeply
- Refraining from touch
- Keeping hands in front of you in an open, non-threatening manner
- Making no sudden movements
- Listening to the individual's concerns

- Empathizing and validating concerns
- Using positive feedback
- Offering reassurance
- Being willing to step away and disengage if not getting the desired response
- Setting expectations and boundaries for acceptable behavior
- Utilizing all available resources
- Providing information when appropriate
- Providing choices whenever possible

If the individual's disruptive behavior continues and intervention skills have failed, call security for backup and support. Inform the security officers of the situation and communicate what needs to occur. Notify the nursing management team, physician, and risk manager for assistance. If this intervention has been successful, continue to monitor the situation and maintain limits. Document the behaviors and communicate effective interventions by adding them to the nursing care plan, problem list, or treatment plan. If the disruptive behavior continues, have the treatment team evaluate for limited visitation or restricted visitation. Evaluate the need for escorting from the premises. If this is necessary, security will determine if this can be accomplished, or they may request police intervention.

Individual Strategies to Counter Workplace Violence

Nurses should always be on the lookout for signs of stress in patients or family members and recognize the need for intervention (Barthel, 2004). Signs of stress and possible escalation of anger and aggression may include (Petit, 2005):

- Increased volume of speaking
- Excessive demands
- Pacing, psychomotor agitation
- Fidgeting
- Wringing the hands
- Demanding attention
- Verbal or non-verbal expression of anger
- Signs of intoxication
- Threatening statements
- Paranoia or suspiciousness

- Emotional lability
- Irritability

Intervening early can prevent violence and prevent a hostile work environment from occurring. Individual intervention strategies to minimize violence can be varied and, depending on the situation, may include (Crisis Prevention Institute, 2005; NIOSH, 2002; Petit, 2005):

- Take the family member to a quiet location so he or she can calm down.
- Present a calm, caring manner.
- Avoid getting too close or touching.
- Give the family member your full attention and actively listen to concerns.
- Validate the family member who is upset.
- Ask what they think would be helpful in the situation: What goal would they like to achieve?
- Avoid arguing or becoming defensive with the family member.
- Use calming language: "This must be very difficult for you and your family. What would be helpful?"
- Be aware of non-verbal communication, both on your part and that of the family member.
- Find common ground where you can both agree: "Under what conditions can we [insert shared goal, e.g., proceed with discharge plans]?"
- Set limits with family members when necessary: Describe behaviors that are needed to support their loved one and the other patients.
- Use a team approach: Call in colleagues who may have a long-standing relationship with the family.
- Ask a supervisor or manager to answer a family member's question or address a concern if you do not have the information.
- Develop a behavioral contract or plan of care for what the family may do and what the staff will do.
- Keep the door open when interviewing patients or family members that you anticipate may become angry.
- If you anticipate that a family member or patient may become threatening or violent, alert a colleague that you will be having this conversation beforehand.
- Always have an exit to avoid getting trapped in a room.
- Know how to get help quickly.
- Call security if the situation becomes threatening.

- Before security officers enter the patient's room, communicate the situation and what you would like them to do.

- Ask security to search rooms for dangerous objects.

- Know where panic alarms are located.

- Consider every experience a learning experience.

- Reflect on how well the situation was handled: What could be done differently to improve the team's future responses?

- Request feedback from colleagues on how well the situation was handled.

Setting Limits

Setting limits is an important skill for nurses to learn when encountering patients or family members who act inappropriately toward others in a socially unacceptable manner. This could include cursing or yelling loudly at others, pushing, shoving, or going into other patients' rooms. Again, as part of the assessment, the nurse must assess for any underlying physiological basis for the behavior and, if so, that condition must be treated by the medical provider. In all situations, the judicious use of limit setting is a helpful strategy that forms boundaries within which individuals assume responsibility for the management of their behavior. There are three purposes for setting limits: (1) to establish boundaries, (2) to prevent escalation of the conflict, and (3) to counteract resistance and gain cooperation.

The intent of limit setting is not to control another person but rather to provide consistent expectations and guidelines for self-management. Interventions that provide structure also add security to the situation by limiting the possibility of behavioral escalation to violence. Clear expectations reduce ambiguity and minimize anxiety. Establishing trust and rapport reduces opportunities for manipulation and increases cooperation. Allowing options whenever possible and giving positive feedback for making appropriate choices will decrease resistance to limits. It is never acceptable for any individual to threaten the safety and security of others in the environment.

Some general principles when setting limits are:

- The top priority is preventing violent behavior.

- External control over another person is temporary.

- Only the degree of change that is essential should be expected.

- Natural consequences are the best motivators for change.

- Limit setting takes time and consistency.

Disruptive behaviors are unacceptable in the hospital setting because they jeopardize the health, security, and safety of patients, family, visitors, and healthcare providers in the environment and should not be tolerated. The most important goal is safety, so utilize all available resources and call security for support when necessary.

Treatment Team Strategies

Each multidisciplinary team member is affected by a violent episode whether he or she was directly or indirectly involved. However, there are strategies that the treatment team or nursing management team can implement to prevent or minimize violent episodes and to lessen the impact of a traumatic event.

Behavioral Contracts

Behavioral contracts or letters of agreement are used in some healthcare facilities to modify specific patient, family, and visitor behaviors. These types of contracts or agreements specify that both parties agree to certain conditions or limits on specific behaviors (e.g., refusal to get out of bed, spitting, yelling, verbal abuse) and outline consequences for violations. Contracts or agreements can be helpful in some situations to establish acceptable behavior for all stakeholders. For example, the nurse will arrange for the hospital chaplain to visit twice daily, and the patient will agree to refrain from calling the spiritual care department five or six times per day requesting visits. Contracts or agreements must honor the patient's rights and must be agreed upon by all treatment team members and the patient/family. Including a risk manager in the development of the behavioral contract or agreement should also be considered. The patient should sign the contract or agreement and be given a copy. Each nurse should sign the contract or agreement and recommit to his or her part of the contract. A contract or agreement is useful to ensure a consistent and unified approach among staff members. Behavioral contracts or agreements should be treatment focused and may occasionally be used with family members. Behavioral contracts or agreements are not legally binding and are used as part of the treatment plan to negotiate for appropriate and acceptable behaviors.

Debriefing

Critical situations that may occur in healthcare can create a great deal of stress among nurses and other healthcare providers that may exhaust normal coping mechanisms, especially when colleagues get injured or there are actual or potential threats to personal safety and well-being. Stress is associated with a variety of physiological and psychological symptoms. Debriefing by a trained professional provides an opportunity to express feelings and receive stress education, emotional support, and reassurance. Referral to an Employee Assistance Program (EAP) representative or counselor can also be made if necessary. A quick debriefing within 1 to 4 hours following a crisis can mitigate acute symptoms and stabilize the involved employees to determine which employees can return to work, which employees need to go to Occupational Health, and which employees should be released to home (Everly & Mitchell, 2010). A more formal debriefing can occur within 1 to 10 days post-crisis to mitigate any acute symptoms, assess the need for ongoing followup care and treatment, and to provide some closure on the incident (Everly & Mitchell, 2010). All debriefings must be confidential.

Conclusion

To manage challenging patient, family member, and visitor behaviors and prevent workplace violence, education for all nursing staff is essential. Several key points should be highlighted:

- Violence threatens our fundamental human right to security and safety (Paterson, Leadbetter & Miller, 2005).

- Early signs of anxiety and agitation can often be identified before the behavior escalates (Crisis Prevention Institute, 2005).

- Many factors that contribute to disruptive behaviors are beyond the control of the nurse.

- Debriefings can mitigate the negative physiological and psychological effects of traumatic events.

- Healthcare organizations have a responsibility to create environments that protect patients, families, and healthcare providers from violence and abuse.

It is critical to empower nurses to build confidence in their ability to manage potentially disruptive situations. Furthermore, organizations need to (1) provide adequate resources to equip nurses for dealing with challenging situations; (2) institute institutional programs and support services to help healthcare providers de-escalate violent behavior; (3) implement comprehensive reporting programs to view trends and intervene where necessary; and (4) create a culture where violence is not tolerated and where employees feel empowered to speak up. Accurate documentation and reporting of incidents for tracking and trending purposes are an invaluable method to substantiate the need for programs to prevent workplace violence and to identify action plans. Evaluating outcomes over time and making employee safety a hospital or healthcare system initiative will ensure program success. Hospitals that adopt an organizational approach to promote a healthy work environment will allow nurses to focus on delivering high-quality care that is rewarding and satisfying. Nurses are valuable assets to the organization and should not have to work in abusive environments nor tolerate violence as part of their job (Barthel, 2004).

References

Allen, P. B. (2009). *Violence in the emergency department: Tools and strategies to create a violence-free ED.* New York, NY: Springer.

American Association of Occupational Health Nurses (AAOHN). (2012). *Preventing workplace violence: The occupational and environmental health nurse role.* [Position Statement.] Retrieved from www.aaohn.org/practice/position-statements.html

American Nurses Association (ANA). (n.d.). Model "state" bill: "The violence prevention in health care facilities act." Retrieved from http://nursingworld.org/MainMenuCategories/Policy-Advocacy/State/Legislative-Agenda-Reports/State-WorkplaceViolence/ModelWorkplaceViolenceBill.pdf

American Nurses Association (ANA). (2006). *Preventing workplace violence.* Retrieved from http://www.nursingworld.org/MainMenuCategories/WorkplaceSafety/Healthy-Nurse/bullyingworkplaceviolence/PreventingWorkplaceViolence.pdf

Barthel, V. A. (2004). We stop aggression as soon as it starts. *RN, 67*(10), 33-36.

Bureau of Labor Statistics (2013, August 22). *National census of fatal occupational injuries in 2012.* News Release. Retrieved from www.bls.gov/news.release/archives/cfoi_08222013.pdf

Crisis Prevention Institute. (2005). *Nonviolent crisis intervention training program participant workbook.* Brookfield, WI: Author.

Emergency Nurses Association (ENA). (2010). *Violence in the emergency care setting* [Position Statement]. Retrieved from http://www.ena.org/SiteCollectionDocuments/ Position%20Statements/Violence_in_the_Emergency_ Care_Setting_-_ENA_PS.pdf

Emergency Nurses Association (ENA). (2011, November). Emergency department violence surveillance study. Retrieved from www.ena.org/practice-research/research/ Documents/ENAEDVSReportNovember2011.pdf

Emergency Nurses Association (ENA). (2013). *50 state survey criminal laws protecting health professionals.* Retrieved from https://www.ena.org/government/State/Documents/ StateLawsWorkplaceViolenceSheet.pdf

Everly, G. S. & Mitchell, J. T. (2010). *A primer on critical incident stress management (CISM).* Retrieved from www.icisf.org/who-we-are/what-is-cism

Gillespie, G. L., Gates, D. M., Miller, M. & Howard, P. K. (2010). Workplace violence in healthcare settings: Risk factors and protective strategies. *Rehabilitation Nursing, 35*(5), 177-184.

Gulinello, J. J. (1998). A systematic approach to identify, assess and address workplace violence. *Journal of Healthcare Protection Management, 14*(2), 8-15.

Hollinworth, H., Clark, C., Harland, R., Johnson, L., & Partington, G. (2005). Understanding the arousal of anger: A patient-centered approach. *Nursing Standard, 19*(37), 41-47.

Longo, J. (2007). Horizontal violence among nursing students. *Archives of Psychiatric Nursing, 21*(3), 177-178.

National Institute for Occupational Safety and Health (NIOSH). (1996). *Violence in the workplace.* DHHS (NIOSH) Publication Number 96-100. Current Intelligence Bulletin 57. Retrieved from www.cdc.gov/ niosh/docs/96-100/introduction.html

National Institute for Occupational Safety and Health (NIOSH). (2002). *Occupational hazards in hospitals.* DHHS (NIOSH). Publication Number 2002-101. Retrieved from www.cdc.gov/niosh/docs/2002-101/

National Institute on Drug Abuse (NIDA). (2012). *Drug facts: Nationwide trends.* Retrieved from http://www.drugabuse. gov/publications/drugfacts/nationwide-trends

Paterson, B., Leadbetter, D., & Miller, G. (2005). Beyond zero tolerance: A varied approach to workplace violence. *British Journal of Nursing, 14*(15), 810-815.

Petit, J. R. (2005). Management of the acutely violent patient. *Psychiatric Clinics of North America, 28*(3), 701-711.

Phillips, S. (2007). Countering workplace aggression: An urban tertiary care institutional exemplar. *Nursing Administration Quarterly, 31*(3), 209-218.

Smith, L., Medves, J., Harrison, M. B., Tranmer, J., & Waytuck, B. (2009). The impact of hospital visiting hours policies on paediatric and adult patients and their visitors. *Journal of Advanced Nursing, 65*(11), 2293-2298.

Thompson, P. M., Hayashi, K. M., Simon, S. L., Geaga, J. A., Hong, M. S., Sui, Y.,…London, E. D. (2004). Structural abnormalities in the brains of human subjects who use methamphetamine. *The Journal of Neuroscience, 24*(26), 6028-6036.

Weiss, A. P. (2012). Disruptive patient behavior as a quality and safety concern. *Focus on Patient Safety* [Newsletter], *15*(2), 1-5. Retrieved from www.npsf.org/wp-content/ uploads/2013/04/Focus-v15-2-2012.pdf

Zuzelo, P. R. (2007). *The clinical nurse specialist handbook.* Sudbury, MA: Jones and Bartlett.

Chapter 19

Narrative Approaches to Understanding Patient and Family Perspectives

Lance Wahlert, PhD
Meghan Thornton O'Brien, MBE

Hopeful first-time parents Sharon and Darius are at once enthusiastic and apprehensive about attending their latest consultation with their obstetric healthcare team. A year prior, they encountered a similar consultation, only to be informed after an ultrasound that the fetus in their first pregnancy was deemed nonviable, with Sharon ultimately suffering a miscarriage 2 weeks later. Visiting the OB/GYN's office for the first ultrasound of this second pregnancy, Sharon and Darius are consumed by feelings of disquietude, excitement, and uncertainty. And yet the consultation goes without incident: The intake process is swift and cordial; the nurse technician performing the ultrasound provides standard procedural explanation of the process in a timely fashion; the obstetrician physician gladly tells the couple that their pregnancy is progressing wonderfully and that the fetus in in excellent health. Sharon and Darius soon leave the clinic feeling elated that their pregnancy is sound and that their dream of becoming parents is more surely secured. Yet they also feel a nudging sense of dissatisfaction about the obstetrical consultation itself. The service provided was positively competent and the outcome of that consultation was nothing short of good news. But the efficiency of the procedure has left the couple feeling as though the clinical moment they just experienced was just that—a merely "clinical" one. For Sharon and Darius, it feels as though the biographical significance of this recent consultation has been rendered incommensurate with the narrative that they will now be forced to tell to family and friends about how it went.

Such a scenario speaks to the stakes of narrative medicine and the topics to be outlined in this chapter. How can we say that the medical needs of Sharon and Darius have been merely partially met by their serving clinical team, in spite of the efficacy of the healthcare team's work and the positive outcome that resulted? Could the intake professionals, the nurse technician, and the obstetrician have done a richer job of invoking the parent-planning history and present feelings of the couple? Could their fear, apprehension, enthusiasm, and uncertainty as future parents (articulated in a narrative framework) have been just as valuable to this consultation as the results of, for example, a fetal echocardiogram? Can engaging with the medical stories of a patient be just as important as the clinical details that are exchanged in a consultation?

Reviewing the Broadway adaptation of Joan Didion's best-selling memoir *The Year of Magical Thinking* (2007)—a book in which an author, wife, and mother simultaneously lingers on each of these roles in light of being a newfound caregiver and griever in the medical realm—*The New York Times* critic Ben Brantley wrote of the play's narrative impact (in the opening line of his review) as follows: "The substance is in the silences." Ironically (or appropriately), the title of Brantley's review of the play was "The Sound of One Heart Breaking" (2007). The implication on Brantley's part, and by extension the message of Didion's narrative memoir on healthcare, is thus: Silence and sound are often synonymous.

While almost 100 years apart, the sentiments of canonical English author Virginia Woolf and narrative medicine scholar Arthur Kleinman speak to a trans-historical and, thereby, still persistent need for the appreciation of narratives and stories in healthcare:

> Considering how common illness is, how tremendous the spiritual change that it brings, how astonishing, when the lights of health go down, the undiscovered countries that are then disclosed, what wastes and deserts of the soul a slight attack of influenza brings to view...when we think of this, as we are so frequently forced to think of it, it becomes strange indeed that illness has not taken its place with love and battle and jealousy among the prime themes of literature. (Woolf, 2002, pp. 3-5)

> Each patient brings to the practitioner a story. That story enmeshes the disease in a web of meanings that make sense only in the context of a particular life. (Kleinman, 1989, p. 96)

While Woolf ponders why illness has been underaddressed in the canon of literary studies, Kleinman invokes a similar dilemma by reminding us of the importance of narrative structures and forms of storytelling—as not mere embellishments in terms of how healthcare is actualized, but as the very core of healthcare itself.

This chapter on narrative approaches to understanding patient- and family-centered perspectives on medicine undertakes a similar appreciation of the values of saying and not saying (and hearing and not hearing) stories in healthcare practice, in the clinic, and beyond. There is immense power and incredible responsibility that comes with the tasks of eliciting, receiving, engaging in, recording, and returning testimonials from persons in healthcare. Accordingly, whether patient, provider, caregiver, nurse practitioner, family member, general clinician, or hospital ministry personnel (to name but a few potential storytellers and story-listeners), caregivers are called to pay great attention to the very important and very vital ways in which stories function in combination with healthcare practices for patients and families.

Throughout this chapter, the stakes, dilemmas, and honors of being privy to and participant in moments of storytelling and story sharing in healthcare are covered. Invoking theoretical and methodological approaches to the interactive storytelling moments in healthcare, this chapter asks us to think of narrative approaches to medical and healthcare practices as at once vital, complicated, and essential.

The Relationship Between Storytelling and Healthcare

Historically and contemporarily, the relationships between storytelling (or narrative) and medicine (or healthcare) have been understood in three ways:

- **As a supplementary model**: Storytelling has been appreciated as a way to enhance clinical practice or expand the narrative of normative clinical practice. How do stories contribute to traditional healthcare practice? How do they bolster already in-place clinical relationships?

- **As a reciprocal model**: Storytelling has been appreciated as a way to think about how medicine influences the ways we talk about healthcare, but also how nonprovider discourses on healthcare affect clinical discourses. There is a negotiated conversation that exists between clinical and nonclinical appreciations of health moments. What do medical narratives from the provider have to say about patient and family healthcare experiences? And what do healthcare narratives from patients and families have to say about medicine? As literary and historical scholar of medicine G. S. Rousseau (1981) has addressed these dilemmas, he asks us to consider how there is a shared sense of intimacy that can come from this reciprocity of narratives to and from medicine.

- **As a model of centrality**: Storytelling exists neither outside of nor in conversation with medicine, but actually operates within medical and clinical discourses. Storytelling is a form of healthcare practice. Historically this has been most resonant in fields such as psychoanalysis, group therapy, and addiction recovery, where the acts of sharing stories, reading stories, and writing stories have long-standing therapeutic underpinnings. Storytelling is also at the heart of clinical practice, for it is through the patient's relation of symptoms and their corresponding beliefs that the healthcare provider gains the knowledge necessary to diagnose and treat. To share and to read stories collectively is to heal, or to enable healing.

This chapter embraces and operates in an appreciation of the supplementary, reciprocal, and centrality models of narrative medicine outlined above. In truth, all are viable models. Collectively, all of these models speak to the disparate ways in which patients, families, caregivers, and providers appreciate their storytelling connections to healthcare practice, medicine, the clinic, and one another.

How Stories Work and Why They Are Important in Clinical Settings

The scientific breakthroughs of medicine have long been rooted in the soils of creative imagination. Yet medical practitioners are taught to assess patients with an increasingly standardized and formulaic approach. This is necessary, in part, for expediency and consistency of case-history taking. However, in a realm where stories are the currency of medical exchange, understanding the power of narrative can unearth subtleties, connections, and details that enrich the individual therapeutic experiences of patients and providers alike. How we choose to think about and linger on the ways we communicate with and among patients, families, and providers are often some of the most important aspects of healthcare.

Consider the following clinical example in which narrative played a vital role. A once medically compliant diabetic and hypertensive patient stopped talking all of his medications and infrequently visited his medical team for the last 10 years. The patient bounced between providers, all frustrated with the patient's "non-compliance" that allowed his diabetes and high blood pressure to rage out of control despite their attempts to medicate him. Only after a stroke that left him with severe left-sided weakness did the patient tell his story about why he stopped taking his medication. Ten years earlier, his sister who also suffered from diabetes and hypertension and who was rigorously compliant with her medications died in a car accident. Her blood sugar at the time her body was pried from the vehicle was 10 times the normal limit. Racked with grief at the loss of his primary familial support, the patient was left with a sense that medical treatment for his disease was futile. Only through the patient's narrative did the medical team learn about these critical emotional barriers to the patient's ability to take care of himself and his disease.

Healthcare professionals, in particular clinical nurses, call on patients to tell stories about their illness for multiple reasons. Not only do narratives elicit important clinical details that inform diagnosis and treatment plans, but they also serve the patient-provider relationship with a host of potential benefits, including deeper feelings of intimacy, comfort, trust, honor, and confidence for all parties. Narrative savvy and narrative appreciation are, therefore, valuable not only to providers, but also to families, patients, and other persons involved in healthcare settings. The commitment to think about communication within healthcare settings as not just about information exchange, but also about story exchange is, therefore, an invaluable distinction. As we share personal details in healthcare, so we offer somatic and psychological details germane to the clinical case at hand. But we also simultaneously share attitudes, opinions, beliefs, fears, and expectations of equal importance.

Storytelling, therefore, is as vital a part of the clinical team as clinical care. And in many ways, storytelling is emblematic of clinical care itself.

And yet, patients vary widely in their storytelling abilities and styles—for example, in their senses of chronology, understandings of causality, and appreciations for relevant details—making the provider's ability to actively listen all the more important. Likewise, practitioners vary in their abilities to both elicit and actively listen to patients', families', and caregiver's narrative expressions of their healthcare experiences.

Active Listening

Active listening refers to the intentional and purposeful act of listening, not merely as a passive acceptance of narrative content, but also as an engaged, sustained, and dutiful attention to details of narrative context, tone, subtlety, and word choice. There is listening to gather facts and then there is active listening, which strives to do more than merely gather facts. Active listening is an attuned sense of listening (or reading). Physician Dr. Jon Kabat-Zinn, founding director of the Center for Mindfulness, Health Care, and Society at the University of Massachusetts, characterizes mindfulness as paying attention in a particular way: " on purpose, in the present moment and nonjudgmentally" (1994, p. 4).

The skills employed by an active listener are the same as those employed by a close reader.

Close Reading

As described by noted New Criticism literary scholar M. H. Abrams (1999), *close reading* involves one who explicates "the work itself" (p. 14)—which is to say, one who honors the word choice of a narrative and focuses on its intrinsic value as having nuance and tension. Rephrased: Close reading asks us to linger, and to listen and read more closely, because (as storytellers) what we say has meaning beyond the mere facts of the story itself.

Narrative medicine pioneer Dr. Rita Charon (2005), a physician and literary scholar by training, has explained this responsibility of reading as follows:

> [B]eing a close reader equips one to perform some of the most difficult tasks of the health care professionals: attentive listening, simultaneously being transported by a text while analyzing it most meticulously and critically…, adopting alien perspectives, following the narrative thread of the story of another, being curious about other people's motives and experiences, and tolerating the uncertainty of stories. (p. 262)

Close reading provides a method of engaging another's narrative, building bridges between reader and author, and forging deeper and more nuanced understandings than merely following prescribed and predictable medical relationships.

Close Listening

Similarly, close listening affords healthcare professionals a way to engage their patients more deeply by offering an approach to engaging patient stories. Through close listening, providers gather information, build empathy, and explore character—all of which are critical to forming the therapeutic alliance. An understanding of how narrative functions both in clinical and personal settings is critical to developing the relationships that keep healthcare patient-centered in the face of the push toward evidence-based standardization. Practicing close reading, then, can hone a clinician's ability to listen closely. Or, as Charon (2011) has stated in a recent TED Talk: "Clinical practice is fortified by the knowledge of what to do with stories."

Telling Stories

Not only does the ability to read closely translate into a clinician's ability to listen closely, to explore and understand character motivations, and to nurture empathy for the patient, but practicing telling stories affords nursing and healthcare practitioners an essential moral testing ground. Charon offers the example of the early-twentieth-century German philosopher and literary critic Walter Benjamin who, in his seminal essay "The Storyteller," argued that storytelling is valuable as an art of reproduction—which is to say, we receive stories because we are called upon to repeat them to other audiences, to the initial storyteller, and to ourselves (2006). How well we listen to stories in medicine is authenticated by our ability to pass them on to others.

Telling stories also provides healthcare workers an essential space in which to explore and confront difficult clinical and social situations, for example, those in which an emotional response incited by the patient or his/her circumstances conflicts with a morally sound decision. As physician-storyteller Jay Baruch (2010) writes:

> Narrative serves as an ideal medium for wrestling with intense incongruity: a patient insults the very person trying to help him, and a physician finds himself on empathy's chilly ledge. Consider John Gardner's thoughts on the value of fiction: "[It] helps us to know what we believe, reinforces those qualities that are noblest in us, leads us to feel uneasy about our faults and limitations." (pp. 9-10)

Such a testing ground is vital to nurses' and physicians' well-being and (by extension) to patient care. It offers practitioners the tools and the space to evaluate what has happened, what might have happened, and what they wished had happened in a specific clinical moment. In short, narrative combats apathy.

Furthermore, engaging with the patient's narrative, understanding his or her own role as healthcare provider in the patient's narrative, and giving voice to his or her own narrative as provider allows the healthcare provider to create a space for what Charon calls "reciprocal recognition" (Charon, 2012, p. 1880). "We come to realize," she writes, "that narrative writing in clinical settings makes audible and visible that which otherwise would pass without notice" (Charon, 2007, p. 1266).

Taking the time to linger on the words used in clinical encounters allows nurses, patients, caregivers, and other healthcare members to both cherish the sanctity of these words and appreciate that modes of communication (such as conversations, case histories, storytelling moments, and discursive exercises) can forge potent connections in healthcare dynamics. As we share perspectives, so we are reciprocally enhancing (or not) the relationships that are vital to frontline clinical care. Accordingly, the byproduct of a shared engagement in narrative is ideally deeper trust and deeper communication—both critical relational elements necessary for navigating pathways around clinical dead ends.

The Healing Power of Hearing

For patients who are already asked to engage in various kinds of storytelling at each clinical encounter—whether those be patient history intakes, moments of prayer or counsel at the bed-side, or casual conversations in the clinic—changing the way an audience engages the patient-storyteller serves to broaden the scope of what a narrative can and should include. Therefore, when sharing with an audience who is especially attuned to receiving his or her narrative, the act of storytelling is transformed into a tool for patients to understand their illness, suffering, treatment, and recovery. Given this magnitude, we are called upon to linger in storytelling moments. We are asked, if not to spend more time sharing and hearing details on stories, then at least to listen to those stories better. Quality of words is as important as quantity of words in narrative exchanges in healthcare practice.

If we are mindful of the abilities to both listen better and listen longer, we can perhaps do at least one of these in the service of the other. Accordingly, the attending nurses and other clinicians can still gain salient clinical details to help guide healthcare management, but they can also afford the patient a narrative experience that provides the catharsis of being heard. Healing is as much a narrative exercise as it is a clinical one—often in the same moments and often in the same ways.

Finally, storytelling is an essential component to patient advocacy. Without a reliant, competent, and compelling retelling of a patient's story, the patient advocate (whether that is a caregiver, social worker, clinical ethics mediator, provider, chaplain, or the patient him/herself) loses the most persuasive element of their position—the self-specific, human element. The story is not a mere template or trope, for example, in cancer care narratives. Rather, the story of cancer care that is specific to this patient, this family, this caregiving team, and this clinical moment is essential. Such narrative specificity is a reward for all parties involved.

Types of Narrative

Healthcare narratives are often understood as the stories told or written by the ill and by those who care for the ill. From the case study to the medical history to the talking cure, storytelling has been a central component in the diagnostic, therapeutic, and pastoral strategies of medical cosmologies for centuries. Social historian of medicine Roy Porter (1985) has written extensively about the intrinsic and scholastic value of studying medicine "from below." His claim is that without an appreciation of medicine and healthcare practice from the perspectives of laypersons, patients, caregivers, family members, and even those "not yet deemed a patient" (p. 175), we cannot fully appreciate the narrative landscape of medicine itself.

However, medical narratives also exist in less traditional forms, for example, in the movement of bodies, in images of bodies, numerical interpretations of bodies, and in prayer. Some questions that elucidate the panoply of forms that medical narratives can take include:

- How do sick bodies move differently?
- How do radiographs and scans capture progression?

- How do lab analyses, probabilities, and odds ratios portend a future?
- How do personal conversations with a higher power sculpt a landscape of hope, gratitude, or fear?
- How does the genre in which a medical narrative is couched (as memoir, as YouTube testimony, as official patient complaint, as prayer, or as conversation with a pastoral caregiver) alter its meaning, impact, and appreciation?

Consequently, a patient's narrative may take on new meanings depending on who is "telling" a version of the patient's story, who the audience is, and which version of a patient's narrative is given authority. As frontline nurses and healthcare providers, we engage with patients and ourselves, often in different versions of the same narrative. With appropriate mindfulness of how these narratives intersect with one another and the authority bestowed upon our interpretations as care providers, we can better harness the power of narrative in the service of patient care.

Often, this asks us to consider questions such as:

- Who is the protagonist in one version of a healthcare narrative?
- How does the healthcare team have a vested interest in the outcome of a medical narrative in tandem with the patient and caregiving family?
- Can the clinical stakes of the medical moment be altered by the revision of a medical narrative?
- By altering the third-person ("he," "she," "they," "their") in one narrative to the first-person ("I," "we," "us"), can we see drastically different levels and stakes of somatic, emotional, spiritual, or communal need?

By understanding the many forms of patient narratives and the anatomical structure of narratives, close listeners and storytellers effectively harness narrative power in the clinical setting by making themselves mindful of how the various elements of narrative (plot, narration, character motivation, audience, etc.) come together to create narrative shape, significance, and cohesion.

What to Do With Stories
We, and our patients, use stories in a number of ways.

To Bear Witness
Leading medical humanities scholar Howard Brody (2002), in his seminal text *Stories of Sickness*, makes the wise, palindromic claims that "healing is storytelling" and that "storytelling is healing" (p. 8). At the cornerstone of his treatise is the belief that a primary role of healthcare providers (e.g., nurses, doctors, and chaplains) and healthcare participants (e.g., patients, caregivers, and loved ones) is the expectation (not just the desire) to be an active participant in the medical world via medical narratives. And although this would seem to be a straightforward task, Brody

asks us to pause and consider the great complexities and great responsibilities that come with such expectations.

Accordingly, to elicit a patient's story, the nurse clinician and clinical team must ask questions, informed by both their clinical and personal curiosities. The architecture of their curiosities guides their attentions. "It is why and how we attend to others," explains Rachel Hamer, an MFA and medical student. "Questions are touchstones for affiliation. In the end, the questions themselves are what make room for self-discovery, not the search for answers" (Hamer, 2013).

Thus, we can ask:

- What questions guide our attention and direct how we bear witness?
- How do we ask patients questions?
- How do our questions shape the stories they tell?
- When do we lead; when do we probe for more?
- What is the value in what is left unsaid?
- Are we an active audience or a passive one?
- Which audience is appropriate for this patient?

The healthcare practitioner must combine mindfulness, self-awareness, and the powers of observation and attuned attention to receive what the patient communicates in story, through body, and in silence. If in illness, patients are isolated from their healthy selves (as Susan Sontag has famously written in *Illness as Metaphor*, 2001), then they are often dislocated from others—family, society, loved ones, clinical care providers, faith-based communities, and even from their own bodies. By being a willing receiver of the patient's story, the nurse practitioner has the duty and privilege to offer relief from the isolation that can accompany illness.

To Share

The acts of writing, listening, reading, and recording are all forms of sharing—and they transform the nurse practitioner and general clinician into a narrator. Through oral, written, and aural methods, by acquainting oneself with the importance of one's own story's details, one discovers questions and engages in the self-discovery unearthed by the acts of "writing." A narrative writer or receiver can hone his or her attunement to the importance of details and the self-discovery at work in another's narrative process. In this way, the clinician-writer enhances his or her relational perspective and patient appreciation.

In practicing writing, the healthcare provider–writer comes to understand first-hand the role and power of different narrative elements. Writing the details of an experience automatically attunes one to the details of one's surroundings. Smells once overpowered by disinfectant and sounds once lost in the din of beeping machines become pivotal narrative details. Deliberate omissions sensitize the healthcare provider–writer to the significance of the patient's choice to leave something unsaid and the depth of what may lurk unspoken.

Character casting during the act of writing affords exploratory tools into the motivations and interpersonal dilemmas directing others' actions that might otherwise seem unrelatable. Developing the patient's and the practitioner's character provides a depersonalized pathway to empathy by promoting understanding of how one character experiences the other. In short, engaging our own story is an exercise in self-exploration that strengthens the tools with which we can assist patients in their own self-exploration. The writer is a closer reader; so too is the storyteller a more attentive audience.

Healthcare narratives can take many forms:

- The sexual history one shares with a clinical nurse or other healthcare provider
- The letter one writes to a loved one or a clinician
- The phone call consultation that manifests between a chaplain and a patient
- The group prayer that may take place with hospital ministry services, a clinical care team, or family members
- The decoration, strategy, and explanation of a patient's hospital-bed setting
- The documentation of a patient's healthcare experiences in a diary, on a blog, on Twitter feeds, on Facebook posts, and in email exchanges (both public and private)
- The history, physical, and progress notes documented by physicians or shared on daily rounds
- The clinical documentation of patient care and patient status by nurses at the bedside
- The stories shared between providers about the patient
- The sharing of a patient's healthcare story on other platforms

Stories can also be shared in forms other than the written and spoken word. For example, choreographer and MacArthur Genius Award recipient Liz Lerman has been using choreographic techniques in the healthcare setting to promote healing and strengthen relationships between providers and relationships between providers and their patients. Using choreographic exercises and relational theater games, she and her dancers engage people not conventionally considered dancers in the choreographic creative process, asking them to share their story through movement (Lerman, 2003). As with shared narrative, shared movement (especially when informed by an individual's life experience) can be a choreographed invitation for reciprocal recognition, relationship building, and narrative healing.

To Interpret and Authenticate

In addition to cultivating a narrative practice with one's own story, either real or fictionalized, the physician- or nurse-writer may also use the patient's story as narrative substrate. This is routinely done through chart documentation—verbally while calling consultations or in writing, via the case report or the progress note. By retelling, incorporating parallel narratives of images and lab data, and asking questions, the provider interprets and authenticates the salient details. However, relevance, in this instance of inter-provider communication, is largely audience specific.

The healthcare practitioner can also use written narrative as a clinical tool. With permission, the attending nurse or physician may write the patient's story for the patient. The act of writing, sharing, or reinterpreting the patient's story with the patient centers the narrative on the individual, letting her know that she has been heard and restoring her agency to the details of her illness story. Regarding the act of representing the patient in narrative in such a moment, Charon (2007) writes that it "requires the expressive force and creativity of the writer along with the contained meaning of that which is now in view, unifying seer and seen in the creation of the text" (p. 1266). It carves the space for mutual definition, reinterpretation, and evolution of the patient within her own narrative and in the eyes of her healthcare practitioners.

The Narrative in Clinical Practice

The role of narrative in the clinical setting is several-fold. As writers, readers, and listeners in the world, we all engage with language to understand our experiences. Narrative practices can, therefore, hone clinician skills, such as character exploration, attention to detail, and the catharsis that comes from restorative processing. Soliciting narratives (formal or informal) can, in turn, be a healthcare tool that practitioners use to promote the trust and relationship-building necessary to navigating clinically problematic moments.

Disability studies scholar Rosemarie Garland-Thomson (2009), for example, has offered great insights on the ways in which narrative studies can better enhance our discourses on disabled identities and persons. In her book *Staring: How We Look*, she argues that speaking with and about the disabled need not be predicated on the polite, euphemistic rationale of "It's impolite to stare at the disabled." By contrast, she suggests that acts of staring, talking about, and blatantly engaging in narration about disabled bodies and (by extension) disabled persons are infinitely more humanizing. Although the politically correct standard of not narrating on and not drawing attention to disabled bodies can be understood as culturally competent, Garland-Thomson asks that we take the bold and precarious act of engaging in storytelling about sensitive issues such as disability.

Of course, in addition to disability, we could make such bold recommendations on the narrative elasticity to speak blatantly on other valuable or sensitive topics such as gender identity, sexuality, race, ethnicity, religion, and veteran status. And we should be mindful of and eager to include these topics in the healthcare narrative fold. But we should embrace this expansion of the medical narrative discourse by also appreciating that nurse practitioners, medical students, and clinicians should undergo regimens of narrative training so that they are able to strengthen their therapeutic alliances with patients and deepen their ability to empathize.

As such, considerations of narrative power and awareness of the variety of narrative possibilities can sensitize healthcare practitioners to the affect parallel narratives (images, lab data, a patient chart) can have on the patient experience. Often we give these parallel narratives clinical authority, and understanding how narratives layer in the clinical setting will shape a clinician's interpretation of the clinical evidence in service of a more patient-centered therapeutic interaction.

How do we practically incorporate narrative into clinical practice? First, we become practicing writers and readers. We cultivate an awareness of the ways in which we are already telling stories and vesting them with clinical authority over the patient's narrative authority. We can then bring narrative into the clinical setting as a tool. Here's how:

Close Reading

Set aside time each week devoted to engaging the narrative expressions of others. Whether a work of literature, a newspaper article, a poem, or even a TV episode, examples of narrative expression on healthcare are plentiful. Our responsibilities are to be both inclusive of and sensitive to the nuances in medical stories.

Accordingly, pay attention to the details:

- Why did the author choose the words, phrasing, or context she did?
- How has the structure of a story affected its interpretation and appreciation?
- Who are the characters in a particular medical narrative?
- Do you see ways in which the story might be told or read differently if you recast one character as a protagonist rather than a secondary character?
- What are the motivations of a particular character, and how do you isolate those motivations?
- Can you imagine how you might retell, rewrite, or just pass along this narrative?
- Can you imagine how the skills you've just practiced might help you become a better close listener?

Telling Stories

Set aside time each week to write or create. Many have a hard time facing a blank page, so here are some exercises to help you transition into writing mode:

- What questions do you have? Write down all of your questions for a minute. Were you surprised about where these questions led you? Now pick a question and answer yourself. Are you answers kind? What have you learned? (From Rachel Hamer)
- Take a line from a poem and use it as a starting point for your own story or poem. See where this kernel allows your mind to travel.
- Choose something with emotional salience that happened this week. Write about what happened in the third person. Was this easy or difficult to do?

- Pick a person you came across this week—someone who did something kind, perhaps, or unkind. Write a character sketch of this person that delves into their motivations, fears, inconsistencies, hopes, etc.

- Try focusing on sensual details. Describe a moment and explore how the five senses were at play.

- Consider a time when you were frustrated with a patient or a patient's family member. Write the same story with several endings. It's okay to keep it short. Pay attention to your character and the patient's character. How did the characters change with each ending? Which ending ultimately resonated with you?

- Tell a patient's story with just the numbers (lab data, etc.). What is the tone that develops? Punctuate the story with an emotional response (the patient's, his partner's, her child's, his parent's, etc.). How does the juxtaposition of the sterile authority of the numbers intensify the emotional reaction of the characters?

- Write a *parallel chart*. Take a patient and write the story that happens outside and around the story of the medical data.

Eliciting the Patient's Story

In his essay "On Caregiving," in which he articulates the ethical and moral stakes of providing care and comfort to loved ones in enduring healthcare scenarios, Arthur Kleinman (2010) talks about the value of "experiential language." He describes this concept as both a method and an awareness of how the act of rendering into words the experiences of pain, suffering, caregiving, comfort, and treatment are linguistically and narratively entrenched. Kleinman (2010) writes:

> To use the close experiential language of actually doing it, caregiving is also a defining moral practice. It is a practice of empathetic imagination, responsibility, witnessing, and solidarity with those in great need. It is a moral practice that makes caregivers, and at times care-receivers, more present and thereby fully human. (p. 29)

Healthcare professionals (frontline nurses, in particular) are like caregivers, and the ailing and infirmed in their close proximity give access to the "experiential language" that Kleinman identifies as a very sacred and valuable form of clinical discourse. Consequently, an ability to appreciate the gravitas of these storytelling moments is as important as the stories themselves.

In eliciting stories from patients and families, then, start with something open-ended that sets expectations for what the patient should include in his or her story. Charon (2006) offers an open-ended introduction to her patients to set the stage for information gathering and storytelling: "I will be your doctor, and so I have to learn a great deal about your body and your health and your life. Please tell me what you think I should know about your situation" (p. 177). Then she does her best to be quiet until the patient stops talking.

The story that follows reflects the patient's understanding of what is important. The empty spaces offer added depth; missing elements to the narrative may reflect the patient's reservations, mistrust, fear, shame, ignorance, or oversight. What do they choose to share and how do they share it? Sit and absorb what is being said. What does the story reveal about the patient's character? What is lurking in the unshared story around the shared story? Often patients begin their story at the time of onset of physical symptoms. For most, however, the story precedes the patient's presence in the clinical setting. What is known about the unknown?

Writing the Patient's Story

Introducing narrative into the clinical setting may seem a bit unorthodox, but the relational power it affords is unparalleled. Asking patients if you may write a narrative about them honors them, restores their agency, and affords them an opportunity to understand how they are being heard. "Hearing" can take on many meanings in such healthcare moments: literally listening to every word, recording the words of persons, maintaining eye contact in a way that connotes attentive investment, or using the acts of touch or gesture to reinforce one's commitment to demonstrating narrative receptivity. Medical Humanities scholar and philosopher Arthur Frank (1997) has referred to "illness as a call for stories" (p. 54). His use of the term "call" is a testament to the ways in which spoken, unspoken, silent, and blatant forms of "voicing" are vital to healthcare discourses.

Charon (2007) writes that medical narrative takes on "the force of both creation and clinical intervention. The writing renders the doctor audible, the patient visible, and the treatment a healing conversation between them" (pp. 1266–1267). Frank (1997) asks us to be mindful of the ways in which unattended stories in healthcare can produce "narrative wreckage" (p. 53). Like a ship beached on the shore and not safely moored to the deck, healthcare stories not appropriately listened to, recorded, or heard are (to take Frank's metaphor to its logical conclusion) left as wreckage. In other words, they are not afloat.

By both reading and writing stories in healthcare settings, we set them "afloat"; the patient has the opportunity to correct or expand on the captured themes, sparking new clinical insights and paths for therapeutic intervention. Writing and witnessing promotes essential affiliation between patient and provider, a remaking and re-experiencing of the writer and subject through co-creation—sailing together, not as narrative wreckage.

When writing the narrative, sit and absorb what the patient says. Note what is left unsaid and consider why. Which parts of the story occur outside of the clinic and before the illness? Examine the character's motivations. Share the story with the patient and ask for feedback. What discussion ensues and how does the patient react to being the subject of your time and attention? Did you get his or her story right?

Writing With Patients and Their Families

Literally writing with a patient or family can be just as valuable as storytelling in the oral context. Therefore, think about asking the patient to write a parallel chart to the one you keep. Will they share their story with you? What was revealed that you didn't know before? Why had one detail not come up in one context versus another?

Ask the patient if it is permissible for the family to write about the patient's illness. If so, have the family member share writing with the patient. Consider reimagining the clinical and healthcare encounters you have with patients as correspondence. How would I write this medical moment to you in a letter? Via a tweet? In an email? Via a text message? Or even in skywriting? Does the platform on which we choose to write healthcare stories and share healthcare details to one another matter as much as the details themselves?

Narrative Pitfalls

Although there are many strengths and possibilities of narrative for personal and clinical practice, the narrative medicine approach is not without its pitfalls. Many patients may be reluctant to engage in a practice that is not conventionally found in the clinical setting. For example, as much as a patient or caregiver might welcome the possibility to share at length or be listened to at length within a healthcare moment, ironically, such narrative attentiveness might be understood as patronizing. One must, therefore, be mindful that a person's investment in the storytelling aspects of healthcare are not received by patients and caregivers as "window dressing" moments—suggesting that nurses, doctors, and other providers are compromising their clinical care on other somatic fronts. Such suspicions might not only jeopardize the trust of patients and families, but they may also risk undermining the perceived competence of the clinical team. The authenticity, sincerity, and transparency of narrative and storytelling approaches to healthcare can avoid these pitfalls.

Moreover, for those patients who choose to engage in the narrative process, writing and sharing may risk feelings of oversentimentalization, romanticization, or a false sense of closure. Just as narrative and storytelling approaches to healthcare moments can provide lucidity and catharsis to patients, caregivers, and families, they (of course) have the possibility to make such persons' autobiographically specific details feel scripted or "fictional" in their appreciation.

Medical Humanities scholar and narrative theorist Tod Chambers has written extensively about the dangers of the "fiction of bioethics"—which is to say that medical narratives, as all narratives, have a latent tendency to purport to share "realness" when they are in fact drafted versions of narratives, subject to the same pitfalls of bias, exaggeration, or misinterpretation (Chambers, 1999). In receiving, writing, recording, and returning medical stories to patients and families in healthcare settings, therefore, one must be very mindful of the perilous potential to couch an individual's story in a stock scenario or to record one's story as the absolute truth of the case at hand. Healthcare stories can vary drastically based on who, when, where, and to what ends they are shared. A consistent mindfulness of these perspective- and circumstance-based stakes is obligatory.

With the great power and great gifts that come from listening to, receiving, recording, and returning healthcare narratives to patients and families, there is also the potential that we can misinterpret or appropriate such stories for our own ends. Let us appreciate the power of stories in healthcare settings, by reminding ourselves that their composition, revision, and evaluation are always a collective exercise across the patient, provider, caregiver, and communal divides.

Case Scenarios

The following three case studies are designed to offer practical, real-world examples of how narrative can be therapeutically incorporated into clinical practice. In addition to the scenarios themselves, a series of discussion questions follows each to assist you facilitate of discussion about the cases.

Healthcare Scenario 1: Narrative in an Emergency Care Setting

> *Melissa Johnson is a 16-year-old young woman who presents to the emergency department for the second time in 4 days. On her first visit, she was diagnosed with bacterial vaginosis and given an antibiotic prescription. Today, she returns complaining of lower abdominal cramping and vaginal bleeding that feels like her usual period pain and asks for another antibiotic prescription because she never got the first prescription filled. During the history taking, Melissa reveals that she is having unprotected sex with her male partner (who she thinks has other partners), but with whom she is monogamous and not using any form of birth control. You also learn that she has a primary care physician and a gynecologist, and that she has decided to come to the emergency room "just because." In addition, you learn that she is a high school student and intends to go to college, so you decide to initiate a discussion about birth control and safe(r) sex practices. When you bring up birth control, Melissa gets visibly agitated, exclaiming: "I will be a good mother, and if I get pregnant, I get pregnant!" She begins preparing her things to leave the emergency department. You convince her to stay, and she is ultimately diagnosed with normal menstrual period and discharged with the same prescription she never initially got filled.*

Questions and practice for storytelling and sharing:

- Imagine yourself closely listening to the patient. What seems to trigger Melissa's anger? What words does she use that stand out?

- Take a line that Melissa said and use it as a starting point for a free-writing moment on your part.

- Write about Melissa's day at school.

- Write about Melissa's interaction with her boyfriend when she leaves the hospital.

- Write about Melissa's last appointment at her primary care doctor's office.

- Write about how Melissa understands her body.

- Write a rant about the trigger, from the perspective of a 16-year-old woman.

- As a healthcare practitioner, you are frustrated that patients use emergency services inappropriately and waste resources. Write a rant to the patient.

- Make a list of the questions you would like to ask this patient but would never ask. Make a list of questions you would ask this patient.

- How can you use these stories and rants writing exercises to help you to "take a step back" in your clinical care of Melissa?

- How can they help you to redirect the conversation with the patient?

Healthcare Scenario 2: Narrative in a Chronic Care Setting

Michael Baker is a 48-year-old obese man with hypertension and diabetes. He presents to the clinic for follow-up to discuss his lab results. Despite multiple counseling visits, he continues to have poorly controlled hypertension, and his recent hemoglobin A1c has been creeping up. You really don't want to put Mr. Baker on insulin, but you are afraid he is headed down that path unless he makes some radical changes in his diet and exercise practices. Plus, you recently started him on his third blood-pressure medication, which seems to have had little effect. He is waiting for you in your office; you plan on exploring why his blood pressure (BP) and diabetes is so out of control. When you inform him that his BP and lab values indicate that his diabetes and blood pressure are out of control, he says, "You keep giving me all these pills, and they aren't working!"

Questions and practice for storytelling and sharing:

- Prior to your next consult, free-write for 1 to 2 minutes and make a list of questions that you have for Mr. Baker.

- Pick three of the open-ended questions and three of the more targeted questions. Imagine Mr. Baker's answers to each of them. Spend 30 seconds writing each answer. Which answer is most revealing and why?

- Which kinds of questions elicited the most revealing answers for you? Can you imagine asking these questions to Mr. Baker in practice? What are your concerns about asking them?

- What frustrations do you have with the patient? Write a rant about them.

- Write a counter-rant from the perspective of Mr. Baker.

- Spend 1 minute writing about Mr. Baker's trip to his doctor's office.

- Imagine you are Mr. Baker. Write about his day from the moment he gets up to the moment he goes to sleep. Write this story on an optimistic day. Then, write this story on a pessimistic day.

- Describe the experience of waiting in Mr. Baker's exam room. Spend 30 seconds exploring this waiting experience using the five senses (taste, touch, hearing, sight, and sound).

- Describe the experience of eating breakfast in Mr. Baker's home. Spend 30 seconds on each of the same five senses.

- Did you imagine Mr. Baker as rich or poor? If so, repeat the sensory description exercise as though Mr. Baker came from the other class.

- From Mr. Baker's perspective, write about his previous visit to the doctor's office.

- Collectively, how have these writing exercises shaped or changed your appreciations of Mr. Baker's healthcare scenario?

Healthcare Scenario 3: Narrative in a Pastoral Care Setting

Michael Kilpatrick has been in a loving relationship with his life partner, Kevin Thomas, since 1985, shortly after he was first diagnosed as HIV positive. Over the past 3 decades, Michael and Kevin have frequently visited their healthcare providers together as a couple, taking great pride in their ability to be viewed as a decision-making team about one another's health needs. This is a quality that each has regularly stressed to their clinical care team, in particular to their nurse practitioner, Barbara Johnson, who has been Michael's primary point-person in healthcare for more than 15 years. Both Michael and Kevin also have a long history of being significant contributors to the AIDS activist programs in their local community—organizing fundraising events, disseminating educational material on AIDS and safe sex in LGBT spaces, and volunteering at area healthcare outreach centers for the LGBT community. Of equal importance to Michael and Kevin, they are very active members of their Unitarian Church, taking great comfort in the solidarity and spirituality that comes from their faith-based community.

In recent weeks, Michael has been diagnosed with an opportunistic respiratory infection that has left him homebound for the next 6 weeks. Although he is expected to rebound from this latest infection, Michael says he feels saddened to be disconnected from his long-standing, regular interactions with his AIDS-activist community, LGBT volunteer network, healthcare team, and his faith community. Kevin has spoken to Barbara Johnson to see if she has any recommendations on how to help Michael (individually) and them (as a couple) during this period of extended home respite. He asks, "Can you think of ways Michael and I can stay in touch with our wider healthcare network? Or ways that Michael doesn't feel isolated, as it's been decades since he was homebound for a health scare? How can we stay in contact with you for his clinical needs, my caregiver needs, and our morale as a couple over the next several weeks?"

Questions and practice for storytelling and sharing:

- How can Barbara Johnson be an advocate for Michael and Kevin, helping them to stay in regular communication with their wider community of support?

- Can she encourage and remind them that regular conversations and storytelling with friends, clinical care team, and parishioners at their church are just as valuable in the success of Michael's treatment these next 6 weeks as the regimens of medicine he is taking?

- In what ways can Barbara provide an example for Michael and Kevin on how to keep the narrative exchange between the couple and their community of support viable during this period?

- In lieu of regular face-to-face meetings, which have been the standard of communication for many years now, can Barbara suggest that they have their regular consultations over telephone or video chat?

- How would these mediums affect and change the typical narrative exchange processes that patient and provider have experienced up until now?

- Is there a pastoral resource available to the couple (either through their healthcare network or their church), whereby their spiritual needs are preserved?

- Rephrased, how can Barbara be an advocate for the need of prayer as a very important form of narrative for this couple?

- Should Michael and Kevin be encouraged to think about this period of homestay as an opportunity for them to do activism on AIDS that requires a written form of narrative testimonial?

- Would this be a perfect time for them to undertake a writing project that pays tribute to their years of work in the AIDS and LGBT communities? Not in the spirit of closure, but (given Michael's excellent prognosis) as a narrative exercise that literally and figuratively can feel like the writing of a new chapter in their lives as a loving couple and HIV activists going forward?

- What kinds of written, recorded, reflective, or storytelling exercises could Nurse Barbara recommend for them to do, in anticipation for when Michael is next able to attend the clinic in person?

- Can Barbara, herself, offer to do a small form of writing on her behalf to share with them when they are next in the clinic as a couple?

Conclusion

This chapter has examined the uses and power of the narrative in giving voice to the person engaged in healthcare, in providing an opportunity for connection between the person and the caregiver, and in helping the caregiver be a more effective source of healing. To optimally use the narrative requires appreciation of and commitment to several core concepts:

- **Narrative medicine:** The appreciation of and the inclusion of stories and various forms of storytelling in healthcare practice, including how healthcare providers can be better listeners of, recorders of, participants in, and agents in the fostering of storytelling in medical care.

- **Active listening:** A commitment to a most heightened, sensitive, and nuanced listening to health-related experiences of patients and providers within and beyond clinical settings, so as to foster greater attentiveness to the patient narrative and the patient/ provider relationship.

- **Close reading:** On the page and in conversation, paying special attention to the language, tone, voice, context, and meanings (liminal and subliminal) that persons use when sharing stories. More succinctly, (1) "close reading" is reading in ways both aural and literal; (2) "close reading" is the act of rereading, or lingering on the words we use.

- **Cultural competency:** An appreciation of the panoply of perspectives that inform the practices and cultural appreciations of healthcare in action—including categories of identity, such as race, gender, class, sexuality, disability, ethnicity, and other demographics; as well as proximities and castings in the healthcare system, such as patient, provider, family member, surrogate, advocate, caregiver, spiritual counselor, and beyond.

Through the use of the narrative tools detailed in this chapter, healthcare providers can enrich and complement the ways in which they forge connections with their patients, strengthening therapeutic relationships. By telling stories, writing imagined stories, and receiving the stories of others, frontline nurses and other healthcare workers can carve out important spaces for imagination, empathy building, and "reciprocal engagement" in an increasingly reductive clinical context. Patients, caregivers, and clinicians alike *all* benefit from the narrative exercises that honor their shared senses of humanity in the reciprocal engagement of healing.

References

Abrams, M. H. (1999). *A glossary of literary terms* (7th ed.). New York, NY: Harcourt Brace.

Baruch, J. (2010). Dr. Douchebag: A tale of the emergency department. *The Hastings Center Report, 42*(1), 9-10.

Benjamin, W. (2006). The storyteller: Reflections on the work of Nikolai Leskov. In D. J. Hale (Ed.), *The novel: An anthology of criticism and theory, 1900–2000* (pp. 362-378). Malden, MA: Blackwell Publishing.

Brantley, B. (2007, March 30). The sound of one heart breaking. *The New York Times*. Retrieved from http://www.nytimes.com/2007/03/30/theater/reviews/30magi.html?pagewanted=print

Brody, H. (2002). *Stories of sickness*. New York, NY: Oxford University Press.

Chambers, T. (1999). *The fiction of bioethics*. New York, NY: Routledge Press.

Charon, R. (2005). Narrative medicine: Attention, representation and affiliation. *Narrative, 13*(3), 261-270.

Charon, R. (2006). *Narrative medicine: Honoring the stories of illness.* New York, NY: Oxford University Press.

Charon, R. (2007). What to do with stories: The sciences of narrative medicine. *Canadian Family Physician, 53*(8), 1265-1267.

Charon, R. (2011, November 4). *Honoring the stories of illness: Dr. Rita Charon at TEDxAtlanta* [Video file]. Retrieved from http://www.youtube.com/watch?v=24kHX2HtU3o

Charon, R. (2012). The reciprocity of recognition—What medicine exposes about self and other. *New England Journal of Medicine, 367*(20), 1878-1881.

Didion, J. (2007). *The year of magical thinking.* New York, NY: Viking Press.

Frank, A. W. (1997). *The wounded storyteller: Body, illness, and ethics.* Chicago, IL: University of Chicago Press.

Garland-Thomson, R. (2009). *Staring: How we look.* New York, NY: Oxford University Press.

Hamer, R. (2013). Workshop: Writing as traction for spinning wheels. *2013 American Medical School Association (AMSA) Humanities Institute 2013 Conference.* Sterling, VA.

Kabat-Zinn, J. (1994). *Wherever you go, there you are—Mindfulness mediation in everyday life.* New York, NY: MJF Books.

Kleinman, A. (1989). *The illness narratives: Suffering, healing, and the human condition.* New York, NY: Basic Books.

Kleinman A. (2010, July-August). On caregiving. *Harvard Magazine,* 25-29.

Lerman, L. (2003). *Liz Lerman's critical response process: A method for getting useful feedback on anything you make, from dance to dessert.* New York, NY: Dance Exchange, Inc.

Porter, R. (1985). The patient's view: Doing medical history from below. *Theory and Society, 14*(2), 175-198.

Rousseau, G. S. (1981). Literature and medicine: The state of the field. *ISIS, 69*(4), 583-591.

Sontag, S. (2001). *Illness as metaphor* and *AIDS and its metaphors.* New York, NY: Picador Press.

Woolf, V. (2002). *On being ill.* New York, NY: Paris Press.

Chapter 20

Managing Compassion Fatigue, Burnout, and Moral Distress

Françoise Mathieu, MEd, CCC
Leslie McLean, MScN, RN

Jana is a registered nurse (RN) working in a hemodialysis unit. She has been there for 15 years and takes pride in knowing all of her patient's special needs and idiosyncrasies. She looks forward to going to work and enjoys most of the patients and families she works with. In the past 2 years, however, the volume of work on the unit has dramatically increased. There are fewer nurses on the floor, and as a result, Jana has to monitor more patients than before. She spends most of her time rushing from one bed to the next, checking on patients' dialyzers and vitals.

Recently, she had to spoon-feed lunch to two of her patients, which took a great deal of time, and she had to frequently interrupt what she was doing to respond to alarm bells. One of the patients she was feeding was experiencing difficulty swallowing, and Jana found herself becoming very impatient with the patient's slowness in eating her meal. Later, on her way home, Jana felt very guilty about this and regretted being so irritable with this lovely elderly patient.

Over the past 2 decades, the healthcare system in the United States has been in a state of flux: We have experienced numerous budgetary cutbacks that, in turn, have led to a reduction in staffing, more hospital mergers (Small & Small, 2011), and a decrease in resources to care for patients:

> During the 5 years ending December 31, 2009, there were at least 278 hospital mergers covering 639 hospitals with 108,711 beds. This represents 11% of the American Hospital Association estimate of the 944,277 total staffed hospital beds in the United States. (Small & Small, 2011, p. 3)

Nurses all over North America report that they are being asked to do more with less (Duxbury, Higgins & Lyons, 2010) and are having to care for a larger number of sicker patients who require more complex care than in the past (American Hospital Association, 2012; Canada Census, 2011; Schoen et al., 2011; U.S. Census Bureau, 2010).

In acute-care settings, family members are now more involved in decisions about the care of their loved ones. This can present new challenges for nurses and physicians around sharing decision-making, communication, and control. In addition, as a result of more family presence at the bedside, healthcare workers must not only provide care and support to their patients but also offer comfort and bear witness to traumatized and, at times, highly distressed family members (Egging et al., 2011).

Nurses are now having to meet the multiple and sometimes competing demands of those to whom they are accountable: their employer, supervisor, physician colleagues, professional association, patients and their families, the public at large, the government, and, in instances when things go wrong, the media and judicial courts. In the midst of this complex and evolving landscape, higher expectations have been set to improve quality of patient care by focusing on "safety, effectiveness, timeliness, efficiency, equity and patient-centeredness" (Institute of Medicine [IOM], 2001). The requirement to provide patient-centered care, in particular, highlights the ongoing tension that nurses face: They must provide top-quality care to patients while contending with insufficient resources and work overload, just as Jana faced in the vignette at the beginning of this chapter. Without adequate resources, nurses are placed in an untenable situation in which they are at increased risk of developing stress-related illnesses—which paradoxically jeopardizes quality patient care.

Is it possible to offer high-quality patient-centered care while preserving the health of staff? Rising rates of sick leave, workplace grievances, complaints from patients and families, and lowered work satisfaction among hospital staff have fueled an interest in gaining a better understanding of the forms of occupational stress that can affect healthcare workers, particularly nurses. Burnout, compassion fatigue, and moral distress are distinct but inter-related concepts that refer to the various ways in which the work affects care providers (Mathieu, 2012). The first step in developing an effective strategy to ensure that nurses can provide high-quality care while staying healthy is to understand the complex consequences of work overload and repeated exposure to patients and families in pain and in distress.

Research in the fields of compassion fatigue and burnout in healthcare workers has grown tremendously in the past decade—we now have access to new data to assist us in recommending best practices to support staff in their rewarding but challenging work. In this chapter, we will discuss the relationship between compassion fatigue, burnout, and moral distress and offer strategies at both the individual and organizational level which will help prevent and/or mitigate their effects and ultimately support nurses in being able to provide high-quality patient-centered care. We will also discuss the concept of "role overload," provide a self-assessment tool for the warning signs of compassion fatigue, discuss the impact of compassion fatigue and burnout on patient-centered care, suggest strategies for developing and maintaining an ethical climate in the workplace, and provide an action plan for self-care for individuals, teams, and organizations.

Burnout

Bernard works as a nurse in a long-term care facility that primarily cares for patients with Alzheimer's disease and other types of dementia. A new owner recently purchased the facility, and the climate at work has changed drastically: Staff members have lost control over their shift schedules, their workload has increased significantly, and the unit manager seems punitive and intimidating. There are rumors that the new owner will be cutting those who don't seem to be "pulling their weight." Bernard enjoys caring for the patients, but feels stressed and anxious about the workplace climate. With his new shift schedule, he is also struggling to balance home and work life and feels like he is "walking on eggshells" whenever the manager is near him.

The concept of burnout is not new to healthcare. It was first mentioned in the late 1970s and early 1980s by psychologists Herbert Freudenberger (1980) and Christina Maslach (1978, 1982), who were studying the effects of professional exhaustion. Since that time, the term burnout "has been widely used to describe the physical and emotional exhaustion that workers can experience when they have low job satisfaction and feel powerless and overwhelmed at work" (Mathieu, 2012, p. 10). Burnout can affect non-healthcare workers as well: Being employed in a high-stress, low-reward factory or a frenetic law office can lead to burnout just as easily as working in a challenging hospital ward.

In 2006, Statistics Canada published their first National Survey of the Work and Health of Nurses. They found that "close to one-fifth of nurses reported that their mental health had made their workload difficult to handle during the previous month" (para. 37). In the year preceding the study, more than half of the nurses surveyed had taken time off work because of a physical illness, and 10% had been away for mental health reasons. Access to EAP (employee assistance program) was a shocking 80%, which is more than twice as high as EAP use by the total employed population (Mathieu, 2012).

Burnout in Physicians Affects Patient Care

Numerous global studies involving nearly every medical and surgical specialty indicate that approximately 1 of every 3 physicians is experiencing burnout at any given time—in this case, burnout being defined as "emotional exhaustion" "depersonalization" and "low personal accomplishment" (Shanafelt, 2009, p. 1338). Dr. Tait Shanafelt, one of the leaders in physician wellness research in the United States, recently published a series of findings that compares U.S. physician health with the overall American population. In this 2012 study, Shanafelt and colleagues (2012) found that 45% of physicians experienced symptoms of burnout with differences depending on the medical specialty: "[…] the highest rates among physicians [were] at the front line of care access (family medicine, general internal medicine, and emergency medicine)" (p. 1377). Shanafelt then juxtaposed the findings against the general population and found that physicians were more likely to experience burnout than the average American citizen: "Compared with […] US adults, physicians were more likely to have symptoms of burnout (37.9% vs 27.8%) and to be dissatisfied with work-life balance (40.2% vs 23.2%)" (p. 1377).

This study, as well as a prior 2009 paper by Shanafelt, both indicate that burnout has a direct impact on the quality of care delivered by physicians and on the relationship between physicians and their patients. Strikingly, Shanafelt (2009) also found that it affected treatment compliance:

> Physicians' degree of burnout and professional satisfaction are related to physician empathy and compassion, prescribing habits, referral practices, professionalism, and the likelihood of making medical errors. Physician burnout also appears to influence patient adherence to recommended therapy, the degree of trust and confidence patients have in their physician, and patients' satisfaction with their medical care. (p. 1338)

Although it was not a finding of the Shanafelt studies, it is not difficult to imagine that burnout in physicians will in turn contribute to increased stress among nurses.

The Challenge of Increased Interaction With Family Members

Although it has been shown to be beneficial to most patients (Egging et al., 2011), the push for more family presence 24/7 in acute-care settings and their involvement in patient care (The Joint Commission, 2010) can pose challenges to nursing staff. Some families are extremely vocal and strong advocates for their loved ones, which can be challenging when nurses are struggling with role overload and time compression. Unfortunately, when resources are limited, one of the first casualties is quality communication between staff and family members (Azoulay et al., 2000; Heyland et al., 2002).

Addressing burnout in healthcare workers is clearly a crucial aspect of improving patient-centered care, but we also need to gain a better understanding of two other threats to the delivery of quality patient-centered care: compassion fatigue and moral distress.

Reflection Activity

You are now invited to go back and re-read Bernard's story. Then consider the follow-ing questions:

- *Did you have any thoughts about or reactions to this story?*

- *Have you ever worked (or do you currently work) in an environment where burn-out is present for you? Is it present in your colleagues? What key features stand out for you?*

- *What options, if any, do you feel that Bernard has at this time?*

- *Have you ever been physically assaulted or verbally abused on the job? Were you surprised by the incidence rates of abuse reported in this section?*

Role Overload

To combat compassion fatigue and burnout, agency administrators and therapists may also wish to ask themselves "How many cases are too many?" (Killian, 2008, p. 42)

Hurried and stressed physicians order tests or referrals and prescribe medicines in an attempt to appease and give the illusion of high quality care. (Rickert, 2012, para. 16)

Although employees of all walks of life can experience *work* overload, which can be defined as having too much work to do in a certain span of time, *role* overload specifically refers to the accumulation of too many competing duties. A 2010 study commissioned by the Workplace Safety and Insurance Board of Ontario revealed that 60% of healthcare workers were suffering from "role overload," which they defined as "having too many responsibilities and too little time in which to attend to them" (Duxbury et al., p. 2). Nurses sometimes refer to it as "having too many hats to wear." In their report, the authors paint a picture of healthcare workers struggling to juggle all the demands on their time and energy:

[Role] overload at work is caused by a lack of time (too many commitments, time constraints, and unrealistic work deadlines and work expectations), multiple compet-ing priorities, a lack of help and support, understaffing, an inability to control the situ-ation, and a non-supportive organizational culture. [Role] overload at home is related to expectations at work, a lack of time, competing demands and priorities, a lack of help and support, life cycle stage (eldercare, children at a difficult age) and an inability to control the situation. (Duxbury et al., 2010, p. 3)

The study found a direct correlation between role overload and poor outcomes, including "negative emotions, […] poorer physical and mental health, increased work-life conflict, poorer relationships at work and at home, greater intent to turnover, increased absenteeism, greater use of EAP, and lower commitment and productivity" (Duxbury & Higgins, 2013, p. 3). The investigators also found that healthcare workers were in poorer physical and mental health than staff surveyed in other sectors of the population: In healthcare, "59% report high levels of stress and 36% report high levels of depressed mood and […] one in five are in poor physical health" (Duxbury & Higgins, 2013, p. 56).

NOTE

An additional phenomenon that can amplify the stress of role overload is unpredictability. In a 2007 study, Krichbaum and colleagues referred to "complexity compression" which they defined as "what nurses experience when expected to assume additional, unplanned responsibilities while simultaneously conducting their multiple responsibilities in a condensed time frame" (p. 86).

In addition to role overload, nurses report regular workplace violence. A 2008 position statement from the Registered Nurses' Association of Ontario (RNAO) stated that "nurses are three times more likely to experience violence than any other professional group" (RNAO, 2008). The Statistics Canada National Survey of the Work and Health of Nurses, mentioned earlier, found that "… [O]ne-third of all nurses had been physically assaulted in the past year" (Statistics Canada, 2006, para. 35). A national survey carried out in 2006 by the American Association of Critical-Care Nurses showed that 64.6% of their respondents had experienced verbal abuse in the past year (from various sources such as patients, family members, other nurses, and physicians) and 22.2% had been physically abused at least once, primarily by patients (Ulrich et al., 2006). One recent study on verbal abuse in the workplace among registered nurses in the U.S. found that "about 49% experienced verbal abuse from nurse colleagues at least once during the past 3 months" (Budin, Brewer, Chao, & Kovner, 2013, p. 4).

Warning Signs of Burnout

- *Feeling hopeless and discouraged in dealing with work*

- *Feeling like your efforts at work do not make a difference*

- *Not feeling connected to others at work*

- *Feeling trapped by your job as a nurse*

- *Often feeling worn out because of your job as a nurse*

- *Often feeling overwhelmed because your caseload seems endless*

- *Feeling bogged down by the system*
- *Feeling that you are no longer a very caring person*

Source: Adapted from the Professional Quality of Life—Proqol Self-Test (Stamm, n.d.)

Compassion Fatigue

Amina is a student nurse on placement in a busy emergency department. She is job-shadowing Louise, a seasoned ED nurse with more than 20 years of experience in the field. They are called to attend to a patient who has been sexually assaulted during a party following a local college football game. "Here we go," says Louise, "Another drunk girl who is going to cry in our ED because she can't remember who she went home with." Amina is shocked by Louise's comments and by her lack of empathy toward the patient.

What Is Compassion Fatigue?

The term *compassion fatigue* is a more recent concept than burnout. It was first mentioned in the literature in the early 1990s. Carla Joinson referred to "compassion fatigue" in a 1992 paper exploring the impact of work-related stress among emergency room nurses. Subsequently, psychologists such as Dr. Charles Figley (1995) found that helping professionals of all stripes such as nurses, social workers, physicians, and child welfare workers were exhibiting symptoms of profound emotional exhaustion, poor work engagement, hopelessness, and a decrease in feelings of empathy and compassion toward patients. In addition, professionals who worked in high-trauma situations (such as child welfare workers and emergency department nurses) were showing symptoms similar to post-traumatic stress disorder (PTSD) without ever having been in the line of fire themselves.

Unlike burnout, which is related to challenges within the work environment such as role overload, lack of control, and lack of reward, this new form of work-related stress was connected to the empathic engagement between the healthcare provider and the patient. This gave rise to a new field of research and the creation of new terminology as experts began to try and better understand this complex form of burnout that seemed to affect only caregivers and helping professionals rather than the general public.

As discussed in detail in Mathieu's 2012 book *The Compassion Fatigue Workbook*, compassion fatigue refers to the profound emotional and physical exhaustion that a caregiver or helping professional can experience over time. Unlike burnout, which can happen to anyone who is struggling with unsatisfactory workplace conditions, compassion fatigue is specific to being in a caregiving relationship.

> Compassion fatigue refers to the gradual erosion of all the things that keep us connected to others in our caregiver role: our empathy, our hope, and of course our compassion—not only for others but also for ourselves. When we are suffering from compassion fatigue, we start seeing changes in our personal and professional lives: We can become dispirited and increasingly bitter at work; we may contribute to a toxic work environment; we are more prone to clinical errors; we may violate patient boundaries and lose a respectful stance towards our patients. We become short-tempered toward our loved ones and feel constant guilt or resentment at the never-ending demands on our personal time. (Mathieu, 2012, p. 8-9)

As previously mentioned, in acute-care settings, families now participate increasingly in decision-making and are more frequently present at the bedside. As a result, nurses may be exposed to more traumatic details and may, at times, develop a deeper understanding of the suffering of patients and families as they bear witness to the grief and distress around them. For example, one pediatric cancer ward recently expressed difficulty retaining their recreational staff for more than 1 to 2 years. The causes of the attrition varied, but one frequently stated reason was the staff's inability to cope with the pain and suffering of the families and children with terminal cancer (B. Muskat & A. Robertson, personal communication, 2013).

Mathieu (2012) quotes the following incidence rates:

> Depending on the studies, between 40 to 85% of helping professionals were found to have compassion fatigue and/or high rates of traumatic symptoms. For example, a … study carried out by Abendroth and Flannery in 2006 among Florida hospice nurses found that 79% of them had moderate to high rates of compassion fatigue and 83% of those who did not have debriefing/support after a patient's death, had symptoms of compassion fatigue. (p. 34)

Mathieu (2012) continues:

> The level of compassion fatigue that a helper experiences can ebb and flow from one day to the next, and even very healthy helpers with optimal work/life balance and self-care strategies can experience a higher than normal level of compassion fatigue when they are overloaded, are working with a lot of traumatic content or find their case load suddenly heavy with patients and families who are all chronically in crisis. (p. 9)

Compassion fatigue is a normal consequence of prolonged exposure to difficult stories and individuals in pain and in crisis. It is not a disease or a mental illness. The warning signs can vary from person to person depending on several factors such as your personality, coping style, prior life history, current life circumstances, the quality of social support that is available to you at work and at home, and the quality of training you have received (Gentry, 2002; Pearlman & Saakvitne, 1995).

Self-Assessment—Warning Signs of Compassion Fatigue

The following self-assessment is not intended to be a diagnostic test, but rather an exercise in "taking stock," to help you identify what areas in your life are currently contributing to making you more vulnerable to developing compassion fatigue. We invite you to take the test when you have some time to reflect on your current home and work situation, and when it is done, to take a step back and look at the overall picture: Are there areas that need more attention than others? Would it be possible for you to change some of your coping styles, to get access to more training, or to ask some colleagues to create a support group at work or outside of work?

What Is Your Coping Style?

When you are overwhelmed with difficult stories from work do you frequently...

❏ *Have several stiff alcoholic drinks or use drugs to numb out when you get home*

❏ *Watch hours of television until you fall asleep in front of the set*

❏ *Spend hours surfing the Web*

❏ *Numb yourself with overwork*

❏ *Binge on sugary, salty, or fatty foods*

❏ *Shop even though you can't afford it*

❏ *Gamble online or in a casino*

How often do you...

❏ *Exercise or meditate*

❏ *Play with children*

❏ *Play with pets*

❏ *Find someone to debrief*

❏ *Journal*

Personality

❏ *Are you a very sensitive person? Do you take on other people's suffering?*

❏ *Is your volunteer job exactly the same as your day job?*

❏ *Do you ever get a break from being in a caregiver role?*

❏ *Were you a caregiver in your personal life long before you became a nurse?*

❏ *Do you have a hard time delegating? Saying no?*

Prior Life History

❑ Do you have a history of trauma, abuse, neglect and/or domestic violence in your personal life?

❑ Do you have a history of drug or alcohol abuse, compulsive gambling, or other addictions?

❑ Do you have a history of depression or an anxiety disorder?

❑ Have you ever been physically assaulted on the job?

Current Life Circumstances

❑ Are you currently going through a divorce or separation?

❑ Are you currently caregiving for a person in your own family (a child, spouse, or other relative with a long-term illness or disability)?

❑ Are you currently dealing with financial difficulties?

❑ Are you currently struggling with an addiction?

❑ Are you currently suffering from clinical depression or an anxiety disorder?

Quality of Social Support

❑ Do you have access to good emotional support at home or among your friendships?

❑ Do you have access to someone who can help you with daily chores at home (errands, cleaning, cooking, home repairs, finances, etc.)?

❑ Do you have access to good emotional support at work?

Training

❑ Do you feel that you are adequately trained to care for the patients on your current caseload?

❑ Do you have access to regular professional development to learn new techniques and stay on top of your nursing skills?

❑ Is there any training you wish you could receive at this time? What kind of training is it? Write it down here:

Supervision

❑ Do you have access to good quality supervision and debriefing at work?

❑ If you do not have access to good quality supervision and debriefing at work, is it something you can access outside of work?

The goal of this self-assessment is not to tally up your check marks in order to get a score. Rather, we invite you to take a look at the themes that emerged from your inventory. Where do you need to focus your energy? What is working well for you at the moment? If you are comfortable doing so, this is an exercise you may want to do with a close friend or colleague, so you can discuss your results and reactions to the self-assessment. If you find yourself overwhelmed by your responses, you may want to contact a mental health practitioner to discuss your feelings and reactions.

The Impact of Compassion Fatigue and Burnout on Patient-Centered Care

In her 2009 book *Trauma Stewardship*, Laura van Dernoot Lipsky, a Seattle-based social worker with many years of experience working in hospital emergency departments, reflects on one frequent consequence of compassion fatigue in healthcare staff—minimization and desensitization to other peoples' suffering:

> We may start out being moved by each person's story, but over time it may take more and more intense or horrific expressions of suffering to deeply move us. We may consider less extreme experiences of trauma as less "real" and therefore less deserving of our time and support. … Minimizing is not triaging and it is not prioritizing. This coping strategy is at its worst when you've witnessed so much that you begin to downplay anything that doesn't fall into the most extreme category of hardship. Although you may still be able to nod and do active listening and feign true empathy, internally you are thinking something like, "I cannot believe this conversation is taking 20 minutes of my time. There wasn't even a weapon involved." (van Dernoot Lipsky & Burke, 2009, pp. 78-79)

Anyone who works in a trauma unit or a similar high-stress setting for any length of time will be familiar with this phenomenon, and a certain amount of desensitization is not, in and of itself, necessarily a bad thing—we cannot perform effectively as healthcare workers if we are reeling at every patient's story. The problem arises when our detachment starts interfering with our empathy and with the quality of care we offer patients and their families. There are, unfortunately, too many stories of poor bedside manners in hospitals, of patients and families being ignored or treated disrespectfully by staff who have lost their compassion and become numb to human suffering.

But rather than laying the blame on individual helping professionals, recent research clearly demonstrates that the problem also lies at a systems level; therefore, our solutions must not solely focus on the individual but must also address the organization as a whole. Given this, one key element at the organizational level that needs to be addressed is the issue of how institutions can foster an ethical work environment that will support patients and staff alike.

An "Ethical Climate"

The concept of an "ethical climate" first emerged in the business literature approximately 50 years ago (Schluter, Winch, Holzhauser, & Henderson, 2008). Since that time, the concept has expanded into the healthcare domain, and an *ethical climate* can be described as the organizational conditions and practices that affect how ethical patient care issues are discussed and decided (Hart, 2005). Lützén and Kvist (2012) propose that "a safe environment that supports ethical action and allows messy ethical questions to be raised and discussed is absolutely essential to a morally habitable healthcare environment" (p. 36).

According to Olson, five conditions need to be met in order for staff to engage in ethical reflection. Staff should (Olson, 1998, p. 346):

- Have the right to relevant information and be free to express what needs to be said about an issue (power)

- Be free to disagree with one another in order to increase their understanding of an issue (trust)

- Be included in the decision-making process if they have a stake in the outcome of the decision (inclusion)

- Be allowed to take different positions on issues or to change their views (role flexibility)

- Be encouraged to ask questions, participate in decision-making, and have access to the information necessary to make informed decisions (inquiry)

Research has shown that a restrictive ethical climate is related to moral distress and is a factor in nurses leaving their positions and profession (Hart, 2005). However, factors such as ethics education; control over the practice environment; and improvements in workload, staffing, and resources have been demonstrated to be related to nurses staying in their positions (Austin, Bergum, & Goldberg, 2003; Corley, Minick, Elswick, & Jacobs, 2005; Hart, 2005; Pauly, Varcoe, Storch, & Newton, 2009).

Moral Distress

Melinda, a 22-year-old with a history of congenital heart disease and multiple comorbidities, recently underwent a valve repair and was subsequently admitted to the CVICU with a diagnosis of sepsis. Melinda's father, a recent immigrant from Greece with limited English language skills, refused to leave his daughter's bedside, despite urging from the unit staff. Within 2 days of her admission, Melinda's status rapidly deteriorated, and she went into cardiac arrest. Nancy, the nurse caring for Melinda, had previously questioned the attending physician about the patient's code status, feeling she should not be resuscitated, but the physician disagreed. Consequently, Nancy initiated CPR while the father pleaded with her not to hurt his daughter.

Melinda eventually died in the early morning hours, and the father's cries of anguish could be heard throughout the unit. This was the fourth death in the unit within a week. Nancy felt she had failed both the patient and her father that night. She believed she had caused the patient and her father undue suffering by administering CPR that she felt to be futile. In addition, she felt she was not able to provide the degree of support to Melinda's father that he needed, in part due to being short staffed in the unit, but also because she did not have access late at night to interpretive services to address the language barrier or to pastoral care services to support his spiritual needs. As days passed, Nancy described feeling an overwhelming sense of guilt and failure for not meeting her standard of care and found herself to be tearful and unable to rid herself of the sound of the father's anguished cries for his daughter.

Andrew Jameton (1984), a professor of Philosophy and Ethics in Public Health at the University of Nebraska Medical Center, is credited with first coining the term "moral distress" in 1984 in a book on nursing ethics. In it he states, "[M]oral distress arises when one knows the right thing to do, but institutional constraints make it nearly impossible to pursue the right course of action" (p. 6). According to Epstein & Delgado (2010), moral distress involves a threat to one's *moral integrity*, which is defined as "the sense of wholeness and self-worth that comes from having clearly defined values that are congruent with one's actions and perceptions" (p. 3).

What Is Moral Distress?

The American Association of Critical-Care Nurses (AACN) defines moral distress as "[something that] occurs when you know the ethically appropriate action to take, but are unable to act upon it [and when] you act in a manner contrary to your personal and professional values, which undermines your integrity and authenticity" (AACN, n.d., p. 1). The Canadian Nurses Association (CNA) *Code of Ethics for Registered Nurses* defines moral distress as arising

> in situations where nurses know or believe they know the right thing to do, but for various reasons (including fear or circumstances beyond their control) do not or cannot take the right action or prevent a particular harm. When values and commitments are compromised in this way, nurses' identity and integrity as moral agents are affected and they feel moral distress. (CNA, 2008, p. 6)

Three Causes of Moral Distress

The research literature defines three root causes of moral distress (Hamric, Borchers, & Epstein, 2012):

- Problematic clinical situations
- Internal constraints
- External constraints

Examples of problematic clinical situations include aggressive treatment that is considered futile, working with providers who do not have the required level of competence, inadequate informed consent, inadequate pain relief, using resources inappropriately, disregard for patient's wishes, lack of truth-telling, and providing false hope to patients and families (Corley, 2002; Hamric et al., 2012; Pauly et al., 2009).

Internal constraints include personal characteristics of the healthcare professional that limit his or her ability to affect the situation, for example, a lack of assertiveness or confidence, perceived powerlessness, an error in judgment, lack of understanding the full situation or of alternative treatment options, socialization to follow orders, fear of losing one's job, or anxiety about creating conflict (Hamric et al., 2012; Hamric, Davis, & Childress, 2006; Wilkinson, 1987).

External constraints include the broader organizational and contextual constraints, such as hierarchies and power imbalances within the healthcare system, lack of collaboration, lack of resources, pressures to cut costs, inadequate team communication, policies that conflict with patient care needs, following family wishes regarding patient care for fear of litigation, tolerance within team of disruptive and/or abusive behavior, and a negative ethical climate (Elpern, Covert, & Kleinpell, 2005; Epstein & Hamric, 2009; Gutierrez, 2005; Hamric et al., 2012; Kälvemark, Höglund, Hansson, Westerholm, & Arnetz, 2004; Ludwick & Silva, 2003; Papathanassoglou et al., 2012; Zuzelo, 2007).

Reflection Activity

You are now invited to go back and reread Nancy's story with patient Melinda. Then consider the following questions:

- *Did you have any thoughts about or reactions to this story?*

- *Can you identify the problematic clinical situation?*

- *What internal constraints were present, in your opinion?*

- *What external constraints were present, in your opinion?*

- *If Nancy worked in your workplace, what resources would she have available to address her moral distress during and after the event?*

- *In terms of managing your own moral distress, is there a resource you wish was available to you at your workplace, but currently isn't?*

- *Can you think of one or two outside sources of support to help you manage this stressor? (You may wish to read on and return to this question once you have completed this section.)*

The negative effects of moral distress have been well established and include both psychological and physical effects (Pauly, Varcoe, & Storch, 2012). The psychological reactions often involve feelings of frustration, sadness, isolation, guilt, anxiety, tearfulness, depression, nightmares, helplessness, powerlessness, and anger (Elpern et al., 2005; Wilkinson, 1987). The experience of moral distress increases the risk of poor coping, low self-esteem, loss of personal integrity, and avoidance or withdrawal from patients (Epstein & Delgado, 2010).

Physical responses include sweating, trembling, headaches, gastrointestinal upset, and insomnia. The effects on the workplace include lack of trust, poor collaboration, poor pain management, health professional burnout, and high turnover rates (Austin et al., 2003; Austin, Lemermeyer, Goldberg, Bergum, & Johnson, 2005; Corley, et al., 2005; Elpern, et al., 2005; Gutierrez, 2005; Hamric, 2000; Hamric & Blackhall, 2007; Jameton, 1993; Meltzer & Huckabay, 2004; Nathaniel, 2006; Sundin-Huard & Fahy, 1999; Wilkinson, 1987).

Studies have also highlighted the powerful lingering effects of moral distress, termed "moral residue" by Webster and Baylis (2000). In organizations where moral distress is unaddressed, the moral residue builds over time in what is referred to as a "crescendo effect" (Epstein & Hamric, 2009). As noted by Epstein & Hamric (2009), there are three potential consequences of moral distress and moral residue:

- The first consequence is that nurses may become desensitized to the moral aspects of care and see their disregard of their ethical obligations as normal.

- Second, nurses may engage in different ways of conscientiously objecting to an ethically challenging situation, which may be either productive (e.g., calling an ethics consult) or disruptive (e.g., documenting a disagreement in a patient's chart) (Epstein & Delgado, 2010).

- The third consequence is burnout.

Research shows a correlation between moral distress and burnout (Epstein & Delgado, 2010; Meltzer & Huckabay, 2004) with some studies identifying moral distress as a reason nurses choose to leave their position or even their profession (Corley, 1995; Hamric & Blackhall, 2007).

Wendy Austin, in the Faculty of Nursing and the John Dossetor Health Ethics Centre at the University of Alberta, argues that healthcare restructuring and cutbacks are demoralizing. She believes the shift to a corporate model of healthcare and the streamlining of services places health professionals at greater risk of being in conflict with their ethical obligation to those in their care. According to Austin (2012):

> [H]ealth care practice needs to be grounded in a capacity for compassion and empathy, as evident in standards of practice and codes of ethics. Such grounding allows for humane response to the availability of unprecedented advances in biotechnology treatment, for genuine dialogue and the raising of difficult, necessary ethical questions and for the mutual support of health professionals themselves. If healthcare environments are not understood as moral communities but rather as simulated market places, then the healthcare professionals' moral agency is diminished and their vulnerability to moral distress is exacerbated. (p. 27)

The 4As—An Approach to Address and Reduce Moral Distress

- *Ask: Review the definition and symptoms of moral distress and ask yourself whether what you are feeling is moral distress. Are your colleagues exhibiting signs of moral distress as well?*

- *Affirm: Affirm your feelings about the issue. What aspect of your moral integrity is being threatened? What role could you (and should you) play?*

- *Assess: Begin to put some facts together. What is the source of your moral distress? What do you think is the "right," action and why is it so? What is being done currently and why? Who are the players in this situation? Are you ready to act?*

- *Act: Create a plan for action and implement it. Think about potential pitfalls and strategies to get around these pitfalls.*

Source: AACN, 2005, n.d; Rushton, 2006.

The Connection Between Compassion Fatigue and Moral Distress

To date, there is limited research that explores how these types of occupational stressors are interrelated. Evidence exists to demonstrate the validity of each as distinct concepts, but what is not known is the role each may play in the development of the other (Sabo, 2011). What is known, however, is that moral distress is the result of a "perceived violation of one's core values and duties, concurrent with a feeling of being constrained from taking ethically appropriate action" (Epstein & Hamric, 2009, p. 331). It is this challenge to one's personal and professional values and moral integrity that distinguishes moral distress from psychological distress and compassion fatigue (Epstein & Hamric, 2009). Psychological distress describes emotional reactions to situations, but does not necessarily involve a violation of core values and obligations (Epstein & Hamric, 2009; McCarthy & Deady, 2008).

Strategies for Creating a Positive Ethical Climate

Several authors have discussed strategies for addressing moral distress (Austin et al., 2005; Badger & O'Connor, 2006; Bell & Breslin, 2008; Corley et al., 2005; Epstein & Hamric, 2009; Hamric et al., 2006; Hamric & Blackhall, 2007; Hart, 2005; McDaniel, 1997; Olson, 1998; Papathanassoglou et al., 2012; Pauly et al., 2009; Pauly et al., 2012).

Their suggestions for creating a positive ethical climate are compiled here:

- Speak up: Identify the problem, gather the facts, and voice your opinion.

- Be deliberate: Know whom you need to speak with and know what you need to speak about.

- Be accountable: Sometimes our actions are not quite right. Be ready to acknowledge this and accept the consequences.

- Build support networks: Align yourself with colleagues who support you. Speak with one authoritative voice. Foster caring colleagues and a zero-tolerance policy on lateral violence.

- Focus on changes in the work environment: Focusing on the environment is more productive than focusing on one individual patient. Similar problems tend to re-occur. It's not usually the patient that needs changing, but the system.

- Participate in moral distress education: Attend forums and discussions about moral distress. Learn all you can.

- Make it interdisciplinary: Multiple views are needed to determine the common causes of moral distress in your unit. Target those. Facilitate open interdisciplinary communication.

- Develop policies: Develop policies to encourage open discussion, interdisciplinary collaboration, and the initiation of ethics consults.

- Design a workshop: Train staff to recognize moral distress, identify barriers to change, and create a plan for action.

- Make sure everyone knows how to utilize the hospital Ethics Committee.

- Provide an opportunity for those less powerful to be heard.

- Seek out effective role models for novice nurses.

- Provide an adequate orientation for new staff.

- Establish an environment that supports professional autonomy.

- Consider ethics rounds.

- Self-reflection may help people develop the courage needed to change circumstances that they view as morally wrong.

- Make use of well-established ethical decision-making frameworks to facilitate dialogue and balanced application of various relevant values among stakeholders.

- Support caring for self.

Source: Adapted in part from Epstein & Delgado, 2010, p. 7

Reducing Compassion Fatigue and Burnout— What Works?

Mathieu (2012) discusses strategies to reduce compassion fatigue and burnout. In summary, research in the field shows that the following key strategies reduce compassion fatigue and burnout in healthcare professionals:

- Strong social support both at home and at work (Bober & Regehr, 2005; Killian, 2008)
- More control over work schedule (Duxbury et al., 2010; Killian, 2008)
- Rebalancing caseload and workload reduction (Bober & Regehr, 2005; Killian, 2008)
- Timely access to good quality debriefing and supervision (Killian, 2008; Saakvitne & Pearlman, 1996)
- Reduced number of hours spent working directly with traumatized individuals (Bober & Regehr, 2005)
- Access to regular professional development and ongoing training (Killian, 2008)
- Increased self-awareness through mindfulness meditation and narrative work such as journaling (Cohen-Katz et al., 2005; Kearney, Weininger, Vachon, Harrison, & Mount, 2009; Shapiro, Brown, & Biegel, 2007)
- Good self-care (Gentry, 2002; Saakvitne & Pearlman, 1996)
- Improved work/life balance
- High job satisfaction
- Access to counseling and/or coaching as needed
- Increased recognition of the work done by nurses (Saakvitne & Pearlman, 1996)

Duxbury, Higgins, and Lyons' 2010 study also found that most of the strategies used by healthcare workers to manage overload were self-initiated and few of them came from the hospital offering flexibility and support: "It appears that supportive management, being prepared emotionally, having a plan, setting priorities and having a good support team and access to help are the best ways to cope" (p. 2). Budin et al. (2013) recently showed that nurses working at magnet hospitals were less likely to report verbal abuse by colleagues.

Strategies to reduce compassion fatigue, burnout, and moral distress and to improve quality patient care need to be implemented at all levels simultaneously (Saakvitne & Pearlman, 1996):

- Individually (nurses deciding to improve their self-care and work-life balance)
- Professionally (nurses accessing additional training, championing positive team engagement, choosing not to participate in gossip or lateral violence at work)
- Organizationally (hospitals providing adequate staffing, access to good quality supervision, and ongoing education and training)
- With the system as a whole (recognizing that person-centered care, which includes the health of the caregivers, is a priority to ensure high-quality patient care; more funding being provided to healthcare and social services; improved salaries and working conditions for healthcare professionals)

Individual Strategies

The advantage of individual strategies is that they can be implemented by the healthcare practitioner at any time, no matter *where* they work, with *whom* they work or how healthy or toxic their workplace is. Individual strategies begin with the self through a process called self-awareness, through the practice of mindfulness, and finally by identifying one's own early warning signals of burnout and compassion fatigue.

Develop Self-Awareness

As explained in *The Compassion Fatigue Workbook*:

> Self-awareness means being in tune with your stress signals. Do you have a good sense of how your body communicates to you when it is overwhelmed? Do you get sick as soon as you go on vacation, develop hives, or get a migraine when you are stressed? Many of us live in a state of permanent overload and are dimly aware of it. What happens when you feel angry? Do you explode or do you swallow your rage? Where in your body do you feel your anger? (Mathieu, 2012, p. 81)

Self-awareness also means being aware of our current feelings and behaviors, understanding the choices we make, being aware of the reasons why we act or react the way we do and how this is connected to our past history, perhaps, or a trauma we experienced. Do you live in a constant state of overwhelm? Many healthcare workers, when pressed, will admit that they have become "hooked" on stress and tend to live in crisis mode most of the time.

In her book *Trauma Stewardship*, Laura van Dernoot Lipsky addresses the risk of living in a constant state of tension and urgency: "When we keep ourselves numbed out on adrenaline or overworking or cynicism, we don't have an accurate internal gauge of ourselves and our needs" (van Dernoot Lipsky & Burke, 2009, p. 110). The best way to develop self-awareness is to practice mindfulness, which is our second strategy for individuals in healthcare.

Practice Mindfulness

Mindfulness is an ancient Buddhist practice that invites participants to meditate while being in the present moment, without judgment. Mindfulness-Based Stress Reduction (MBSR) is a mind-body approach that was originally developed by Jon Kabat-Zinn in the late 1970s and was popularized by the publication of his book *Full Catastrophe Living* (1990) and by a very successful stress-reduction program taught by Kabat-Zinn and colleagues at the University of Massachusetts Medical Center (Kabat-Zinn, 1982). MBSR has become extremely popular since: Many hospitals and mental health services provide MBSR training to their staff and patients alike.

Among many health benefits, MBSR has been found to effectively reduce relapse in depression and help chronic-pain patients manage their symptoms (Kabat-Zinn, 1982; Teasdale, Segal & Williams, 1995). Additional work exploring the effectiveness of MBSR in reducing compassion fatigue has shown some very positive results: "One study of clinical nurses found that MBSR helped to significantly reduce symptoms of compassion fatigue [...and] helped subjects be calmer and more grounded during their rounds and interactions with patients and colleagues" (Cohen-Katz, et al., 2005 as cited in Mathieu, 2012, p. 123). In 2005, a randomized control trial exploring the effectiveness of MBSR in reducing stress in healthcare professionals found that "those who participated in the MBSR intervention reported decreased perceived stress and greater self-compassion when compared with controls" (Shapiro, Astin, Bishop & Cordova, 2005, p. 170).

Develop an Early Warning System

Compassion fatigue and burnout are cumulative effects of working in high-stress, high-volume workplaces, but they do not manifest themselves in the same way in each person. The best strategy is for each helping professional to get to know his or her own warning signs. If we were to place your stress and overload symptoms on a continuum from green to yellow to red (green being when you are least symptomatic, red being when you are close to stress leave, for example), what would your yellow zone look like? What would be your main behavioral, emotional, and physical symptoms (Mathieu, 2012)?

Examples of Self-Care Activities

- *Participate in non–work related hobbies where you are not in a helping role*
- *Exercise regularly*
- *Eat healthy, nourishing foods during your shifts*
- *Have a transition ritual to leave work behind when you get home*
- *Spend time with friends and family who are not in your field, without talking shop*
- *Have access to regular debriefing or counseling, as needed*
- *Journal, meditate, connect with nature*
- *Read non–work related books during your downtime*
- *Spend time with pets*

Professional Strategies

Professional strategies are tools that each healthcare professional can use to enhance their resiliency such as ensuring that their clinical skills are well-honed and up-to-date; developing healthy boundaries; enhancing presence; and finally, assessing one's interaction with work colleagues to avoid toxicity and gossip and instead foster positive professional connections.

Identify Areas of Work Where You Need Additional Training

When hospitals and other healthcare agencies have to compress budgets, one of the first areas affected is often education and training; staff report no longer having access to as many continuing education programs as they did in the past, or departments find themselves unable to fund backfill while nurses are away at training courses, and, as a result, requests for educational leave are denied (Gentry, 2002). One of the very first studies on treating compassion fatigue identified "skill acquisition" as one of the five key pillars of wellness for helping professionals (Gentry, Baranowsky, & Dunning, 1997). In another later paper, J. Eric Gentry refers to situations in which staff is "working beyond levels of competency" and explains that this is often a result of role overload and lack of training (Gentry, 2002, p. 49).

You are invited to ask yourself the following questions:

- Are there areas of your work that are new to you, and where you feel unskilled and worried about your lack of training and/or experience?

- Are there areas of your work where you feel rusty? Are there techniques you have not used in a long time, and do you feel that you would benefit from some additional training/practice?

- Have you been "volunteered" to perform some clinical techniques that are outside your scope of practice without having access to further training?

Practice "Exquisite Empathy"

Richard Harrison and Marv Westwood, two psychologists in the field of compassion fatigue, have coined a beautiful term to describe our ultimate goal: *exquisite empathy*. They define exquisite empathy as a key characteristic of highly resilient helping professionals.

The key features of these helpers are that they experience, in their work with patients, "highly present, sensitively attuned, well-boundaried, heartfelt empathic engagement" (Harrison & Westwood, 2009, p. 213). Harrison and Westwood explain that these are practitioners who are "invigorated rather than depleted by their intimate professional connections with traumatized clients" (p. 213) Another way to put this: On the continuum between feeling completely numb and desensitized at one end of the spectrum and being devastated and weeping at every patient story at the other end, there is this "sweet spot" in the middle that allows helping professionals to care "just the right amount" while remaining grounded and present for our patients.

The challenge is that our compassion, although it may have been at an optimal level when we started working in the field, is constantly challenged by workplace burnout, competing demands on our time, and a sometimes less than ideal organizational context.

Connect with Colleagues on Your Team

In a 2008 study, York University researcher Kyle Killian found that social support at work was "the most significant factor associated with higher scores on compassion satisfaction" (p. 40).

Compassion satisfaction is defined by Beth Stamm as the "pleasure you derive from being able to do your work well" (Stamm, n.d., para. 1).

Unfortunately, one of the first casualties of burnout and compassion fatigue is workplace collegiality. Ample data on what is often referred to as lateral violence demonstrates that nurses, in particular, tend to be very hard on each other when they are stressed and overloaded; in an atmosphere of role overload, staff members in a hospital often turn on each other and develop what has been called a "poverty mentality" (Sheridan-Leos, 2008; Stanley, Martin, Michel, Welton, & Nemeth, 2007).

As a strategy, we recommend that you identify the most positive staff members on your team and foster constructive alliances with them: Take lunch breaks together and embrace a "no-gossip" policy. Encourage staff members to have open discussions about their yellow zones of compassion fatigue and burnout, and share strategies on the best ways that your colleagues can support you when you are in the yellow zone.

Beware of Getting Stuck in a Negative Spiral

Mathieu (2012) discusses strategies to manage negativity in the workplace: "When a workplace is toxic, several things happen: The atmosphere becomes one of mistrust (with the suspicion often directed at upper management). Many of us get locked into a negative frame of mind" (pp. 71–72).

Laura van Dernoot Lipsky (2009) has written about the dangers of gossip and negativity in the workplace:

> We become convinced that others are responsible for our well-being and that we lack the personal agency to transform our circumstances. This notion has less to do with our physical surroundings than with our internal states. We may believe that we deserve better pay, safer work environments, more respect, adequate time away from work, and greater resources, and this all may be true, [...but] we can succumb to a belief that we have no capacity to influence any outcome. (p. 93)

You are invited to take an honest look at your current attitude toward work and office gossip, and see whether you are surrounding yourself with colleagues who are likely in the red zone, and who promote cynicism and negative talk.

Examples of Professional Strategies for the Team

- *Avoid office gossip.*
- *Form positive strategic alliances: Identify your colleagues who are still in the green or light yellow zone and spend more time with them.*

- *Advocate for change in a constructive manner: Use business language to make your case (e.g., showing that compassion fatigue and burnout lead to increased rates of sick leave and attrition—retention statistics may have more sway with senior leadership than speaking about how staff is feeling about the workload).*

- *Join or form a wellness committee.*

- *Invite a few colleagues to participate in a lunch sharing program where each person makes lunches for everyone in the group one day a week and then receives a meal from a different person during the rest of the week.*

Organizational Strategies

Research demonstrates that rates of burnout and compassion fatigue are lowered when staff perceives that their organization is supportive (Bober & Regehr, 2005; Duxbury & Higgins, 2012; Killian, 2008). Over the past 2 decades, work-life balance specialists Duxbury and Higgins have carried out several extensive surveys on employee work-life balance, caregiver duties, and role overload, interviewing more than 100,000 subjects since 1991. Their latest reports, released in 2012–2013, present a shocking decline in the quality of work-life balance among their survey sample: At this present time, only 23% of their subjects say that they are satisfied with their work-life balance compared to 46% in 1991; 57% reported high levels of stress; and 40% said that were experiencing role overload, which is defined as "a type of role conflict that results from excessive demands on the time and energy supply of an individual such that satisfactory performance is improbable" (Duxbury & Higgins, 2012, p. 7).

They also found that employees who cannot balance work and home tend to miss more work, have lower productivity, and be heavier users of employee benefits than those who are coping well (Duxbury & Higgins, 2012; Duxbury & Higgins, 2013).

What can organizations do? Duxbury and Higgins (2012) offer concrete recommendations for organizations, and name "3 key determinants of employee mental health, work-life balance and absenteeism":

- "Being able to vary arrival and departure times"
- "Arrang[ing] work schedule to accommodate family demands"
- "Being able to interrupt work day to deal with personal matters and then return to work" (p. 12)

They also demonstrate that what makes the biggest difference is the quality of management— "who you work for vs where you work"—and recommend that managers be offered the training they need with enough time to "grow into their role" (Duxbury & Higgins, 2012, p. 12).

Conclusion

It is a gray and cold Tuesday in the middle of the Minnesota winter, and Jana is working at her usual fast pace in the dialysis unit, trying to keep on top of the call bells and beeping monitors. One of her patients, Mr. Simmons, who has been coming three times a week for 12 years, was recently admitted as an inpatient for end stage renal failure, and doctors gave him a few days left to live. He is receiving dialysis nonetheless as per his and his wife's wishes. At some point during her busy day, Jana notices that this man's vitals are fading fast. The physician comes and declares there is nothing left to be done except to keep him comfortable. His dialyzer is unplugged, and his wife is called to his side.

Jana is upset that the doctor has not ordered for this patient to be wheeled to a more discreet space for his last moments on earth. There he is, dying in a noisy, brightly lit unit among 30 other patients. All that Jana can do is pull the curtain around Mr. Simmons and ask the family visiting the patient beside him to be quieter, given the circumstances. Mrs. Simmons is left alone sitting next to her husband holding his hand. After about an hour, when Mr. Simmons has breathed his last breath, Jana pops her head in briefly and asks whether there is anyone she can call for Mrs. Simmons. She also asks her, as per protocol, to fill out the required forms for the removal of the body. At the end of her shift, Jana feels exhausted and sad. This isn't what she would want for her loved ones.

Reflection Activity

- *What are your thoughts about and reactions to this story?*

- *Based on what you have read in this chapter, please identify three resources that Jana could harness in helping her manage this stressful situation:*

    a. *Personal:*

    b. *Professional:*

    c. *Organizational:*

In his 2012 blog article "Patient-Centered Care: What It Means and How to Get There," James Rickert writes, "[P]atient-centered care is a method of care that relies upon effective communication, empathy, and a feeling of partnership between doctor and patient to improve patient care outcomes and satisfaction, to lessen patient symptoms, and to reduce unnecessary costs." It stands to reason that nurses, many of whom are suffering from some level of work-related exhaustion and are working with depleted physicians and other allied health professionals, may find that their effective communication skills with families and patients erode over time. We believe that patient safety and quality of care can be improved by providing units with adequate staffing, reducing role overload, providing staff with regular educational training on complex issues (such as psychiatric illnesses and the impact of trauma on patient and family behaviors), and by addressing other factors related to burnout, compassion fatigue, and moral distress.

It is clear that if we are going to successfully navigate the upcoming surging demographic tide of aging patients while delivering high-quality care, healthcare workers need more support, better working conditions, and better training. True patient-centered care cannot be implemented without taking the full organizational picture into account. We cannot expect nurses to provide high-quality care without supplying them with the tools necessary to do their work in a way that is sustainable for both individual helping professionals and institutions as a whole.

References

Abendroth, M., & Flannery, J. (2006). Predicting the risk of compassion fatigue: A study of hospice nurses. *Journal of Hospice and Palliative Nursing, 8*(6), 346-356.

American Association of Critical-Care Nurses (AACN). (n.d.). *The 4As to rise above moral distress.* Retrieved from http://www.aacn.org/moraldistress4As

American Association of Critical-Care Nurses (AACN). (2005). AACN standards for establishing and sustaining healthy work environments: A journey to excellence. *American Journal of Critical Care, 14*(3), 187-197.

American Hospital Association. (2012, December). Are Medicare patients getting sicker? *Trendwatch.* Retrieved from http://www.aha.org/research/reports/tw/12dec-tw-ptacuity.pdf

Austin, W. (2012). Moral distress and the contemporary plight of health professionals. *HealthCare Ethics Committee Forum, 1*(24), 27-38.

Austin, W., Bergum, V., & Goldberg, L. (2003). Unable to answer the call of our patients: Mental health nurses' experiences of moral distress. *Nursing Inquiry, 10*(3), 177-183.

Austin, W., Lemermeyer, G., Goldberg, L. Bergum, V., & Johnson, M. S. (2005). Moral distress in healthcare practices: The situation of nurses. *HealthCare Ethics Committee Forum, 17*(1), 33-48.

Azoulay, E., Chevret, S., Leleu, G., Pochard, F., Barboteu, M., Adrie, C.,…Schlemmer, B. (2000). Half the families of intensive care unit patients experience inadequate communication with physicians. *Critical Care Medicine, 28*(8), 3044-3049.

Badger, J. M., & O'Connor, B. (2006). Moral discord, cognitive coping strategies, and medical intensive care unit nurses: Insights from a focus group study. *Critical Care Nursing Quarterly, 29*(2), 147-151.

Bell, J., & Breslin, J. M. (2008). Healthcare provider moral distress as a leadership challenge. *Journal of Nursing Administration's Healthcare Law, Ethics and Regulation, 10*(4), 94-97.

Bober, T., & Regehr, C. (2005). Strategies for reducing secondary or vicarious trauma: Do they work? *Brief Treatment and Crisis Intervention, 6*(1), 1-9.

Budin, W. C., Brewer, C. S., Chao, Y-Y., & Kovner, C. (2013). Verbal abuse from nurse colleagues and work environment of early career registered nurses. *Journal of Nursing Scholarship, 45*(3), 308-316. doi: 10.1111/jnu.12033

Canada Census, (2011). The Canadian population in 2011: Age and sex. Retrieved from http://www12.statcan.ca/census-recensement/2011/as-sa/98-311-x/98-311-x2011001-eng.cfm

Canadian Nurses Association (CNA). (2008). *Code of ethics for registered nurses.* Retrieved from http://www.cna-aiic.ca/~/media/cna/files/en/codeofethics.pdf

Cohen-Katz, J., Wiley, S. D., Capuano, T., Bakers, D. M., Kimmel, S., & Shapiro, S. (2005). The effects of mindfulness-based stress reduction on nurse stress and burnout, Part II: A quantitative and qualitative study. *Holistic Nursing Practice, 19*(1), 26-35.

Corley, M. C. (1995). Moral distress of critical care nurses. *American Journal of Critical Care, 4*(4), 280-285.

Corley, M. C. (2002). Nurse moral distress: A proposed theory and research agenda. *Nursing Ethics, 9*(6), 636-650.

Corley, M. C., Minick, P., Elswick, R. K., & Jacobs, M. (2005). Nurse moral distress and ethical work environment. *Nursing Ethics, 12*(4), 381-390.

Duxbury, L., & Higgins, C. (2012). *National study on balancing work and caregiving in Canada.* Carleton University: Sprott School of Business. Retrieved from http://newsroom.carleton.ca/wp-content/files/2012-National-Work-Long-Summary.pdf

Duxbury, L. & Higgins, C. (2013). *Balancing work, childcare and eldercare: A view from the trenches.* Carleton University: Sprott School of Business.

Duxbury, L., Higgins, C., & Lyons, S. (2010). *The etiology and reduction of role overload in Canada's health care sector.* Carleton University: Sprott School of Business. Retrieved from http://sprott.carleton.co/wp-content/files/complete-report.pdf

Egging, D., Crowley, M., Arruda, T., Proehl, J., Walker-Cillor, G., Papa, A.,…Bokholdt, M. L. (2011). Does family presence have a positive or negative influence on the patient, family and staff during invasive procedures and resuscitation? *Journal of Emergency Nursing, 37*(5) 469-473.

Elpern, E. H., Covert, B., & Kleinpell, R. (2005). Moral distress of staff nurses in a medical intensive care unit. *American Journal of Critical Care, 14*(6), 523-530.

Epstein, E. G., & Delgado, S. (2010). Understanding and addressing moral distress. *The Online Journal of Issues in Nursing, 15*(3). Retrieved from http://gm6.nursingworld. org/Main MenuCategories/ANAMarketplace/ ANAPeriodicals/OJIN/TableofContents/Vol152010/No3-Sept-2010/Understanding-Moral-Distress.aspx

Epstein, E. G., & Hamric, A. B. (2009). Moral distress, moral residue, and the crescendo effect. *The Journal of Clinical Ethics, 20,* 330-342.

Figley, C. R. (Ed.). (1995). *Compassion fatigue: Coping with secondary traumatic stress disorder in those who treat the traumatized.* New York, NY: Brunner/Mazel.

Freudenberger, H. J. (1980). *Burn-Out: The high cost of high achievement.* Norwell, MA: Anchor Press.

Gentry, J. E. (2002). Compassion fatigue: A crucible of transformation. *Journal of Trauma Practice, 1*(3/4), 37-61.

Gentry, J. E., Baranowsky, A., & Dunning, K. (1997, November). *Accelerated recovery program for compassion fatigue.* Paper presented at the meeting of the International Society for Traumatic Stress Studies, Montreal, Canada.

Gutierrez, K. (2005). Critical care nurses' perceptions of and responses to moral distress. *Dimensions of Critical Care Nursing, 24*(5), 229-241.

Hamric, A. B. (2000). Moral distress in everyday ethics. *Nursing Outlook, 48*(5), 199-201.

Hamric, A. B., & Blackhall, L. J. (2007). Nurse-physician perspectives on the care of dying patients in intensive care units: Collaboration, moral distress, and ethical climate. *Critical Care Medicine, 35*(2), 422-429

Hamric, A. B., Borchers, C. T., & Epstein, E. G. (2012). Development and testing of an instrument to measure moral distress in healthcare professionals. *AJOB Primary Research, 3*(2), 1-9.

Hamric, A. B., Davis, W. S., & Childress, M. D. (2006). Moral distress in health care professionals. *Pharos, 69*(1), 16-23.

Harrison, R. L., & Westwood, M. J. (2009). Preventing vicarious traumatization of mental health therapists: Identifying protective practices. *Psychotherapy: Theory, Research, Practice Training, 46*(2), 203-219.

Hart, S. E. (2005). Hospital ethical climates and registered nurses' turnover intentions. *Journal of Nursing Scholarship, 37*(2), 173-177.

Heyland, D. K., Rocker, G. M., Dodek, P. M., Kutsogiannis, D. J., Konopad, E., Cook, D. J.,…O'Callaghan, C. J. (2002). Family satisfaction with care in the intensive care unit: Results of a multiple centre study. *Critical Care Medicine, 30*(7), 1413-1418.

Institute of Medicine (IOM). (2001). *Crossing the quality chasm: A new health system for the 21st century.* Washington, DC: National Academy Press.

Jameton, A. (1984). *Nursing practice: The ethical issues.* Upper Saddle River, NJ: Prentice-Hall.

Jameton, A. (1993). Dilemmas of moral distress: Moral responsibility and nursing practice. *Clinical Issues in Perinatal and Women's Health Nursing, 4*(4), 542-551.

Joinson, C. (1992). Coping with compassion fatigue. *Nursing, 22*(4), 116-121.

The Joint Commission (TJC). (2010). *Advancing effective communication, cultural competence, and patient- and family-centered care: A roadmap for hospitals.* Oakbrook Terrace, IL: Author.

Kabat-Zinn, J. (1982). An outpatient program in behavioural medicine for chronic pain patients based on the practice of mindfulness meditation: Theoretical considerations and preliminary results. *General Hospital Psychiatry, 4*(1), 33-42.

Kabat-Zinn, J. (1990). *Full catastrophe living: Using the wisdom of your body and mind to face stress, pain, and illness.* New York, NY: Delta.

Kälvemark, S., Höglund, A. T., Hansson, M. G., Westerholm, P., & Arnetz, B. (2004). Living with conflicts: Ethical dilemmas and moral distress in the health care system. *Social Science & Medicine, 58*(6), 1075-1084.

Kearney, M. K., Weininger, R. B., Vachon, L. S., Harrison, R. L., Mount, B. M. (2009). Self-care of physicians caring for patients at the end of life. *Journal of the American Medical Association, 301*(11), 1155-1164.

Killian, K. (2008). Helping till it hurts? A multimethod study of compassion fatigue, burnout, and self care in clinicians working with trauma survivors. *Traumatology, 14*(2), 32-44.

Krichbaum, K., Diemert, C., Jacox, L., Jones, A., Koenig, P. Mueller, C., & Disch, J. (2007). Complexity compression: Nurses under fire. *Nursing Forum, 42*(2), 86-94.

Ludwick, R., & Silva, M. C. (2003). Errors, the nursing shortage, and ethics: Survey results. *Online Journal of Issues in Nursing, 8*(2). Retrieved from www.nursingworld.org/MainMenuCategories/ ANAMarketplace/ANAPeriodicals/OJIN/Columns/ Ethics/ShortageSurveyResults.aspx

Lützén, K., & Kvist, B. E. (2012). Moral distress: A comparative analysis of theoretical understandings and inter-related concepts. *HealthCare Ethics Committee Forum, 1*(24), 13-25.

Maslach, C. (1978). Job burn-out: How people cope. *Public Welfare, 36,* 56-58.

Maslach, C. (1982). Understanding burnout: Definitional issues in analyzing a complex phenomenon. In W. S. Paine (Ed.), *Job stress and burnout* (pp. 29-40). Beverly Hills, CA: Sage.

Mathieu, F. (2012). *The compassion fatigue workbook.* New York, NY: Routledge.

McCarthy, J., & Deady, R. (2008). Moral distress reconsidered. *Nursing Ethics, 15*(2), 254-262.

McDaniel, C. (1997). Development of psychometric properties of the ethics environment questionnaire. *Medical Care, 35*(9), 901-914.

Meltzer, L. S., & Huckabay, L. M. (2004). Critical care nurses' perceptions of futile care and its effect on burnout. *American Journal of Critical Care, 13*(3), 202-208.

Nathaniel, A. K. (2006). Moral reckoning in nursing. *Western Journal of Nursing Research, 28*(4), 419-438.

Olson. L. L. (1998). Hospital nurses' perceptions of the ethical climate of their work setting. *Journal of Nursing Scholarship, 30*(4), 345-349.

Papathanassoglou, E. D .E., Karanikola, M. N .K., Kalafati, M., Giannakopoulou, M., Lemonidou, C., & Albarran, J. W. (2012). Professional autonomy, collaboration with physicians, and moral distress among European intensive care nurses. *American Journal of Critical Care, 21*(2), e41-e52.

Pauly, B. M., Varcoe, C., & Storch, J. (2012). Framing the issues: Moral distress in health care. *HealthCare Ethics Committee Forum, 1*(24), 1-11.

Pauly, B. M., Varcoe, C., Storch, J. & Newton, L. (2009). Registered nurses' perceptions of moral distress and ethical climate. *Nursing Ethics, 16*(5), 561-573.

Pearlman, L. A., & Saakvitne, K. W. (1995). *Trauma and the therapist: Countertransference and vicarious traumatization in psychotherapy with incest survivors.* New York, NY: W.W. Norton.

Registered Nurses' Association of Ontario (RNAO). (2008). *Violence against nurses—"Zero" tolerance for violence against nurses and nursing students.* Retrieved from http://rnao.ca/policy/position-statements

Rickert, J. (2012, January 24). Patient-centered care: What it means and how to get there [blog post]. Retrieved from http://healthaffairs.org/blog/2012/01/24/patient-centered-care-what-it-means-and-how-to-get-there/

Rushton, C. H. (2006). Defining and addressing moral distress: Tools for critical care nursing leaders. *AACN Advanced Critical Care, 17*(2), 161-168.

Saakvitne, K. W., & Pearlman, L. A. (1995). Treating therapists with vicarious traumatization and secondary traumatic stress disorders. In C. Figley (Ed.), *Compassion fatigue: Coping with secondary traumatic stress disorder in those who treat the traumatized* (pp. 150-177). New York, NY: Brunner/Mazel.

Saakvitne, K .W., Pearlman, L. A., & the Staff of the Traumatic Stress Institute (1996). *Transforming the pain: A workbook on vicarious traumatization.* New York, NY: W.W. Norton.

Sabo, B., (2011). Reflecting on the concept of compassion fatigue. *Online Journal of Issues in Nursing, 16*(1), Manuscript 1. doi: 10.3912/OJIN.Vol16No01Man01

Schluter, J., Winch, S., Holzhauser, K., & Henderson, A. (2008). Nurses' moral sensitivity and hospital ethical climate: A literature review. *Nursing Ethics, 15*(3), 304-321.

Schoen, C., Osborn, R., Squires, D., Doty, M., Pierson, R., & Appelbaum, S. (2011). New 2011 survey of patients with complex care needs in eleven countries finds that care is often poorly coordinated. [Commonwealth Fund] *Health Affairs, 30*(12), 2437-2448.

Shanafelt, T. D. (2009). Enhancing meaning in work: A prescription for preventing physician burnout and promoting patient-centered care. *Journal of the American Medical Association, 302*(12), 1338-1340.

Shanafelt, T. D., Boone, S., Tam, L., Dyrbye, L. N., Sotile, W., Satele, D.,…Oreskovich, M. R. (2012). Burnout and satisfaction with work-life balance among U.S. physicians relative to the general U.S. population. *Archives of Internal Medicine, 172*(18), 1377-1386.

Shapiro, S., Astin, J., Bishop, S., & Cordova, M. (2005). Mindfulness-based stress reduction for health care professionals: Results from a randomized trial. *International Journal of Stress Management, 12*(2), 164-176.

Shapiro, S., Brown, K. W, & Biegel, G. M. (2007). Teaching self-care to caregivers: Effects of mindfulness-based stress reduction on the mental health of therapists in training. *Training and Education in Professional Psychology, 1*(2), 105-115.

Sheridan-Leos, N. (2008). Understanding lateral violence in nursing. *Clinical Journal of Oncology Nursing, 12*(3), 339-403.

Small, D. C. & Small, R. M. (2011). Patients first! Engaging the hearts and minds of nurses with a patient-centered practice model. *Online Journal of Issues in Nursing, 16*(2), Manuscript 2.

Stamm, B. H. (n.d.). Beth Hudnall Stamm website. Retrieved at http://www.isu.edu/~bhstamm/

Stanley, K. M., Martin, M. M., Michel, Y., Welton, J. M., & Nemeth, L. S. (2007). Examining lateral violence in the nursing workforce. *Issues in Mental Health Nursing, 28*(11), 1247-1265.

Statistics Canada. (2006, December 11). National survey of the work and health of nurses. Retrieved from http://www.statcan.gc.ca/daily-quotidien/061211/dq061211b-eng.htm

Sundin-Huard, D. & Fahy, K. (1999). Moral distress, advocacy and burnout: Theorising the relationship. *International Journal of Nursing Practice, 5*(1), 8-13.

Teasdale, J. D., Segal, Z. V., & Williams, J. M. G. (1995). How does cognitive therapy prevent depressive relapse and why should attentional control (mindfulness) training help. *Behaviour Research and Therapy, 33*(1), 25-39.

Ulrich, B. T., Lavandero, R., Hart, K. A., Woods, D., Leggett, J., & Taylor, D. (2006). Critical care nurses' work environments: A baseline status report. *Critical Care Nurse, 26*(5), 46-50, 52-57.

U.S. Census Bureau. (2010). Older population in the United States: 2009. Retrieved from https://www.census.gov/newsroom/releases/archives/miscellaneous/2010-12-09_miscellaneous.html

van Dernoot Lipsky, L., & Burke, C. (2009). *Trauma stewardship: An everyday guide to caring for self while caring for others.* San Francisco, CA: Berrett-Koehler.

Webster, G. C., & Baylis, F. E. (2000). Moral residue. In S. B. Rubin & L. Zoloth (Eds.), *Margin of error: The ethics of mistakes in the practice of medicine* (pp. 217-230). Hagerstown, MD: University Publishing Group.

Wilkinson, J. M. (1987). Moral distress in nursing practice: Experience and effects. *Nursing Forum, 23*(1), 16-29.

Zuzelo, P. R. (2007). Exploring the moral distress of registered nurses. *Nursing Ethics, 14*(3), 344-359.

Chapter 21

Patient- and Family-Centered Care and the Interprofessional Team

Gail E. Armstrong, DNP, ACNS-BC, CNE

Amy J. Barton, PhD, RN, FAAN

Wesley Nuffer, PharmD, BCPS, CDE

Lynne Yancey, MD

Mr. Yeager is a 70-year-old man with a history of an aortic valve replacement, rheumatoid arthritis, and recurrent sinusitis. He lives independently with his wife. His medications include warfarin, metoprolol, gabapentin, infliximab, and acetaminophen. He is followed by a nurse practitioner at his primary care clinic, a cardiologist in his cardiology clinic, a physician assistant in his rheumatology clinic, an otolaryngologist in his ENT clinic, and a pharmacist at the hospital's anticoagulation clinic. He also attends twice weekly physical therapy as part of his continuing recovery from recent spinal surgery. His cardiologist adjusts his blood pressure medications, his orthopedic surgeon managers his postoperative care, his rheumatology PA monitors his pain and anti-inflammatory medications, and the pharmacist adjusts his warfarin. At no point in time do these care providers communicate with one another.

Over the weekend, Mr. Yeager develops symptoms of a recurrent sinus infection. He calls the nurse practitioner who is on call for his ENT. She has access to his ENT clinic records, but not his primary care records. Based on his symptoms, she prescribes him amoxicillin/clavulanate for a presumed sinus infection. She is unaware of the increased risk of bleeding for Mr. Yeager with the medication interaction of these two medications. Mr. Yeager's wife asks the NP if she would contact Mr. Yeager's cardiologist, as she is aware that Mr. Yeager is on several cardiac medications, and the NP responds with "I'm sure this antibiotic will be fine."

The following week Mr. Yeager presents for his regular physical therapy. The therapist notes that he seems fatigued and decides to cut his therapy short for the day. As Mr. Yeager is finishing his exercises, he trips on the edge of the treadmill and falls, striking his face and causing a nosebleed. Despite repeated attempts by clinic staff, they are unable to stop the bleeding and eventually transport him by ambulance to the emergency department (ED), where he continues to bleed. At the ED, his blood pressure is 88/40, with a heart rate of 55. His nose is packed to stop the bleeding, and his hematocrit is found to be 23 with an INR of 9.5. He is admitted to the intensive care unit, where he receives a transfusion of fresh frozen plasma to reverse his coagulopathy and red blood cells for his severe blood loss. He is discharged from the hospital 8 days later with diagnoses of a fall due to postoperative weakness combined with hypotension secondary to his blood pressure medication, and severe nasal hemorrhage secondary to nasal trauma. At no point before Mr. Yeager's discharge are there any discussions about altering any of the medications that Mr. Yeager will resume taking upon his return to home.

Patient- and family-centered care (P&FCC) and teamwork enjoy generous overlap in shared concepts. Both competencies are aimed at improving patient safety, quality, and efficiency, yet there is a significant gap in translating overlapping values and concepts into practice, as shown in the preceding vignette. Instead of being complementary competencies, many healthcare professionals experience P&FCC and teamwork as competing competencies. Little is written about how healthcare teams can use a team-based approach in providing P&FCC.

How do members of the healthcare teams ensure that they are patient-centered? How might interprofessional healthcare teams assess whether they are patient- and family-centered in their communication, work processes, and decision-making? This chapter addresses the often complex reality of healthcare teams, and the various factors that contribute to healthcare teams losing sight of the provision of P&FCC. Additionally, this chapter offers team-based strategies and tools to effectively maintain the important aim of P&FCC as a common team priority.

P&FCC and the Interprofessional Mandate for All Healthcare Professions

In *Crossing the Quality Chasm* (Institute of Medicine [IOM], 2001), published more than a decade ago, the need to create a patient-centered care environment in which health professionals use evidence-based interventions and "knowledge is shared and information flows freely" (p. 67) was cited as an important approach to improving patient safety. This notion was further accentuated in a later report, *Health Professions Education: A Bridge to Quality* (Greiner & Knebel, 2003), in which educators and accreditation, licensing, and certification organizations were charged with the mandate that students and working professionals develop and maintain proficiency in five core areas (see Table 21.1). The national initiative Quality and Safety Education for Nurses (QSEN) built on this 2003 IOM report provides competency definitions and requisite knowledge, skill, and attitude elements to operationalize each competency. QSEN's definition of patient-centered care is: "Recognize the patient or designee as the source of control and full partner in providing compassionate and coordinated care based on respect for patient's preferences, values, and needs" (Cronenwett et al., 2007, p. 123).

TABLE 21.1   Five Core Competencies for Students of All Health Professions

Delivering patient-centered care

Working as part of interdisciplinary teams

Practicing evidence-based medicine

Focusing on quality improvement

Using information technology

Source: IOM, 2003

The link between patient-centered care and an interprofessional approach to that care has remained in the forefront of recommendations to reform both the healthcare system and the educational system producing the future workforce. The World Health Organization (WHO) created a *Framework for Action on Interprofessional Education and Collaborative Practice*. "Collaborative practice in healthcare occurs when multiple health workers from different professional backgrounds provide comprehensive services by working with patients, their families, careers and communities to deliver the highest quality of care across settings" (WHO, 2010, p. 13). The belief is that a collaborative health workforce is required to achieve successful outcomes with patients who need complex care.

To create this collaborative-practice ready workforce, participants in The Lancet Commission of Education of Health Professionals for the 21st Century (Frenk et al., 2010) propose the following vision:

> All health professionals in all countries should be educated to mobilize knowledge and to engage in critical reasoning and ethical conduct so that they are competent to participate in patient and population-centered health systems as members of locally responsive and globally connected teams. (p. 1924)

The report recommends a number of instructional reforms, most notably adoption of a competency-based curriculum that features patient-centered care and promotion of interprofessional education to enhance collaborative skills in creating effective healthcare teams. In the vignette that opens this chapter, there is a total lack of coordination of Mr. Yeager's care or his engagement as he moves across outpatient and inpatient settings. Thus, care providers are unable to accurately ascertain causes of Mr. Yeager's symptoms and healthcare needs and fail to coordinate their approaches to his multiple problems. And in the absence of teamwork and P&FCC, there is the high likelihood that Mr. Yeager may experience dangerous medication interactions in his future.

Another well-disseminated set of standards for practice for interprofessional teams comes from the Interprofessional Educational Collaborative (IPEC), an initiative sponsored by professional organizations in nursing, osteopathic medicine, pharmacy, dental education, medical educators, and public health. The IPEC Expert Panel identified patient- and family-centered care as a core competency for the functioning of a healthcare team (2011). Recognizing the multidisciplinary nature of health delivery systems, one of the core ethical principles for all clinicians to hold in common is "cooperation with those who receive care" (IPEC, 2011, p. 18). Additionally, the IPEC competencies are based on the relationship that the healthcare team holds with the patient and family, as this relationship undergirds all aspects of the care that team provides (IPEC, 2011).

Strategies to Enhance Team Functioning

Clinicians are educated with similar values around P&FCC, although practical approaches among disciplines vary. Moreover, among the resources for P&FCC and for teamwork, few integrate the two concepts, that is, actively incorporating patients and families while strengthening the team. The following strategies are not specific to any discipline and are effective when used by interdisciplinary healthcare teams. Supportive strategies for interdisciplinary healthcare teams include open and direct communication, shared values and principles, shared decision-making, collegial trust, swift trust, and a shared value of humility.

Open and Direct Communication

For healthcare teams to perform as high-functioning teams, communication must be a core concern. Communication among healthcare team members influences patient outcomes as well as provider satisfaction. Research with high-reliability organizations has demonstrated the vital importance of communication in complex work environments. An abundance of evidence-based tools exist for teams to improve their communication, including:

- TeamSTEPPS provides team-based communication tools for healthcare teams to increase clarity, accuracy, and efficiency of communication within and between healthcare teams (Agency for Healthcare Research and Quality [AHRQ], 2008).

- SBAR (Situation, Background, Assessment, Recommendation) is a structured approach for hand-offs and inquiries between healthcare providers. Principles of Crew Resource Management (CRM) have been used very effectively in improving patient outcomes by addressing team communication (Leonard, Graham, & Bonucom, 2004).

Similarly, several P&FCC models exist to assist individual clinicians in providing P&FCC, including:

- One model encourages clinicians to respond "With HEART" (**H**ear the story, **E**mpathize, **A**pologize, **R**espond to the Problem, and **T**hank the Patient) (Planetree & Picker Institute, 2008).

- Donald Berwick has written about using a P&FCC model based on "Nothing about me, without me," (p. w560) emphasizing how all care planning and discussions of care must include the patient and family (Berwick, 2009; Delbanco & Berwick, 2001).

As important as these two focal areas of evidence-based practice are, there is little overlap in the execution of how to provide P&FCC on teams. Open and direct communication tools are common to both teamwork strategies and P&FCC strategies, yet very little literature addresses the provision of team-based P&FCC. Wynia, VonKohorn, and Mitchell (2012) examine the important overlap of teamwork and P&FCC by providing useful team-based values and principles to illuminate high-functioning healthcare teams. For patients interacting with teams where members are transitory, there must be "structured processes to both introduce and refine the roles, expectations and norms of the team to meet the patient's needs" (p. 1327).

Additionally, high-functioning teams that provide P&FCC place a high value on open and direct communication as evidenced by the team's transparency and common language. Therefore, inclusion of patients and families into teams requires uniform use of "plain language," strategies to confirm understanding and access to information (Wynia et al., 2012). Table 21.2 outlines shared values among team members and shared principles to guide patient-centered, team-based care, and offers (in italics) team questions that will focus these values and principles on the provision of P&FCC. A common thread throughout both the values and principles is that whatever structure is created for interprofessional interactions must always include the patient. The added team questions highlight this theme.

TABLE 21.2 Values and Principles of High-Functioning Healthcare Teams

SHARED VALUES AMONG TEAM MEMBERS	SHARED PRINCIPLES TO GUIDE TEAM-BASED CARE
Honesty	**Clear Roles**
Put a high value on open communication within the team, including transparency about aims, decisions, uncertainty, and mistakes.	Have clear expectations for each member's function, responsibilities, and accountabilities.
Do the patient/family experience the team communication as transparent? Has the team asked the patient/family what transparency would look like to them?	*Are the patient/family included in outlining responsibilities?*
Discipline	**Mutual Trust**
Carry out roles and responsibilities even when inconvenient and seek out and share information to improve even when it is uncomfortable.	Earn each other's trust, creating strong norms of reciprocity and greater opportunities for shared achievement.
How are the patient/family included in team responsibilities?	*How are the patient/family included in understanding reciprocity among team members?*

continues

TABLE 21.2 *continued*

SHARED VALUES AMONG TEAM MEMBERS	SHARED PRINCIPLES TO GUIDE TEAM-BASED CARE
Creativity	**Effective Communication**
Be excited by the possibility of tackling new or emerging problems, seeing errors and unanticipated bad outcomes as potential opportunities to learn and improve.	Prioritize and continuously refine communication skills using consistent channels for candid and complete communication.
Are suboptimal outcomes shared with the patient/family? Are plans to improve systems or processes communicated to the patient/family?	*How are sporadically involved family members included in consistent channels for communication?*
Humility	**Shared Goals**
Recognize differences in training but do not believe that one type of training or perspective is uniformly superior; recognize that team members are human and will make mistakes.	Work to establish shared goals that reflect patient and family priorities and that all members can clearly articulate, understand, and support.
Do the patient/family know the primary function of the professions represented by individuals on the healthcare team?	*What is the mechanism to track patient/family goals that evolve over time?*
Curiosity	**Measurable Processes and Outcomes**
Delight in seeking out and reflecting on lessons learned and using those insights for continuous improvement.	Agree on and implement reliable and timely feedback on success and failures in both the overall functioning of the team and achievement of specific goals.
Are the patient/family included in harvesting ideas for improvement?	*Do the patient/family have differing definitions of "timely feedback" than the other members of the healthcare team?*

Source: Adapted from Wynia et al., 2012

Shared Decision-Making

Légaré and colleagues (2011) created a new conceptual model to explore a process in which patients are engaged in decision-making about their care with a team of health professionals. The model consists of an individual (or micro) level as well as two healthcare system levels (designated as meso and macro). At the individual level, a patient with a health condition experiences a decision point with options that require the weighing of potential risks and benefits for each one. Table 21.3 outlines the six steps of this model.

TABLE 21.3   The Six Steps of Shared Decision-Making

STEP	DESCRIPTION	DEFINITION
One	Sharing of knowledge	The key to the interprofessional nature of this model is that the health professionals are required to share their knowledge with the patient. This sharing may occur simultaneously or sequentially as the patient gathers data.
Two	Information exchange	The second step of the model involves an information exchange between the health professionals and the patient, along with information about potential risks and benefits, using evidence and educational materials.
Three	Values clarification	The third step requires values clarification. This step is especially important because lifestyle effects that may be of paramount importance to the patient may not hold the same priority with the professionals. Healthcare professionals must make care decisions based on the patient's preferences, values, and needs.
Four	Feasibility	The factual information for each option, along with risks and benefits, are considered within the context of the patient's value system.
Five	Actual decision	A decision is made about the patient's care.
Six	Ongoing support	The professionals support the patient's choice in order to have a favorable impact on the health outcomes that the patient values most.

Some patients are unable to fully participate in shared decision-making, and still others would rather defer to the judgment of their providers. In a study of mental health providers, Chong, Aslani, and Chen (2013) emphasized the importance of patients being informed about their illness and treatment plan, but there was less consensus concerning the involvement of these patients in decision-making. For patients who are reluctant to participate in decisions about their care, including health professionals who act as a decision coach and work through values, clarification can help the patient to participate at a higher level of decision control.

Collegial Trust

Another critical factor in effective team function is the degree of trust among team members. Ring and van de Ven (1992) describe trust simply as "confidence in another's goodwill," (p. 488) which implies that one's own behavior will be influenced by expectations of cooperation from others. Trust can then be indirectly measured by one's behavior toward others. Adler (2001) describes three sources of trust: a calculated trust derived from an assessment of costs and benefits, trust derived from familiarity through continuing interaction, and trust based on shared values and norms.

Trust on healthcare teams builds slowly over time, as members have repeated interactions and get to know each other. Tuckman and Jensen's (1977) stages of team development reflect the growth of trust among team members:

- **Forming:** During the forming stage, relationships are fairly formal and guarded, and the emotional climate is one of uncertainty.

- **Storming:** As team members get to know each other and their tasks and roles, conflicts begin to arise (the storming stage). Relationships are negotiated to fit the needs of the team's goals.

- **Norming:** In the norming stage, team members settle into patterns of interaction and begin to resolve earlier differences. A new sense of cohesion grows as team members get to know and trust each other. Members begin to defer to each other's relevant experience, and leadership may be shared or situational based on previously demonstrated expertise.

- **Performing:** When a team reaches the performing stage (which not all do), team members now have good working relationships and a positive sense of group identity. Conflict can be managed, because team members trust each other's commitment to team goals and have a history of shared successful interactions.

The climate of trust and safety allows for innovation and creativity, which are crucial to the team's growth and continued productivity. This trust also allows team members to voice disagreements and manage conflict in ways that strengthen rather than undermine the team (Jones & Jones, 2011).

"Swift" Trust

What happens when a healthcare team does not have the luxury of time and repeated experiences to progress through Tuckman's stages and develop trust among team members? Many teams in healthcare have constantly changing membership, physical separation between team members, and multiple competing demands on members' energy and time. Teams may form and disband on an ad hoc basis, working together for only one shift, or even one task, such as a surgical case or a critical resuscitation. These teams often face exceptionally complex tasks, with high-risk and high-stakes outcomes. They must perform at a high level, despite their lack of previous experience with one another.

Meyerson, Weick, and Kramer (1995) argue that teams under these circumstances must develop "swift" trust in order to function effectively. Team members under these circumstances have little data to support person-based interactions; they must rely instead on role-based interactions. These interactions, in turn, serve to reinforce the roles, which allows for less uncertainty and more rapid development of trust. This trust is further facilitated by having a salient, high-stakes purpose, such as happens in an emergency department or intensive care unit.

In the P&FCC model, the team includes the patient and family. Therefore, these team members must also develop swift trust. Because patients and families have traditionally been excluded from the care team, they may not expect or even realize that they have a role on the team. As discussed previously, swift trust is often initially based on role interactions. Clinical care providers can facilitate swift trust by explicitly designating patients and family as team members and by clarifying their role expectations for all members of the team. Alternately, it is important to clarify roles of the clinical team to the patient and family. For example, a family member's role might be to report any subtle changes they notice in a patient's clinical condition, which might be missed by clinical staff. A patient's role might include taking responsibility for an outpatient medication regimen and reporting any symptoms that might be medication side effects.

Likewise, clinical care providers must trust the patient and family members in order to optimize their contributions to the team. Often family members can provide some of the most important safety data in avoiding adverse events. Again, clarifying role expectations up front will be key to developing swift trust. Issues that might complicate trust, such as Health Insurance Portability and Accountability Act (HIPAA) concerns or perceived conflicts of interest among family members, must be addressed directly with the entire team as early as possible.

Virtual Teams and Trust

Healthcare teams may only interact via telephone, electronic health records, or telemedical consult. Because "swift" trust is based more on behaviors than on interpersonal interactions, it can still allow a temporary or virtual team to function as a team, rather than as a group of individuals. Under these circumstances, frequent and clear two-way communication forms the cornerstone for developing trust (Iacono & Weisband, 1997). The need for effective communication is especially important in the virtual environment to effectively integrate patients and families as care team members. Interactions among patients, families, and clinical staff may occur primarily by telephone or email. It will be incumbent on clinical staff to make sure that virtual communications with patients and families are shared with the rest of the clinical team.

Humility

Humility is an attribute of effective teams that have P&FCC as an explicit priority in the team's norms (Wynia et al., 2012). Several definitions of humility exist in the literature. One definition specific for teams is to recognize differences in training without believing that one type of training or perspective is uniformly superior, and to recognize that team members are humans and make errors (Wynia et al., 2012). Other research in this area operationalizes humility as a trait of leaders who demonstrate inclusiveness. *Inclusiveness* is operationally defined as words and deeds exhibited by leaders that invite and appreciate others' contributions. Humility and inclusiveness in a team leader can help teams overcome the detrimental effects of status differences, allowing members to provide care in a manner that is effectively focused on the patient (Nembhard & Edmondson, 2006).

Within the area of cultural diversity, humility is defined as a continuous process of self-reflection and self-awareness to identify one's own preconceptions and worldview as compared to that of the patient (Alsharif, 2012). This increasingly familiar ideal, when applied to the individual clinician, is a private process and an expression of that individual's professional values. However, applying this concept to a healthcare team, the model demands an explicit process, dialogue, and consideration by the team with the patient and family. What are the team's preconceptions? What is the team's worldview? How does this worldview compare to the patient's? What recurring process or dialogue allows the team to continuously reflect on these issues?

Barriers to Effective Team Functioning

The effectiveness of strategies to maximize teamwork and P&FCC are amplified when teams can remain cognizant of common barriers that impede effective team functioning. The familiar barriers identified are not specific to a discipline and are best neutralized when teams have a shared understanding of them. Interdisciplinary teams are more successful in providing P&FCC when they understand and respect members' strengths, can effectively address team conflict, can adapt to the dynamic nature of the healthcare team, remain mindful of authority gradients inherent to healthcare, and understand the common inclination to avoid confrontation.

Failure to Understand and Respect Each Other's Strengths

Healthcare professionals are educated in the tradition and silo of their own disciplines. Although interprofessional education in health professions education is strongly supported (Greiner & Knebel, 2003), effective interprofessional educational models for healthcare professions students are only recently emerging. As a result of this segregation, clinicians do not understand and appreciate the practice, scope, and strengths of other disciplines. Nurses are not well informed of the breadth of pharmacy education, nor are physical therapists well aware of the extent of nursing education, and so on. A lack of knowledge about collegial disciplines contributes to a lack of respect for other team members' strengths and capacity. Introducing patients and families as members of the team requires organizational support and usually significant cultural change to address this barrier.

Team Conflict

Conflict is intimately connected to a team's ability to provide P&FCC. Unresolved discord among team members will limit a patient or family's ability to trust their care team or dialogue in candid ways with individuals or the entire team. Booij defines conflict on healthcare teams as a disagreement or difference of opinion related to the management of a patient, involving more than one individual and requiring some decision or action (Booij, 2007). Conflict that is not effectively managed can negatively affect patient safety, quality of care, and satisfaction for both patients and healthcare workers in the provision of P&FCC.

It is important to recognize that conflict is a normal part of interaction on any healthcare team. In fact, conflict can serve to help a team grow and provide opportunities for creative problem-solving, which can lead to higher productivity (Lencioni, 2002). One marker of a team's effectiveness is its ability to manage conflict in a constructive manner (Hakanen & Soudunsaari, 2012). Teams with no apparent conflict may lack the trust between team members that is necessary to allow the conflict to surface. Over time, this unacknowledged or unresolved conflict corrodes a team's ability to work together.

Sources of conflict can exist on many levels. For example, on the micro (individual) level, conflict may arise from different personality styles or overlapping scopes of practice. At the meso or macro level, sources might include scheduling and volume of patients, financial pressures, or clinical practice guidelines (Brown et al., 2011). Sources of conflict can also be described in terms of substantive issues (e.g., clinical judgment regarding patient care) versus emotional issues (personality differences or power differentials) (Payne, 2000). Unresolved or unaddressed team conflict always impedes the provision of P&FCC.

Brown and colleagues (2011) describe common sources of conflict on interprofessional primary care teams as falling into three main thematic categories. These include:

- **Role boundary issues:** In this case, there may be a lack of understanding or appreciation for a team member's role and responsibilities. For example, a team member may not communicate an important piece of information to another team member, not realizing the other team member needs or uses this information to perform his role.

- **Scope of practice:** This issue identifies overlap or lack of clarity regarding team members' scopes of practice. This can be especially evident when a new team member is added to a previously established team. It may manifest as conflict between two healthcare workers, or between a patient/family member and a healthcare worker.

- **Accountability:** Team members may fail to take responsibility for their actions, but just as often, conflict arises regarding more than one team member feeling solely responsible for a given aspect of patient care. The existing culture of individual blame, as opposed to a systems approach to medical error, may magnify the feeling of individual responsibility and discourage collaboration among team members. This is reinforced by the punitive stance of the medicolegal and risk-management processes in most healthcare settings. Indeed, patients and their family members often share this culture of blame. A care team member may think, "If something goes wrong, I'm the one who gets sued," or "It's my license that's on the line."

The Persistently Dynamic Makeup of Healthcare Teams

One common challenge to effective patient-centered care and healthy team dynamics is the dynamic nature of the healthcare team. Clinical environments are constantly changing and increasingly complex, and this fluidity is a challenge for clinicians, patients, and families (Dayton & Henrikson, 2007). Increasing specialization in healthcare has contributed to increased fragmentation in the provision of care and an increase in the number of individuals on the healthcare team, and results in a lack of stability in the team's composition (Volpp & Grande, 2003). With care dependent on the input of multiple healthcare team members—and those teams' participants are constantly changing—the potential for conflict is high and impedes teamwork, collaboration, and an effective focus on the patient and family (Drinka & Clark, 2000). In the opening clinical scenario at the beginning of this chapter, the absence of coordination of Mr. Yeager's care across settings and across providers creates a hazardous situation for a vulnerable patient.

This fluidity in team makeup has deleterious effects on a team's ability to provide P&FCC in three evident ways:

- Most frequently examined in research is team members' lack of familiarity with each other. In the hospital, a team's composition changes each day as teams are formed and reformed. High functioning teams create, maintain, improve, and adapt informal rules and customs over time (Wynia et al., 2012). The dynamic nature of teams in healthcare challenges these processes.

- Changing team members create challenges for patients and families. To best direct inquiries, patients and families must be familiar with the individuals on their healthcare team. An inability to identify changing team members and not knowing which team member to contact about deteriorating patient conditions were vital facets of the medical error tragedy that killed Lewis Blackman (Raymond, 2009). This challenge focuses on patients and families merely being able to identify team members and know team members' roles.

- Finally, effective P&FCC occurs over time and is dependent on developing relationships upon which trust can be built. Changing team members create obstacles to effective team-based P&FCC as it is difficult for patients and families to develop trust and be vulnerable when the makeup of the healthcare team is persistently dynamic. Beyond just confusion about the identities of team members, the fluidity of team membership complicates the development of trust in team members by patients and families.

Authority Gradients

The concept of authority gradients has its etiology in aviation science, when it was discovered that pilots and copilots may not effectively share information in stressful circumstances if there is a notable difference in experience, expertise, or authority (Alkov, Borowsky, Williamson, & Yacavone, 1992). A strong hierarchical structure is very beneficial in high-stakes, time-pressured healthcare situations in which decisions must be made efficiently and care delegated cleanly and clearly. However, only a small percentage of healthcare is delivered in such circumstances. Research indicates that authority gradients are a hazardous dynamic on healthcare teams (Cosby & Croskerry, 2004). The presence of authority gradients in interdisciplinary healthcare teams can contribute to struggles with interpersonal power and conflict (Sutcliffe, Lewton, & Rosenthal, 2004). Leaders in both nursing and medicine have long proposed strategies for increased cooperation on healthcare teams rather than competition (Fagin, 1992; Prescott & Bowen, 1985).

Patients can also fall prey to authority gradients when dealing with their healthcare team, especially if there are authority dynamics occurring between the team members. Patients and families are very sensitive to these dynamics and can easily feel like the least empowered member of the team. Recent definitions of P&FCC employ language with the patient being the source of control and full partner in planning of care. Yet many healthcare teams fall short of this aim. Healthcare teams must take extra care to be aware of authority gradients that affect their communication and ability to be authentically patient-centered. These deleterious dynamics can affect the full exchange of information among team members and always profoundly affect the patient's and family's ability to candidly interact with their healthcare team.

Avoiding Confrontation

Avoiding confrontation can lead to fear-based, problematic communication between team members and also affects the delivery of P&FCC. Communication is more likely to be inaccurate or incomplete in situations where there are hierarchical differences, especially when one party is concerned about appearing competent or is afraid of confrontation (O'Daniel & Rosenstein, 2008).

Avoiding confrontation can lead to significantly adverse patient outcomes. In 2005, AACN and VitalSmarts conducted a study that found that 84% of doctors identified colleagues who took dangerous shortcuts when caring for patients and 88% of the study's participants worked with people who demonstrated poor clinical judgment (Maxfield, Grenny, McMillan, Patterson & Switzler, 2005). Despite the risks to patients, there was a preponderance of avoiding confrontation, as fewer than 10% of physicians, nurses, and other clinical staff directly confronted their colleagues about their concerns (Maxfield et al., 2005). Maxfield and colleagues repeated the study in 2010, where 84% of respondents reported that 10% or more of their colleagues take dangerous shortcuts. Despite these risks, only 31% of the study participants shared their full concerns with the person (Maxfield, Grenny, Lavandero, & Groah, 2010). Even when clinicians see inaccurate or dangerous care, they place a higher value on avoiding confrontation than protecting patients.

Any dynamic present on a healthcare team directly affects that team's ability to provide P&FCC. Additionally, any poor communication pattern on a team limits a patient's and family's ability to be honest, vulnerable, and exposed with that healthcare team. To the degree that team members are setting team standards to avoid confrontation, patients will follow this lead and may withhold vital information integral to care planning from those providing care.

Is the Difficult Patient Really the Complex Patient?

One of the hardest challenges to healthcare teams is the patient who is identified as "difficult." The dynamics of teamwork and collaboration and provision of P&FCC quickly break down in these situations. These patients necessitate much more time and individualized care in order to meet their needs, and they often come across as unappreciative or even rude toward their caregivers. These dynamics often result in compromised care. Utilizing complexity science to reframe the perspective on these patients is useful in recognizing the specific challenges these patients present and how interdisciplinary healthcare teams might best approach these complex situations so as to provide P&FCC. Fiester in Chapter 5 of this book examines in detail some of the issues surrounding the difficult patient.

Complexity science looks at models in which highly intricate systems with multiple interplaying factors interact together to produce widely varied results (Allen, Maguire, & McKelvey, 2011). This contrasts with the simple linear model, in which there is a clear cause and effect: A given intervention should predictably yield a consistent result. An example of this would be mandating helmets for motorcyclists; regardless of the specific driver or the geographic location, in an accident a helmet predictively protects the head and saves lives. For more advanced systems, it is much more difficult to establish a direct cause and effect relationship; there are too many interplaying factors that interact with each other that can result in many different outcomes.

Complexity science has coined these as "complex adaptive systems" (CAS) (Jayasinghe, 2011). *Complex adaptive systems* are defined as "a dynamic network of many diverse agents…constantly acting and reacting to what the other agents are doing" (van Beurden, Kia, Zask, Dietrich, & Rose, 2013, p. 74). This results in varied, often unpredictable results (Cilliers, 1998). An example of this in patient care would be smoking cessation programs, in which success rates vary tremendously despite well-established interventions. An individual's ability to stop smoking depends on a number of different interplaying factors, including the person's past history with smoking, support system, stress level at work, personal characteristics, etc. It can be quite difficult to predict who will be successful with smoking cessation at the start of the program.

Using this framework to understand patient and family behavior, it is easy to see how the complexity of healthcare can be informed by many concepts of CAS. Five people who experience the same stressful event will each respond differently, based on myriad factors that influence their perceptions and reactions. In regard to the "difficult" patient, using complexity science allows the clinician team to reframe their perspective on this person to that of an objectively challenging situation. Recognizing that the model is nonlinear implies that no one intervention is likely to consistently produce the most beneficial result. Patients should be approached as individuals, recognizing that small situational differences can greatly influence any intervention's success. By critically examining all the various interplaying factors that together have generated these unwanted behaviors, it becomes possible to identify areas for the team to address.

A thorough patient interview is critical in guiding the team toward various interventions. What is the person's chief complaint? What symptoms are most prevalent and troubling? Are medications contributing to these symptoms? How is the pain management? Is there a loss of independence? What social support systems are present? Are there cultural elements informing the patient's or family's experience of the provision of care? Identifying these interplaying factors and engaging key personnel within the team best equipped to address each factor provides a comprehensive approach to these patients without placing blame or further isolating the patient or family. The team now views the elements of the patient's situation as a challenging "puzzle" that can motivate them to seek and find solutions.

Contemporary Models for Care Provision with the Patient and Family as Integral Partners

Healthcare teams need to be simultaneously focused on their team dynamics, inclusive of the patient and family in these dynamics, and responsive to patient and family priorities. Early models are emerging that integrate these equally important priorities. Example of models in the outpatient and inpatient setting are discussed in this section.

Outpatient Patient-Centered Medical Home Model

The patient-centered medical home model, first advanced by primary care professional organizations in 2007, has enjoyed growing support within the medical profession. In this model, an interprofessional team with a physician lead provides primary care that addresses a patient's physical, emotional, and social issues in an evidence-based fashion and incorporates patients and their families into the care team to tailor care to their needs and preferences (Rittenhouse & Shortell, 2009). Part of the physician's responsibility in this role is to support care coordination and to ensure that the interprofessional team addresses acute, chronic, and preventive care for patients. As this model has evolved, the possibility of nonphysician providers (e.g. nurse practitioners or physician assistants) serving as lead clinician has emerged and is supported.

The joint principles of the patient-centered medical home (PCMH) promote a clinician-led coordination of patients' primary healthcare needs, utilizing a healthcare team to provide patient-centered care (Landon, Gill, Antonelli, & Rich, 2010). The Nursing Alliance for Quality Care (NAQC) developed standards in 2008 for recognizing these PCMH practices and has expanded this evaluation program (Sofaer & Schumann, 2013). The PCMH model has six major attributes or functions that are outlined in Table 21.4.

TABLE 21.4   Six Attributes of the Patient-Centered Medical Home

ATTRIBUTE	DEFINITION
Patient-centered	One strength of this model is the focus on the patient, largely encompassing the "whole person." A partnership is made with the patient and his or her family, with efforts taken to understand unique cultural values and personal treatment preferences.
Comprehensive care	The medical home should take care of most of the patient's primary care needs, both physical and mental. This includes preventive care and wellness, acute care, and chronic disease management. To best achieve this comprehensive care, the model utilizes a physician-led, coordinated, integrated team approach, with a team that may include advanced practice nurses and physician assistants, pharmacists, physical therapists, nurses, mental health specialists, nutritionists, educators, and care team coordinators, as well as other services based on the individual patient's needs.
Coordinated care	The PCMH relies on coordination across all of the different elements within the healthcare system, including hospitals, home care, specialist services, and community support programs. This coordination is critical during transitions across different sites of care, such as a hospital discharge. Coordinated care leads to open communication across the team of healthcare providers and includes the patient and family within this communication.
Accessible service	The model provides access to care for the patient, with routine communications catered to each patient's preference, providing support through email and telephone communications as well as face to face. Urgent care needs should be addressed without prolonged delays, and some member of the healthcare team should be accessible to the patient around the clock.
Safety and quality	The primary care medical home team utilizes evidence-based medicine and treatment guidelines while engaging with patients and their families to make sound decisions regarding medical treatment. Patient satisfaction is a priority within this model and is measured with questionnaires and other feedback. Improvements to health information technology are essential for sharing and reviewing patient health information across the medical home team.
Payment	Reimbursement for the PCMH integrates pay-for-performance, fee-for-service, and reimbursement for coordinated care. Payment should be value driven with successful patient management resulting in cost savings. There is an emphasis on enhanced technologies that lead to better coordinated care.

Source: Sofaer & Schumann, 2013

This model clearly has several strengths, with the patient's preferences, values, and needs serving as the center of focus and all the different healthcare team members coordinating together with the patient to optimize the care received and manage the "whole patient."

Inpatient P&FCC Models

As with outpatient care in the PCMH model, P&FCC in the inpatient setting requires that members of all professions involved in the care of a patient collaborate to develop a unified care plan. The cornerstone of this approach has been the inclusion of patient and family planning care, such as through regular interprofessional rounds or care team meetings. Such meetings may occur at the bedside on daily rounds, in a regularly scheduled care team meeting, or some combination of these. Because the care team treating the patient in the hospital will normally not be the same as the people taking care of the patient after discharge, a critical element of inpatient P&FCC must be communication and coordination with the patient's outpatient care providers.

The inclusion of patients and family members in planning care is most widely established in pediatric units. The experience of hospitalization is highly stressful for children and their parents, and the emotional benefit to parents of being included in the care team is readily apparent. Despite this, a recent Cochrane collaboration review noted that there are few randomized trials which assess the effects of P&FCC in the pediatric inpatient setting on outcomes such as morbidity and mortality, length of inpatient stay, and cost (Shields et al., 2012).

P&FCC has gained some popularity in adult inpatient specialty units (e.g., ICU, rehabilitation, palliative care, transplant). Emerging visitation policies include a patient having the right to a support person at the bedside around the clock (Whitcomb, 2010). There have been some qualitative and retrospective studies of the perceptions of patients, family, and clinicians to P&FCC, and these have been mostly positive. Bechel, Myers, and Smith (2000) found that a patient-centered care approach was associated with fewer complications and unexpected mortality in Michigan hospitals, but was also associated with higher cost. More research into outcomes is desperately needed.

Case Scenario 1: At the Pharmacy

Mrs. Morales is a 56-year-old Hispanic woman who steps up to hand her new prescription for a second blood pressure medication to her local pharmacist, John, whom she's known and worked with for a few years. She is a little upset over having yet another medication added to her regimen, but her blood pressure has been spiking quite a bit recently, and the doctor is concerned, particularly with her family history. He did note that her cholesterol has been well controlled with the simvastatin 40mg she is taking. John smiles at her and begins to put her prescription into the computer when he stops and frowns at the screen, then at Mrs. Morales.

"Did you just get this prescription, Mrs. Morales?"

"Yes, John, I just came from my doctor's office. He's concerned about my blood pressure getting higher." John begins shaking his head, waving the prescription for verapamil 240mg in the air.

"Well, I'm concerned too…" the pharmacist begins. "I'm concerned that your doctor doesn't know what he's doing!" Mrs. Morales just stares at him, clearly not understanding. "There's a pretty severe reaction between this medication and your cholesterol one. It could lead to some pretty bad muscle wasting, or worse!"

"But…but I just left his office," Mrs. Morales stammers. "Surely he wouldn't give me something that would hurt me…"

"C'mon, now, Mrs. Morales!" John states emphatically. "We all know that doctors just don't know their medications!"

This example shows how different health professionals can be counterproductive in their patient care and undermine the trust patients have in their healthcare team.

- How could this health professional better deal with the situation without placing blame?

  The pharmacist should have explained that there could be an interaction between medications and that he wanted to clarify this problem with the physician to see if a different medication may be a better alternative. The actual interaction, though significant, is not life threatening and is commonly seen at the pharmacy. Some physicians know medications in their field as well as (if not better than) other healthcare providers, including pharmacists.

- How would this scenario differ in the P&FCC provision model?

  Interprofessional P&FCC assumes that the healthcare team is already working together with the patient as the central focus. With established relationships between the pharmacist and physician, open communication would have resolved this interaction easily; the pharmacist would have voiced his concerns directly to the physician and an alternative therapy would have been chosen. This type of intervention falls within the pharmacist's role, but he also has a responsibility to support the team, not build silos between professions by highlighting what is perceived to be a mistake. Calling and changing the prescription minimizes the risk to the patient while demonstrating the relationship between providers and showing how they worked together to optimize the patient's health.

- What might be needed for the patient or family to be a full partner in the care process?

  Interprofessional P&FCC is optimal when it is the understood model shared by all members of the healthcare team. Most importantly, the patient and family should consistently experience this model across settings. If the primary care physician and pharmacist have developed a rapport with Mrs. Morales over time where her input is regularly requested and valued, she would be able to comfortably ask the pharmacist to clarify her BP medication with her primary care physician. In healthcare teams where P&FCC is valued and addressed, patients do not have to worry about offending any of their providers, and everyone's focus is safe, effective, timely P&FCC.

Case Scenario 2: Palliative Care

You are the nurse caring for Mr. Phillips. Mr. Phillips is a 57-year-old man just admitted to your med/surg unit for pain control and failure to thrive. He is on a hydromorphone PCA as well as oral doses of oxycodone. Based on Mr. Phillips's chart, he has been seen by his oncologist in the ED and the hospitalist as he was admitted to your unit.

HX: Recent diagnosis of pancreatic cancer, stage 4. Has been receiving chemotherapy for 3 weeks, as ordered by oncologist. Prognosis is poor. Hx of gastric bypass 4 years ago with a history of dumping syndrome that took 12 months to resolve. Prior to hospitalization, Mr. Phillips has called oncologist's office frequently for pain crises, and his oral dose of oxycodone has been continually increased to oxycodone 40mg 3X/day. Patient has not been compliant in attending chemotherapy infusion appointments, citing lack of support and inability to get to appointments.

Physical Exam: BP 108/68, HR 68, RR 10, Temp 98.8, Pulse ox 90%. Increased dependent edema, 18% weight loss in the last 3 weeks with loss of lean muscle. Recurring episodes of watery diarrhea each day (6–8/day) during hospitalization. Currently patient is minimally responsive and extremely somnolent.

You are called out of your morning nursing report by Mr. Phillips's daughter, Rose, who is angry about her father's care. She asks to speak to the charge nurse. Rose lives across the country and sees her father once or twice per year. She arrived in town late last night. Rose does not understand why her father has been hospitalized and wants him discharged. However, before his discharge, there are some problems to resolve. Rose cites poor pain control reported by her father and new onset of intermittent delirium. Rose seems unaware of the poor prognosis for her father's cancer and is referencing plans for her father 2 years in the future. As you review Mr. Phillips's chart, there is no documentation of Mr. Phillips's wishes for his care.

You assess Mr. Phillips as being respiratorily depressed, and attribute his decreased level of consciousness as a result of excessive narcotics because of his hyrdomorphone PCA and oral doses of oxycodone.

This case study demonstrates how the priority of P&FCC can get lost in how clinicians address competing needs in a complex clinical situation.

- How could the healthcare team for Mr. Phillips better deal with the emerging situation?

Assuring Mr. Phillips's safety is most important. The team will want to immediately address Mr. Phillips's apparently deteriorating respiratory status. Additionally, as Mr. Phillips becomes more lucid, it will be important to center his care discussions on Mr. Phillips's values, preferences, and needs. It will also be vital to assess and address the values and needs of his identified support/family members. Engaging Rose in this moment of care and shift in care will be vital. Acknowledging Rose's concerns, summarizing her questions, and outlining next steps to get problems resolved will bring her more effectively into her father's care. It will be helpful for members of the healthcare team to ask what Rose understands or has been told about her father's condition. How does she understand her father's hospitalization? Rose arrived at her father's bedside for a reason and is working from some framework of her father's problems and needs. If the nurse can elicit this information, it will give the team a good starting point to collaborate with Rose so that she feels heard and understood. She might then be more willing to engage with the team more readily.

Next you will want to look at whether the hospitalist or oncologist will be leading Mr. Phillips' plan of care during his hospitalization and post discharge. There are several immediate care priorities and longer range care priorities that you will want to address with Rose and Mr. Phillips once Mr. Phillips is more coherent.

- How would this scenario differ in the P&FCC provision model?

A difficult aspect of Mr. Phillips's situation is that the patient is nonresponsive. The patient's only accessible family is a daughter whose visits are sporadic. There are immediate care needs (Mr. Phillips's pain, his dehydration, his diarrhea, his nutrition needs) and then more long-term care needs (option of palliative care team, assistance at home, long-term pain control needs, advanced directives) that need to be addressed.

Employing the P&FCC model, Rose will be included in the healthcare team as described. Additionally, Mr. Phillips and Rose will be consulted about additional family or support people to include in team planning. Mr. Phillips and his family will be included as the healthcare team expands to include more members who may contribute to short-term and long-term care goals of Mr. Phillips and his family. Beyond the patient and family, some members of the team for this clinical scenario may include a hospitalist, an oncologist, a pain specialist, a palliative care team, and a case manager.

- What might be needed for the patient or family to be a full partner in the care processes?

Communication has been lacking in planning and organizing Mr. Phillips's care. Consistent interprofessional rounds will be necessary to keep all team members abreast of Mr. Phillips's situation and emerging short-term and long-term needs. Inclusion of local support people as well as communication strategies to include family who are at a distance (e.g., video chat or conference calls) are all valuable in this situation.

The QSEN competency of Teamwork & Collaboration identifies requisite knowledge, skills, and attitudes necessary for effective team functioning (Cronenwett et al, 2007). The reader will find additional knowledge, skills, and attitudes related to teamwork at www.qsen.org. The key points that follow stem from this competency:

- **Describe own strengths, limitations, and values in functioning as a member of a team.** It is more common for healthcare professionals on the healthcare team to discuss their strengths and limitations as a team member, but how often do healthcare teams ask patients and families about their strengths, limitations, and values as team members? When this discussion is initiated with the patient and family, the team will want to discuss strategies for sharing this information with rotating members of the team. Are the patient and family comfortable with their answers becoming part of the electronic health record (EHR), where future team members will have access to the same information?

- **Analyze differences in communication style preferences among patients, families, nurses, and other members of the healthcare team.** Include a regular check-in with all members of the healthcare team about whether team communication is meeting each member's needs. Routine questions might be: Are you receiving the information that you need about the plan of care through current team communication? Do you have adequate opportunities to contribute to team communication? Do you have any recommendations on improving team communication?

- **Choose communication styles that diminish the risks associated with authority gradients among team members.** Include explicit team communication about authority gradients. Healthcare occurs in a hierarchical system, with some members of the team having more authority than others. Explicitly ask traditionally lower ranking individuals (e.g., patient, family, nursing aide, respiratory therapist, occupational therapist) whether they feel comfortable contributing to team communication and team processes. If individuals identify a reluctance to speak up because of authority gradients, engage the team in a conversation about strategies to remedy this averseness.

- **Contribute to resolution of conflict and disagreement.** When conflict occurs between any two members of the team, set up a meeting to discuss the cause, consequences, and potential impact on team functioning. Allow all involved, including the patient and family, to discuss their concerns about the conflict and to provide commitment to strategies to avoid a recurrence of a similar conflict in the future.

- **Appreciate the risks associated with handoffs among providers and across transitions in care.** Include the patient and family in daily rounding. Using a standardized checklist for team rounds that includes the patient and family can decrease variability in including the patient and family in handoffs. A well-informed patient can reduce the likelihood of needed orders or aspects of a plan of care being overlooked. An example of a standardized checklist is included in this chapter's section in the Resources appendix at the back of the book.

Conclusion

In the emerging science of quality and safety competencies, there is a critical need for clearer definitions in the overlap in competencies. Although physicians, nurses, pharmacists, physical therapists, and dentists learn about P&FCC and teamwork as discrete competencies, these competencies share significant overlap. The patient and family are the crux of the healthcare team, and strategies to improve teamwork must always include them. When P&FCC and teamwork are competing necessities, a healthcare team's ability to provide safe, quality care is diminished.

Common educational priorities are clear for health professions students in interdisciplinary training in teamwork, P&FCC, and other quality and safety competencies (IPEC, 2011). These educational priorities offer promise for healthcare teams that are just entering healthcare. However, what is currently needed is effective team training that extends to existing healthcare professionals who were not explicitly trained in interdisciplinary team functioning in their formative education. Although there was a historical belief that P&FCC and teamwork were "soft skills" that health professionals would "pick up" in their practice, quality and safety data support that there is a tremendous need for explicit training in these distinct skill sets.

References

Adler, P. S. (2001). Market, hierarchy, and trust: The knowledge economy and the future of capitalism. *Organization Science, 12*(2), 215-34.

Agency for Healthcare Research and Quality (AHRQ). (2008). *TeamStepps: Team strategies and tools to enhance performance and patient safety.* Rockville, MD: Author. Retrieved from http://teamstepps.ahrq.gov/abouttoolsmaterials.htm

Alkov, R. A., Borowsky, M. S., Williamson, D. W., & Yacavone, D. W. (1992). The effect of trans-cockpit authority gradient on navy/marine helicopter mishaps. *Aviation, Space, Environment and Medicine, 63*(8), 659-661.

Allen, P., Maguire, S., & McKelvey, B. (2011). *The sage handbook of complexity and management.* Los Angeles, CA: Sage Publishing.

Alsharif, N. Z. (2012). Cultural humility and interprofessional education and practice: A winning combination. *American Journal of Pharmaceutical Education, 76*(7), 120. doi: 10.5688/ajpe767120

Bechel, D., Myers, W., & Smith, D. (2000). Does patient-centered care pay off? *Joint Commission Journal on Quality and Patient Safety, 26*(7), 400-409.

Berwick, D. M. (2009). What "patient-centered" should mean: Confessions of an extremist. *Health Affairs, 28*(4), w555-w565.

Booij, L. (2007). Conflicts in the operating theatre. *Current Opinions in Anaesthesiology, 20*(2), 152-156.

Brown, J., Lewis, L., Ellis, K., Stewart, M., Freeman, T., & Kasperski, M. (2011). Conflict on interprofessional primary health care teams—Can it be resolved? *Journal of Interprofessional Care, 25*(1), 4-10.

Chong, W. W., Aslani, P., & Chen, T. F. (2013). Multiple perspectives on shared decision-making and interprofessional collaboration in mental healthcare. *Journal of Interprofessional Care, 27*(3), 1356-1820.

Cilliers, P. (1998). *Complexity and postmodernism: Understanding complex systems.* New York, NY: Routledge.

Cosby, K. S., & Croskerry, P. (2004). Profiles in patient safety: authority gradients in medical error. *Academic Emergency Medicine, 11*(12), 1341-1345.

Cronenwett, L., Sherwood, G., Barnsteiner, J., Disch, J., Johnson, J., Mitchell, P., ... Warren, J. (2007). Quality and safety education for nurses. *Nursing Outlook, 55*(3), 122-31.

Dayton, E., & Henrikson, K. (2007). Communication failure: Basic components, contributing factors and the call for structure. *Joint Commission Journal on Quality and Patient Safety, 33*(1), 34-47.

Delbanco, T., & Berwick, D. M. (2001). Healthcare in a land called People-Power: Nothing about me without me. *Health Expectations, 4*(3), 144-150.

Drinka, T. J. K., & Clark, P. G. (2000). Developing and maintaining interdisciplinary health care teams. In T. J. K. Drinka & P. G. Clark (Eds.), *Health care teamwork: Interdisciplinary health care practice and teachings* (pp. 11-49). Westport, CT: Auburn House.

Fagin, C. M. (1992). Collaboration between nurses and physicians: No longer a choice. *Nursing and Health Care, 13*(7), 354-362.

Frenk, J., Chen, L., Bhutta, Z. A., Cohen, J., Crisp, N., Evans, T.,…Zurayk, H. (2010). Health professions for a new century: Transforming education to strengthen heath systems in an interdependent world. *The Lancet, 376*(9756), 1923-1958.

Greiner, A. C., & Knebel E. (Eds.). (2003). *IOM health professions education: A bridge to quality* [IOM report]. Washington, DC: National Academy Press.

Hakanen, M., & Soudunsaari, A. (2012, June). Building trust in high-performing teams. *Technology Innovation Management Review*, 38-41.

Iacono, C., & Weisband, S. (1997). Developing trust in virtual teams. *System Sciences, Proceedings of the Thirtieth Hawaii International Conference, 2*, 412-420.

Institute of Medicine (IOM). (2001). *Crossing the quality chasm: A new health system for the 21st century*. Washington, DC: National Academy Press.

Interprofessional Education Collaborative Expert Panel (IPEC). (2011). Core competencies for interprofessional collaborative practice: Report of an expert panel. Washington, DC: Author.

Jayasinghe, S. (2011). Conceptualising population health: From mechanistic thinking to complexity science. *Emerging Themes in Epidemiology, 8*(1), 2. doi: 10.1186/1742-7622-8-2

Jones, A., & Jones, D. (2011). Improving teamwork, trust and safety: An ethnographic study of an interprofessional initiative. *Journal of Interprofessional Care, 25*(3), 175-181.

Landon, B. E., Gill, J. M., Antonelli, R. C., & Rich, E. C. (2010). Prospects for rebuilding primary care using the patient-centered medical home. [Research Support, U.S. Gov't, P.H.S.]. *Health Affairs, 29*(5), 827-834. doi: 10.1377/hlthaff.2010.0016

Légaré, F., Stacey, D., Pouliot, S., Gauvin, F-P, Desroches, S., Kryworuchko, J., … Graham, I .D. (2011). Interprofessionalism and shared decision-making in primary care: A stepwise approach towards a new model. *Journal of Interprofessional Care, 25*(1), 18-25.

Lencioni, P. (2002). *The five dysfunctions of a team*. San Francisco, CA: Jossey-Bass.

Leonard, M., Graham, S., & Bonucom, D. (2004). The human factor: the critical importance of effective teamwork and communication in providing safe care. *Quality and Safety in Healthcare, 13*(Suppl 1), 185-190.

Maxfield, D., Grenny, J., Lavandero, R., & Groah, L. (2010). *The silent treatment*. Aliso Viejo, CA: AACN. Retrieved from www.silenttreatmentstudy.com

Maxfield, D., Grenny, J., McMillan, R., Patterson, K., & Switzler, A. (2005). Silence kills. Retrieved from http://www.silenttreatmentstudy.com/silencekills/SilenceKills.pdf

Meyerson, D., Weick, K., & Kramer, R. (1995). Swift trust in temporary groups. In R. M. Kramer & T. R. Tyler (Eds.), *Trust in organizations: Frontiers of theory and research* (pp. 166-195). Thousand Oaks, CA: Sage Publications.

Nembhard, I., & Edmondson, A. C. (2006). Making it safe: The effects of leader inclusiveness and professional status on psychological safety and improvement efforts in health care teams. *Journal of Organizational Behavior, 27*(7), 941-966.

O'Daniel, M., & Rosenstein, A. (2008). Professional communication and team collaboration. In R. G. Hughes (Ed.), *Patient safety and quality: An evidence-based handbook for nurses* (Chapter 33). AHRQ Publication No. 08-0043. Rockville, MD: Agency for Healthcare Research and Quality.

Payne, M. (2000). *Teamwork in multiprofessional care*. Chicago, IL: Lyceum Books.

Planetree & Picker Institute. (2008). *Patient-centered care improvement guide: Introduction*. Retrieved from www.patient-centeredcare.org/chapters/introduction.pdf

Prescott, P. A., & Bowen, S. A. (1985). Physician-nurse relationships. *Annals of Internal Medicine, 103*(1), 127-133.

Raymond, J. (2009). South Carolina patient safety legislation: The impact of the Lewis Blackman Hospital Patient Safety Act on a large teaching hospital. *The Journal of the South Carolina Medical Association, 105*(1), 12-5.

Ring, P. S., & van de Ven, A. H. (1992). Structuring cooperative relationships between organizations. *Strategic Management Journal, 13*(7), 483-498.

Rittenhouse, D. R., & Shortell, S. M. (2009). The patient-centered medical home: Will it stand the test of health reform? *Journal of the American Medical Association, 301*(19), 2038-2040.

Shields, L., Zhou, H., Pratt, J., Taylor, M., Hunter, J., & Pascoe, E. (2012). Family-centred care for hospitalised children aged 0-12 years. *Cochrane Database of Systematic Reviews, 10*, Art. No.: CD004811. doi: 10.1002/14651858.CD004811.pub3

Sofaer, S., & Schumann, M. J. (2013). *Fostering successful patient and family engagement: Nursing's critical role* [White paper]. Retrieved from Nursing Alliance for Quality Care website: http://www.naqc.org/WhitePaper-PatientEngagement

Sutcliffe, K., Lewton, E., & Rosenthal, M. (2004). Communication failures: An insidious contributor to medical mishaps. *Academic Medicine, 79*(2), 186-194.

Tuckman, B. W., & Jensen, M. A. (1977). Stages of small group development revisited. *Group and Organization Studies, 2*(4), 419-427.

van Beurden, E. K., Kia, A. M., Zask, A., Dietrich, U., & Rose, L. (2013). Making sense in a complex landscape: How the Cynefin framework from Complex Adaptive Systems Theory can inform health promotion practice. *Health Promotion International, 28*(1), 73-83. doi:10.1093/heapro/dar089

Volpp, K. G., & Grande, D. (2003). Residents' suggestions for reducing errors in teaching hospitals. *New England Journal of Medicine, 348*(9), 851-855.

Whitcomb, J. A. (2010). Evidence-based practice in a military intensive care unit family visitation. *Nursing Research, 59*(1 Suppl), S32-S39.

World Health Organization (WHO). (2010). *Framework for action on interprofessional education & collaborative practice.* Geneva, Switzerland: World Health Organization Press.

Wynia, M. K., VonKohorn, I., & Mitchell, P. M. (2012). Challenges at the intersection of team-based and patient-centered health care. *Journal of the American Medical Association, 308*(13), 1327-1328.

Chapter 22

Healing Environments

Shirley M. Moore, PhD, RN, FAAN
Ann S. Williams, PhD, RN, CDE
Jennifer E. Wason, BA, MLIS

Jennifer Smith is a 43-year-old woman who is receiving chemotherapy infusion treatments for breast cancer. Jennifer is arriving for her third infusion treatment at a large cancer center. Her sister, Jill, who has come with Jennifer to her two previous treatment sessions, is accompanying her. As they arrive at the entrance to the medical center, they leave their car with the free valet service and decide to take a stroll through the garden just outside the entrance. Jennifer wants to check on some flowers that were close to blooming when they were here 2 weeks ago. She remembers that the flowers were near the waterfall, so they follow the garden path toward the gentle sounds of falling water. Jennifer notes that the flowers are now in bloom and that the colors of the garden are vivid and beautiful.

It is now nearing the time of the treatment session, so Jennifer and Jill enter the lobby of the treatment center. The lobby is full of sunlight, and has warm wooden floors and nature-inspired wall colors. There is a fireplace at one end of the lobby and comfortable sofas and chairs around it. Jennifer checks in at a reception desk and knows that her physician, nurses, and laboratory technicians who will be caring for her during this visit will now be automatically notified that she has arrived. As they enter the infusion treatment area, Jennifer and Jill are greeted by Jennifer's primary nurse who asks Jennifer about her preferences today regarding the type of infusion space in which she will spend the next few hours getting her treatment. Jennifer can select either a private room or a treatment nook. She will be able to choose whether she wants to be seated by windows, where she will have direct sunlight and views of the outdoors, or in a more subdued light-filtered area. If she selects a nook, she also will be able to arrange a set of privacy panels to enclose her space or open it up, allowing her to control how much she can see and talk with others. The infusion treatment nook has a comfortable oversized reclining chair with temperature controls. Jennifer chooses a nook with a view of the outside garden that also has panels she can use to close out the light if she wants to sleep at some point during today's treatment.

Before going to the treatment nook, Jennifer and Jill stop at the infusion-treatment patient library that contains lendable books and DVDs as well as patient-education pamphlets and materials. They select a DVD and two iPads loaded with games Jennifer and Jill like to play during the treatment sessions. Jennifer's nook also has Internet access, which is a relief to her because she has a pressing issue at work that she would like to check on while she is here today. The nook also has television and options for listening to music. Jennifer's nook has a digital artwork wall that will display different types of artwork (landscape, whimsical, modern, nature) according to her preferences. She chooses whimsical artwork today. As the nurse comes in to begin the infusion treatment, Jill goes to the patient and family area and gets some freshly made coffee and a fruit snack for them both and returns to sit in the comfortable chair provided for family members in each nook. There is a locked cabinet in the nook in which Jennifer and Jill can safely store their purses or other valuables during the visit.

At the completion of the treatment, the nurse shares with Jennifer and Jill that there will be a piano recital in the lobby of the hospital beginning soon if they wish to attend. Jennifer decides instead to walk through the garden again, this time to stroll through the outdoor labyrinth. She states, "It helps me keep a balance through all of this."

This chapter provides information about factors that make up healing environments to enhance P&FCC. Examples that illustrate specific design elements comprising healing environments are provided, as well as current literature about evidence-based design of physical environments and care processes to promote healing, including enhancing patient control, privacy, dignity, comfort, and support from family, friends, and providers. We also describe the impact of evidence-based design in healthcare systems to promote safety and reduce errors. Additionally, we present information about designing more optimal environments and care processes for persons with disabilities. Lastly, the importance of patients, families, and care providers as members of healthcare system design teams is discussed.

What Is a Healing Environment?

A healing environment is a place where the interaction between patient and staff produces positive health outcomes within the physical environment (Huisman, Morales, van Hoof, & Kort, 2012). A healing environment can help make a stressful time a positive experience. As you can see from the preceding vignette, numerous facility design elements were approached from the patient's perspective. Healing environments include physical design details, patient-centered philosophies, and human interaction (Stichler, 2008). Healing environments promote a positive, pleasurable, and safe experience.

The Use of Evidence-Based Design to Promote Healing Environments

The importance of environment as a concept central to healing is not new. Both Hippocrates (Codinhoto, Tzortzopoulos, Kagioglou, Aouad, & Cooper, 2009) and, later, Florence Nightingale (Nightingale, 1992) emphasized the centrality of the physical environment in the care of the sick. More recently, the Institute of Medicine's reports on the safety and quality of care in the United States—*To Err is Human* (Kohn, Corrigan, & Donaldson, 1999) and *Crossing the Quality Chasm: A New Health Care System for the 21st Century* (Institute of Medicine [IOM], 2001)—highlighted the need for redesign of healthcare delivery systems to reduce hospital errors and improve patient outcomes and patient satisfaction.

In the last 2 decades, a body of research has produced considerable knowledge about evidence-based design of physical environments to promote healing (Aaron et al., 1996; Beauchemin & Hays, 1996; Bracco, Dubois, Bouali, & Eggimann, 2007; Clancy, 2008; Huisman et al., 2012; Walch et al., 2005; Wilson & Ridgway, 2006). Design elements of healing environments most likely to affect human health and well-being are:

- Comfort factors related to privacy, temperature, lighting, noise, and visual serenity
- Access to nature (views of nature and opportunities to interact with nature)
- Positive distractions
- Access to social support
- Allowing for choice

Healing environments consist of both a philosophy of care and design attributes that create better outcomes and experiences for patients and their families. Philosophically, healing environments focus on P&FCC in which a high priority is placed on patient preferences and patient choice. Healing environments promote wellness and comfort in all dimensions—mind, body, and spirit.

Contributing to our understanding of evidence-based designs for healing environments is an emerging area of science, neuroarchitecture, which consists of knowledge from studies of the psychoneuroimmunological responses of human beings to the built environment. Evidence-based design also considers how patients move through the healthcare facility and interact with the environment in different phases of illness. It addresses the psychological, physical, and spiritual needs of patients, as well as their levels of stress during the illness experience. An added bonus is that healing environments can also positively affect staff efficiency, stress, and satisfaction (Huisman et al., 2012).

Patient Comfort and Control

Control of temperature, lighting, blinds, placement of personal belongings, bed control, sound, and natural light have all been shown to be important to patients and their families. The single- patient room is a major design feature that permits patients to control the room temperature, lights, and window blinds (Reiling, Hughes, & Murphy, 2008). Current hospital designs include window blinds that allow several levels of light filtering. Single-patient rooms also promote privacy and, to some extent, noise reduction. Noise has been shown to affect patients' quality of sleep and overall satisfaction with the hospital experience (Aaron et al., 1996; Huisman et al., 2012; Parthasarathy & Tobin, 2012). The ability of hospitalized patients to personalize their space, such as by being able to display family pictures and personal artwork, rearrange room furniture, and have personal items close by, has been shown to increase patient comfort and feelings of security (Hoybye, 2013) as well as help hospital staff understand more about the "person" within the "patient."

Access to natural light and nature have also been shown to be important elements of healing environments. Several studies have examined the relationship of access to natural sunlight in hospital rooms and comfort. For example, in a study of abdominal-surgery patients, those who had windows with views of nature experienced faster recovery times and required less medication compared with those who looked out at a brick wall (Ulrich, 1984). In another study, patients who had outside views of nature took 22% fewer medications for pain and had 21% lower medication costs. When given a choice, patients preferred daylight to artificial light and preferred to be close to windows (Walch et al., 2005).

Another important choice for patients is whether or not to wear hospital clothing. Patients vary in their preferences for wearing a hospital gown or robe. In a study by Hoybye and colleagues (2013), some patients reported that wearing the hospital gown was a transformational experience in that they lost their normal identity as soon as they put on the gown. These patients said that the ability to wear their own clothes would make them feel more like themselves and more dignified. However, some patients reported that they found the hospital clothing more comfortable or that it was a way to separate their sick self from their well self. It is important, therefore, that care providers be sensitive to patients' sense of identity during illness and offer choices about wearing hospital clothing. If patients choose to wear their own clothing, there may be a need to provide laundry facilities for personal items if there is a lengthy stay. No evidence could be found in the literature about the risk of infection from soiled personal clothes.

NOTE

There are new hospital gown designs that are more comfortable and less revealing. Sometimes referred to as *dignity robes*, these hospital gowns cover patients warmly and fully while still allowing medical staff to treat patients (DeNarvaez, 2012).

Involving patients in their care is another way to consider patient preferences and offer care choices. A design feature to support patient involvement in their care is for patients to have easy access to their medical information, especially medication records and plans of care. In some acute-care settings, patients can access these records in their hospital room using the same computers nurses use (Reiling et al., 2008). Internet access is also increasingly available in patient rooms, allowing for patients' remote access to medical records. Involving patients in their care and decision-making, however, is a philosophy of care, and technology alone will not be sufficient to make it an effective element of a healing environment.

Offering patients control over medical regimens, while hospitalized that they had control over at home is another way of involving patients in their care and supporting independence. Patient use of insulin pumps when hospitalized is a good example of offering patients control of a health regimen that they controlled at home. Insulin pumps were designed for use by persons with diabetes in ambulatory settings and often are removed when these individuals are hospitalized. Studies of patient use of insulin pumps while hospitalized showed no differences in mean glucose levels among patients who remained on pumps during hospitalization as compared to those for whom it was discontinued (Cook et al., 2012), however episodes of severe hyperglycemia and hypoglycemia were significantly less among pump users than those who had their pumps removed on hospitalization (Cook et al., 2012; Nassar et al., 2010). No pump site infection, pump machine failures, or episodes of ketoacidosis were found.

Reduction of Stress Through Environmental Features

One goal of healing environments is to reduce the stress of illness and restore wholeness through design features that address the thoughts and emotions of patients (Stichler, 2008). What one views through the window can make a difference. Bedridden patients show a strong preference for having a hospital window with a view of nature (Henriksen, Isaacson, Sadler, & Zimring, 2007), and views to the outside have been associated with reduced anxiety levels (Clancy, 2008).

Restful places, such as meditation rooms and gardens, offer the opportunity to enhance and refresh the spirit. These restful spaces often have a water feature, such as a waterfall or fountain, and may encourage and include methods for expressing feelings, as through writing in notebooks, leaving computer messages, or creating art.

Attending to a patent's need for distraction and filling idle time is another important element of healing environments. Interactive art in the room, as made available by selections on a television, can be a positive diversion from stressful illness experiences and fill idle hours, as can access to computers, patient libraries, and outdoor spaces (Diette, Lechtzin, Haponik, Devrotes, & Rubin, 2003).

Access to Social Support From Family and Friends

Access to social support from family and friends is an important factor in healing environments. Space for patients to be with family and friends reduces patient social isolation, provides distraction, and helps pass time (Diette et al., 2003). An important environmental feature to encourage family and friend support is the availability of quiet retreat spaces close to the patient's room where members of a family can be alone together. These spaces often contain healthy snacks, places for families to store their own food, and activities and materials for diversion, such as televisions, DVDs, and games. A patient library that offers fiction and nonfiction books, as well as patient education materials for patients and families, also helps families to pass time together. The ability for families to bring in pets and have easy access to the outdoors with patients during visits also has been shown to be an important component of healing environments.

Several facility design elements can reduce patient and family stress associated with interacting with unfamiliar, large, and complex healthcare institutions, such as having easy access to low-cost parking, good signage for finding the way among and in buildings, and entranceways that are home-like, warm, and inviting (warm colors, comfortable furniture) (Brown, Wright, & Brown, 1997). Family members also have described their need for Internet access in patient rooms and waiting rooms, locked drawers for storage of valuables, overnight accommodations, laundry, and access to showering. In addition to physical design elements, healthcare professionals can promote healing partnerships with families by being mindful of a family's physical, psychological, and spiritual needs.

> **NOTE**
>
> There is a growing body of literature on the design of hospital environments for children (Abbas & Ghazali, 2012; Lambert, Coad, Hicks, & Glacken, 2013; Turner, Newman-Bennett, Fralic, & Skinner, 2009). Children want to be socially connected to both the internal hospital community as well as to the outside community. This includes access to technology to support social interaction; visits from siblings, friends, and family; and spaces for age- and developmentally appropriate play, gaming, and social interactions (Abbas & Ghazali, 2012; Lambert et al., 2013).

Healing Environments Are Safe Environments

Considerable research has been done in recent years to address the relationship between the design of healthcare environments and the quality and safety of care (Henriksen et al., 2007; Reiling et al., 2008). Evidence supports that specific elements in the design of physical environments can reduce patient falls, hospital-acquired infections, and errors by healthcare professionals. Facility design features to decrease patient falls include having a short bed-to-bathroom distance, the availability of hand rails along the way, and adequate lighting (Reiling et al., 2008). Additionally, new hospital room designs are being developed that use infrared technology to notify staff if a patient sits up and moves to the edge of the bed or enters the bathroom (Salonen et al., 2013).

Physical design elements to reduce infections consist of having single rooms for patients (Bracco et al., 2007; Wilson & Ridgway, 2006), hand washing facilities in each room and treatment area (Bracco et al., 2007), and consideration for latent environmental factors such as ventilation, dust, humidity, and air quality (Huisman et al., 2012). Considerable evidence supports the importance of single patient rooms, not only to reduce infections but also to reduce patient transfers, length of stay, and noise. Increased access to natural light reduces patient depression (Beauchemin & Hays, 1996) and enhances satisfaction (Huisman et al., 2012; Salonen et al., 2013).

Design elements to reduce errors by clinicians include making all rooms identical in the placement of furniture, supplies, and equipment; sufficient lighting to assist healthcare professionals in reading patient records, using equipment dials, and administering medications; decentralized nursing stations; and reduction in handoffs required by patient transfers (Huisman et al., 2012; Reiling et al., 2008; Salonen et al., 2013; Trochelman, Albert, Spence, Murray, & Slifcak, 2012). Hospitals can decrease patient transfers by having headwalls that are adaptable to different levels of acuity so that patients can stay in the same room as the acuity level changes (Brown & Gallant, 2006). The close proximity of patient charts to their hospital room (such as in a decentralized nursing station alcove adjacent to a set of patient rooms or in the patient's room) not only allows nurses quick access to information but also allows patient proximity to this information so that they can be more involved in their care decisions. In general, the design principles for patient safety include automating and standardizing physical spaces and processes whenever possible (Reiling et al., 2008).

Design for Inclusion

Consider the following scenario:

Jim Grady is 58 years of age and has been blind since birth. Jim has just found out that he has type 2 diabetes and has been referred to a series of diabetes self-management education classes. Because his wife, Mary, does the cooking at home, Jim would like Mary to go with him to the classes to learn about diabetes self-management with him. Jim and Mary are pleased to learn that the diabetes education sessions in their community are designed to include persons who are blind or deaf in the same classes with seeing and hearing persons.

After Jim has signed up for the classes, the diabetes nurse educator phones him and asks how he accomplishes his usual daily living activities. He states that he is a braille reader, independently gets to work each day to his job as director of a recreation department where he has a text-to-speech reader on his computer, and he likes to listen to books on tape. The next week, when Jim and Mary arrive at the diabetes education center, they find that the nurse educator verbally describes the graphical elements in the class audiovisual presentations and has handouts prepared in braille for Jim and printed English for Mary. Jim and Mary are invited to audiotape the diabetes education classes so that they can listen to the information again when they are at home.

Jim is taught to use an insulin pen to deliver his insulin injections. The dose-setting mechanism on the pen provides audible and tactile feedback to Jim so that he can independently administer his own insulin. He also learns to use a fully accessible talking blood glucose meter to check his blood glucose levels and a tactile method for getting the blood drop on the strip. Jim is taught a method of foot self-examination that uses touch and smell instead of sight, sparing him the embarrassment of having to rely on someone else to routinely examine his feet. Jim and Mary take home a handout that lists several good websites containing diabetes self-management information that Jim can access at home using the text-to-speech feature on his computer.

This scenario illustrates how the patient education process can be designed to meet the needs of a broad spectrum of abilities present in a typical population of patients, including those with disabilities. For example, a typical population of people with diabetes includes people with sensory disabilities (sight, hearing, and tactile) and motor impairments. The design of products, environments, and services to be usable by all people, including those with disabilities, without the need for adaptation or specialized design is named "universal design" (UD) (Connell et al., 1997; National Center on Universal Design for Learning, 2013; Welch, 1995). Rather than focusing on design for typical *individual* users (average person design), UD focuses on design for typical *populations* of users (in this case, persons with diabetes).

UD creates simple, nonstigmatizing access for the large minority of the population that has disabilities. In general, UD also has an unintended benefit—a universal design often makes products, environments, and services easier and more convenient for *everyone*. Classic examples include curb cuts, recorded books, elevated wall plugs, elbow-assisted faucets and door handles, and closed captioning, all originally intended for use by persons with disabilities and now commonly used by everyone.

The principles of UD and a brief description of each are listed in the following sidebar.

Principles of Universal Design

- *Equitable use: The design is useful and marketable to people with diverse abilities.* The same design should be usable by all persons, regardless of ability or disability. The design should be useful to everyone and ensure privacy, security, and safety for all users.

- *Flexibility in use: The design accommodates a wide range of individual preferences and abilities.* Users are provided with a choice of a variety of methods to use the design, including left- or right-handed use, and adaptability in pace of use.

- *Simple and intuitive use: Use of the design is easy to understand, regardless of the user's experience, knowledge, language skills, or current concentration level.* The design is simple, consistent with user expectations, and not dependent on literacy or a high level of language skills.

- *Perceptible information: The design communicates necessary information effectively to the user, regardless of ambient conditions or the user's sensory abilities.*

Multiple sensory inputs (auditory, tactile, and visual) present essential information in a variety of ways, perceptible by people with a variety of abilities. The design is compatible with approaches and techniques commonly used by people with sensory limitations.

- *Tolerance for error: The design minimizes hazards and the adverse consequences of accidental or unintended actions.* The arrangement of the design reduces the likelihood of hazards and errors by highlighting elements most prominent and eliminating predictable mistakes. Hazards and errors have built-in warnings and fail-safe features. When possible, the design allows the user to undo mistakes.

- *Low physical effort: The design can be used efficiently and comfortably with a minimum of fatigue.* The user can maintain a natural body position in all phases of use. The design minimizes repetitive actions and sustained physical effort.

- *Size and space for approach and use: Appropriate size and space is provided for approach, reach, manipulation, and use regardless of the user's body size, posture, or mobility.* The design has enough space for commonly used assistive devices or personal assistance. The design allows a seated or standing user to have a clear line of visual and tactile approach, with all essential components for operation easily reached. The design is easy to use for people with a wide variety of hand size, dexterity, and grip strength.

Source: Adapted from Williams, 2009

Diabetes self-management education in the U.S. is typically delivered in classes and conversations, with slide presentations, printed handouts, and demonstrations requiring the ability to hear, see, and read. Fortunately, these access and communication challenges can be overcome with the design and provision of diabetes self-management education using the principles of UD in Universal Design for Learning (UDL). UDL is a set of principles for curriculum development that give all individuals equal opportunities to learn in a single curriculum that is flexible enough for easy inclusion of people with a wide range of abilities in the same classroom (Kurzweil Educational Systems, 2009). In the case of diabetes education, a typical group learning situation designed according to UDL could include all necessary information presented in both visual and auditory formats with participatory activities (Williams, 2009; Williams, 2012). Thus, persons with hearing, visual, and cognitive impairments can perceive all that is presented, engage with the material, and learn effectively.

The use of UDL principles in designing educational programs produces an enriched learning environment that benefits all learners. Nondisabled persons with a variety of learning styles, as well as persons with low literacy or English as a second language, can all benefit from multisensory, participatory learning activities. In the example of Jim described at the beginning of this section, the presentation of essential materials in multiple formats can help to make educational processes more comfortable for learners from diverse ethnic backgrounds, more convenient for learners with time pressures, and more effective for nondisabled learners with a variety of learning styles (such as auditory, visual, or kinesthetic).

Although school teachers frequently put into use the principles of UDL, healthcare professionals have been slow to learn about and use this person-centered approach to patient education. Case Western Reserve University in Cleveland, Ohio has established a laboratory to provide resources to care providers and researchers about the design of care approaches and interventions to facilitate fuller inclusion of persons with disabilities in mainstream healthcare. The FIND Lab (Full INclusion of persons with Disabilities) provides consultation, equipment loans, and hands-on workstations where care providers and research investigators can develop teaching materials and assessment techniques to accommodate persons with disabilities.

Healthcare professionals also should be more involved in the design of new products that promote increased accessibility and usability for patients with a wide range of abilities. The insulin pen described in the earlier scenario is an example of a product that incorporates the principles of UD, offering multisensory feedback to the user and containing few steps for optimal use.

Healthcare professionals and potential users with a wide range of abilities not only should be included on new product design teams, but new products should be subject to practical, cost-effective techniques for evaluating product usability in a manner that is consistent with the tenets of UD and traditional usability heuristics. One such evaluation tool is the Rapid Assessment of Product Usability and Universal Design (RAPUUD) tool (Lenker, Nasarwanji, Paquet, & Feathers, 2011) that is constructed to support product designers and developers to identify products and product features that are problematic for those with physical, sensory, or cognitive impairments due to aging or disability. The following sidebar displays the items assessed using a Likert-type scale by users of a product.

Items Assessed in Rapid Assessment of Product Usability and Universal Design (RAPUUD)

- *This product is easy to set up or prepare to use.*

- *This product is easy to use.*

- *This product is easy to clean up and place into storage.*

- *For me, using this product poses a personal safety risk.*

- *I often need assistance to use this product.*

- *When using this product I make mistakes or errors that require me to "do over" some steps.*

- *I get the information I need to use the product efficiently.*

- *Using this product takes more time than it should.*

Source: Lenker, Nasarwanji, Paquet, & Feathers, 2011

It is important that patient and family self-management education be accessible across varied geographical locations and settings throughout the nation—in large cities and small towns, specialists' offices and primary care offices, large medical centers and small clinics. The use of UD principles in the design of patient education in general, and diabetes education in particular, has the potential to increase the accessibility to information, skills, and behavior change vital to maintaining and improving health. Furthermore, use of UD principles may benefit people who have no identified disabilities. It is design for everyone.

Key Points for Practice

Evidence-based design of healthcare physical environments and care processes affect patient outcomes, reduce adverse events, and promote patient and family satisfaction. Key points for clinicians to promote evidence-based healing environments are:

- Provide patients and families with choice and control over as many elements in the environment as possible, including privacy, light, temperature, noise, room views, and diversion activities.

- Place patients in private rooms when possible.

- Involve patients and their identified support persons in their care.

- Establish a patient and family advisory council to advise about environmental and care processes design features—not just when designing a new space or building, but on an ongoing basis.

- Provide flexible care options using UD principles to promote access and usability of healthcare services for persons with motor, sensory, or cognitive impairments.

- Incorporate the principles of evidence-based environmental designs to prevent adverse events, especially falls and hospital-acquired infections.

- Participate in committees to design healthcare spaces, devices, products, and delivery systems.

- Attend to the everyday things that you can do to promote healing environments, such as honoring patient privacy; creating spaces for patients and families to be comfortable together; reducing noise levels; maintaining general order and cleanliness of the patient and family areas; instructing patients on how to get out of bed and use the bathroom safely; seeking patient preferences about temperature, light, room views, and scheduling of procedures; identifying patient need for distraction or to fill idle time; sharing information with patients in a timely way; and hand washing.

- Remember that healthcare providers themselves are an essential element of healing environments.

Table 22.1 provides a list of additional resources for learning more about healing environments and evidence-based healthcare design.

TABLE 22.1   Resources for Healing Environments and Evidenced-Based Design

TOPIC	RESOURCE
Planetree (healing environment model)	The Planetree Model Hospital Project: An example of the patient as partner (Martin, Hunt, Hughes-Stone, & Conrad, 1989)
	www.planetree.org
Universal Design	www2.ed.gov/about/offices/list/ovae/pi/AdultEd/disaccess.html
Universal Design of Learning	www.udlcenter.org/aboutudl/udlguidelines/
	www.cast.org/udl/
Healing Environments	www.hfmmagazine.com/hfmmagazine/
	www.healinglandscapes.org
Center for Health Design	www.healthdesign.org/edac
FIND Lab (Full INclusion of Persons with Disabilities), Case Western Reserve University	fpb.case.edu/FINDLab/index.shtm

Conclusion

The design and provision of healing environments can facilitate the provision of P&FCC. However, more studies are needed about the effects of healing design features on patient outcomes and experiences to continue developing the evidence base in this area. Specifically, more information is needed on how the design of care environments and processes can increase the quality of communication and information sharing between patients or families and clinicians. For example, there are, unfortunately, unintended consequences that are now emerging on staff efficiency and sense of teamwork and collaboration due to single patient rooms, decentralized nursing stations, individual reports at the bedside, and computers/charts in patients' rooms (Zborowsky, Bunker-Hellmich, Morelli, & O'Neill, 2010). With further study will come a greater understanding of the impact of healing environments on patient satisfaction, care outcomes, staff satisfaction, and the cost-effectiveness of healthcare. Expanding the current knowledge of healing environments will also export their effectiveness beyond the settings in which it has been traditionally applied (acute care, hospice, and pediatric settings) to primary care, nursing home, and rehabilitation settings. More knowledge also is needed about the everyday things healthcare professionals can do to promote healing environments in their own practice settings.

References

Aaron, J. N., Carlisle, C. C., Carskadon, M. A., Meyer, T. J., Hill, N. S., & Millman, R. P. (1996). Environmental noise as a cause of sleep disruption in an intermediate respiratory care unit. *Sleep, 19*(9), 707-710.

Abbas, M. Y., & Ghazali, R. (2012). Healing environment: Paediatric wards—Status and design trend. *Procedia-Social and Behavioral Sciences, 49*, 28-38.

Beauchemin, K. M., & Hays, P. (1996). Sunny hospital rooms expedite recovery from severe and refractory depressions. *Journal of Affective Disorders, 40*(1), 49-51.

Bracco, D., Dubois, M. J., Bouali, R., & Eggimann, P. (2007). Single rooms may help to prevent nosocomial bloodstream infection and cross-transmission of methicillin-resistant Staphylococcus aureus in intensive care units. *Intensive Care Medicine, 33*(5), 836-840.

Brown, B., Wright, H., & Brown, C. (1997). A post-occupancy evaluation of wayfinding in a pediatric hospital: Research findings and implications for instruction. *Journal of Architectural and Planning Research, 14*(1), 35-51.

Brown, K. K., & Gallant, D. (2006). Impacting patient outcomes through design: Acuity adaptable care/universal room design. *Critical Care Nursing Quarterly, 29*(4), 326-341.

Clancy, C. M. (2008). Designing for safety: Evidence-based design and hospitals. *American Journal of Medical Quality, 23*(1), 66-69.

Codinhoto, R., Tzortzopoulos, P., Kagioglou, M., Aouad, G., & Cooper, R. (2009). The impacts of the built environment on health outcomes. *Facilities, 27*(3/4), 138-151.

Connell B. R., Jones, M., Mace, R., Mueller, J., Mullick, A., Ostroff, E., ...Vanderheiden, G. (1997). *The principles of universal design.* Retrieved from http://www.ncsu.edu/ncsu/design/cud/about_ud/udprinciplestext.htm

Cook, C. B., Beer, K. A., Seifert, K. M., Boyle, M. E., Mackey, P. A., & Castro, J. C. (2012). Transitioning insulin pump therapy from the outpatient to the inpatient setting: A review of 6 years' experience with 253 cases. *Journal of Diabetes Science and Technology, 6*(5), 995-1002.

DeNarvaez, D. (2012, February). Healing Environment newsletter. Kingsport, TN, Wellmont Health System: Hudson Valley Medical Center.

Diette, G. B., Lechtzin, N., Haponik, E., Devrotes, A., & Rubin, H. R. (2003). Distraction therapy with nature sights and sounds reduces pain during flexible bronchoscopy: A complementary approach to routine analgesia. *Chest Journal, 123*(3), 941-948.

Henriksen, K., Isaacson, S., Sadler, B. L., & Zimring, C. M. (2007). The role of the physical environment in crossing the quality chasm. *Joint Commission Journal on Quality and Patient Safety, 33*(Suppl 1), 68-80.

Hoybye, M. T. (2013). Healing environments in cancer treatment and care: Relations of space and practice in hematological cancer treatment. *Acta Oncologica, 52*(2), 440-446.

Huisman, E. R. C. M., Morales, M., van Hoof, J., & Kort, H. S. M. (2012). Healing environment: A review of the impact of the physical environmental factors on users. *Building and Environment, 58*, 70-80.

Institute of Medicine (IOM). (2001). *Crossing the quality chasm: A new health system for the 21st century.* Washington, DC: National Academies Press.

Kohn, L. T., Corrigan, J. M., & Donaldson, M. S. (1999). *To err is human: Building a safer health system* [IOM report]. Washington, DC: National Academies Press.

Kurzweil Educational Systems. (2009). *Kurzweil 3000 supports universal design for learning.* Retrieved from http://www.kurzweiledu.com/files/udl.pdf

Lambert, V., Coad, J., Hicks, P., & Glacken, M. (2013). Social spaces for young children in hospital. *Child: Care, Health and Development.* Advance online publication. doi: 10.1111/cch.12016

Lenker, J. A., Nasarwanji, M., Paquet, V., & Feathers, D. (2011). A tool for rapid assessment of product usability and universal design: Development and preliminary psychometric testing. *Work, 39*(2), 141-150.

Martin, D. P., Hunt, J. R., Hughes-Stone, M., & Conrad, D. A. (1989). The Planetree Model Hospital Project: An example of the patient as partner. *Hospital & Health Services Administration, 35*(4), 591-601.

Nassar, A. A., Partlow, B. J., Boyle, M. E., Castro, J. C., Bourgeois, P. B., & Cook, C. B. (2010). Outpatient-to-inpatient transition of insulin pump therapy: Successes and continuing challenges. *Journal of Diabetes Science and Technology, 4*(4), 863.

National Center on Universal Design for Learning. (2013). *UDL guidelines—Version 2.0.* Retrieved from http://www.udlcenter.org/aboutudl/udlguidelines

Nightingale, F. (1992). *Notes on nursing: What it is and what it is not.* Philadelphia, PA: Lippincott Williams & Wilkins.

Parthasarathy, S., & Tobin, M. J. (2012). Sleep in the intensive care unit. In M. R. Pinsky, L. Brochard, J. Mancebo, & M. Antonelli (Eds.), *Applied physiology in intensive care medicine 2* (pp. 61-70). Berlin, Germany: Springer-Verlag.

Planetree (2013). *Planetree.* Retrieved from http://planetree.org

Reiling, J., Hughes, R. G., & Murphy, M. R. (2008). The impact of facility design on patient safety. In *Patient safety and quality: An evidence-based handbook for nursing* (Chapter 28). Rockville, MD: Agency for Healthcare Research & Quality.

Salonen, H., Lahtinen, M., Lappalainen, S., Nevala, N., Knibbs, L. D., Morawska, L., & Reijula, K. (2013). Design approaches for promoting beneficial indoor environments in healthcare facilities: A review. *Intelligent Buildings International, 5*(1), 26-50.

Stichler, J. F. (2008). Healing by design. *Journal of Nursing Administration, 38*(12), 505-509.

Trochelman, K., Albert, N., Spence, J., Murray, T., & Slifcak, E. (2012). Patients and their families weigh in on evidence-based hospital design. *Critical Care Nurse, 32*(1), e1-e10.

Turner, J., Newman-Bennett, K., Fralic, J., & Skinner, L. (2009). Everybody needs a break! Responses to a playgarden survey. *Pediatric Nursing, 35*(1), 27-34.

Ulrich, R. S. (1984). View through a window may influence recovery from surgery. *Science, 224*(4647)**,** 420-421.

Walch, J. M., Rabin, B. S., Day, R., Williams, J. N., Choi, K., & Kang, J. D. (2005). The effect of sunlight on postoperative analgesic medication use: A prospective study of patients undergoing spinal surgery. *Psychosomatic Medicine, 67*(1), 156-163.

Welch, P. (1995). *What is universal design?* Retrieved from http://udeducation.org/resources.html

Williams, A. S. (2009). Universal design in diabetes care: An idea whose time has come. *The Diabetes Educator, 35*(1), 45-57.

Williams, A. S. (2012). Human factors for diabetes devices: Creating low vision and nonvisual instructions for diabetes technology: An empirically validated process. *Journal of Diabetes Science and Technology*, 6(2), 252.

Wilson, A. P. R., & Ridgway, G. L. (2006). Reducing hospital-acquired infection by design: The new University College London Hospital. *Journal of Hospital Infection, 62*(3), 264-269.

Zborowsky, T., Bunker-Hellmich, L., Morelli, A., & O'Neill, M. (2010). Centralized vs. decentralized nursing stations: Effects on nurses' functional use of space and work environment. *Health Environments Research & Design Journal, 3*(4), 19.

Chapter 23

System Change for Patient- and Family-Centered Care

Juliette Schlucter, BS

As it was written, the policy was clear:

"No Siblings under the Age of 12 Permitted in the NICU"

What was far from clear was how the policy was interpreted and implemented!

Over the years, the policy was open to wide interpretation depending on the nurse manager on duty, the shift, or in some cases the family. Discussion about the policy sparked impassioned debate among staff members. The topic was polarizing, with steadfast opinions being offered by infection control, administration, and nursing. Families scored the NICU poorly on patient satisfaction surveys for questions related to the experience of care and support of the family. The policy for sibling visitation in the NICU had become a lightning rod for families and staff. As a result, there were huge inconsistencies in the application of the policy, not to mention often disgruntled families and many times disengaged staff as confusion and inconsistency in practice continued.

Through a recent shared governance committee, formed to advance a culture of patient- and family-centered care, nursing leadership believed a solution was possible. The committee began by first bringing together a team of traditional and nontraditional stakeholders. Unlike previous hospital committees, which typically included only senior physicians, nurses on this new committee also included frontline staff, a resident, infection control, the unit clerk, a member of the security staff, the unit housekeeper, a member of the patient relations team, the head of facilities, and two family members who recently had their newborns cared for in the NICU. The committee's goal was to lead with a commitment to the core values of patient- and family-centered care and to look at the current impact of the sibling visitation policy. The committee's shared vision was to first understand the current realities from the points of view of each of the stakeholders, including the families, and then to commit to changes and decisions that reflected a patient- and family-centered culture.

Members of the committee contacted peer hospitals, examined the research available, and benchmarked a variety of approaches and then shared those best practices with the committee. Having all of the stakeholders together was essential to working through options and proposing a solution that considered the varied points-of-view of those who work and receive care in the NICU. The solution the committee recommended was to pilot sibling visitation and monitor concerns about increased infection rates and unsupervised children on the unit, and evaluate before implementing an open visitation policy. This approach had everyone's support because stakeholder voices were heard and their concerns addressed in the change process.

The vignette just described was based on a collaborative model for system-level change, which supports designing healthcare systems *with* patients and families as opposed to *for* them. This collaborative model forms the basis for patient- and family-centered system change. The above scenario describes four key elements necessary for sustained, system-level patient- and family-centered change:

- Leadership commitment
- Engaged patients and families
- Empowered staff
- A collaborative model

The purpose of this chapter is to explore each of these key elements in detail and offer pragmatic suggestions for achieving a patient- and family-centered environment through system change.

Leadership Commitment

The urgency for leaders to advance cultures of care that are safe, effective, of the highest quality, and place patients and families at the center of care decision-making has never been greater. A crescendo of voices from the Institute of Medicine (IOM, 2001), The Joint Commission (TJC, 2010), the National Patient Safety Foundation (NPSF, 2008), Quality and Safety Education for Nurses (QSEN) (Cronenwett et al., 2007), and the Agency for Healthcare Research and Quality (AHRQ, 2013), among many others, have been clear about the mandates to transform healthcare delivery and the experience of care. A move toward transparency has exposed system-level flaws; skyrocketing costs; inefficiencies; a lack of standardization of the best, evidence-based, clinical care; and alarming care delivery error rates.

Patient and family voices, individually and collectively through advocacy groups, have joined the chorus. Individuals are empowered with information about their or their loved ones' diagnosis and have access to the latest research. They enter the healthcare system with a sincere expectation of respect, dignity, access to information, and partnership for care decisions.

Though the mandates are clear and plentiful, sustainable system-level change can be stymied and complicated by the complexity of the care environment, the silos caregivers work in, and competing priorities that keep them from translating the philosophy of P&FCC to actionable change. These changes also can be compromised by several beliefs or assumptions. System-level challenges for implementing a culture of P&FCC include:

- P&FCC is often viewed as one of many other competing initiatives as opposed to an organization's core value system or culture of care.

- P&FCC as a concept may be viewed as the "flavor of the day" in a healthcare environment that changes rapidly.

- P&FCC may be mistakenly viewed as the domain of one department or discipline and viewed as a "departmental" (nursing, social work) initiative as opposed to the value system for all who work within the healthcare organization.

- P&FCC is viewed as "amenities," a patient satisfaction–driven initiative, good customer service, or just being nice to patients and families.

- The priority to engage patients and families in meaningful ways as partners in system design as well as in moments of care delivery is not resourced or supported sufficiently.

To meet these challenges, healthcare organizations need:

- Sustained and visible commitment from senior leadership including CEOs and other senior administrators as well as local unit, clinic, or department leaders

- Engagement of patients and families as advisors and the infrastructure and resources to support their involvement

- A shared vision for improvement between patients and families and healthcare professionals

- A multidisciplinary patient- and family-centered care team that includes representation from stakeholders across the system, including patients and families and frontline staff

- Empowerment of local leaders to advance a culture of P&FCC by acknowledging that the best problem-solving happens when those who work and receive care in a specific area are empowered to work collaboratively

- An action plan that moves the vision to practice, is owned and managed by local leaders, and is linked to the operational goals of the organization

With the mandates and urgency well-articulated by numerous and respected agencies, as described at the beginning of this section, leaders have an obligation to share a vision for P&FCC that is (1) linked to the mission of the organization, (2) visible in the operational plan, (3) part of the organization's core measures, and (4) evident in the expectations of managers and staff.

Patient and Family Engagement: A Call to Action

Few experiences in life elicit the level of vulnerability, fear, and anxiety that individuals feel when they or their loved ones become patients. For many, that vulnerability and anxiety soon serves as a force to mobilize them as advocates for themselves or their loved ones, empowered to receive the best possible care and outcome. This is patient and family engagement at its finest—it is the natural human desire to partner with those providing care—whether at a private practice visit, in a busy emergency department, a critical care unit, or at the bedside on a medical surgical floor—patients and their loved ones are engaged in the care process because they care deeply about the experience and the outcome.

With this as the motivation, the stage is set for leaders to promote a culture in which staff from all disciplines value engaged patients and families; partner with them to learn from their observations, hear their concerns, and respond to their questions; share information with them openly; and encourage their participation in care at the level they choose.

In the experience of care across all settings, the best practices for engaging patients and families are:

- Open visiting hours and removal of any policies that limit the ability of patients to stay united with their loved ones while in the hospital (Obama, 2010)
- Clinical, medical, and teaching rounds that include patients and families in care plan decisions
- Patient and family participation in change of shift report
- Family presence at resuscitation or during invasive procedures
- Transparency of patient safety risks and patient and family education and participation in checklists to minimize risk
- Open access to all healthcare information about the patient, including the electronic health record through a patient portal

These best practices affect the direct care experience and are significant indications of successful system-level change. Implementation of these best practices is evidence of a healthcare system that supports an activated or engaged patient and family. Furthermore, researchers are beginning to establish evidence that supports a link between patient engagement and improved care plan adherence, safety, quality, and the experience of care (AHRQ, 2013; James, 2013).

Such practices support the vital partnership with patient, and families in the moments of care delivery. For sustained system-level change to be effective, formal collaboration with patient and family advisors as partners in the design of care is also essential.

Formal Patient and Family Advisory Roles

Healthcare organizations embedding P&FCC into their organizations have developed formal partnerships with patients and families as advisors. These partnerships can be set up in a variety of ways. Presented here are several strategies that have been proven not only to be effective but also sustainable over the long term. As part of this partnership, patient and family advisors are recruited and provided orientation and training to partner effectively for their particular roles or responsibilities.

Patient, Family, and Youth Advisory Councils

Advisors are recruited and trained to serve on councils and committees to work with clinical staff and administrators on strategic planning initiatives, patient safety committees, facility design, and policies and programs. In some children's hospitals, youth advisors serve on councils to provide the unique perspective of the adolescents receiving care.

Many hospitals are harnessing the power of technology, social media, and the Internet and have developed ways to have advisors who cannot physically be at the hospital for a meeting offer their perspective as "eAdvisors" via video chat, or in a virtual electronic meeting portal. These technological options give organizations the ability to connect with larger, more diverse populations of patients and families, all of whom are committed to improving the experience of care.

Patient and Family Faculty

Patients and families partner with healthcare educators to teach nurses, physicians, and non-clinical staff about the experience of illness from the lens of those receiving care. Often the patient and family faculty are included as teachers in new employee orientation programs to set the stage for P&FCC for new hires. Patients and families also present at Grand Rounds, serve as guest lecturers in nursing and medical schools, and mentor new medical residents and fellows.

Peer-to-Peer Mentors

Patients and families are trained in active and therapeutic listening skills and share their firsthand knowledge about navigating a specific care environment or illness with newly diagnosed patients and families. As with the patient advisor programs, peer-to-peer support programs have also harnessed technology and the Internet for greater access and flexibility to forums where patients and families can connect with one another and provide expertise.

Patients and Families in Paid Professional Roles

Many hospitals have created paid professional roles for experienced patient and family advisors to manage the P&FCC programs, serve as liaisons to patient and family advisors, and bring the voice of the patient and family to hospital-wide committees. To stay wedded to the fundamental principle that patient- and family-centered system-level change happens through planning and implementation *with* patients and families and not *for* them, creating programmatic infrastructure that supports the formal advisory roles is essential. Sources for recruitment and training and toolkits that cover all of the elements of developing patient and family advisor roles can be found in the back of this book in this chapter's section in the Resources appendix.

Leaders who set the expectation for partnerships with patients and families in care delivery and as advisors begin the journey toward system-level P&FCC, but many organizations are challenged with how to translate that expectation to sustainable action. For many organizations the patient and family advisor roles and councils become "window dressing" for P&FCC because the system does not have an infrastructure that supports collaborative decision-making.

A Model of Collaboration

For system-level change to be effective, a model of collaborative decision-making must be supported. One such model is that developed by the author of this chapter (Schlucter, 2010) and depicted in Figure 23.1. In a collaborative model, the goal is to find the overlapping interests and priorities of each of the stakeholder groups, as represented by the star in the center.

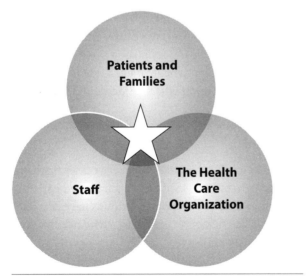

FIGURE 23.1

A collaborative model of decision-making.

This model acknowledges that each of the interest groups has a unique set of pressures and priorities that may exist outside of the center but they are working together toward a common goal—in this case P&FCC—to develop solutions that each of them can support. P&FCC places emphasis on *mutually beneficial partnerships* between patients, families, and healthcare professionals. Those three words, "mutually beneficial partnerships," serve as the cornerstone of P&FCC, but mutually beneficial partnerships require a new framework for system change.

Historically, patients and families were absent from system-level conversations or decision-making in healthcare. Many employees or healthcare providers themselves would suggest that patients and families were not the only ones left out. System-level changes often happened within departmental silos or in a culture that valued autonomy and traditional medical hierarchy, or it was headed by leaders or managers who were removed from the actual care experience. Often these forums did not include frontline staff, nonclinical staff, or staff from other disciplines.

In addition to not always having the right stakeholders in the room, many healthcare professionals have shared that the skill set needed to collaborate effectively in partnership with stakeholders from different disciplines was not always emphasized or taught in nursing, medical, or professional schools. The P&FCC model is collaborative; it values the diversity of roles and opinions of everyone at the table and is committed to including the unique perspective of the patients and families receiving care.

Within the model, the keys to successful collaboration include:

- **Sharing a common purpose or goal that is well articulated:** For patient- and family-centered system change, a collaborative team unites around the collective vision that care safety, quality, and experience improves when patients and families share in decision-making with healthcare professionals.

- **Including the right mix of stakeholders:** It is easy to invite our allies, but effective collaboration requires us to step outside of our comfort zone and invite stakeholders that may challenge our thinking. For collaboration to be successful, it is important to invite decision-makers *and* non-supervisory staff. Invite champions *and* objectors, supporters *and* influencers, and patients *and* families that represent the diversity of the healthcare system.

- **Giving equal voice that is fair and balanced:** Collaborative efforts can be stalled or ineffective if we have invited the stakeholders but neglect to manage the process to ensure there is an even playing field and that every voice is heard. This concept is as important for staff as it is for patients and families. It is easy to imagine how, without the best facilitation, a lone patient or family contribution could be ignored by a clinically dominated team, but this happens all the time to fellow healthcare professionals invited to the table as well. Many examples exist of a recently hired frontline nurse or resident invited to work on a new initiative, but their insight or voice is buried because of group dynamics that value years of experience more.

- **A commitment to labor together:** This concept for successful collaboration comes directly from the root of the word *collaboration*—to "co-labor" for the best solution. The co-laboring should respect diverse points of view and challenge the participants to labor together to seek solutions that are as close as possible to the overlapping interest or the shared interest of the group. This co-laboring challenges the group to think differently and seek common ground, and it is what drives innovation and sustainable solutions.

Table 23.1 outlines some examples of different realities, pressures, and priorities for each of the stakeholders in a P&FCC workgroup: patients and families, staff, and leadership. By listing these pressures as part of each stakeholder's reality, it legitimizes that the organization, individual staff members, and patients and families have unique needs, pressures, and reasonable goals that lie outside of the overlapping center and must be acknowledged and factored into the equation for a collaborative decision to be sustainable.

TABLE 23.1   Separate Realities of Key Stakeholders in Decision-Making

PATIENTS AND FAMILIES	STAFF	TOP LEADERSHIP
Diagnosis	Time	Budget constraints
Lack of sleep	Resources	Staffing
Worry	Education	Juggling multiple priorities
Medical jargon	Safety	Community needs vs. individual patient needs
Uncertainty of illness and outcomes	Partnering with families	Long- vs. short-term strategies
Partnering with staff	Administrative responsibilities	Regulations
Hospital environment	Internal staff/unit dynamics	Payer and reimbursement pressures

An Example to Appreciate Separate Realities

As highlighted in Table 23.1, each person brings his or her own bias, perspectives, and unique pressures to the table. We can imagine that if we brought together a group to work on a new patient flow design for the day medicine unit of a busy oncology center, we would need to begin by understanding the points of view of each of the stakeholders.

In the case of a young husband, newly diagnosed with cancer and asked to participate in the newly formed Oncology Advisory Council, he brings an overwhelming amount of stress of living with cancer and the uncertainty of his prognosis. From his first admission on, he knows all too well how hard it is to sort through the medical jargon and learn how to navigate a complicated healthcare system. His perspective on the experience of waiting for his next appointment or for an exam room to open is colored now by his reality that his life may be shortened. When he comes to the day medicine unit and he is asked to wait, seemingly endlessly, in waiting rooms and exam rooms for treatments and clinicians, his sense of frustration is heightened; he wants to be home spending time with his loved ones, not wasting time waiting for treatment. He is empowered by this sense of impatience to find answers and make changes quickly to a broken system. These are his realities.

In the case of the new hematology-oncology nurse, a recent nursing school graduate, she comes to the committee frustrated by how little time she actually has with individual patients and families. She is adjusting to the internal dynamics of the unit and is burdened with the pressure to complete a series of online course modules to be compliant with the latest safety standards. She is surprised and frustrated by barriers to spending time and connecting with patients and families, and sometimes she wonders if this is the kind of nursing care she expected to deliver when she chose her profession. As a junior level staff member, she is concerned that her perspective will not be credible to more senior staff members on the team.

Also at the table is the vice president for operations. As an administrator committed to P&FCC, she is challenged to find resources in the budget to do more with less as reimbursement models contract and expenses increase. A constant internal struggle is balancing the cries for improving patient flow in the immediate future while staying wedded to a long-term strategic facility improvement plan that will not affect the day medicine unit for 4 years. She is a seasoned leader and has come to accept and not challenge that change takes time in healthcare. With her many years of experience, she believes that she knows the realities of the patients and families in her healthcare system.

Each of these stakeholders' realities is valid. They come to the table with the common goal: To do the right thing and make improvements on the oncology unit. Through a model of collaboration they will labor together, be informed by each other's separate realities, and compromise to create a solution that everyone can support.

With a systems approach to understanding stakeholders separate realities, conflict is viewed not as a negative but as a provocative challenge for the group to develop creative ideas that are, in fact, more sustainable because the conflict was worked through and addressed. It acknowledges that no stakeholder holds greater power or the best answer. Supporting this effectively requires the members of the team to use "relational thinking"—the ability to expand their own point-of-view and consider the realities of their fellow collaborators.

Effective collaborative teams begin by inquiring about the diverse perspectives and realities around the table and spend time listening to the issues and unique demands of others. The team leader repeatedly asks questions of everyone at the table to promote relational thinking: Tell us how this will feel/work/be perceived by you or others on the team?

As the team listens and responds to the barriers or issues that surface, they are required to suspend judgment and to leverage the reality of the other stakeholders. Working through topics using a collaborative model of change with all of the stakeholders present—including patients and families—supports patient- and family-centered system change.

With this collaborative model in place, the patient- and family-centered care team, supported by leaders, must look across the core system components that drive and embody a culture of care and inclusion and develop an action plan that asks key questions to continually advance the journey toward P&FCC.

Domains of System Change and Key Questions

To successfully achieve system change that supports and sustains patient- and family-centered care, attention has to be paid to the creation of core system components to support the work. Presented here are five of these components, with questions that prompt consideration and action.

Vision, Mission, and Strategy

The vision, mission, and strategy are important opportunities for an organization to communicate their commitment to patient- and family-centered care. When defined by key stakeholders, including patients and families, the mission vision and strategy should reflect the value the organization places on a culture of partnership between patients and families and healthcare professionals.

- Do we have a clearly articulated vision for P&FCC?
- How is our vision linked to the hospital strategy and operational plan?
- Are national best practices for P&FCC implemented or part of operational goals?
- Have we invited all stakeholders, including patients and families, to contribute ideas to the vision, mission, strategy, and operational priorities of the hospital?

Communication

The complexity of healthcare organizations, the fragmentation of care, and the volume of information available to be shared have increased the demand for all organizations to have a clearly defined communication strategy for patient- and family-centered care. Internal and external communication plans need to continually reinforce a culture of care that emphasizes respect and dignity, information sharing, and participating in care to the level a patient chooses.

- Are there communications that are highly visible to patients, families, and staff at all levels of the organization that articulate clearly the values and priorities for patient- and family-centered care?

- Have we incorporated the use of multiple media resources including the external facing website, the intranet, video, YouTube channel, digital signage, social media, and print to reach diverse learners and populations?
- Do we regularly share staff, caregiver, and patient stories that illustrate the core concepts of P&FCC?

Training, Tools, and Resources

If P&FCC is a system-level priority, its philosophy, competencies, and behaviors must be a part of staff orientation, training, and continuing education.

- Have we implemented high-impact adult learning modules that translate the philosophy of P&FCC to behavior-based tools?
- Have we embedded practices of P&FCC in nursing and physician clinical education? As examples: When we teach a new nurse how to place an IV, are we teaching in ways that support family members' being present and communicating with patients the risks and safety precautions? When we mentor new residents in the delivery of a difficult diagnosis, does the approach value the environment in which the news is shared and give considerations to honor the dignity of the patient, respect cultural differences, and provide ample time for the physician to listen and learn from the patient and for the patient or family to ask questions?
- Have patients and family members been invited and mentored to offer their perspective to teach healthcare professionals about the experience of care?
- Are there visible cues, signage, and communication tips and tools in patient care areas that support healthcare information sharing and transparency?

Human Resources

Human Resource professionals are often missing from the early discussion for system-level adoption of P&FCC but are key to an organization's success in hiring the ideal candidates and establishing organizational development programs and accountability strategies.

- Do recruitment and career opportunity messages on websites and in printed materials share with candidates the P&FCC values of the organization?
- Does new employee orientation establish expectations of supporting a culture of patient- and family-centered care and for working with patients and families throughout the care experience?
- Are position descriptions revised to include expectations of P&FCC? For example, a traditional job description may list the nurse's role to develop, implement, and evaluate the plan of care. A patient- and family-centered job description might read: With the patient and family, and in partnership with other team members, the nurse develops, implements, and evaluates a coordinated plan of care.

- Are core competencies for patient- and family-centered care embedded in performance appraisal tools?
- Are patient and family advisors invited onto search committees to evaluate and interview candidates for key roles across the healthcare organization?

Honoring Excellence

An ideal strategy to reinforce system-level adoption of patient- and family-centered care is the honoring of the specific best practices of individual staff, departments, and teams and the contributions of patient and family advisors that advance a culture of P&FCC.

- Are staff, nursing, and physician awards for excellence grounded in principles for P&FCC?
- Does administration use frequent opportunities to highlight the work of individuals, teams and patient and family advisors who advance the work of patient and family-centered care?

Conclusion

For system-level P&FCC, the analogy of a journey, not a destination has long been shared. Healthcare organizations are complex, and the internal and external environments are continually changing. To be successful, leaders, staff, patients, and families must embrace this concept of journeying together to sustain system-level change. They must maintain the commitment to the fundamental principle of P&FCC: to lead and do *with* patients and families rather than *to* or *for* them. With this as the guiding principle, engaging patients and families to share in the collaborative process across all of the domains of an organization establishes a sustainable culture that ultimately supports improvements in safety, quality, and the experience of care.

References

Agency for Healthcare Research and Quality (AHRQ). (2013). *Guide to patient and family engagement in hospital quality and safety.* Retrieved from http://www.ahrq.gov/professionals/systems/hospital/engagingfamilies/index.html

Cronenwett, L., Sherwood, G., Barnsteiner, J., Disch J., Johnson, J., Mitchell, P., ...Warren, J. (2007). Quality and safety education for nurses. *Nursing Outlook, 55,* 122-31.

Institute of Medicine (IOM). (2001). *Crossing the quality chasm: A new health system for the 21st century.* Washington, DC: National Academy Press.

James, J. (2013, February 14). Health policy briefs: Patient engagement. *Health Affairs.* Retrieved from https://www.healthaffairs.org/healthpolicybriefs/brief.php?brief_id=86

The Joint Commission (TJC). (2010). *Advancing effective communication, cultural competence, and patient and family-centered care: A roadmap for hospitals.* Oakbrook Terrace IL: The Joint Commision.

National Patient Safety Foundation (NPSF). (2008). *National agenda for action: Patients and families in patient safety: Nothing about me, without me.* Chicago, IL. Retrieved from http://www.npsf.org/wp-content/uploads/2011/10/Nothing_About_Me.pdf

Obama, B. (2010, April 15). Presidential memorandum—Hospital visitation. Retrieved from http://www.whitehouse.gov/the-press-office/presidential-memorandum-hospital-visitation

Schlucter, J. (2010). Supporting and mentoring the collaborative process between patient advisors and health care professionals to advance patient- and family-centered care. Webinar and workshop. Retrieved from BRIDGEKEEPER website: www.bridgekeeper.org

Chapter 24

The Role of Leaders in Assuring Person- and Family-Centered Care

Joanne Disch, PhD, RN, FAAN

Michael is a 24-year-old graduate student who has had type 1 diabetes since he was 9 years old. Over the years he has had a number of hospitalizations to bring his glucose into control. He has also spent a number of sessions with his diabetes nurse educator to learn how to choose foods that work for him and how to use his insulin pump. For the most part, he has had an active life and done well. However, last week he came down with the flu, with 2 days of vomiting and diarrhea. He was hospitalized last night to regulate his fluids, intake, and insulin. Shortly after being admitted to the inpatient medical unit, he was informed by his nurse that they were placing him on a different insulin pump so that they could better control his glucose levels. Michael's response was "I want to use my own pump. I've been successful at regulating my glucose levels for over 10 years, and I know what works and doesn't." His nurse, Anisha, replied: "We need to do that for you here. Our policy is that patients cannot use their own equipment from home—there is too much risk involved, and what if something happened?" Something did happen—because of the use of a different kind of pump and a different titration protocol that the nursing staff used, Michael's blood glucose soared to 450 mg/dL, and he needed adjuvant drug therapy to bring his glucose into acceptable levels, requiring 3 extra days in the hospital.

The role of the leader in promoting person- and family-centered care is to create systems, processes, and structures for providing care that is respectful of and responsive to individual patient preferences, needs, and values and ensuring that patient values guide all clinical decisions. This involves working with and through others to achieve active, authentic person and family engagement. Although it seems an obvious goal to pursue, it offers one of the greatest challenges to healthcare leaders at all levels. What is at stake is the traditional model of healthcare delivery: the bureaucratic structures and practices, historical reward systems, and perceived or actual power differentials. Fortunately, there are powerful societal pressures to move in this direction from consumers, patients, families, many healthcare providers, and numerous influential organizations. Moreover, there is a vast array of resources that can help organizational leaders get started or progress further along their own path.

The purpose of this chapter is to help leaders apply their understanding of the characteristics of a person- and family-centered organization with strategies and tools for accomplishing this goal. Practical strategies will be offered for conducting an organizational assessment, setting up a person/family advisory council, developing key organizational documents to reflect this philosophy, establishing person-centered policies and guidelines for operationalizing a person-centered organization, and providing other ways in which individuals and their families (or significant others) can become full partners and allies in designing and executing holistic, individualized care.

The Role of Leaders in Promoting Person-Centered Care

A fair amount of research has been done to link the leader's role and patient safety. Some of this is from the industrial sector (Cooper, 2000; Geller, 2000; Grubbs, 1999; Hofmann & Morgeson, 1999; Mullen & Kelloway, 2009; Tomas, Melia, & Oliver, 1999; Zohar, 2002), while more recent work is from the healthcare sector, with strategies such as implementation of rapid response teams (Conway et al., 2006; Jones, Bleyer, & Petree, 2010), rounds (Frankel et al., 2008), patient safety audits (Ursprung et al., 2005), checklists (Gawande, 2009; Tanner, 2010), and patient safety officers (Frankel, Gandhi, & Bates, 2003). In a comprehensive review of the literature, Manser (2009) found that:

1. Teamwork plays a key role in preventing adverse events.
2. Staff perceptions about teamwork and attitudes about the team's safety-related behavior influence the quality and safety of care.
3. Staff well-being is associated with perceptions of both teamwork and leadership.
4. Leadership, communication, and coordination all affect clinical performance.

Wong and Cummings (2007) conducted a systematic review of seven studies examining the relationship between nursing leadership and patient outcomes. Moving toward a transformational leadership style was associated with improved patient satisfaction and a reduction in adverse patient outcomes in nursing homes. In 2010, Richardson and Storr (2010) examined 11 studies that had used various methodologies, and they concluded that the great variability in the quality of the studies and their findings limited clear conclusions on the relationship between nursing leadership and patient outcomes. The Joint Commission (2013), through its review of root cause analyses of sentinel events from years 2011–2013, has identified leadership as one of the three most frequently cited contributory factors in the sentinel events.

Little research has been done to assess the impact of the leader on creating and sustaining person-centered environments of care that consistently deliver person- and family-centered care. In 2007, Shaller conducted a set of interviews with leaders of patient-centered organizations and initiatives to explore what it would take to achieve "more rapid and widespread implementation of patient-centered care in both inpatient and ambulatory health care settings" (p. v.) In this study, commissioned by The Picker Institute and funded by the Commonwealth Fund, Shaller conducted 17 phone interviews. Leaders' opinions varied as to how well organizations were doing, with one noting, "We've made a lot of progress," and another saying, "We're not even close to a tipping point. I've never seen us so far from our customers" (p. 5). A consistent perspective was that a relatively few organizations are doing extremely well, but the vast majority fall far short of achieving high-level, consistent P&FCC. The seven factors that they identified as contributing to P&FCC at the organizational level were:

1. Leadership
2. A strategic vision clearly and constantly communicated
3. Involvement of patients and families
4. Care for the caregivers through a supportive work environment
5. Systematic measurement and feedback
6. Quality of the built environment
7. Supportive technology

NOTE

In spite of their being relatively little research, there is no dearth of opinion on what constitutes P&FCC. Chapters 2 and 6 in this text provide an overview of the concept from the perspective of several influential national and international organizations.

As to the role of the leader in promoting P&FCC, The Joint Commission (TJC) provides the following set of expectations for leaders in healthcare organizations in general, which can be adapted as appropriate for specific expectations related to P&FCC:

It is the leaders who can together establish and promulgate the organization's mission, vision, and goals. It is the leaders who can strategically plan for the provision of services, acquire and allocate resources, and set priorities for improved performance. And it is the leaders who establish the organization's culture through their words, expectations for action, and behavior—a culture that values high-quality, safe patient care, responsible use of resources, community service, and ethical behavior; or a culture in which these goals are not valued. (TJC, 2009, p. 3)

When applying this set of responsibilities to the specific concept of P&FCC, the Institute of Medicine (IOM) outlined four levels of care that need to be addressed by healthcare leaders:

At the *experience* level: Care should be provided in a manner that is respectful, ensures the candid sharing of useful information in an ongoing manner, and supports and encourages the participation of patients and families. Patients and families can contribute to the process of gathering information about patient and family perceptions of care as well as analyzing and responding to collected data.

At the *clinical microsystem* level: Patients and family advisors should participate as full members of quality improvement and redesign teams, participating from the beginning in planning, implementing, and evaluating change. Design of the experience of care should respect the patient and family, optimize access to that care, allow for participation, and support and stimulate activation and commitment to achieving their clinical goals.

At the *organizational* level: The perspectives and voices of patients and families are vital to quality improvement, planning, and policy and programmatic development at the organizational level. Patients and families should participate as full members of key committees such as patient safety, facility design, quality improvement, patient/family education, ethics, and research. Patient and family faculty programs should be an integral part of all schools and clinical programs preparing health professionals and administrative leaders. Patient and family advisory councils should report to senior leadership, and patient and family faculty programs should function in a way that assists academic institutions in achieving their academic mission.

At the *environment* level: The perspectives of patients and families can inform local, state, federal, and international agency policy and program development. These agencies, along with accrediting and licensing bodies, are in a position to set the expectations and develop reimbursement incentives that encourage and support the engagement of patients and families in healthcare decision-making at all levels. Policies developed and issued by these agencies also affect programs in graduate and undergraduate schools for the health professions and healthcare administration. For these reasons, these agencies are in an excellent position to support initiatives that build the collaborative skills of patients, families, healthcare professionals, and agency personnel. (Conway et al., 2006, pp. 8-9)

Batalden et al. (2003) explored the issue of leadership in microsystems, the essential building blocks of all organizations. As Table 24.1 suggests, leaders must exert influence upward to the macrosystem and society as well as to the individual clinician at the patient's side. Batalden and his team identified three core processes of leading that can guide action at all of these levels:

1. *Building knowledge* about the necessary structure, processes, and outcomes
2. *Taking action,* which involves executing plans, developing people, and creating teams
3. *Reviewing and reflecting,* which relates to creating the vision, evaluating processes and outcomes, and revising the plan

Integrating the different perspectives on leadership with the IOM's definition of patient-centered care (IOM, 2001, p. 40), the following goal seems appropriate: *to create systems, processes, and structures for providing care that is respectful of and responsive to individual patient preferences, needs, and values and ensuring that patient values guide all clinical decisions.*

Greene, Tuzzio, and Cherkin (2012) have proposed a model for interpersonal, clinical, and structural dimensions and attributions of a P&FCC healthcare system:

- Examples of the *interpersonal*, or relationship, dimension include communication, knowing the patient, and teams.

- The *clinical* dimensions address elements such as clinical decision support, coordination and continuity, and types of encounters (clinics, virtual visits, reimbursements).

- The *structural* elements to be addressed by healthcare leaders in creating a P&FCC system are the built environment, access to care, and information technology.

The relevant aspect of this model for leaders is to identify the actions for which they are accountable in creating systems, processes, and structures for each of the dimensions. For example, changes at Group Health (which coordinates healthcare and coverage for more than 660,000 individuals in Washington state) that were put in place to deliver on these dimensions included establishing online self-management programs and virtual visits; providing smartphone apps to give patients online access to their records; providing way-finding signs and maps to help patients and visitors navigate; remodeling clinics; and tracking patient preferences.

Gaining Organizational Buy-In for P&FCC

A key first step for organizational leaders in pursuing P&FCC is to obtain organizational buy-in. Given the national push for P&FCC from so many different sources, it might seem unnecessary to spend time on this step, but it is crucial. Transitioning an organization to one that is fully and fundamentally person- and family-centered is an enormous undertaking because it will challenge many assumptions that exist within an organization and require change from so many directions.

According to the American Hospital Association (AHA):

> The traditional model calls for patients and families to give blind obedience to the expertise of paternalistic health care professionals. The patient- and family-centered model calls for an equal partnership. This is not about advocacy, although advocacy is important. It is not about enhancing case management, which is also very important. It is not about holding focus groups or occasionally asking for opinions and feedback from patients. In the patient- and family-centered care model patients and families are viewed as essential allies and treated as true partners. (Sodomka, 2006, p. 9)

Table 24.1 outlines some of the changes that must occur when changing an organization from a traditional one to one that embodies P&FCC.

TABLE 24.1 Differences Between Traditional Organizations and Those Operating Under a P&FCC Philosophy

TRADITIONAL	P&FCC
Healthcare provider (HCP) is the expert	HCP is expert in diagnosis and treatment options; patient and family are experts in the patient's history and experience
Patient is seen as a recipient of care	Patient/family are seen as partners in the design, implementation, and evaluation of care
One size fits all	Plan and preferences are individualized to the person and family
Uniformity	Flexibility
Rules and regulations serve as boundaries for decision-making	Rules and regulations serve as a baseline
Access to information is tightly controlled	There is free sharing of information with the patient and his/her designee
Decisions are made by administrators, physicians, and/or hospital staff	Decisions are made in collaboration with patients and families

In pursuing buy-in, it is helpful to use the *business/legal/quality (BLQ)* approach in identifying compelling reasons to embrace the concept of P&FCC. First are *business* considerations that make this a desirable option. Charmel and Frampton (2008) point out that P&FCC has the potential to reduce costs through several mechanisms, including a reduced length of stay, lower costs per stay, a decreased number of adverse events, reduced operating costs, employee retention, increased market share (a competitive advantage), and decreased malpractice costs. Charmel and Frampton cite several concrete examples of organizations that embraced P&FCC and experienced significant savings. Recently, the AHA (2013) identified five business reasons why hospitals should pursue a P&FCC strategy:

- Contributes to better clinical outcomes
- Reduces institutional and individual costs of care
- Increases adherence to recommended treatment regimens, which can lead to fewer complications and re-hospitalizations
- Improves patient satisfaction with care coordination and other patient experience measures that affect the hospital's reimbursement rates from Medicare and other payers
- Enables compliance with patient engagement requirements included in HITEC meaningful use and patient-centered medical home payment models (AHA, 2013, p. 2)

For the *legal* (and regulatory) case, regulatory agencies are increasingly including standards related to patient and family involvement. Examples include The Joint Commission (TJC) (2009, p. 25) with one specific standard: *Standard LD.03.04.01:The hospital communicates information related to safety and quality to those who need it, including staff, licensed independent practitioners, patients, families, and external interested parties.* The Joint Commission also includes several, more specific Elements of Performance in their set of standards, but it has to be noted that these represent a very small proportion of the dozens of Elements of Performance required by TJC:

- Leaders communicate the mission, vision, and goals to staff and the population(s) the hospital serves. (TJC, 2009, p. 15)

- Leaders discuss issues that affect the hospital and the population(s) it serves, including input from the population(s) served. (TJC, 2009, p. 16)

- Leaders define how members of the population(s) served can help identify and manage issues of safety and quality within the hospital. (TJC, 2009, p. 20)

- The hospital has a process that allows staff, patients, and families to address ethical issues or issues prone to conflict. (TJC, 2009, p. 28)

- Leaders provide the resources required for communication, based on the needs of patients, the community, physicians, staff, and management. (TJC, 2009, p. 25)

- Patients receive information about charges for which they will be responsible. (TJC, 2009, p. 28)

- Leaders involve staff and patients in the design of new or modified services or processes. (TJC, 2009, p. 32)

For the *quality* case, Jim Conway, a nationally known expert in patient safety and quality, has observed, "It's just the right thing to do" (Maurer, Dardess, Carman, Frazier, & Smeeding, 2012, p. 34). Additionally, recognition programs such as the Baldrige Award and the AHA-McKesson Award for Quality incorporate grading criteria that explicitly emphasize the inclusion of patients, families, and significant others in actively participating in care and care decisions to the extent they choose. For example, one of the Baldrige Award criteria focuses on customer support and includes questions such as the following:

> How do you enable customers to seek information and support? How do you enable them to conduct business with you and give feedback on your products and customer support? What are your key means of customer support, including your key communication mechanisms? How do they vary for different customers, customer groups, or market segments? How do you determine your customers' key support requirements? How do you ensure that these requirements are deployed to all people and processes involved in customer support? (Baldrige Performance Excellence Program, 2013, p. 14)

Furthermore, leaders are expected to model effective communication, information-sharing, and collaboration with all colleagues, employees, patients and families, other healthcare organizations, and health-related organizations.

The AHA recently issued a mandate for pursuing P&FCC:

> Hospitals have many systems and processes in place to ensure that patients receive safe, high-quality and efficient care. But unlike processes designed to manufacture products, which use standardized and inert raw materials, hospital processes must be adaptable to the needs of patients and families that differ with respect to what they know and have experienced in the past. Patients and families have different beliefs, preferences and values that can affect their choices for end-of-life care, communication with providers, diet and family presence. Creating an organization with systems and processes that can identify and adapt to diverse patient needs and with staff trained to effectively use these systems is a priority and responsibility of every hospital leader. Many hospitals do not fully engage patients and their families. (2013, p. 3)

Additional encouragement for including the patient and family perspective comes from the national Hospital Consumer Assessment of Healthcare Providers and Systems (HCAHPS), Pediatric Hospital CAHPS (Pediatric HCAHPS), Home Health CAHPS (HHCAHPS), Nursing Home CAHPS (NHCAHPS), and Clinician and Group CAHPS (CGCAHPS). These national surveys provide a standardized assessment tool for reporting patients' perspective on care in the relevant groupings (HCAHPS, 2013).

Strategies for Achieving P&FCC

The Institute for Patient- and Family-Centered Care (IPFCC) provides a wealth of resources on its website for creating a P&FCC environment and for helping employees, patients, and families develop the necessary knowledge, skills, and attitudes for accomplishing this. They suggest that the following eight steps can serve as a framework for getting started (IPFCC, 2011, pp. 4-5):

"1. Implement a process for all senior leaders to learn about patient- and family-centered care. Include patients, families, and staff from all disciplines in this process.

2. Appoint a patient- and family-centered steering committee comprised of patients and families and formal and informal leaders of the organization.

3. Assess the extent to which the concepts and principles of patient- and family-centered care are currently implemented within your hospital or health system.

4. On the basis of the assessment, set priorities and develop an action plan for establishing patient- and family-centered care at your institution.

5. Using the action plan as a guide, begin to incorporate patient- and family-centered concepts and strategies into the hospital's strategic priorities. Make sure that these concepts are integrated into your organization's mission, philosophy of care, and definition of quality.

6. Invite patients and families to serve as advisors in a variety of ways. Appoint some of these individuals to key committees and task forces.

7. Provide education and support to patients, families, and staff on patient- and family-centered care and on how to collaborate effectively in quality improvement and health care redesign. For example, provide opportunities for administrators and clinical staff to hear patients and family members share stories of their health care experiences during orientation and continuing education programs.

8. Monitor changes made, evaluate processes, measure the impact, continue to advance practice, and celebrate and recognize success."

Because the goal is for the whole organization to incorporate these principles and fully engage people and their families in their care in the ways in which they prefer, a few points need to be emphasized for leaders:

- Identify an organizational champion who will guide and coordinate organizational activities. This person is not solely responsible for achieving an environment that promotes P&FCC but is the one administrative lead who will ensure that efforts are coordinated and progress is measured. The IPFCC (2013) offers factors that should be considered in identifying an individual for this key role.

- In addition to educating the traditional caregivers and administrators, include all employees, such as housekeeping, dietary staff, secretaries, and security. Every interaction should convey a sense of inclusion and welcoming, not just those with care providers.

- Education of staff is an ongoing process, not only with new staff coming on board but also with those who have been in the organization for a while. Change of this magnitude requires a great deal of reinforcement.

- Communicate, communicate, communicate: Communicate the importance of a P&FCC culture, how to do this, how to correct old patterns.

- Make sure that senior leaders are consistently and actively modeling the desired behaviors. Activities here could include making rounds and speaking with patients and families; inviting patients or family members to share their stories at board meetings; assuring that all hospital or system committees have some form of patient/family involvement.

- Build in ongoing measurement of progress from several directions: Celebrate successes, learn from failures.

Activities for Incorporating Patients and Families

Once an organization has committed to truly becoming patient- and family-centered, there are a number of activities or initiatives leaders can undertake to operationalize the commitment to P&FCC at all levels in the organization.

Conduct an Organizational Assessment

Assessing the organization's current views and values related to person and family involvement is an essential first step. There are a number of resources available to help in this process (Conway, 2008; IPFCC, 2011; IPFCC, 2013). Key elements that most tools include are questions like these:

- Do the organization's primary documents (mission, vision, values, strategic plan) speak to P&FCC?
- Is there currently some form of advisory council?
- Does the environment reflect a person-centered orientation?
- Are family members welcome according to the patient's wishes?
- Are there restrictive visiting policies?
- Are there systems in place to ensure that individuals and their families have ready access to information that is complete, unbiased, and in a usable format?
- Do staff and physician evaluation forms include components related to their ability to deliver P&FCC?

Invite Clinicians and Leaders to Conduct Self-Assessments

Spath (2004), in her helpful text *Engaging Patients as Safety Partners,* reminds us that "the attitudes and beliefs of individual caregivers can greatly impact an organization's ability to create safety partnerships with patients and family members. Before embarking on a culture change initiative intended to increase patient involvement in safety, it is important to understand the prevailing culture" (Spath, 2004, pp. 72–73). She encourages caregivers to conduct a self-assessment to determine readiness to support this major organization initiative. She suggests statements for evaluation such as the following, with ratings expressing agreement on a scale of 1–5:

- I believe it is important to engage patients and families in preventing medical errors and adverse events.
- I believe that patients and families bring a safety viewpoint to the care team that no one else can provide.
- I listen respectfully to the safety concerns of patients and their family members.
- I know that all patients and family members cannot serve as safeguards in their care, and I do not place unrealistic expectations on individuals unable to participate in preventing medical errors and adverse events. (Spath, 2004, p. 73)

Establish a Person and Family Advisory Council

In Chapter 23 of this book, Schlucter describes the importance of establishing person-family advisory councils (PFAC). Action steps for leaders to consider in establishing a well-functioning, effective PFAC include:

- Invite individuals who have been patients, family members, or caregivers to participate.

- Create a blend of members, some who are staff from within the organization and some who reflect the patient and family perspective.

- Educate the members on the purpose of the PFAC, its role and responsibilities, and the organization and help them develop the particular knowledge, skills, and attitudes necessary to effectively function as an active member on this council.

- Establish the frequency and structure of meetings. Some groups meet monthly, others bimonthly or quarterly. Reid-Ponte et al. (2003) suggest that agendas are established by council co-chairs and staff liaisons, focusing on items suggested by council members or relating to issues raised by others. As sub-committees are formed, reports on their activities and progress should also be included.

- Develop activities and initiatives to which members can be appointed that capitalize on their knowledge and strengths. Examples include conducting patient rounds; serving on general standing committees, or something as specific as the Joint Quality Improvement and Risk Management Committee; participating in interviews for senior executive appointments; and serving on capital committees. Eventually, as acceptance of the concept unfolds, and the belief that patients and families are allies and members of the team solidifies, the presence of a member of the PFAC on most committees becomes the standard.

- Encourage council members to hold casual get-togethers or coffee hours with patients, families, staff, and physicians to gather their recommendations and ideas on making the environment more person-centered and to hear issues that need resolving. (Henneman & Cardin, 2002; IPFCC, 2013; Meyers, 2008; Reid-Ponte et al., 2003)

Create a Healthy, Person-Centered Environment

The Picker/Planetree website also provides a wealth of resources to help leaders operationalize a commitment to P&FCC, including creating healing environments that benefit persons, families, and employees. According to these thought leaders:

> A patient-centered environment of care is one that is safe and clean, and that guards patient privacy. It also engages all the human senses with color, texture, artwork, music, aromatherapy, views of nature, and comfortable lighting, and considers the experience of the body, mind and spirit of all who use the facility. Space is provided

for loved ones to congregate, as well as for peaceful contemplation, meditation or prayer, and patients, families and staff have access to a variety of arts and entertainment that serve as positive diversions. At the heart of the environment of care, however, are the human interactions that occur within the physical structure to calm, comfort and support those who inhabit it. Together the design, aesthetics, and these interactions can transform an institutional, impersonal and alien setting into one that is truly healing. (Planetree & the Picker Institute, 2008, p. 170)

These leaders speak to the need for all leaders to pay attention to several dimensions that are particularly important to individuals and their families, such as first impressions, way-finding, guarding privacy, elimination of physical and symbolic barriers, designs that encourage family participation, views and access to nature, the auditory and olfactory environments, gathering spaces, and the need for adequate attention to staff and work areas.

Reiling, Hughes, and Murphy (2008) apply the concept of P&FCC to the built environment and recommend that human factors need to be considered when designing new (or renovating old) facilities with the intent of improving the quality, safety, and patient-centeredness of care. Among these are using variable-acuity rooms and single-bed rooms; ensuring sufficient space to accommodate family members; facilitating access to healthcare information; having clearly marked signs to navigate the hospital; using assistive devices to avert patient falls; using ventilation and filtration systems to control and prevent the spread of infections; using surfaces that can be easily decontaminated; and facilitating hand washing with the availability of sinks and alcohol hand rubs.

Obviously, the culture of the environment is immensely important in creating a space which is healing for patients, families, employees, and others. In Chapter 8 of this book, Koloroutis and Trout outline several factors that need to be considered when creating a healing culture and learning environment. The leader's role in co-creating this culture with his or her subordinates is critically important. Kreitzer (2014) calls for *whole systems leadership,* which requires traits different from those seen in many healthcare leaders today. She cites the following as necessary: deep listening, awareness of systems, awareness of self, seeking diverse perspectives, suspending certainty/embracing uncertainty, and taking adaptive actions.

Models of Whole System Leadership

There are many leaders today at the system, organizational, and local levels modeling whole systems leadership, resulting in whole systems change and, in particular, the inclusion of patients and families as active partners. For example, trustees at Cincinnati Children's Hospital sit on patient/faculty advisory groups. At Springfield Hospital in Vermont, the CEO and board chair meet monthly with the patient experience team. CEOs and senior staff in many organizations participate in Executive Walk-Rounds, and at Kaiser Permanente, this includes speaking with patients and families about their thoughts and concerns. At Maine Medical Center, patients and families contribute to the development of the strategic plan, and in some organizations, a vice president for patient affairs has been created (IPFCC, 2011). Other examples of ways in which patients and families have been successfully engaged can be found at the Planetree and Picker Institute website (2008).

Select and Implement Specific Programs and Initiatives

In many organizations, patients and families are being invited to become actively involved in efforts to improve the quality and safety of care, whether through providing input and feedback or through active participation. These initiatives include rapid response teams, medication reconciliation, resuscitation efforts, root cause analyses, house staff, and new employee orientation. The IPFCC (2013) suggests that they can also provide a helpful perspective on the design of the organization's website so that it reflects the active participation of patients and families in patient safety; on the development of a satisfaction survey that would resonate with the issues faced by patients and families; and in the education of students (medical, nursing, and other health professionals) about medical errors, their sources, and how to discuss the occurrence of an error or near-miss with a patient or family member. One very helpful way in which an advisory council can provide immense help is in providing feedback into policies that directly affect patient rights and responsibilities.

Analysis of the Vignette

The practice of allowing patients to bring in their own equipment to use in the hospital is one that is still largely discouraged. Some organizations will only allow the practice if the equipment is not available in their institution (Duke, 2013; University of Texas Medical Branch [UTMB], 2013). Faxton St. Luke's Healthcare (ECRI, n.d.) analyzes cases individually. Standard-setting organizations such as the ECRI Institute (2008) recommend that this practice generally be prohibited, although exceptions can be made if the hospital has taken safety precautions.

Fortunately, in the spirit of person-centered care, a growing number of organizations are revising their approaches and developing policies to support the thoughtful, planned use by patients of their own equipment in the hospital, such as Seattle Children's Hospital (CHMC, 2006), Christus Health (2007), and the University Hospital of Newark New Jersey (UHNJ, n.d.). This makes sense in situations where the individual has operated this equipment for a period of time, is familiar with its functioning and its impact on his or her body, and when disruption due to new equipment could pose problems, such as we saw in the example that opened the chapter. In promoting truly person-centered care, if the patient is able and prefers to use his or her own equipment, efforts should be made to support this. This does, however, pose a direct challenge to staff, physicians, or administrators who have practiced within a patriarchal and bureaucratic mode of care that is based on the beliefs that "we know best" and "our equipment is safest."

For institutions who wish to pursue this course, the following steps are recommended:

1. Develop a policy statement that outlines restrictions and allowances
2. Educate staff, providers and patients on use
3. Ensure that physician approval is obtained
4. Work with legal counsel to develop forms and waivers

Subsequent to the situation in the example, Diana, the nurse manager, brought the issue of safe patient use of their own equipment to the Joint Practice Committee (JPC) at her organization. At first, several of the members expressed concern about the safety of this practice and rejected the idea. However, Diana contacted clinical leaders and legal counsel at three organizations that had adopted this practice, asking for information about their experiences and copies of their policies. She made sure that legal counsel at her hospital was actively included in generating the policy, as was Michael, the patient who had the bad experience. One approach that was helpful was to ask, "Under what conditions could we introduce a policy that would allow patients to use their own equipment?" This allowed JPC members to identify situations where all agreed it was not safe (e.g., the patient was sedated) and those situations where it was feasible. The committee proposed a 2-month pilot on the general medical unit where Michael had been a patient, and a work plan and timeline were developed. The nurse manager from one of the hospitals Diana had originally contacted served as a resource to the project. At the end of 2 months, a review of the pilot was conducted. Four patients had asked to use their own equipment; in three situations it worked well. After a thorough review of the fourth situation, it became clear that the patient wasn't as familiar with his equipment as he had claimed. This, then, led to a revision of the criteria for assessing patient competence.

Establish Ways to Contribute to Policy Development

As indicated previously, the input of persons, families, and caregivers into the development of organizational policies that affect the person(s) receiving care is a helpful addition to the process, whether it relates to direct care delivery, a supportive environment, adequate access to information, visiting guidelines, or other relevant areas. Leaders at all levels of the organization must assure that patients and families, through a formal advisory council or otherwise, can have input.

What is less clear, however, is the involvement in, and impact of, lay individuals and their families or caregivers in shaping broader national policy. The International Alliance of Patients' Organizations (IAPO) issued a policy statement in 2005, citing a practical, moral, and ethical responsibility for patients and families to be involved. Citing the fact that healthcare decisions will affect people's lives, they said that patients and families must be engaged to ensure that the policies reflect patient and caregiver needs, preferences, and capabilities. "Patient involvement is often tokenism…It should not be dependent on the good will of individuals but institutionalised in policy frameworks in order to become the rule, rather than the exception" (IAPO, 2005, p. 1). They issued four recommendations for action:

1. Stakeholders should review mechanisms and structures to ensure that patient involvement occurs throughout the process, from start to finish.

2. Patient involvement initiatives should follow IAPO guidelines, which include attention to aspects such as reaching underrepresented groups and providing adequate financial and educational resources.

3. Patient involvement should occur in a wide array of situations, such as regulatory processes, facility design, education, and training programs.

4. All patients' organizations should insist on involvement in the full range of policy efforts (e.g., social, health, economic). (IAPO, 2005)

In 2008, the National Patient Safety Foundation (NPSF) issued its Universal Patient Compact with its Principles of Partnership. This document outlines what healthcare providers pledge to patients and what patients should pledge. The pledge to patients includes items such as including the patient as a member of the team, treating him or her with respect, being responsive, and providing information in a way that the patient can understand (NPSF, 2008). This document would be a helpful template to use for an organization in setting up guiding principles or a philosophy statement about patient/family involvement. Although it does speak to providing information that can help a patient make decisions, there is little about pledging to actively include patients or their families in participating in policy development.

In its 2012 Annual Progress Report to Congress, the U.S. Department of Health and Human Services (DHHS) presented the National Strategy for Quality Improvement in Health Care (the National Quality Strategy). This strategy includes six priorities, one of which relates to including patients and families:

1. Making care safer by reducing harm caused in the delivery of care

2. Ensuring that each person and family are engaged as partners in their care

3. Promoting effective communication and coordination of care

4. Promoting the most effective prevention and treatment practices for the leading causes of mortality, starting with cardiovascular disease

5. Working with communities to promote wide use of best practices to enable healthy living

6. Making quality care more affordable for individuals, families, employers, and governments by developing and spreading new healthcare delivery models (U.S. DHHS, 2012, p. 1)

A wide range of organizations are working together to address these priorities: the National Quality Forum, the National Priorities Partnership (NPP), the Measure Applications Partnership, the Interagency Working Group on Health Care Quality, and the Agency for Healthcare Research and Quality (AHRQ). Of these organizations, the NPP is a collaborative of stakeholders that include purchasers, providers, consumers, physicians, nurses, hospitals, and health research organizations. The voice of the consumer is particularly advanced through this organization.

Conclusion

As healthcare is moving toward a greater commitment to person- and family-centered care, the role of the leader has to dramatically shift. Previously, the leader was seen as the person with the answers, to whom others brought their problems. Now the leader's role is to engage others to achieve the Triple Aim, that is, improving healthcare outcomes, improving the care experience, and reducing the costs of care. Particular to this book, the role of the leader is to *create systems, processes, and structures for providing care that is respectful of and responsive to individual patient preferences, needs, and values and ensuring that patient values guide all clinical decisions.* This requires leaders to listen to and learn from the experiences of individual patients and their families, to avoid a defensive stature and sincerely examine what could be improved, to work with colleagues to ensure that the appropriate changes are put into place, and to incorporate new learnings into ongoing quality improvement efforts. It also requires leaders to stay current on new approaches and to work within new teams of employees, colleagues, and persons and their families.

References

American Hospital Association (AHA). (2013). *A leadership resource for patient and family engagement strategies.* Chicago IL: Health Research & Educational Trust.

Baldrige Performance Excellence Program. (2013). 2013-2014 Criteria for Performance Excellence. Retrieved from http://www.nist.gov/baldrige/publications/upload/2013-2014_Business_Nonprofit_Criteria_Free-Sample.pdf

Batalden, P. B., Nelson, E. C., Mohr, J. J., Godfrey, M. M., Huber, T. P., Kosnick, L., & Ashling, K. (2003). Microsystems in health care: Part 5. How leaders are leading. *Joint Commission Journal on Quality and Safety, 29*(6), 297–308.

Charmel, P. A., & Frampton, S. B. (2008, March). Building the business case for patient-centered care. *Healthcare Financial Management.* Retrieved from http://planetree.org/wp-content/uploads/2012/01/HFM-business-case-for-Planetree.pdf

Children's Hospital and Medical Center. (CHMC). (2006). Use of patient owned/rented medical equipment during hospitalization. Retrieved from http://www.seattlechildrens.org/pdf/use_patient_owned_rented_medical_equipment.pdf

Christus Health. (2007). Christus Health clinical policy: Privately-owned medical equipment. Retrieved from http://uthscsa.edu/gme/documents/ClinicalPolicy-Privately-OwnedMedicalEquipment.pdf

Conway, J., Johnson, B., Edgman-Levitan, S., Schlucter, J., Ford, D., Sodomka, P., & Simmons, L. (2006). *Partnering with patients and families to design a patient- and family-centered health care system: A roadmap for the future.* Bethesda, MD: Institute for Family-Centered Care. Retrieved from http://www.hsi.gatech.edu/erfuture/images/c/c2/Family.pdf

Conway, J. (2008). Patients and families: Powerful new partners for healthcare and for caregivers. In *Advancing the practice of patient- and family-centered care in hospitals: How to get started* (pp. 11–12). Bethesda MD: IPFCC. Retrieved from http://www.ipfcc.org/pdf/getting_started.pdf

Cooper, M. D. (2000). Towards a model of safety culture. *Safety Science, 36*(2), 111-136.

Duke Medical Center. (2013). Non-Duke owned medical equipment. Retrieved from http://clinicalengineering.duhs.duke.edu/wysiwyg/downloads/Non_Duke_Owned_Medical_Equipment_Policy_Draft_Jan_20_2010.pdf

ECRI Institute. (n.d.). Hazard alert stimulates new policy on patient-owned equipment. Retrieved from https://www.ecri.org/Documents/Brochures/AlertsTracker_Faxton_St.Luke_Case_Study.pdf

ECRI Institute. (2008). Patient-supplied equipment. Retrieved from https://www.ecri.org/Documents/RM/HRC_TOC/MedTech8ES.pdf

Frankel, A., Gandhi, T. K., & Bates, D. W. (2003). Improving patient safety across a large integrated healthcare delivery system. *International Journal for Quality in Health Care, 15*(Suppl 1), i31-i40.

Frankel, A., Grillo, S. P., Pittman, M., Thomas, E. J., Horowitz, L., Page, M., & Sexton, B. (2008). Revealing and resolving patient safety defects: The impact of leadership WalkRounds on frontline caregiver assessments of patient safety. *Health Services Research, 43*(6), 2050-2066.

Gawande, A. (2009). *The checklist manifesto: How to get things right.* New York, NY: Metropolitan Books.

Geller, E. S. (2000). 10 leadership qualities for a total safety culture. *Professional Safety, 45*, 38-41.

Greene, S. M., Tuzzio, L, & Cherkin, D. (2012). A framework for making patient-centered care front and center. *The Permanente Journal, 16*(3). Retrieved from http://www.thepermanentejournal.org/issues/2012/summer/4809-patient-centered-care.html

Grubbs, J. R. (1999). A transformational leader. *Occupational Health and Safety, 68*(8), 22-26.

Henneman, E. A., & Cardin, W. (2002). Family-centered critical care: A practical approach to making it happen. *Critical Care Nurse, 22*(6), 12-19.

Hofmann, D. A., & Morgeson, E. P. (1999). Safety-related behavior as a social exchange: The role of perceived organizational support and leader-member exchange. *Journal of Applied Psychology, 84*(2), 286-296.

Hospital Consumer Assessment of Healthcare Providers and Systems (HCAHPS). (2013). Hospital care quality information from the consumer perspective. [Background]. Retrieved from http://www.hcahpsonline.org/home.aspx

Institute for Patient- and Family-Centered Care (IPFCC). (2011). *Advancing the practice of patient- and family-centered care in hospitals: How to get started.* Bethesda, MD: Author. Retrieved from http://www.ipfcc.org/pdf/getting_started.pdf

Institute for Patient- and Family-Centered Care (IPFCC). (2013). *Partnering with patients and families to enhance quality and safety: A mini toolkit.* Retrieved from http://www.ipfcc.org/tools/Patient-Safety-Toolkit-04.pdf

Institute of Medicine (IOM). (2001). *Crossing the quality chasm: A new health system for the 21st century.* Washington, DC: The National Academies Press.

International Alliance of Patients' Organizations (IAPO). (2005). *Patient involvement* [Policy statement], pp 1-2. Retrieved from http://www.patientsorganizations.org/attach.pl/312/182/IAPO%20Policy%20Statement%20on%20Patient%20Involvement.pdf

The Joint Commission (TJC). (2009). *Leadership in healthcare organizations: A guide to Joint Commission leadership standards.* San Diego, CA: The Governance Institute.

The Joint Commission (TJC). (2013). *Sentinel event data: Root causes by event type.* Retrieved from http://www.jointcommission.org/assets/1/18/Root_Causes_by_Event_Type_2004-2Q2013.pdf

Jones, C. M., Bleyer, A. J., & Petree, B. (2010). Evolution of a rapid response system from voluntary to mandatory activation. *Joint Commission Journal on Quality and Patient Safety, 36*(6), 266-270.

Kreitzer, M. J. (2014). Whole systems healing: A new leadership path. In M. J. Kreitzer & M. Koithan (Eds.), *Integrative nursing* (pp. 47-55). New York, NY: Oxford University Press.

Manser, T. (2009). Teamwork and patient safety in dynamic domains of healthcare: A review of the literature. *Acta Anaesthesiologica Scandinavica, 53*(2), 143-151.

Maurer, M., Dardess, P., Carman, K. L., Frazier, K., & Smeeding, L. (2012). *Guide to patient and family engagement: Environmental scan report.* (AHRQ Publication No. 12-0042-EF). (Prepared by the American Institutes for Research under contract HHSA 290-200-600019.) Rockville, MD: Agency for Healthcare Research and Quality.

Meyers, S. (2008). Take heed: How patient and family advisors can improve quality. *Trustee, 61*(4), 14-22.

Mullen, J. E., & Kelloway, E. K. (2009). Safety leadership: A longitudinal study of the effects of transformational leadership on safety outcomes. *Journal of Occupational and Organizational Psychology, 82*(2), 253-272.

National Patient Safety Foundation (NPSF). (2008). *The universal patient compact: Principles for partnership.* Retrieved from http://www.npsf.org/wp-content/uploads/2011/10/UniversalPatientCompact.pdf

Planetree & the Picker Institute. (2008). *Patient-centered care improvement guide: V11.F Environment of care.* Retrieved from http://www.patient-centeredcare.org/chapters/chapter7f.pdf

Reid-Ponte, P., Conlin, G., Conway, J. B., Grant, S., Medeiros, C., Nies, J., …Conley, K. (2003). Making patient-centered care come alive: Achieving full integration of the patient's perspective. *Journal of Nursing Administration, 33*(2), 82-90.

Reiling, J., Hughes, R. G., & Murphy, M. R. (2008). The impact of facility design on patient safety. In R. G. Hughes (Ed.), *Patient safety and quality: An evidence-based handbook for nurses* (Chapter 28). Rockville, MD; Agency for Healthcare Research and Quality. Retrieved from http://www.ncbi.nlm.nih.gov/books/NBK2633/

Richardson, A., & Storr, J. (2010). Patient safety: A literature review on the impact of nursing empowerment, leadership and collaboration. *International Nursing Review, 57*(1), 12-21.

Shaller, D. (2007). *Patient-centered care: What does it take?* New York, NY: The Commonwealth Fund.

Sodomka, P. (2006). Engaging patients and families: A high leverage tool for health care leaders. In *Advancing the practice of patient- and family-centered care in hospitals: How to get started* (pp. 8–9). Bethesda, MD: Author. Retrieved from http://www.ipfcc.org/pdf/getting_started.pdf

Spath, P. (2004). *Engaging patients as safety partners: A guide for reducing errors and improving satisfaction.* Chicago, IL: Health Forum, Inc.

Tanner, K. (2010). Patient safety: Checklists and teamwork lower number of surgery deaths. *Huffpost Healthy Living.* Retrieved from http://www.huffingtonpost.com/2010/10/20/study-lives-saved-by-surg_n_769421.html

Tomas, J. M., Melia, J. L., & Oliver, A. (1999). A cross-validation of a structural equation model of accidents: Organizational and psychological variables as predictors of work safety. *Work and Stress, 13*(1), 49-58.

University Hospital of Newark New Jersey (UHNJ). (n.d.). University hospital environment of care: Medical equipment. Retrieved from http://www.uhnj.org/eocweb/medequip/

University of Texas Medical Branch (UTMB). (2013). Patient-owned medical equipment/devices. Retrieved from http://www.utmb.edu/policies_and_procedures/IHOP/Clinical/General_Clinical_Procedures_and_Care/IHOP%20-%2009.13.03%20-%20Patient-Owned%20Medical%20Equipment%20or%20Devices.pdf

Ursprung, R., Gray, J. E., Edwards, W. H., Horvar, J. D., Nickerson, J., Plsek, P., …Goldmann, D. A. (2005). Real time patient safety audits: Improving safety every day. *Quality and Safety in Health Care, 14*(4), 284-289.

U.S. Department of Health and Human Services (DHHS). (2012). *2012 Annual progress report to Congress: National strategy for quality improvement in health care.* Retrieved from http://www.ahrq.gov/workingforquality/nqs/nqs2012annlrpt.pdf

Wong, C. A., & Cummings, G. G. (2007). The relationship between nursing leadership and patient outcomes: A systematic review. *Journal of Nursing Management, 15*(5), 508-521. doi: 10.1111/j.1365-2834.2007.00723.x

Zohar, D. (2000). Modifying supervisory practices to improve sub-unit safety: A leadership-based intervention model. *Journal of Applied Psychology, 87*(1), 156-163.

Chapter 25

The Call for a Change to Person- and Family-Centered Care

Jane H. Barnsteiner, PhD, RN, FAAN

Joanne Disch, PhD, RN, FAAN

Mary K. Walton, MSN, MBE, RN

"You cannot blame your patients for lower patient satisfaction scores. Blame justifies inaction." (Press, 2006, p. 163)

"Engaged, empowered patients are one of the six characteristics of an effective, efficient, and continuously improving health system." (Institute of Medicine [IOM], 2012, p. 7)

Providing care in today's healthcare environment is challenging at best. Pressures such as insufficient staffing, continuous cries to improve patient satisfaction scores, decreasing costs, staying current with the literature, being a good colleague to distracted and exhausted colleagues, and ministering to suffering patients and family members are just a few of the challenges faced on a daily basis. However, the goal of providing quality care most efficiently while valuing patient preferences and values cannot be lost amid the challenges. The preceding chapters in this book have attempted to address the challenges, benefits, and joys in identifying and providing person- and family-centered care (P&FCC). This chapter will explore the future horizon of P&FCC.

New Ways of Thinking

Perhaps the most fundamental change is that we have to learn to think differently. As Einstein noted: "We cannot solve our problems with the same thinking we used when we created them" (BrainyQuote, 2013). For the past several decades, the American healthcare system has been acuity-oriented, hospital-based, and physician-dominant. Now, as the authors in this book have noted, we need to move toward a system that provides care "that is respectful of and responsive to individual patient preferences, needs, and values and ensuring that the patient values guide all clinical decisions" (IOM, 2001, p. 40). The intent of this book has been to provide frameworks and models for thinking about this seismic shift, as well as strategies for helping deliver this model of care. The purpose of this chapter is to highlight several perspectives that, we propose, need to change as well.

A Move From Patient-Centered Care to Person- and Family-Centered Care

The earlier Institute of Medicine (IOM) reports, beginning with *Crossing the Quality Chasm* (2001), emphasized the centrality of the patient as a full partner and source of control for care decisions. Patient-centered care became one of the dimensions of quality espoused by the IOM, along with safe, timely, effective, efficient, and equitable. The concept of the family was also emphasized as a recipient of, and partner in, care, with the idea of "family" broadly defined as those individuals designated by the patient as being close to him or her.

Over the past 10 years, there has been growing recognition that our system of care has to not only treat illness, but also promote health and prevent disease. With that orientation, it has become apparent that the provision of healthcare is far broader than what occurs in hospitals or even clinics. Actually, all Americans need to be engaged in healthcare; the vast majority are not patients in hospitals. Attention is turning toward upstream factors and social determinants of health (Robert Wood Johnson Foundation [RWJF], 2009) that require totally different approaches to care—and the recognition that not everyone is a patient. Koloroutis and Trout, in Chapter 8 of this book, emphasize that individuals want to be seen as people, not patients, and Schenck and Churchill remind us that, even in the hospital setting, we need to "engage the person to treat the patient" (2012, p. 138).

P&FCC Is Not an "Add-On"

We need to change the view of P&FCC; it is not an "add-on" but a way of being. To obtain buy-in from our nursing and medicine partners, we need to be able to illustrate how elements of P&FCC lessen the burden and improve patient outcomes. For example, Chapter 10 on family systems theory illustrates how getting to know family patterns of relationships and communication styles can help us make our care interventions more successful and, ultimately, more efficient.

At times, families may request assistance that they feel is important for the patient but that may be inconvenient for staff or outside the scope of staff members' perceived job definitions. These requests may upset organizational or unit routines. Some of these requests may be reasonable; some may not be. Healthcare providers need to recognize any frustration that these requests may engender, and separate out frustrations that they may feel from their busy assignments, from those which are appropriate yet might require time, from those which may be inappropriate. Working effectively with families means developing skills in negotiation and accommodation.

Patients and Families as Partners With the Healthcare Team

While we are moving in the direction of patients having increased roles in decision-making and improved access to health information that can be understood and used by them and their families, we need to guard against pushing decisions onto individuals who may not be able to effectively make them or who choose not to participate in the decision-making and prefer to leave healthcare decisions to the provider. This may seem contradictory to the themes in this book. However, patient participation in decision-making is a personal thing, and some people choose not to participate or choose varying levels of participation. P&FCC means customizing care for individual preferences and providing user-friendly, reliable information about clinical choices.

The Presidential Commission for the Study of Bioethical Issues recently released a report offering recommendations for the management of incidental and secondary findings in clinical, research, and direct-to-consumer settings (2013). With emerging technologies such as gene sequencing and evolving cost structures and health practices, the likelihood of discovering incidental and secondary findings will increase. Although some of the findings may be lifesaving, they may also result in identifying conditions for which there is no effective treatment, resulting in distress to patients and families. The commission recommends that clinicians anticipate and plan for incidental findings and communicate that plan to patients, research participants, and consumers so they are informed ahead of time about what findings may be discovered. They can then consent to be told the incidental and secondary findings or refuse the procedure.

We need to acknowledge that patients and families come with their own expertise. We are experts at delivering care; patients are experts at their own experiences with care and managing their health, and some are better at this than others. Numerous studies indicate that patients are more satisfied when their healthcare provider engages them in decision-making than if they do not (Alston et al., 2012; Bechtal, & Ness, 2010).

Moving From the Notion of a Family Spokesperson to a Spokesgroup

To be person- and family-centered is to recognize that family members serve a variety of roles, including advocate, care provider, trusted companion, and surrogate decision-maker (Levine & Zuckerman, 1999). They may want, or not want, to be present at all times to explain the patient's needs to staff and to ensure delivery of correct and sensitive care. Benner and colleagues speak of family member presence to ensure "trustworthy watchfulness" given the "fragility of practice" due to the often large patient assignments and competing demands on nurses (Benner, Hooper Kyriakidis, & Stannard, 2011).

We have been moving in the direction of asking the family to name a spokesperson when a patient is unable to speak for himself. This may be for caregiver expediency. Recent evidence, however, indicates that this may be disruptive to family communication and relational patterns (Quinn et al., 2012). Roles of the family may include primary caregiver, primary decision-maker, family spokesperson, out-of-towner, patient wishes expert, and healthcare expert, among others. Furthermore, family members may have their own family or employment responsibilities that prohibit them from coming to the care encounter as they might wish. These informal roles and responsibilities may require that a family spokesgroup be utilized rather than one spokesperson (Quinn et al., 2012). This calls for application of family systems theory, as described in Chapter 10, as well as the ability to navigate among the various relationships to ensure discussions result in the best decision-making relevant to the person's needs.

Understanding Culture and Diversity

In order to move to P&FCC, we need to also focus on health literacy and educating people as to how they may assume a greater role in healthcare issues and in managing their own health. This entails providing the tools, strategies, and support to help them become informed and engaged healthcare consumers who are able to make a positive impact on their own and their family members' healthcare quality and safety (Dickens & Piano, 2013).

Person- and family-centered care requires recognizing and addressing racial, ethnic, and socio-economic disparities in care and outcomes. Patients who are ill, have low health literacy and numeracy, are members of marginalized groups, or who have cognitive deficits tend to ask fewer questions and get less information than their peers without these obstacles (Epstein, Fiscella, Lesser, & Stange, 2010). They are also less likely to understand technical and nontechnical language. The practice of patient-centered care, sharing information, sharing deliberation, and reaching a shared mind helps to bridge the differences among clinicians and patients in health beliefs, race, ethnicity, and culture and promotes equality in prevention and treatment (Epstein, Fiscella, Lesser, & Stange, 2010).

Although an understanding of culture is essential, we need to guard against stereotypes and generalizations to ensure our care is individualized. Providers often make generalizations about the attitudes, preferences, beliefs, and behaviors of an ethnic or racial group rather than the individual. Although knowledge about particular populations may be informative, we need to avoid generalizations and elicit the unique values and preferences of the individual and his or her family. Use of translators for patients who have a preferred language other than English is essential, not only for language translation but also to serve as "cultural translators" as well (Silow-Carroll, Altera, & Stepnick, 2006).

Reconceptualizing Work Processes

Many of the ways we organize our care processes, such as our rounds, medication, and meal schedules, are routine and ritualistic. Although this often promotes efficiency, we also "need routines that initiate, integrate and safeguard patient centered care in daily clinical practice" (Ekman et al., 2011, p. 11). For example, in 2010, Rhode Island passed legislation mandating person-centered care in long-term care facilities. This includes patients having choices about their daily routines, not being awakened at night for routine care, eliminating overhead public address systems, and awakening and eating at their preferred times (changingaging.org, 2010).

We often blame unit or institutional rules for why something cannot be done. We need to analyze the rules and whose needs the rules really meet. For example, signs at the entrance to a unit or clinic or to the unit kitchen often give a message of the patient or family member as an intruder. Is that the intended message? And if not, how could they be improved?

What Messages Are Your Signs Sending?

The following signs are examples of ones that aren't patient- and family-centered.

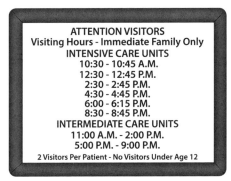
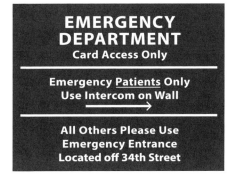

FIGURE 25.1

This shows very prescriptive and limited visiting hours that likely do not meet the needs of patients or families. A policy that discusses the need to individualize visiting and the continuous presence of a support person if the patient wishes would be much more inclusive of the patient as a member of the healthcare team and would acknowledge the patient as a participant in decision-making.

FIGURE 25.2

This emergency department sign indicates that the patient has to enter alone and any family or support person needs to go to another entrance. A sign indicating the patient and a family member/friend may enter would be more patient- and-family centered.

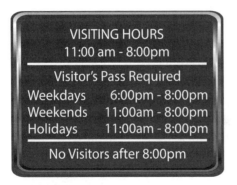

FIGURE 25.3

This visiting hours sign indicates prescriptive and limiting visiting hours, particularly on the weekend. Visitors are not allowed between 8 pm and 11 am. The sign does not differentiate between family/support person and others. A P&FCC friendly–policy would distinguish between a family/support person and other visitors, and the visiting hours would be arranged to meet the patient's wishes.

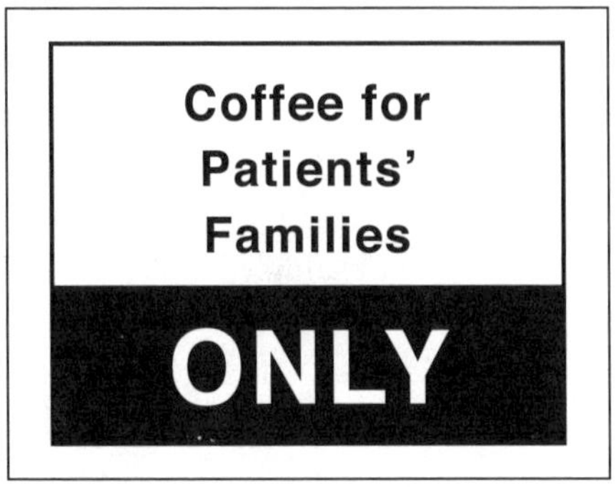

FIGURE 25.4

This sign is over a complimentary coffee area. That is a P&FCC amenity but the sign with the "ONLY" is off-putting and not friendly. It would be a more caring message without the "ONLY" on the sign.

Simply eliminate one word from that last sign pictured and you would have a more welcoming P&FCC message. Other signs require more serious revisitation of institutional or departmental policies. The point is to start being conscious of the messages we are sending to patients and families whom we want as partners in their healthcare decisions.

Person-and Family-Centered Supportive Visiting Policy from the University of Wisconsin Website

The following visiting policy from the UW website embraces P&FCC:

"Hospitalized patients may identify a small number of 'primary support' people who will generally be able to visit at any time during their hospital stay (24 hours a day, 7 days a week). Primary support persons are those who normally provide a patient with significant physical, psychological, or emotional support. Examples might be a close family member, partner, or best friend. Visiting hours (8 am–9 pm) will still apply to a patient's other visitors or guests" (University of Wisconsin Hospitals and Clinics Authority, 2014).

Understanding the Health Insurance Portability and Accountability Act

In a similar vein, healthcare providers often misunderstand and misinterpret the Health Insurance Portability and Accountability Act (HIPAA). They may cite HIPAA regulations as preventing them from answering questions or sharing information about a person. However, the act, which was enacted in 1996, does not totally prevent healthcare professionals from sharing relevant information with family members unless the patient specifically objects. HIPAA protects the patient, not the institution or the healthcare provider. A patient can informally agree to share healthcare information with family, with friends, and with anyone she or he chooses. It doesn't require that there be a written agreement, although some healthcare organizations require that it be in writing; however, that is an organizational requirement, unrelated to HIPAA. The United Hospital Fund's *Next Step in Care* guide (2013) and the U. S. Department of Health and Human Services (U.S. DHHS) website at http://www.hhs.gov/ocr/privacy explain what the act does and doesn't mandate (U.S. DHHS, 2013).

Creating a Culture, Not a Program

Organizational leadership in achieving P&FCC matters a great deal. Leaders must "walk the walk" and not just "talk the talk." Ownership and buy-in for P&FCC must be spread throughout the leadership team as well as across all employees so that if one member of the leadership team leaves the organization, the commitment to P&FCC remains.

A roundtable of CEOs from leading health systems discussed essential strategies for moving to P&FCC (Cosgrove et al., 2013). These include:

- Having foundational elements in place, such as the characteristics of a High Reliability Organization with active leadership from the CEO and board of trustees

- Putting infrastructure fundamentals in place, such as evidence-based practice protocols, the use of best practices, and optimal use of all resources

- Making person- and family-centered care delivery a priority, including shared decision-making with patient and care provider collaboration

- Designing systems for reliability and feedback with transparency in performance, outcomes, and costs

Achieving P&FCC means creating a culture, not just a program. Patients and family members expect competence. They expect warm, tasty meals; prompt answers to call light buttons; easily understood explanations and instructions; appropriate pain control; clean and cheerful rooms; and everyone they meet to be friendly, helpful, and competent (Press, 2006). When employees say there is insufficient staff to do these things, when administrators says there is no money in the budget for sleeping chairs in patient rooms, when nurses say families want to stay because they don't trust them, it speaks to a culture—but not a culture of P&FCC. Achieving the goals of P&FCC requires a full organizational commitment, starting at the top but spreading throughout the organization and community.

A culture of P&FCC requires embedding that culture into organizational values, beliefs, roles, and behaviors that facilitate a special relationship between healthcare providers and persons and their families. For example, words such as *allow, permit, require, our patients,* and *non-compliant* would be eliminated because they speak to a paternalistic, non–person-centered approach. In a P&FCC environment, everyone in the organization knows that this culture is a top priority of senior leadership and that there are expectations and rewards for everyone in the organization for doing it. The culture is worked into the performance appraisal of everyone in the organization, and it is a permanent agenda item from meetings of the board of trustees to those for all care-givers and staff (Press, 2006).

P&FCC is not a project on which to do a small test of change. It needs a total organizational rede-sign. Everyone in the organization needs the same set of values and expectations. Every employee needs to know the patient satisfaction data overall for the organization and for their work areas, and everyone needs access to systems in place for them to participate in discussions of what could be done better and how to improve.

Increasing Use of Technology

Use of electronic systems and user-friendly software programs can promote P&FCC. Electronic health records integrated across the continuum of care provide all pertinent information easily at hand so patients do not need to repeat it at every healthcare encounter. Innovations such as video chat allow persons, providers, and interpreters to interact without all needing to be present in person. Wireless communication can allow individuals and care providers to com-municate regarding health status and for the person receiving care to have access to his or her electronic health record to read the documentation as well as to chart updates and pose questions for clinicians.

Cutting-Edge Initiatives That Illustrate P&FCC

Although the bar of P&FCC is a high one, a number of organizations are achieving it, and a number of legislative bodies are promoting it. Chapters 9 and 24 in this book highlight several success stories, many recognized by the Baldrige and the American Hospital Association (AHA)-McKesson awards. Earlier in this chapter, an example of legislated changes to work processes in long-term care facilities in Rhode Island was described (changingaging.org, 2010). In 2007, Mas-sachusetts passed legislation to promote healthcare transparency and facilitate consumer-pro-vider partnerships. The law mandated every hospital to establish patient advisory boards by 2010 and to allow patients or family members to activate rapid response teams (RRTs) (Massachusetts Coalition for the Prevention of Medical Errors, 2009).

There are a number of global legislative initiatives that mandate changes in P&FCC as well. Sweden has moved as a country to P&FCC, which means a shift away from a model in which the patient is the passive target of a medical intervention to a model in which the patient is an active part in his or her care and the decision-making process. "Person-centered care highlights the importance of knowing the person behind the patient in order to engage the person as an active partner in his/her care and treatment. The starting point is the patient's narrative, which needs to be recorded in a structured manner. From this a mutual care plan may be developed" (Ekman et al., 2011, p. 248). When the Swedish Society of Nursing translated the book *Quality and Safety in Nursing* (Sherwood & Barnsteiner, 2012) into Swedish, they modified the wording of the chapter on patient-centered care to *person-centered care.*

Although organizations, states, and countries can achieve significant results in establishing P&FCC, we can also look to innovative individuals who are achieving significant results in their practice environments. The *Raise the Voice* initiative of the American Academy of Nursing has identified Edge Runners who are practical innovators who have implemented models of care that are person-centered, effective, efficient, pragmatic, and accessible, often to persons and their families in underserved areas. These Edge Runners have developed P&FCC models and interventions that demonstrate significant, sustained clinical and financial outcomes. Examples include the Naylor Transitional Care Program, which incorporates patients and family members into healthcare across the continuum of care, and the 11th Street Family Health Services in Philadelphia (American Academy of Nursing, n.d.).

Conclusion

Achieving person- and family-centered care is a journey, not a destination. It requires a well-coordinated community of healthcare professionals who are passionate about the concept, who see its benefits, who see that it is a mandate for how care should be structured and delivered, and who work together with these goals in mind. (Epstein et al., 2010). The journey is not over after instituting the practices described in this book. We are continually learning through the experiences of individuals (some of whom are patients, some not), family and friends, clinicians, other employees, and administrators. Policies will need to be regularly reviewed and updated. Practices will need to be adapted to new evidence that initiates, integrates, and safeguards P&FCC in daily clinical work. Routines will need to be revisited to ensure that we integrate the evidence with clinician's expertise and the individual's preferences. The ultimate goal in a complex and dynamic healthcare environment is to ensure that P&FCC is systematically and consistently lived in all aspects of healthcare.

References

Alston, C., Paget, L., Halvorson, G., Novelli, B., Guest, J., McCabe, P.,…VonKohorn, I. (2012). *Communicating with patients on health care evidence.* Institute of Medicine, Washington, DC: National Academies Press.

American Academy of Nursing (AAN). (n.d.). *Raise the voice: Edge runner.* Retrieved from http://www.aannet.org/edge-runners

Bechtal, C., & Ness, D. L. (2010). If you build it, will they come? Designing truly patient-centered health care. *Health Affairs, 29*(5), 914-920.

Benner, P., Hooper Kyriakidis, P., & Stannard, D. (2011). *Clinical wisdom and interventions in acute and critical care: A thinking-in-action approach* (2nd ed.). New York, NY: Springer Publishing.

BrainyQuote. (2013). Retrieved from http://www.brainyquote.com/quotes/quotes/a/alberteins121993.html

changingaging.org. (2010). Person-centered culture change sweeps Rhode Island: Rhode Island passes culture change legislation. Retrieved from http://www.pioneernetwork.net/Latest/Detail.aspx?id=224

Cosgrove, D. M., Fisher, M., Gabow, P., Gottlieb, G., Halvorson, G. C., James, B.C.,...Toussant, J. S. (2013). Ten strategies to lower costs, improve quality, and engage patients: The view from leading health system CEOs. *Health Affairs, 32*(2), 321-327.

Dickens, C., & Piano, M. R. (2013). Health literacy and nursing: An update. *American Journal of Nursing, 113*(6), 52-58.

Ekman, I., Swedberg, K., Taft, C., Lindseth, A., Norberg, A., Brink, E.,...Sunnerhagen, K. S. (2011). Person-centered care—Ready for prime time. *European Journal of Cardiovascular Nursing, 11*(4), 248-251.

Epstein, R. M., Fiscella, K., Lesser, C. S., & Stange, K. C. (2010). Why the nation needs a policy push on patient-centered health care. *Health Affairs, 29*(8), 1489-1495.

Institute of Medicine (IOM). (2001). *Crossing the quality chasm: A new health system for the 21st century*. Washington, DC: National Academies Press.

Institute of Medicine (IOM). (2012). *Best care at lower cost: The path to continuously learning health care in America*. Washington, DC: National Academies Press.

Levine, C., & Zuckerman, C. (1999). The trouble with families: Toward an ethic of accommodation. *Annals of Internal Medicine, 130*(2), 148-152.

Massachusetts Coalition for the Prevention of Medical Errors. (2009). Patient and family advisory councils. Retrieved from http://www.macoalition.org/pfac_overview.shtml

Presidential Commission for the Study of Bioethical Issues. (2013). *Privacy and progress in whole genome sequencing*. Retrieved from http://bioethics.gov/node/764

Press, I. (2006). *Patient satisfaction: Understanding and managing the experience of care* (2nd ed.). Chicago IL: Irwin Press.

Quinn, J. R., Schmitt, M., Baggs, J. G., Norton, S. A., Dombeck, M. T., & Sellers, C. R. (2012). Family members' informal roles in end-of-life decision making in adult intensive care units. *American Journal of Critical Care, 21*(1), 43-51.

Robert Wood Johnson Foundation (RWJF). (2009). *Beyond health care: New directions to a healthier America*. Retrieved from http://www.rwjf.org/content/dam/farm/reports/reports/2009/rwjf40483

Schenck, D., & Churchill, L. (2012). *Healers: Extraordinary clinicians at work*. New York, NY: Oxford University Press.

Sherwood, G., & Barnsteiner, J. (Eds.). (2012). *Quality and safety in nursing: A competency approach to improving outcomes*. Ames, IA: Wiley-Blackwell.

Silow-Carroll, S., Altera, T., & Stepnick, L. (2006). Patient-centered care for underserved populations: Definition and best practices. Economic and Social Research Institute. Retrieved from http://www.issuelab.org/resource/patientcentered_care_for_underserved_populations_definition_and_best_practices

United Hospital Fund. (2013). HIPAA: Questions and answers for family caregivers. Retrieved from http://www.nextstepincare.org/next_step_in_care_guides/4/HIPAA/english

University of Wisconsin Hospitals and Clinics Authority. (2014). *UW hospital visiting hours*. UW Hospital Patient Guide. Retrieved from http://www.uwhealth.org/patient-guides/uw-hospital/uw-hospital-visiting-hours/10148

U.S. Department of Health and Human Services (U.S. DHHS). (2013). The Health Insurance Portability and Accountability Act of 1996 (HIPAA) privacy, security and breach notification rules. Retrieved from http://www.hhs.gov/ocr/privacy/

Appendix

Resources

Chapter 1

The Brookings Institute published a report called *Bending the Curve: Person-Centered Health Care Reform: A Framework for Improving Care and Slowing Health Care Cost Growth*. Its intent is to improve the quality of care while slowing down the cost growth curve. It can be accessed at http://www.brookings.edu/research/reports/2013/04/person-centered-health-care-reform#

A non-profit organization, PULSE (or Persons United Limiting Substandards and Errors), is working to improve patient safety and reduce the rate of medical errors using real-life stories and experiences from survivors of medical errors. See http://www.pulseamerica.org/

Similarly, the Empowered Patient Coalition is a group of patient advocates committed to improving quality of care. They can be reached at www.empoweredpatientcoalition.org

Chapter 2

Planetree promotes patient- and family-centered care (P&FCC) through United States and global member organizations for all types of healthcare settings. The website has open access with extensive resources to assist organizations in implementing P&FCC. See these at www.Planetree.org

The Institute for Patient- and Family-Centered Care (IPFCC) offers a toolkit for P&FCC with bibliographies, webinars, presentations, stories, and a hospital assessment survey. These are available at http://www.ipfcc.org

The National Network of Libraries of Medicine provides a comprehensive tutorial on health literacy, including a definition, skills needed for improving health literacy, and several examples of initiatives targeted at improving health literacy. This information can be accessed at http://nnlm.gov/outreach/consumer/hlthlit.html

The Picker Institute at http://pickerinstitute.org/ offers numerous strategies for enhancing person-centered care that have become industry standards.

Hospital Consumer Assessment of Healthcare Providers and Systems (HCAHPS). See http://www.medicare.gov/hospitalcompare/search.html

Chapter 3

A resource that can help elicit the patient's story and questions is *Taking Care of Myself: A Guide for When I Leave the Hospital* at http://www.ahrq.gov/patients-consumers/diagnosis-treatment/hospitals-clinics/goinghome/goinghomeguide.pdf

Chapter 4

The Picker Institute Always Events Initiative reports and toolbox of resources created by grantees are available at http://alwaysevents.pickerinstitute.org/

The Graduate Medical Education Toolbox is available at http://cgp.pickerinstitute.org/?page_id=1230

The *Always Events Blueprint for Action* highlights ways that leaders can use the Always Events concept to improve the patient experience through engaging staff and effectively partnering with patients and families. Retrieved from http://alwaysevents.pickerinstitute.org/wp-content/uploads/2013/01/Always-Events-Blueprint-for-Action-11-2012.pdf

Chapter 5

Read blog entries from patients at the Center for Advancing Help's *Prepared Patient Blog*, especially "When You Fear Being Labeled a 'Difficult' Patient" at http://www.cfah.org/blog/2012/when-you-fear-being-labeled-a-difficult-patient

Chapter 6

The National Health Service Institute for Innovation and Improvement published *The Patient Experience Book* in 2013 (available at http://www.institute.nhs.uk/images/documents/Share%20and%20network/PEN/9340-2900792-TSO-Patient%20Experience_ACCESSIBLE2.pdf). The book highlights the work to improve patient-centered care by improving patient experience through the Patient Experience Learning Program, the Transforming Patient Experience: Essential Guide, and the NHS Patient Feedback Challenge.

View the TEDTalk *The Danger of a Single Story* at http://www.ted.com/talks/chimamanda_adichie_the_danger_of_a_single_story.html

Chapter 7

The website of the Nursing Alliance for Quality Care (NAQC) includes numerous resources related to quality and consumer-centered healthcare, such as the principles of patient engagement and relevant publications such as the whitepaper "Fostering Successful Patient and Family Engagement: Nursing's Critical Role." Retrieved from http://www.naqc.org/Main/Resources/Publications/March2013-FosteringSuccessfulPatientFamilyEngagement.pdf

The Agency for Healthcare Research and Quality (AHRQ) has developed the *Guide to Patient and Family Engagement in Hospital Quality and Safety,* which includes paired resources for patients and providers on four strategies: working with patients and families as advisors, communicating to improve quality, bedside shift report, and "IDEAL" discharge planning. Retrieved from http://www.ahrq.gov/professionals/systems/hospital/engagingfamilies/index.html

AHRQ has also developed *Questions To Ask Your Doctor.* Retrieved from http://www.ahrq.gov/patients-consumers/patient-involvement/index.html

Chapter 8

The Therapeutic Relationship website provides guidance to clinicians in all disciplines in creating, nurturing, and deepening their therapeutic relationships. Included are poems, short essays, Q&As, and reflections from Mary Koloroutis and Michael Trout. Retrieved from www.TheTherapeuticRelationship.com

View the TEDTalk by Brene Brown on *The Power of Vulnerability.* This can be accessed at http://www.ted.com/talks/brene_brown_on_vulnerability.html

Chapter 9

Planetree promotes patient- and family-centered care through U.S. and global member organizations for all types of healthcare settings. The website has open access with extensive resources to assist organizations in implementing patient- and family-centered care. See www.Planetree.org

The Institute for Patient and Family Centered Care offers a tool kit for patient- and family centered-care with bibliographies, webinars, presentations, stories, and a hospital assessment survey. See http://www.ipfcc.org

The *American Journal of Nursing* published a seven-part series on person- and family-centered care in 2009–2010:

- Frampton, S. B., & Guastello, S. (2010). Putting patients first: Patient-centered care: More than the sum of its parts. *AJN, American Journal of Nursing, 110*(9), 49-53.
- Frampton, S. B., Wahl, C., & Cappiello, G. (2010). Putting patients first: Partnering with patients' families. *AJN, American Journal of Nursing, 110*(7), 53-56.
- Michalak, J., Schreiner, N. J., Tennis, W., Szekely, L., Hale, M., & Guastello, S. (2010). The patient will see you now. *AJN, American Journal of Nursing, 110*(1), 61-63.
- Montague, K. N., Blietz, C. M., & Kachur, M. (2009). Ensuring quieter hospital environments. *AJN, American Journal of Nursing, 109*(9), 65-67.
- Frampton, S. B., Horowitz, S., & Stumpo, B. J. (2009). Open medical records. *AJN, American Journal of Nursing, 109*(8), 59-63.

- Spatz, M. A. (2009). Personalized health information. *AJN, American Journal of Nursing, 109*(4), 70-72.

- Frampton, S. B. (2009). Creating a patient-centered system. *AJN, American Journal of Nursing, 109*(3), 30-33.

Chapter 10

American Association of Critical-Care Nurses Synergy Model for Patient Care describes how the needs and characteristics of patients and families influence and drive the characteristics or competencies of nurses. See http://www.aacn.org/wd/certifications/content/synmodel.pcms

View *Family Matters: Navigating the Health System,* a 28-minute video by the Bowen Center for the Study of the Family and the University of the District of Columbia that describes the anxiety many families experience during a health encounter and how this anxiety may affect the relationships within a family. Retrieved from http://www.youtube.com/watch?v=rBd5n7ABDsg

Chapter 11

The Hastings Center hosts a bioethics forum, a diverse commentary on issues in bioethics, at http://www.thehastingscenter.org/BioethicsForum/

Read more about moral courage and distress at http://www.nursingworld.org/MainMenuCategories/EthicsStandards/Courage-and-Distress

Chapter 12

Read Harriet A. Washington's *Medical Apartheid* (Anchor, 2008), and see the Think Cultural Health website (https://www.thinkculturalhealth.hhs.gov/), which has excellent continuing education resources.

Review the Ethnomed website (http://ethnomed.org), which helps healthcare practitioners integrate cultural information into clinical practice.

Quality and Safety Education for Nurses (QSEN) has an 8-week mindfulness program for nursing that can be used by practicing nurses, available at http://qsen.org/eight-week-mindfulness-program-for-nursing-students/

Chapter 13

Read about strategies for personalizing care for the elderly at NICHE (Nurses Improving Care for Healthsystem Elders) website—http://www.nicheprogram.org/niche_solutions_series

Read the new Hastings Center Report: Berlinger, N., Barfield, R., and Fleischman, A.R. (2013, Nov). Facing persistent challenges in pediatric decision-making: New Hastings Center guidelines. *Pediatrics, 132*(5), 789-791. doi: 10.1542/peds.2013-1378. Epub 2013 Oct 7

Chapter 14

For information on vulnerable populations, consult the Centers for Disease Control and Prevention (http://www.cdc.gov/minorityhealth/populations.html); the Robert Wood Johnson Foundation (www.rwjf.org/en/our-work.html); and the Urban Institute Health Policy Center (http://www.urban.org/health_policy/vulnerable_populations/)

Chapter 15

Read about the Federal Mediation and Conciliation Services at http://www.fmcs.gov/internet/

Resources for conflict prevention, resolution, and management can be found at the Conflict Information Consortium, University of Colorado, at http://conflict.colorado.edu/

Chapter 16

Read about the education and improvement of clinical ethics services (by G. J. Agich) at http://www.biomedcentral.com/1472-6920/13/41

Additional information can be found at the National Center for Ethics in Health Care (http://www.ethics.va.gov/ETHICS/integratedethics/index.asp)

Chapter 17

Learn about SPIKES: A Six Step Process for Delivering Bad News (Baile et al., 2000):

- Setting up the interview (S)
- Assessing the patient perception (P)
- Obtaining the patient invitation (I)
- Giving knowledge and information to the patient (K)
- Addressing the patient's emotions with empathic responses (E)
- Strategy and summary (S)

Giving bad news can be a difficult and complex communication task for clinicians. Some planning on how to break bad news can significantly reduce the emotional toll for providers themselves, as well as help the receiver of the news to better accept the reality. Read more about this helpful process: Baile, W. F., Buckman, R., Lenzi, R., Glober, G., Beale, E. A., & Kudelka, A. P. (2000). SPIKES: A six step process for delivering bad news: Application to the patient with cancer. *The Oncologist, 5*(4), 302-311. Retrieved at http://theoncologist.alphamedpress.org/content/5/4/302.full

Online training program/resources for dealing with intractable conflict are available at http://www.colorado.edu/conflict/peace/course.htm

To conduct a self-study of conflict problems and potential solutions and treatments, see http://www.colorado.edu/conflict/peace/online_consulting.htm

And for information on principled negotiation, go to http://www.colorado.edu/conflict/peace/treatment/pricneg.htm

Chapter 18

A training course on Workplace Violence Prevention and Management Course is available from the Centers for Disease Control and Prevention at http://www.cdc.gov/niosh/topics/violence/training_nurses.html

The Emergency Nurses Association Toolkit on workplace violence is available at https://www.ena.org/practice-research/Practice/ViolenceToolKit/Documents/toolkitpg1.htm

Chapter 19

View a TEDTalk by Dr. Rita Charon on *Honoring the Stories of Illness* at http://www.youtube.com/watch?v=24kHX2HtU3o

Hear 16-year-old Trevor's story—*Trevor and the Perks of Diabetes*—on the Institute for Healthcare Improvement (IHI) website: http://www.ihi.org/education/IHIOpenSchool/resources/Pages/Activities/TrevorAndThePerksOfDiabetes.aspx

Chapter 20

Complete the Professional Quality of Life Compassion Fatigue Self-Test at www.proqol.org

For a comprehensive compilation of compassion fatigue research to date in the nursing field, read Tatano Beck, C. (2011, February). Secondary traumatic stress in nurses: A systematic review. *Archives of Psychiatric Nursing, 25*(1), 1-10.

For a discussion of the history of research on lateral violence in nursing, see Sheridan-Leos, N. (2008). Understanding lateral violence in nursing. *Clinical Journal of Oncology Nursing, 12*(3), 399-403.

A memoir on nursing and burnout, moral distress, and compassion fatigue: Barkin, L. (2012). *The comfort garden: tales from the trauma unit.* San Francisco, CA: Fresh Pond Press.

For more on the Mind Body connection, read Maté, G. (2003). *When the body says no.* Toronto, Canada: Knopf.

Read Pfifferling, J. H., & Gilley, K. (2000). Overcoming compassion fatigue. *American Academy of Family Physicians.* Retrieved from http://www.aafp.org/fpm/2000/0400/p39.html

Review the Wellspring Care for the Professional Caregiver program. Available through http://www.cancernetwork.com/nurses/content/article/10165/2008393

Chapter 21

Pharmacy Call to Action: AACP Argus Commission Report 2009-2010. *Call to action: Expansion of pharmacy primary care services in a reformed health system*. Retrieved from http://www.aacp.org/governance/COMMITTEES/argus/Documents/ArgusCommission09_10final.pdf

TeamSTEPPS materials for team training: http://teamstepps.ahrq.gov/

IHI Open School chapter on "Communicating with Patients after an Adverse Event." Retrieved from http://www.ihi.org/offerings/IHIOpenSchool/Courses/Pages/default.aspx

Checklist for documenting team and collaborative behaviors during multidisciplinary bedside rounds:

BEDSIDE ROUNDS CHECKLIST (ELEMENTS THAT ARE P&FCC FOCUSED ARE IN BOLD)

1. Did team give a sign or signal to the patient care team that rounds were starting?

2. Was nurse present during bedside round?

3. Did the nurse participate in the conversation?

4. Did physician acknowledge nurse? Describe

5. **Was team introduced to the patient?**

6. **Was patient invited/included to be part of the conversation?**

7. **Did the patient participate in the conversation?**

8. **Did team interview patient to gather further information?**

9. **Did patient freely volunteer information?**

10. **Did team inform the patient about his/her condition?**

11. Was a care plan developed by the team?

12. **Was the care plan clearly explained to the patient?**

13. **Did team reassure/encourage patient?**

14. **Did team develop a specific role for patient as part of the care plan? If so, please describe:**

15. **Was family present?**

16. **Was family invited/included in the conversation?**

17. **Did family participate in the conversation?**

From Henneman, E. A., Kleppel, R., & Hinchey, K. T. (2013). Development of a checklist for documenting team and collaborative behaviors during multidisciplinary bedside rounds. *Journal of Nursing Administration*, *43*(5), 280-285.

Chapter 22

Review the modules on whole systems healing and healing environments at the Center for Spirituality and Healing's website: www.csh.umn.edu/wsh

The IHI has several resources to guide leaders in creating patient-centered organizations: http://www.ihi.org/explore/PFCC/Pages/default.aspx

The IPFCC has a wealth of resources to assist leaders in assessing their organizations and meaningfully partnering with patients and families: http://ipfcc.org/

Chapter 23

AHRQ's toolkits, one for the redesign of healthcare and one for redesigning healthcare IT, can be found at http://search.ahrq.gov/search?q=Patient+Advisor+Toolkit&entqr=0&output=xml_no_dtd&proxystylesheet=AHRQ_GOV&client=AHRQ_GOV&site=default_collection&x=0&y=0

The PFACnetwork can be accessed at http://ipfcc.org/tools/index.html. The Patient and Family Advisors and Leaders of Advisory Councils network is for anyone interested in the work of patient and family advisory councils and other collaborative efforts in all healthcare settings.

Chapter 24

Read a sentinel event alert that underscores organization's and individual members' responsibilities in eliminating intimidating destructive behaviors or conflicts that can undermine safe, quality healthcare at http://www.jointcommission.org/assets/1/18/SEA_40.PDF

A series of resources from the Joint Commission on meeting the needs of diverse patient populations can be found at http://www.jointcommission.org/assets/1/18/Patient_Centered_Communications_7_3_12.pdf and on patient-centered communication at http://www.jointcommission.org/facts_about_patient-centered_communications/

Review the CNE Leadership Competencies for nurse executives at http://www.aone.org/resources/leadership%20tools/PDFs/AONE_NEC.pdf and those for healthcare leaders in general at the National Center for Healthcare Leadership website at http://www.nchl.org/static.asp?path=2852,3238

Read a recent report from IHI on high-impact leadership at http://www.ihi.org/knowledge/Pages/IHIWhitePapers/HighImpactLeadership.aspx

Chapter 25

The AHRQ 2013 *Guide to Patient and Family Engagement in Hospital Safety and Quality* can be found at http://www.ahrq.gov/downloads/patfamilyengageguide/patfamengagefull.zip

The Beryl Institute offers a wealth of resources at http://www.theberylinstitute.org/?page=DefiningPatientExp

AHRQ's Health Literacy Universal Precautions Toolkit can be found at http://1.usa.gov/ZvChsB

Similarly, the Medical Library Association Health Information Literacy project provides information and resources for healthcare professionals and consumers at http://www.mlanet.org/resources/healthlit/hil_project.html

Index

A

AACN (American Association of Colleges of Nursing)
    Essentials of Baccalaureate Education, 237
    Essentials of Master's Education in Nursing, 237
AACN (American Association of Critical-Care Nurses)
    mental health issues, causes of, 342
    moral distress, 349
    patient advocacy, 233
    study on HCP's poor performance/confrontations
      about, 377
AAN (American Academy of Nursing)
    advocacy resources, 234
    Raise the Voice initiative, 441
AARP
    best-known consumer group, 6
    P&FCC
        definition of, 205
        standards and regulations, 30
Abrams, M. H., 319
ACA (Affordable Care Act)
    long-term impact, 15, 96
    National Quality Strategy, 99, 429
accreditation standards, TJC
    ethics consultation services, 260
    proposals, 29–30
ACSQHC (Australian Commission on Safety and
    Quality in Health Care), 87
active listening, storytelling, 319
admission procedures, reforming, 143–144
*Advancing Effective Communication, Cultural
    Competence and Patient- and Family-Centered Care:
    A Roadmap for Hospitals,* 29, 198
Adwan, Jehad, 85–87
Affordable Care Act (ACA)
    long-term impact, 15, 96
    National Quality Strategy, 99, 429
age and P&FCC
    age-specific strategies, 212–213
        children, 206
        older adults, 206–207
        population relevant statistics, 204–205
        special populations, 210–211

        technology, use of, 213
    family, patients, and providers
        collaboration between, 209–212
        communication with, 207–208, 211–212
        coordination between, 210–212
Agency for Healthcare Research and Quality (AHRQ)
    Guide to Patient and Family Engagement, bedside
        shift change reports, 54, 264–265
    healthcare improvement mandates, 404
    hospital sources of frustration for all, 53
    involvement goals, 430
    TeamSTEPPS, 368
Agency for International Development, U.S., 75
AHA (American Hospital Association), 419
    business advantages of buy-in, 420
    McKesson Award for Quality, 421, 440
    organizational buy-in for P&FCC, 419
AHRQ (Agency for Healthcare Research and Quality)
    Guide to Patient and Family Engagement, bedside
        shift change reports, 54, 264–265
    healthcare improvement mandates, 404
    hospital sources of frustration for all, 53
    involvement goals, 430
    TeamSTEPPS, 368
AIPFCC (Australian Institute for Patient and Family
    Centered Care), 87
alcohol, workplace violence, 300
American Academy of Nursing (AAN)
    advocacy resources, 234
    Raise the Voice initiative, 441
American Academy on Communication in
    Healthcare, 7
American Association of Colleges of Nursing
    Essentials of Baccalaureate Education, 237
    Essentials of Master's Education Nursing, 237
    patient advocacy, 233
American Association of Colleges of Nursing (AACN)
    Essentials of Baccalaureate Education, 237
    Essentials of Master's Education in Nursing, 237
American Association of Critical-Care Nurses (AACN)
    mental health issues, causes of, 342
    moral distress, 349

patient advocacy, 233
    study on HCP's poor performance/confrontations about, 377
American Association of Retired Persons. *See* AARP
American College of Physicians Ethics Manual, 177
American Hospital Association (AHA), 419
    business advantages of buy-in, 420
    McKesson Award for Quality, 421, 440
    organizational buy-in for P&FCC, 419
American Nurses Association (ANA)
    advocacy resources, 234
    Code of Ethics
        ethics consultations, 267
        moral values, 170, 178
        patient advocacy, 237
    Nursing: Scope and Standards of Practice
        family systems theory, 151
        patient advocacy, 232
    Nursing's Social Policy Statement: The Essence of the Profession, 232
American Society of Bioethics and Humanities (ASBH)
    Core Competencies, 68, 262–263
    training of ESC members, 67
ANA (American Nurses Association)
    advocacy resources, 234
    Code of Ethics
        ethics consultations, 267
        moral values, 170, 178
        patient advocacy, 237
    Nursing: Scope and Standards of Practice
        family systems theory, 151
        patient advocacy, 232
    Nursing's Social Policy Statement: The Essence of the Profession, 232
ASBH (American Society of Bioethics and Humanities)
    Core Competencies, 68, 262–263
    training of ESC members, 67
Aurora Health System, 4
Austin, Wendy, 351
Australia
    global concept of P&FCC, 87
    patients' healthcare experiences, 82
Australian Capital Territory, interviews using Wagner model, 76
Australian Commission on Safety and Quality in Health Care (ACSQHC), 87
Australian Institute for Patient and Family Centered Care (AIPFCC), 87

B

balance concept, family systems theory, 155
Baldridge Award, 421, 440
Baruch, Jay, 320
Batalden, Paul, 80
Beacon Award for Excellence, 260

behavioral contracts, 311
Belgium, PCMH model, 84
Benjamin, Walter, 320
Berwick, Don, 80
Berwick, Donald, 368
Beryl Institute survey, 46
bioethics
    American Society of Bioethics and Humanities
        Core Competencies, 68, 262–263
        training of ESC members, 67
    nursing as subcategory of, 171
    theories, 173–174
Blackman, Lewis, 6, 143
Black *versus* White people, history, 186–187
boundaries concept, family systems theory, 154–155
Bowen's model, family systems theory, 154
Brady, Don, 7
Brantley, Ben, 316
Breakthrough Series Collaborative, 81
Brody, Howard, 322
burnout, 339
    causes
        increased interaction with families, 340
        role overload, 341–342
    impact on PCC, 347
    in physicians, 340
    reducing, 353–354
        individual strategies, 355–356
        organizational strategies, 359
        professional strategies, 356–359

C

CAHPS (Consumer Assessment of Healthcare Providers and Systems), 422
Canada
    healthcare improvement, 74
    IHI programs, 80
    patients' healthcare experiences, 82
Canadian Nurses Association (CNA), *Code of Ethics for Registered Nurses,* 349
care settings. *See* healthcare facilities/services
caring processes, therapeutic relationships/practices, 120–121
    applying for healthy work environment, 163–164
    attunement and human attachments, 119–121
    being with, 117–119
    doing for, 117–118
    enabling, 117–118
    following, 117–118, 122
    holding, 117, 122–123
    knowing, 117–118
    listening for understanding, 248–249
    maintaining belief, 117–118
    presence through attunement, 117–118, 119–121
    wondering, 117–118, 121–122

CAS (complex adaptive systems), 153

Case Western Reserve University, FIND Lab, 398, 400

CDC (Centers for Disease Control and Prevention), vulnerable populations, 220

Center for Advancing Health, assessment of participation in care, 38

Center for Health Design, 400

Center for Mindfulness, Health Care, and Society, 319

Centers for Disease Control and Prevention (CDC), vulnerable populations, 220

Centers for Medicare & Medicaid Services. *See* CMS

Chambers, Tod, 329

Charon, Dr. Rita, 319–320

CHC (Cultural Health Capital), 187–189

children
    age-specific strategies, 206
    hospital environments, 394
    movements adopted for adults and families, 24
    National Initiative of Children's Healthcare
        Quality's self-assessment tools, 142
    parents and hospital rules
        overnight stays, 23–24
        visiting hours, 23, 145–146
    population relevant statistics, 204–205

Christus Health, 427

chronic care management
    definition of chronic, 9
    Improving Chronic Illness Care Through Integrated Health Service Delivery Networks, 80
    PCMH model, 84, 379–381
    Wagner model, 76

Cincinnati Children's Hospital, 426

Clinical and Group CAHPS (Consumer Assessment of Healthcare Providers and Systems), 422

clinics. *See* healthcare facilities/services

close reading, 319, 326

CMS (Centers for Medicare & Medicaid Services)
    Conditions of Participation standard, 28, 30
    Electronic Health Records, 103
        incentive programs, 103
        reliability and consistency, 213
    Meaningful Use Program, 103
    Partnership for Patients program, 49
    P&FCC standards and regulations, 28, 30

CNA (Canadian Nurses Association), *Code of Ethics for Registered Nurses,* 349

Code of Ethics, American Nurses Association
    ethics consultations, 267
    moral values, 170, 178
    patient advocacy, 232

Code of Ethics for Nurses, International Council of Nurses
    cultural conflict situations, 186
    moral values, 178

Code of Ethics for Registered Nurses, Canadian Nurses Association, 349

Commonwealth Fund studies
    financial advantages of P&FCC, 98
    healthcare issues, 14
    organizational level requirements, 417

compassion fatigue
    connection with moral distress, 352
    definition of, 343–344
    impact on PCC, 347
    reducing, 353–354
        individual strategies, 355–356
        organizational strategies, 359
        professional strategies, 356–359
    warning signs of, 345–347

The Compassion Fatigue Workbook (Mathieu), 343, 355

complex adaptive systems (CAS), 153

complexity compression, 7

Conditions of Participation standard, 28, 30

conflicts. *See also* difficult patients
    cultural conflicts, 186–187
        averting, 189–191
        based on cultural health capital, 188
        compassionate awareness, 194
        diverse belief systems, 192–194
        education about diversity, 189, 195–196
        focus on commonality, 190
        focus on systems and individuals, 187–189
        journaling about concept of race, 193–194
        Kleinman's framework of questions, 198
        managing serious conflicts, 194–198
        minimizing conflicts, guidelines, 199–200
        moral imagination, 188
        Patient Activation Measure, 191–192
        stereotype-linked bias, 192
        systems for sexual diversity, 198–199
        unconscious bias, 192
    definition of, 280
    The Exchange Strategy for Managing Conflict in Health (Dinkin, et al), 281
    high-intensity conflicts
        causes and sources of, 281–284
        consequences of unresolved conflict, 291–292
        management styles, 290–291
        prevalence of, 280–281
        preventing and solving, 284–292
        principled negotiation, 286–290
        types of conflicts, 281
    on interprofessional teams, 374–375
    mediation
        caucusing, 255
        clinical nurse's role, 246–247
        definition of, 244–245
        developing care proposals, 256
        distinguishing between positions/interests, 250–251
        elevating definition of problems, 254
        eliciting medical facts, 254–255

establishing agreements, 256
techniques during communication, 247–252
connections, mindful and compassionate
attunement and human attachment, 119–120
human caring research and theory
applying, 123
examples, 123–126
RBC (Relationship-Based Care) model, 115–117
therapeutic relationships/practices, 120–121
attunement and human attachments, 119–121
being with, 117–119
doing for, 117–118
enabling, 117–118
following, 117–118, 122
holding, 117, 122–123
knowing, 117–118
maintaining belief, 117–118
presence through attunement, 117–118,
119–121
wondering, 117–118, 121–122
Consumer Advancing Patient Safety, P&FCC standards,
30
Consumer Assessment of Healthcare Providers and
Systems (CAHPS), 422
consumerism, societal factors affecting P&FCC, 5–7
Consumer Reports, healthcare systems information, 14
Consumers Union, 2
Conversation Project, Institute for Healthcare
Improvement, 81
Conway, Jim, 421
Core Competencies, American Society of Bioethics and
Humanities, 262–263
Creative Health Care Management, RBC model, 116
CRM (Crew Resource Management), 368
*Crossing the Quality Chasm: A New Health System for
the 21st Century*
conflict management, 281
healing environments, 391
interprofessional mandates, 366
patient engagement, 130
P&FCC
definition of, 22
promotion of, 2, 434
cultural conflicts, 186–187. *See also* difficult patients;
high-intensity conflicts; mediation
averting, 189–191
based on cultural health capital, 188
compassionate awareness, 194
diverse belief systems, 192–194
education about diversity
of communities, 189
of self, 195–196
focus on commonality, 190
focus on systems and individuals, 187–189
journaling about concept of race, 193–194

managing serious conflicts, 194
example, 196–198
skills required, 195–196
minimizing conflicts, guidelines, 199–200
moral imagination, 188
Patient Activation Measure, 191–192
stereotype-linked bias, 192
systems for sexual diversity, 198–199
unconscious bias, 192
Cultural Health Capital (CHC), 187–189

D

data uses of HCAHPS scores
chasing scores, not goals, 54–55
demoralizing staff, 55
guidelines for effective use and improvement, 56
deBronkart, e-Patient Dave
e-Patient Manifesto, 7
Let Patients Help, 6
Declaration on Patient-Centred Healthcare,
International Alliance of Patients' Organizations,
77–78
Democratic Republic of the Congo (DRC), global
concept of P&FCC, 88
Denmark
IHI programs, 81
PCMH model, 84
DHHS (Department of Health and Human Services)
Affordable Care Act, 15
long-term impact, 15, 96
National Quality Strategy, 99, 429
secretary, Kathleen Sebelius, 2
Didion, Joan, 316
differentiation concept, family systems theory, 155
difficult patients, 60–62. *See also* cultural conflicts;
high-intensity conflicts; mediation
abrasive personality styles, 61, 63
cultural conflicts and solutions, 187–189
difficult circumstances, reactions to, 61
ethical obligations, 60
conflict resolution techniques, 65
five As for dealing with hostile patients, 66
third story, 66
Ethics Consultation Service, 60
Core Competencies, 68
requirement of The Joint Commission, 66–67
skill sets of, 67
inappropriate behaviors of, 62–64
multiple symptoms, 61, 63
predilection for psychosomatic complaints, 61
psychiatric disorders, 61, 63
psychopathologic disorders, 61
somatoform disorders, 61
treatment provoking behaviors, 63
dignity robes, 392

discharge planning, 147
disengagement, 155
Dossetor, John, 351
DRC (Democratic Republic of the Congo), global
    concept of P&FCC, 88

E

ECRI Institute, technology hazards, 12
ECS (Ethics Consultation Service), difficult patients, 60
    Core Competencies, 68
    requirement of The Joint Commission, 66–67
    skill sets of, 67
Edge Runners, 441
effective and efficient, dimensions of quality, 22
EHR (Electronic Health Records)
    incentive programs, 103
    reliability and consistency, 213
Elements of Performance, The Joint Commission, 421
11th Street Family Health Services in Philadelphia, 441
ENA (Emergency Nurses Association), workplace
    violence
        definition of, 298
        statistics, 298–299
Engaging Patients as Safety Partners (Spath), 424
England Journal of Medicine, difficult patients, 65
England/United Kingdom
    HCP's attitudes of healthcare, 76
    IHI programs, 81
    patients' healthcare experiences, 82
    PCMH model, 84
enmeshment, 155
e-Patient Dave (deBronkart)
    e-Patient Manifesto, 7
    Let Patients Help, 6
equitable, dimension of quality, 22
Essentials of Baccalaureate Education, 237
Essentials of Master's Education in Nursing, 237
ethics
    bioethics
        Core Competencies, 68, 262–263
        nursing as subcategory of, 171
        theories, 173–174
        training of ESC members, 67
    Code of Ethics, American Nurses Association
        ethics consultations, 267
        moral values, 170, 178
        patient advocacy, 232
    Code of Ethics for Nurses, International Council of
        Nurses
        cultural conflict situations, 186
        moral values, 178
    consultations, nursing role in
        assisting in process, 273
        identifying key stakeholders, 273–274
        illustrating patient's daily life, 274

initiating consultations, 271–273
        learning from process, 275
        participating in meetings, 274–275
        supporting patients/family, 274
    definitions of
        healthcare ethics consultation, 261
        patient-centeredness, 259
    ethical climates
        creating, 352–353
        definition of, 348
    ethical dilemmas
        definition of, 176
        determining, 175
        versus disagreements, 176
        examples, 176
        resources for handling, 181–182
    ethical dilemmas, values in
        basis of conflicts, 179
        definitions based on diversity and specialty
            areas, 177–178
        personal values, 178–179
        voicing, both by persons and organizations,
            180–181
    Ethic Rounds on advocacy, 225–227
    Ethics Consultation Service, difficult patients, 60
        Core Competencies, 68
        requirement of The Joint Commission, 66–67
        skill sets of, 67
    literature about, 261–262
    moral distress, 172–173
    nursing, definitions of, 170–171
    origins of, 260–261
    overview, 171–172
    person-centered care, 174–175
    promotion of P&FCC
        attention to patient/family voices, 263–264
        quality in consultations, 262–263
        recognition of family role, 264–266
    value-laden concerns
        defining values, 266–268
        formulating ethics questions, 268–270
        informing patients of consultations, 270
Ethics Consultation Service (ECS), difficult patients, 60
    Core Competencies, 68
    requirement of The Joint Commission, 66–67
    skill sets of, 67
Ethics in Public Health, University of Nebraska Medical
    Center, 349
Europe, healthcare improvement, 74
European Observatory on Health Systems and
    Policies, 75
evidence-based design for healing environments
    access to social support, 393–394
    patient comfort and control, 391–393
    promotion of, guidelines, 399

Rapid Assessment of Product Usability and Universal Design, 398–399
resources, 400
stress reduction, 393
universal design, 396–399
Universal Design for Learning, 397–398
use of, 391
The Exchange Strategy for Managing Conflict in Health (Dinkin, et al), 281
exquisite empathy, 357

F

families. *See* FST (family systems theory); patient engagement; patients and families
family systems theory. *See* FST
Federation for Children With Special Needs, 206
f exercise, 48–50
Figley, Dr. Charles, 343
financing healthcare, 4, 13–15
    consumer directed *versus* person-oriented, 14–15
    cost sharing, 14–15
    information asymmetry, 14
    medical interventions *versus* preventive care, 13
    myths concerning, 27
    outcomes of, 25–26
        payment based on outcomes, 39–40
        volume *versus* outcomes, 13
    physician/patient communication, lack of, 15
    United States *versus* other countries, 14
    widening income gap, 4–5
FIND (Full INclusion of Persons with Disabilities) Lab , Case Western Reserve University, 398, 400
5 Million Lives Campaign, 81
Florida Hospital Celebration Health and IPC, 105
for-profit/nonprofit health systems
    distinctions between, 4
    factors affecting P&FCC, 4
Framework for Action on Interprofessional Education and Collaborative Practice, 367
Freudenberger, Herbert, 339
FST (family systems theory). *See also* patient engagement; patients and families; systems theory
    applying for healthy work environment, 162–163
        overfunctioning/underfunctioning in professional roles, 164–166
        self-monitoring, 166
        therapeutic relationships, 163–164
    derived from general systems theory, 153
    disengagement, 155
    enmeshment, 155
    families of origin, 157
    integrating into care strategies, 157–158
        appropriate communication care plans, 159
        communication link for information exchange, 158–159

family meetings, 159–160
family opinions and expectations, 162
sources of anger/strong emotions, 160–161
sources of collateral/historical information, 161
key concepts
    balance, 155
    boundaries, 154–155
    differentiation, 155
    overfunctioning/underfunctioning, 156
    triangles, 156
Full Catastrophe Living (Kabat-Zinn), 355
Full INclusion of Persons with Disabilities (FIND) Lab , CaseWestern Reserve University, 398, 400
"Fundamental Elements of Clinical Ethics ," 67
The Future of Nursing: Leading Change, Advancing Health, 8, 22, 234

G

Gardner, John, 320
Garland-Thomson, Rosemarie, 325
Gentile, Mary C., 180
Gentry, J. Eric, 357
Germany
    patients' healthcare experience, 82
    PCMH model, 84
GetWellNetwork, 104–105
Ghana, IHI programs, 81
Girl Child Education Fund, 81
Giving Voice to Values: How to Speak Your Mind When You Know What's Right (Gentile), 180
global concept of P&FCC
    components of
        general consensus, 74
        from Picker Institute, 75
        from U.S. Agency for International Development, 75
        from World Health Organization, 75
    definitions of, 72–73
    examples
        Australia, 87
        DRC (Democratic Republic of the Congo), 88
        Palestine, 85–87
        Somalia, 88–89
        Sweden, 87
        Uganda, 88
    IAPO's term, patient-centered healthcare, 73
        principles of, 73
    patients' care experiences, 82–84
    personalizing care within different countries, guidelines, 89–92
    perspectives on P&FCC
        Institute for Healthcare Improvement, 80–81
        International Alliance of Patients' Organizations, 77–78

International Council of Nurses, 81–82

Pan American Health Organization, 80

World Health Organization, 78–79

stakeholders in, 76

Gothenburg University Centre for Person-Centered Care, 87

Guide to Patient and Family Engagement, 54, 264–265

Guiding Principles for Patient Engagement, 107–108

H

Hamer, Rachel, 323, 326

Harrison, Richard, 357

Harvard Negotiation Project, 65–66

Haskell, Helen, 6

Hastings Center Report, nurse advocacy, 233

HCAHPS (Hospital Consumer Assessment of Healthcare Providers and Systems) scores

lack of constructive criticism about scores, 47, 55

patient engagement, 99

P&FCC

accepted as core care component, 141

standards and regulations, 28, 422

Planetree, exceeding national scores, 140

practicing in other countries, guidelines, 90–92

public comparing performance, 134

quick-fix/ineffective techniques, 44

sources for frustration, 53

HCPs (healthcare professionals). *See also* interprofessional teams; leaders/leadership

age-specific strategies

collaboration, 209–212

communication, 207–208, 211–212

coordination, 209–212

burnout, 339

causes, 340–342

impact on PCC, 347

in physicians, 340

compassion fatigue

connection with moral distress, 352

definition of, 343–344

impact on PCC, 347

reducing, 353–354

warning signs of, 345–347

ethical climate

creating, 352–353

definition of, 348

HCAHPS scores

demoralizing staff, 55

lack of constructive criticism, 47, 55

moral distress, 348–349

causes of, 349–352

connection with compassion fatigue, 352

definition of, 349

reducing, 354

patient advocacy, 222–225

P&FCC

education and commitment of staff, 133

organizational buy-in required, 421–422

stakeholders in, 76

professional autonomy issue, 11

staff engagement

demoralizing, with value-based purchasing, 55

dismissing staff needs, 52–53

guidelines for effectiveness, 54

reasonable *versus* unreasonable requests, 53

stress reduction strategies, 353–354

exquisite empathy, 357

individual, 355–356

Mindfulness-Based Stress Reduction, 355

organizational, 359

professional, 356–359

stress strap of professionalism, 284

United Kingdom, view as barrier to PCC, 76

workplace violence

factors contributing to negative behavior, 303–304

impact of violence, 303

individual strategies for coping, 308–310

intervention skills, 307–308

reasons for vulnerability, 301

relationships with patients/families, 301–302

setting limits for self-management, 310

treatment team strategies, 311

underreporting of violence, 302–303

violence as part of job, 302

violence management skills needed, 302

healing environments

definition of, 390

evidence-based design

access to social support, 393–394

patient comfort and control, 391–393

promotion of, guidelines, 399

Rapid Assessment of Product Usability and Universal Design, 398–399

resources, 400

stress reduction, 393

universal design, 396–399

Universal Design for Learning, 397–398

use of, 391

hospital cultures, goals, 147

relationship with safe environments, 394–396

The Healing of America (Reid), 13

Health Affairs, understanding healthcare system, 14–15

healthcare facilities/services

education and commitment of staff, 133

models of care

Institute for Healthcare Improvement, 135–136

Institute for Patient- and Family-Centered Care, 136

Patient-Centered Medical Home, 379–381

Picker Institute, 136–137

Planetree, Inc., 137–141
Relationship-Based Care, 115–117
Wagner, 76
reorganizing policies/processes, 36, 39–41,
    130–131, 141–142
    admission/discharge, 143–144, 147
    ancillary department coordination, 147
    bedside shift change reports, 54, 146–147,
        264–265
    care processes, 437–438
    cultural diversity factors, 435–436
    family meetings, 144
    family spokesperson to spokesgroup, 435–436
    flexible schedules, 144
    healing environment, 147
    HIPAA regulations, 439
    information resources, 148
    initiatives promoting P&FCC, 440–441
    interprofessional patient rounds, 144
    new ways of thinking, 433–434
    nutrition resource access, 147
    overnight stays, 23–24
    patient/family advisors, 148
    patient-family partnerships, 146, 435
    philosophy and operations, 131–133
    rapid response teams, 146
    sexual orientation issues, 28–30, 198–199
    spiritual care, 146
    technology use, 440
    total culture, not program concept, 439–440
    visiting hours, 23, 145–146
healthcare professionals. *See* HCPs
Health Ethics Centre, University of Alberta, 351
Health Information Technology (HIT), 99
Health Information Technology for Economic and
    Clinical Health (HITECH) Act, 99
Health Insurance Portability and Accountability Act.
    See HIPAA
Health Insurance Portability and Accountability Act
    (HIPAA)
    health information regulations, 158
    information-sharing regulations, 439
    myth of P&FCC as violation of, 28
*Health Professionals for a New Century: Transforming
    Education to Strengthen Health Systems in an
    Interdependent World* report, 13
Health Professions Education: A Bridge to Quality, 366
Hibbard, Judith, Patient Activation Measure
    cultural conflicts, 191–192
    developer of, 38
    example questions, 101
    use of, 105
high-intensity conflicts. *See also* cultural conflicts;
    difficult patients; mediation
    causes and sources of, 281–282
        data sharing and interpretation, 282

interest tensions, 282
relationships, 282–283
structural, care goals, 283
values, 283–284
consequences of unresolved conflict, 291–292
management styles, 290–291
prevalence of, 280–281
preventing and solving, 284
    with effective communication, 285–290
    with gracious space concept, 285
    P&FCC approach, 292
principled negotiation, 286–290
types of conflicts, 281
HIPAA (Health Insurance Portability and Accoutability
    Act)
    health information regulations, 158
    information-sharing regulations, 439
    myth of P&FCC as violation of, 28
Hippocrates, environment importance, 391
Hippocratic (paternalistic) healthcare model, 217
HIT (Health Information Technology), 99
HITECH (Health Information Technology for
    Economic and Clinical Health) Act, 99
holistic view of medicine, 9
Home Health CAHPS (Consumer Assessment of
    Healthcare Providers and Systems), 422
horizontal violence, 8
Hospital Consumer Assessment of Healthcare
    Providers and Systems scores. *See* HCAHPS scores
hospitals. *See* healthcare facilities/services

I

IAPO (International Alliance of Patients'
    Organizations)
    Declaration on Patient-Centred Healthcare, 77–78
    definition of PCC, 73
    perspectives on P&FCC, 77–78
    policy development involvement, 428–429
    World Health Professions Alliance, 77
ICN (International Council of Nurses)
    Code of Ethics for Nurses, 178, 186
    International Centre for Nurse Migration, 81
    perspectives on P&FCC, 81–82
IHI (Institute for Healthcare Improvement)
    models of care, 135–136
    partnerships between patients and providers, 132
    patients/families on improvement teams, 49
    perspectives on care, 80–81
    self-assessment tools, 142
    shift change bedside reports, 264
Illness as Metaphor (Sontag), 323
IMA World Health, 88
impolite attitude/behavior. *See* incivility
*Improving Chronic Illness Care Through Integrated
    Health Service Delivery Networks,* 80

incivility, societal factors affecting P&FCC, 7–8

information resources, 148

Inpatient P&FCC models, 381

Institute for Healthcare Improvement (IHI), 80–81
- models of care, 135–136
- partnerships between patients and providers, 132
- patients/families on improvement teams, 49
- perspectives on care, 80–81
- self-assessment tools, 142
- shift change bedside reports, 264

Institute for Patient- and Family-Centered Care. *See* IPFCC

Institute of Medicine. *See* IOM

Interactive Heart-Failure Care Plan, 105

Interactive Patient Care (IPC)
- Florida Hospital Celebration Health example, 104–105
- nurses' engagement, 106
- patient engagement, 103–104

Interagency Working Group on Health Care Quality, 430

Inter-American System, PAHO, 80

International Alliance of Patients' Organizations (IAPO)
- Declaration on Patient-Centred Healthcare, 77–78
- definition of PCC, 73
- perspectives on P&FCC, 77–78
- policy development involvement, 428–429
- World Health Professions Alliance, 77

International Centre for Nurse Migration, 81

International Council of Nurses (ICN)
- *Code of Ethics for Nurses,* 178, 186
- International Centre for Nurse Migration, 81
- perspectives on P&FCC, 81–82

Interprofessional Educational Collaborative (IPEC), 367

interprofessional teams. *See also* HCPs (healthcare professionals); leaders/leadership
- barriers to functioning
  - authority gradients, 376–377
  - confrontations, 377
  - dynamic nature of teams, 375–376
  - failures to understand/respect strengths, 374
  - team conflict and sources, 374–375
- care models with patient/family partnerships
  - case scenarios, 381–385
  - Inpatient P&FCC models, 381
  - Outpatient Patient-Centered Medical Home model, 379–381
- core competencies for students, 367
- difficult patients, 378–379
- mandates from professional organizations, 366–368
- patient rounds, 144

strategies for improvement
- collegial trust, 371–372
- humility, 373–374
- open/direct communication, 368–369
- shared decision-making, 370–371
- swift trust, 372–373
- values and principles, 369–370
- virtual teams and trust, 373
- team development stages, 372
- tools and P&FCC models
  - "Nothing about me, without me," 368
  - SBAR (Situation, Background, Assessment, Recommendation), 368
  - TeamSTEPPS, 368
  - "With HEART," 368

IOM (Institute of Medicine)
- *Crossing the Quality Chasm: A New Health System for the 21st Century*
  - conflict management, 281
  - healing environments, 391
  - interprofessional mandates, 366
  - patient engagement, 130
  - promotion of P&FCC, 434
- definitions
  - patient-centeredness, 259
  - P&FCC, 2, 22, 73, 419
- *To Err Is Human,* 391
- *The Future of Nursing: Leading Change, Advancing Health,* 8, 22, 234
- healthcare improvement mandates, 404
- *Health Professions Education: A Bridge to Quality,* 366
- levels of care, 418
- *Preventing Medication Errors,* 10
- teamwork and collaboration, 144
- *Unequal Treatment,* 281

IPC (Interactive Patient Care)
- Florida Hospital Celebration Health example, 104–105
- nurses' engagement, 106
- patient engagement, 103–104

IPEC (Interprofessional Educational Collaborative), 367

IPFCC (Institute for Patient- and Family-Centered Care)
- leadership importance, 423
- models of care, 136
- partnerships of patient/family/staff, 48–49
- P&FCC
  - definitions of, 22
  - standards and regulations, 30
- programs and initiatives, 427
- resources, 422
- self-assessment tools, 142

J

Jameton, Andrew, 349
Joinson, Carla, 343
The Joint Commission (TJC)
    accreditation standards
        ethics consultation services, 260
        proposals, 29–30
    *Advancing Effective Communication, Cultural
        Competence and Patient- and Family-Centered
        Care: A Roadmap for Hospitals,* 29, 198
    conflict management, 281
    Elements of Performance, 421
    ethical issues
        ethical consultation services, 260
        resolving problems, 66
    family involvement as challenge, 340
    healthcare improvement mandates, 404
    nursing leadership expectations, 417
    P&FCC
        definition of IPFCC, 22
        standards and regulations, 29–30
    Sentinel Event Alert
        behaviors undermining safety, 8
        disruptive and inappropriate behaviors, 8

K

Kabat-Zinn, Dr. Jon, 319, 355
Kaiser Permanente, 426
Killian, Kyle, 357
Kleinman, Arthur, 316, 327
Kleinman's framework of questions
    cultural conflicts, 198
    for global view of care, 91–92
    for mediation, 253
KSA (knowledge, skills, attitudes) framework, 30–32

L

Lancet Commission, *Health Professionals for a New
    Century: Transforming Education to Strengthen
    Health Systemsin an Interdependent World* report, 13
The Lancet Commission of Education of Health
    Professionals for the 21st Century, 367
Latin America, IHI programs, 81
leaders/leadership. *See also* HCPs (healthcare
    professionals); interprofessional teams
    characteristics/role of leaders, 44–45, 416–417
    negative sides of, 44–45
        customer-service instead of PCC attitude,
            46–47
        guidelines to improve performance, 47
        lack of constructive criticism about HCAHPS
            scores, 47
        nonclinical amenities for improved PCC, 46

nonpatient priorities as roadblocks, 45
PCC commitments without planning, 45–46
organizational buy-in for P&FCC, 419, 420
    business reasons for, 420
    collaboration with entire staff, 421–422
    Elements of Performance, 421
    P&FCC organizations *versus* traditional, 420
    recognition programs, 421
promoting P&FCC
    changes needed, 418
    with contributions to policy development,
        428–430
    creating healthy environment, 425–427
    establishing advisory council, 425
    with organizational assessment, 424
    selecting/implementing programs/initiatives,
        427
    with self-assessments, 424
    strategies, 418–419, 422–423
Lerman, Liz, 324
Let Patients Help (deBronkart), 6
Lillehel, C. Walton, 12
listening for understanding
    conflict management, 285
    conscious or therapeutic listening, 248–249
    mediation technique, 247–249
    storytelling
        active listening, 319
        close listening, 319

M

Magnet designation, 260
Maine Medical Center, 426
"Make Waves, the Courage to Influence Practice"
    (Thornby), 233
Malawi, IHI programs, 81
Marton, Betty A., 19
Maslach, Christina, 339
MBSR (Mindfulness-Based Stress Reduction), 355–356
McKesson Award for Quality, American Hospital
    Association, 421, 440
Meaningful Use Program, Centers for Medicare &
    Medicaid Services, 103
Measure Applications Partnership, 430
mediation. *See also* cultural conflicts; difficult patients;
    high-intensity conflicts
    caucusing, 255
    clinical nurse's role, 246–247
    definition of, 244–245
    developing care proposals, 256
    distinquishing between positions/interests, 250–
        251
    elevating definition of problems, 254
    eliciting medical facts, 254–255
    establishing agreements, 256

techniques during routine communication
    distinquishing between positions/interests, 250–251
    listening for understanding, 247–249
    preparing, 249
    questioning, 253
    reframing, 251–252
    summarizing, 249–250
  using in healthcare, 245–246
Medical Apartheid: The Dark History of Medical Experimentation on Black Americans from Colonial Times to the Present (Washington), 187
medical-industrial complex
  definition of, 3
  factor affecting P&FCC, 3–4
  societal factors affecting P&FCC, 3
Medicare Current Beneficiary Survey, 2007, 38
medicine, profession of
  physicians
    and team player concept, 10
    views of medicine, *versus* nurses, 9
  specialty dominance, 9
medicine and storytelling
  case scenarios
    chronic care setting, 331–332
    emergency care setting, 330–331
    pastoral care setting, 332–333
  effectiveness and importance of, 318
    active listening, 319
    close listening, 319
    close reading, 319, 326
  healing power of hearing, 321
  medical *versus* patient narratives, 321–322
  patient's stories
    eliciting, 327–328
    parallel charts, 327
    writing, 328–329
  pitfalls, 329–330
  relationship between, 317
  stories in clinical settings, 325–326
    close reading, 326
    regular practice, 326–327
  storytelling practice, 320
  story uses
    bearing witness, 322–323
    interpreting and authenticating, 324–325
    sharing, 323–324
mental health issues. *See also* cultural conflicts; high-intensity conflicts; workplace violence
  workplace climate
    burnout, 339–342, 347
    compassion fatigue, 343–347, 352–354
    ethical climate, 348, 352–353
    Mindfulness-Based Stress Reduction approach, 355
    moral distress, 348–354
    stress reduction strategies, 353–359

Mindfulness-Based Stress Reduction (MBSR), 355–356
moral distress, 348–349
  causes of, 349–352
  connection with compassion fatigue, 352
  definition of, 349
  reducing, 354
    individual strategies, 355–356
    organizational strategies, 359
    professional strategies, 356–359
Multi-Professional Patient Safety Curriculum Guide, 79
Murphy, Margaret, RN, 20
"My Favorite Tips for Engaging the Difficult Patient on Consultation-Liaison Psychiatry Services," 65

N

NAQC (Nursing Alliance for Quality Care)
  Guiding Principles for Patient Engagement, 107–108
  patient advocacy, 232
  patient engagement and cultural diversity, 190, 200
  PCMH model, 379
National Center on Universal Design for Learning, 396
National Committee for Quality Assurance (NCQA)
  patient engagement, 99
  P&FCC standards and regulations, 28
National Initiative of Children's Healthcare Quality (NICHQ), 142
National Institute for Occupational Safety and Health (NIOSH), workplace violence
  definition of, 298
  statistics, 298–299
National Patient Safety Foundation (NPSF)
  healthcare improvement mandates, 404
  Principles of Partnership, 429
  Universal Patient Compact, 429
National Priorities Partnership (NPP)
  Patient and Family Engagement, 29, 97
  standards and regulations, 29
National Quality Forum (NQF), 100
National Quality Strategy, 99, 429
National Strategy for Quality Improvement in Health Care. *See* National Quality Strategy
National Survey of the Work and Health of Nurses, Canada, 339
National Working Group for the Clinical Ethics Credentialing Project, 67
Naylor Transitional Care Program, 441
NCQA (National Committee for Quality Assurance)
  patient engagement, 99
  P&FCC standards and regulations, 28
Netherlands
  chronically ill patients' experiences with PCMH model, 84
  patients' healthcare experiences, 82
Newman, Margaret, 200
New South Wales, Wagner model, 76

New Zealand
    IHI programs, 81
    patients' healthcare experiences, 82
NICHQ (National Initiative of Children's Healthcare
    Quality), 142
Nightingale, Florence
    environment importance, 391
    nursing ethics, 170
NIOSH (National Institute for Occupational Safety and
    Health), workplace violence
    definition of, 298
    statistics, 298–299
nonprofit/for-profit health systems
    distinctions between, 4
    factors affecting P&FCC, 4
"Nothing about me, without me" model (Berwick), 368
NPP (National Priorities Partnership)
    Patient and Family Engagement, 29, 97
    standards and regulations, 29
NPSF (National Patient Safety Foundation)
    healthcare improvement mandates, 404
    Principles of Partnership, 429
    Universal Patient Compact, 429
NQF (National Quality Forum), 100
nurse-to-nurse handoffs. *See* shift change bedside
    reports
Nursing Alliance for Quality Care (NAQC)
    Guiding Principles for Patient Engagement, 107–108
    patient advocacy, 232
    patient engagement and cultural diversity, 190, 200
    PCMH model, 379
Nursing CAHPS (Consumer Assessment of Healthcare
    Providers and Systems), 422
nursing ethics. *See* ethics
Nursing Home CAHPS (Consumer Assessment of
    Healthcare Providers and Systems), 422
nursing homes. *See* healthcare facilities/services
Nursing: Scope and Standards of Practice
    family systems theory, 151
    patient advocacy, 232
*Nursing's Social Policy Statement: The Essence of the
    Profession,* 232

O

Obama, President Barack, comments on healthcare, 29
older adults
    age-specific strategies, 206–207
    population relevant statistics, 205
"On Caregiving" (Kleinman), 327
Open School for HCP students' education, 81
outcomes of P&FCC, 25–26
    financial outcomes, 24–25, 39–40
    patient engagement's role, 100–101
    volume *versus* outcomes, 13

Outpatient Patient-Centered Medical Home model,
    379–381
overfunctioning/underfunctioning concepts, family
    systems theory, 156, 164–166

P

PAHO (Pan American Health Organization)
    *Improving Chronic Illness Care Through Integrated
    Health Service Delivery Networks,* 80
    Inter-American System, 80
Palestine, global concept of P&FCC, 85–87
PAM (Patient Activation Measure)
    cultural conflicts, 191–192
    example questions, 101
    patient engagement, 101, 105, 190
    responses to participation, 38
    use of, 105
Pan American Health Organization (PAHO)
    *Improving Chronic Illness Care Through Integrated
    Health Service Delivery Networks,* 80
    Inter-American System, 80
Partnership for Patients program, 49
paternalistic (Hippocratic) healthcare model, 217
Patient Activation Measure (PAM)
    cultural conflicts, 191–192
    example questions, 101
    patient engagement, 101, 105, 190
    responses to participation, 38
    use of, 105
patient advocacy
    competencies required, 225–227
    definition of, 216–219
    effectiveness
        constraining forces, 235–236
        critiques of, 227–231
        facilitating forces, 236–238
        levels of expertise, 238
        making positive impact on profession, 234
        role in advocacy, 233–234
    implementation methods, 220–221, 221–222
    models of healthcare decision-making
        Hippocratic (paternalistic), 217
        patient sovereignty, 217
        shared, 218
    organizers of, 220
    Protective Nursing Advocacy Scale, 236
    reasons for, 231–233
    reflections
        of agencies/institutions, 224
        of professional caregivers/nurses, 222–224
    situations when needed, 231
    vulnerable populations, 220
Patient and Family Engagement priority, 29, 97, 430
patient-centered care. *See* PCC
Patient-Centered Care Improvement Guide (Planetree),
    142

"Patient-Centered Care: What It Means and How to Get There" (Rickert), 360
Patient-Centered Medical Home (PCMH) model, 84, 379–381
patient engagement, 141. *See also* FST (family systems theory); patients and families
    ACA and National Quality Strategy, 99
    best practices, 406
    challenges and barriers, 108–109
    cultural diversity, 190, 200
    current status, 100
    definition of, 96–97
    importance in hospital experience, 134–135
    influence on patience outcomes, 100–101
    key to P&FCC, 103–105
    nursing's role
        Guiding Principles for Patient Engagement, 107–108
        overview, 106–107
    patient activation
        cultural conflicts, 191–192
        definition of, 101
        interventions for improvement, 102
        Patient Activation Measure, 101, 105
    population health model, 109–110
    priorities and goals, 97–98
    research focus, 102–103
    technology, Interactive Patient Care, 103–105
Patient Experience Seminar and collaboratives, 81
patient navigators, 14
Patient Safety Quiz (WHO), 79
patients and families. *See also* FST (family systems theory); patient engagement
    Advancing Effective Communication, Cultural Competence and Patient- and Family-Centered Care: A Roadmap for Hospitals, 29, 198
    advisory roles, 49, 148, 407, 425
    age-specific strategies
        collaboration, 209–212
        communication, 207–208, 211–212
        coordination, 209–212
    consultations, nursing role in, 274
    definitions of, 22
    Guide to Patient and Family Engagement, 54, 264–265
    Institute for Patient- and Family-Centered Care, 136
    interprofessional teams, care models, 379–385
    Kleinman's framework of questions, 91–92, 198
    Nursing: Scope and Standards of Practice, 151
    partnerships, negative sides of
        doing things to/for instead of with, 48–50
        guidelines for building, 50–51
        inappropriate transfer of responsibility, 50
        reasonable/unreasonable requests, 53
    Patient and Family Engagement priority, 29, 97, 430

patient-centeredness, definition of, 259
promotion of P&FCC
    attention to patient/family voices, 263–264
    initiatives, 440–441
    recognition of family role, 264–266
reorganizing healthcare facilities/services, 36, 39–41, 130–131, 141–142
    admission/discharge, 143–144, 147
    ancillary department coordination, 147
    bedside shift change reports, 54, 146–147, 264–265
    care processes, 437–438
    cultural diversity factors, 435–436
    family meetings, 144
    family spokesperson to spokesgroup, 435–436
    flexible schedules, 144
    healing environment, 147
    HIPAA regulations, 439
    information resources, 148
    interprofessional patient rounds, 144
    new ways of thinking, 433–434
    nutrition resource access, 147
    overnight stays, 23–24
    philosophy and operations, 131–133
    rapid response teams, 146
    sexual orientation issues, 28–30, 198–199
    spiritual care, 146
    technology use, 440
    total culture, not program concept, 439–440
    visiting hours, 23, 145–146
respectful relationships with staff, 146
standards and regulations, 30
Strategies for Leadership: Patient- and Family-Centered Care, a Hospital Self-Assessment Inventory, 142
therapeutic relationships, 123–125
workplace violence
    environmental influences, 303
    reasons for violent behaviors, 299
    relationships with healthcare professionals, 301–302
    staff intervention techniques, 307–308
Patients for Patient Safety (PFPS), 79
patient sovereignty model, healthcare decision-making, 217
Patient Talk website, 82
PCC (person/patient-centered care)
    coining of phrase, 24
    definitions, 22–23
    one dimension of quality care, 22
    versus person-centered, 2, 21
PCMH (Patient-Centered Medical Home) model, 84, 379–381
Pediatric Hospital CAHPS (Consumer Assessment of Healthcare Providers and Systems), 422
person- and family-centered care. *See* P&FCC

person-family advisory councils (PFAC), 425
person/patient-centered care (PCC)
    coining of phrase, 24
    definitions, 22–23
    one dimension of quality care, 22
    versus person-centered, 2, 21
Peru, work of PAHO, 80
PFAC (person-family advisory councils), 425
P&FCC (person- and family-centered care), 20–23.
    See also global concept of P&FCC
    care's scope beyond hospitals, 2–3
    definitions of, 2–3, 152
        AARP, 205
        Institute for Patient- and Family-Centered
            Care, 22
        Institute of Medicine, 2, 22, 73, 259, 419
        Quality and Safety Education for Nurses, 2
    healthcare-related factors affecting, 8–9
        expectations of providers *versus* patients, 10
        financing, 13–15
        medical model of delivery, 9–10
        professionals, autonomy of, 10–11
        professionals, education of, 12–13
        technology, 12
    history of, 23–24
    KSA framework, 30–32
    models of care
        Institute for Healthcare Improvement, 135–136
        Institute for Patient- and Family-Centered
            Care, 136
        Picker Institute, 136–137
        Planetree, Inc., 137–141
    myths related to, 26–28
    participation levels, 37–41
        lack of personalized approach, 2
        person-family advisory councils, 425
    primary drivers of, 20
    societal factors affecting
        consumerism, 5–7
        incivility, 7–8
        medical-industrial complex, 3
        social values, 5, 40
        time, 7
        widening income gap, 4
    standards and regulations
        AARP, 30
        Centers for Medicare & Medicaid Services,
            28, 30
        Consumer Advancing Patient Safety, 30
        Hospital Consumer Assessment of Healthcare
            Providers and Systems, 28, 422
        Institute for Patient- and Family-Centered
            Care, 30
        National Committee for Quality Assurance, 28
        National Priorities Partnership, 29
        World Health Organization, 30
    terminology, patient *versus* person, 2, 21

PFPS (Patients for Patient Safety), 79
Picker, Jean and Harvey, 24
Picker Institute
    Always Events framework, 212
    global concept of, 74–75
    model of care, 136–137
    organizational level requirements, 417
    Picker Commonwealth Program for
        Patient-Centered Care, 137
    "With HEART," 368
Planetree, Inc.
    healing environment model, 400
    measuring effectiveness, 21
        financial outcomes, 24–25, 27
    model of care, 137–141
    "With HEART," 368
PNAS (Protective Nursing Advocacy Scale), 236
polarized views and values, 5
population health model, 109–110
Porter, Roy, 322
President's Commission for the Study of Ethical
    Problems in Medicine and Biomedical and
    Behavioral Research, 24, 260, 435
Preventing Medication Errors, 10
Principles of Biomedical Ethics textbook (Beauchamp
    and Childress), 173
Protective Nursing Advocacy Scale (PNAS), 236
"Provider-Based Patient Engagement: An Essential
    Strategy for Population Health" white paper, 110

Q

QSEN (Quality and Safety Education for Nurses)
    definitions
        patient-centeredness, 259
        of PCC, 22–23
        of P&FCC, 2
    education of healthcare professionals
        goals, 30–32, 130
        shortcomings, 13
    healthcare improvement mandates, 404
    interprofessional mandates, 366
    patient values as emphasis, 73
    teamwork and collaboration, 144
Quality and Safety Education for Nurses. *See* QSEN
Quality and Safety in Nursing (Swedish Society of
    Nursing), 87, 441
Quinlan, Karen, 265

R

Raise the Voice initiative, 441
RAPUUD (Rapid Assessment of Product Usability and
    Universal Design), 398–399
RBC (Relationship-Based Care) model, 115–117
Registered Nurses' Association of Ontario (RNAO), 342

Rickert, James, 360
RNAO (Registered Nurses' Association of Ontario), 342
Robert Wood Johnson Foundation, QSEN, education of professionals, 13, 30
rude attitude/behavior. *See* incivility

S

safety for patients
    dimension of quality, 22
    inappropriate shifts of responsibility by staff, 50
Same Page Transitional Care, 142
SBAR (Situation, Background, Assessment, Recommendation) tool, 368
Scotland, IHI programs, 81
Seattle Children's Hospital, 427
Sebelius, Kathleen, 2
See Me as a Person, 117, 119, 123
self-respect, top value, 5
senior citizens. *See* older adults
Sentinel Event Alert(s)
    behaviors undermining safety, 8
    disruptive and inappropriate behaviors, 8
sexual orientation
    cultural conflicts, 198–199
    representation for same-sex partners, 28–30
Shanafelt, Dr. Tait, 340
shared model, healthcare decision-making, 218
shift change bedside reports
    hospital's needed changes, 146–147
    patient-centered approach, 264–265
    staff engagement challenges, 54
Silence Kills study, 235
The Silent Treatment study, 235
Singapore, IHI programs, 81
Situation, Background, Assessment, Recommendation (SBAR) tool, 368
societal factors affecting care
    consumerism, 5–7
    within different countries, 89–90
    incivility, 7–8
    medical-industrial complex, 3
    social values, 5
    time, 7
    values, 5
        in reorganizing healthcare, 40–41
        top values prioritized, 5
    widening income gap, 4
    workplace violence, 301
Somalia, global concept of P&FCC, 88–89
Sontag, Susan, 323
South Africa, IHI programs, 81
special populations, age-specific strategies, 210–211
spiritual care, 146
Springfield Hospital, Vermont, 426

staff engagement. *See also* patient engagement
    guidelines for effective engagement, 54
    negative side of, 51–52
        dismissing staff needs, 52–53
        reasonable and unreasonable patient/family requests, 53
Stamform (Connecticut) Hospital, 25
Stamm, Beth, 358
standards and regulations
    American Nurses Association
        family systems theory, 151
        patient advocacy, 232
    The Joint Commission, accreditation, 260
    Nursing: Scope and Standards of Practice, 151, 232
    P&FCC
        AARP, 30
        Centers for Medicare & Medicaid Services, 28, 30
        Consumer Advancing Patient Safety, 30
        Hospital Consumer Assessment of Healthcare Providers and Systems, 28, 422
        Institute for Patient- and Family-Centered Care, 30
        National Committee for Quality Assurance, 28
        National Priorities Partnership, 29
        World Health Organization, 30
Staring: How We Look (Garland), 325
Stories of Sickness (Howard), 322
"The Storyteller" (Benjamin), 320
storytelling and medicine
    case scenarios
        chronic care setting, 331–332
        emergency care setting, 330–331
        pastoral care setting, 332–333
    effectiveness and importance of, 318
        active listening, 319
        close listening, 319
        close reading, 319, 326
    healing power of hearing, 321
    medical *versus* patient narratives, 321–322
    patient's stories
        eliciting, 327–328
        parallel charts, 327
        writing, 328–329
    pitfalls, 329–330
    relationship between, 317
    stories in clinical settings, 325–326
        close reading, 326
        regular practice, 326–327
    storytelling practice, 320
    story uses
        bearing witness, 322–323
        interpreting and authenticating, 324–325
        sharing, 323–324
Strategies for Leadership: Patient- and Family-Centered Care, a Hospital Self-Assessment Inventory, 142

stress reduction
    healing environments, 393
    strategies in workplace, 353–354
        exquisite empathy, 357
        individual, 355–356
        Mindfulness-Based Stress Reduction
          approach, 355
        organizational, 359
        professional, 356–359
stress strap of professionalism, 284
substance abuse, workplace violence, 300–301
super-regional healthcare systems, 4
Sweden
    global concept of P&FCC, 87
    IHI programs, 81
    patients' healthcare experiences, 82
Swedish Society of Nursing, 87, 441
Switzerland, patients' healthcare experiences, 82
system change for P&FCC
    collaborative decision-making model, 408–409
        guidelines, 409–410
        mutually beneficial partnerships, 409
        stakeholders' challenges, 410–412
    core support components
        communication, 412–413
        honoring excellence, 414
        human resources, 413–414
        training, tools, and resources, 413
        vision, mission, and strategy, 412
    leadership commitment, 404–405
        challenges/steps to overcome, 405
    patient/family advisory roles
        advisory councils, 407
        faculty, 407
        paid professional roles, 408
        peer-to-peer mentors, 407
    patient/family engagement, best practices, 406
systems theory. *See also* FST (family systems theory)
    complex adaptive systems, 153
    definition, 152–153

T

TeamSTEPPS tool, 368
technology, 103
    EHRs
        incentive programs, 103
        reliability and consistency, 213
    Health Information Technology for Economic and
        Clinical Health Act, 99
    patient engagement, 103
        Interactive Patient Care, 103–104
therapeutic relationships/practices
    applying for healthy work environment, 163–164
    caring processes, 120–121
        attunement and human attachments, 119–121
        being with, 117–119

        doing for, 117–118
        enabling, 117–118
        following, 117–118, 122
        holding, 117, 122–123
        knowing, 117–118
        maintaining belief, 117–118
        presence through attunement, 117–118,
          119–121
        wondering, 117–118, 121–122
    listening for understanding, 248–249
Thibault, George, 13
Thornby, Denise, 233
time, societal factors affecting P&FCC, 7
timely, dimension of quality, 22
TJC (The Joint Commission)
    accreditation standards
        ethics consultation services, 260
        proposals, 29–30
    *Advancing Effective Communication, Cultural
        Competence and Patient- and Family-Centered
        Care: A Roadmap for Hospitals,* 29, 198
    conflict management, 281
    Elements of Performance, 421
    ethical issues
        ethical consultation services, 260
        resolving problems, 66
    family involvement as challenge, 340
    healthcare improvement mandates, 404
    nursing leadership expectations, 417
    P&FCC
        definition of IPFCC, 22
        standards and regulations, 29–30
    Sentinel Event Alert
        behaviors undermining safety, 8
        disruptive and inappropriate behaviors, 8
To Err Is Human—To Delay Is Deadly (Consumers
    Union), 2, 391
Transforming Presence: The Difference Nursing Makes
    (Newman), 200
Trauma Stewardship (van Dernoot Lipsky), 347, 355
triangles concept, family systems theory, 156
Triple Aim framework, 81
Turkal, Nick, 4
A Two-Year-Old Goes To the Hospital (Robertson), 23

U

UD (universal design), 396–400
UDL (Universal Design for Learning), 397–398, 400
Uganda, global concept of P&FCC, 88
UK (United Kingdom)
    HCP's attitudes of healthcare, 76
    IHI programs, 81
    patients' healthcare experiences, 82
    PCMH model, 84
Unequal Treatment, 281

United States. *See* U.S.
universal design (UD), 396–400
Universal Design for Learning (UDL), 397–398, 400
University Hospital of Newark New Jersey, 427
University of Massachusetts Medical Center, 355
University of Wisconsin website, 438
Urban Institute's Health Policy Center, 220
U.S. (United States)
    Agency for International Development, global concept of P&FCC, 75
    DHHS (Department of Health and Human Services)
        Affordable Care Act, 15, 96
        National Quality Strategy, 99, 429
        secretary, Kathleen Sebelius, 2
    healthcare improvement, 74
    HIT (Health Information Technology), 99
    IHI (Institute for Healthcare Improvement)
        models of care, 135–136
        partnerships between patients and providers, 132
        patients/families on improvement teams, 49
        perspectives on care, 80–81
        programs, 80
        self-assessment tools, 142
        shift change bedside reports, 264
    patients' healthcare experiences, 82
    PCMH (Patient-Centered Medical Home) model, 84
    USAID (U.S. Agency for International Development), 88

V

van Dernoot Lipsky, Laura, 347, 355, 358
violence in workplace
    contributing factors, 299–300
        societal influences, 301
        substance abuse, 300–301
    definition of, 298
    healthcare professionals
        factors contributing to negative behavior, 303–304
        impact of violence, 303
        individual strategies for dealing with violence, 308–310
        proactive intervention skills, 307–308
        reasons for vulnerability, 301
        relationships with patients/families, 301–302
        setting limits for self-management, 310
        treatment team strategies, 311
        underreporting of violence, 302–303
        violence as part of job, 302
        violence management skills needed, 302
    organizational strategies to eliminate violence, 305–307

patients/families
    environmental influences, 303
    reasons for violent behaviors, 299
    relationships with healthcare professionals, 301–302
    staff intervention techniques, 307–308
statistics, 298–299
visiting hours in hospitals
    parents and children, 23–24
    patient-directed, 145–146
    same-sex partners, 29

W

Wagner model of chronic care management, 76
Washington, Harriet, 187
Wellness Centres for Health Care Workers, 81
Westwood, Marv, 357
White *versus* Black people, history, 186–187
WHO (World Health Organization)
    European Observatory on Health Systems and Policies, 75
    Framework for Action on Interprofessional Education and Collaborative Practice, 367
    Multi-Professional Patient Safety Curriculum Guide, 79
    Patient Safety Quiz, 79
    Patients for Patient Safety, 79
    perspectives on P&FCC, 78–79
    P&FCC standards and regulations, 30
widening income gap, societal factors affecting P&FCC, 4
"With HEART," 368
Woolf, Virginia, 316
workplace climate
    burnout, 339
        causes, 340–342
        impact on PCC, 347
        in physicians, 340
    compassion fatigue
        connection with moral distress, 352
        definition of, 343–344
        impact on PCC, 347
        reducing, 353–354
        warning signs of, 345–347
    ethical climate
        creating, 352–353
        definition of, 348
    moral distress, 348–349
        causes of, 349–352
        connection with compassion fatigue, 352
        definition of, 349
        reducing, 354
    stress reduction strategies, 353–354
        exquisite empathy, 357
        individual, 355–356

Mindfulness-Based Stress Reduction approach, 355
organizational, 359
professional, 356–359
Workplace Safety and Insurance Board of Ontario, staff mental health issues, 341
workplace violence
contributing factors, 299–300
societal influences, 301
substance abuse, 300–301
definition of, 298
healthcare professionals
factors contributing to negative behavior, 303–304
impact of violence, 303
individual strategies for dealing with violence, 308–310
proactive intervention skills, 307–308
reasons for vulnerability, 301
relationships with patients/families, 301–302
setting limits for self-management, 310
treatment team strategies, 311
underreporting of violence, 302–303
violence as part of job, 302
violence management skills needed, 302
organizational strategies to eliminate violence, 305–307

patients/families
environmental influences, 303
reasons for violent behaviors, 299
relationships with healthcare professionals, 301–302
staff intervention techniques, 307–308
statistics, 298–299
World Health Organization (WHO)
European Observatory on Health Systems and Policies, 75
Framework for Action on Interprofessional Education and Collaborative Practice, 367
Multi-Professional Patient Safety Curriculum Guide, 79
Patient Safety Quiz, 79
Patients for Patient Safety, 79
perspectives on P&FCC, 78–79
P&FCC standards and regulations, 30
World Health Professions Alliance, 77

X-Y-Z

The Year of Magical Thinking (Didion), 316
York University, 357

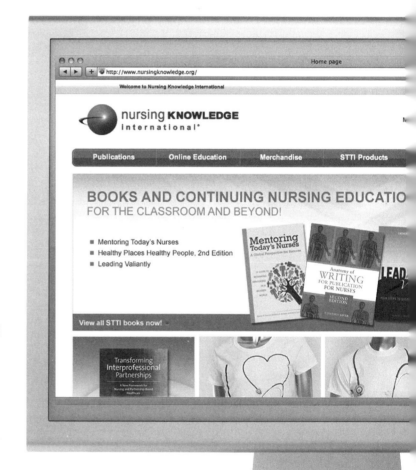

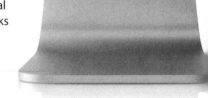